Perspectives on
Nursing Theory

FOURTH EDITION

Perspectives on Nursing Theory

EDITED BY

Pamela G. Reed, PhD, RN, FAAN
Professor
University of Arizona, College of Nursing
Tucson, Arizona

Nelma B. Crawford Shearer, PhD, RN
Assistant Professor
Arizona State University
Tempe, Arizona

Leslie H. Nicoll, PhD, MBA, RN
Editor Emerita

LIPPINCOTT WILLIAMS & WILKINS
A **Wolters Kluwer** Company
Philadelphia · Baltimore · New York · London
Buenos Aires · Hong Kong · Sydney · Tokyo

Acquisitions Editor: Margaret Zuccarini
Managing Editor: Helen Kogut
Editorial Assistant: Carol DeVault
Production Editor: Diane Griffith
Senior Production Manager: Helen Ewan
Managing Editor Production: Erika Kors

Art Director: Carolyn O'Brien
Cover Designer: Melissa Walter
Manufacturing Manager: William Alberti
Indexer: Ellen S. Brennan
Compositor: Lippincott Williams & Wilkins
Printer: RR Donnelley - Crawfordsville

4th Edition

9 8 7 6 5 4 3 2

Library of Congress Cataloging-in-Publication Data

Perspectives on nursing theory / edited by Pamela G. Reed, Nelma B. Crawford Shearer;
  Leslie H. Nicoll, editor-in-chief.--4th ed.
    p.; cm.
Anthology of previously published and articles.
Includes bibliographical references and index.
ISBN 0-7817-4743-0 (alk. paper)
    1. Nursing--Philosophy. 2. Nursing models. I. Reed, Pamela G., 1952- II. Shearer,
Nelma B. Crawford, 1950- III. Nicholl, Leslie H.
    [DNLM: 1. Nursing Theory--Collected Works. WY 86 P467 2003]
RT84.5.P47 2003
610.73'01--dc21

Care has been taken to confirm the accuracy of the information presented and to describe generally accepted practices. However, the authors, editors, and publisher are not responsible for errors or omissions
or for any consequences from application of the information in this book and make no warranty, express
or implied, with respect to the content of the publication.

The authors, editors, and publisher have exerted every effort to ensure that drug selection and dosage
set forth in this text are in accordance with the current recommendations and practice at the time of publication. However, in view of ongoing research, changes in government regulations, and the constant flow
of information relating to drug therapy and drug reactions, the reader is urged to check the package insert
for each drug for any change in indications and dosage and for added warnings and precautions This is
particularly important when the recommended agent is a new or infrequently employed drug.

Some drugs and medical devices presented in this publication have Food and Drug Administration
(FDA) clearance for limited use in restricted research settings. It is the responsibility of the health care
provider to ascertain the FDA status of each drug or device planned for use in his or her clinical practice.

LWW.com

FOURTH EDITION
Perspectives on Nursing Theory

ABOUT THE EDITORS

Pamela G. Reed was born in Detroit, Michigan, in June 1952, and grew up in an environment enriched by the sociopolitical and musical events of Motown, USA. She is a three-time graduate of Wayne State University in Detroit, receiving a BSN in 1974, an MSN in 1976 (with a double major in Child-Adolescent Psychiatric Mental Health Nursing and Teaching), and her PhD with a major in Nursing (focus on Lifespan Development and Aging, Nursing Metatheory) in 1982. She worked as a psychiatric mental health clinical nurse specialist and was an instructor in nursing at Oakland University, Rochester, Michigan from 1976 to 1979. From 1983 to the present, she has been on the faculty at the University of Arizona College of Nursing in Tucson, including 7 years serving as Associate Dean for Academic Affairs. With her doctoral work, she pioneered research into spirituality and its role in well-being. Dr. Reed has developed a theory of self-transcendence and two widely used research instruments, the *Spiritual Perspective Scale* and the *Self-Transcendence Scale*. Her publications reflect her three main passions and contributions to nursing: the conceptual and empirical bases of the significance of spirituality in health experiences; a lifespan developmental perspective of well-being in aging and end of life; and the philosophical dimensions of the development of the discipline. Dr. Reed also enjoys classical music, hiking the Grand Canyon, swimming, and raising her two daughters, Regina and Rebecca, with her husband, Gary.

Nelma B. Crawford Shearer was born in Sioux Falls, South Dakota on August 15, 1950. She was raised on a farm in rural southwestern Minnesota. She received her BS in Nursing from South Dakota State University in 1972, an MEd from University of Missouri-St. Louis in 1977, an MS in Nursing from Southern Illinois University-Edwardsville in 1987, and a PhD with a major in Nursing from the University of Arizona in 2000. It was during her doctoral studies and her work with Dr. Reed that she became interested in metatheory and philosophy of nursing. Dr. Shearer is an Assistant Professor at Arizona State University College of Nursing where she teaches nursing theory and community health courses. She is an ANF Scholar and conducts research into the process of health empowerment in women, most recently homebound older women. Dr. Shearer and her husband, James, have two grown children, Christopher and Sarah. She enjoys entertaining family and friends, baking, antiquing, and traveling.

Leslie H. Nicoll served as Editor for the first three editions of *Perspectives on Nursing Theory*. She received her PhD from CWRU in 1988. In addition, Dr. Nicoll has degrees in Nursing from Russell Sage College (BS, 1977) and the University of Illinois (MS, 1980), plus an MBA from the Whittemore School of Business and Economics at the University of New Hampshire (1991). Since 1990, she has focused her career on research, writing, and publication. In 2001, Dr. Nicoll started her own business, Maine Desk. Maine Desk serves as the editorial office for two journals: *CIN: Computers, Informatics, Nursing* and the *Journal of Hospice and Palliative Nursing*. Dr. Nicoll has been the Editor-in-Chief of CIN since 1995 and of JHPN since 2001. In addition, Dr. Nicoll and the staff of Maine Desk provide professional editorial services and research consultation to aspiring authors and researchers throughout the world. Dr. Nicoll is happily married to Tony Jendrek and has two children, Lance, 14, and Hannah, 11. They also have a retired racing greyhound named Jessie. They live in Westbrook, Maine, in an historic home that celebrated its bicentennial in 2003.

*W*e dedicate this book to the student and teacher in all of us who, in reading and reflecting on its chapters, can become informed and inspired to extend our nursing knowledge.

Pamela G. Reed
Nelma B.C. Shearer

Contributors

Wendy Austin, RN, PhD
Associate Professor
Co-Director, WHO Collaborating Centre in
    Nursing and Mental Health
Faculty of Nursing and The John Dossetor
    Health Ethics Centre
University of Alberta
Edmonton, Alberta, Canada

Alan Gordon Barnard, RN, BA, MA, PhD, MRCNA
Senior Lecturer
School of Nursing
Queensland University of Technology (QUT)
Australia

Elizabeth Ann Manhart Barrett, RN, PhD, FAAN
Professor Emerita of Nursing
Hunter College
City University of New York
New York, New York

Janet Isabel Beaton, RN, BN, MA, PhD
Professor and Dean Emerita
Faculty of Nursing
University of Manitoba
Winnipeg, Manitoba
Canada

Ian Beech, RMN, RGN, BA (hons), PGCE
Senior Lecturer in Mental Health Nursing
School of Care Sciences
University of Glamorgan
Wales, United Kingdom

Anne H. Bishop, EdD
Professor of Nursing Emerita
Lynchburg College
Lynchburg, Virginia

Barbara A. Carper, EdD, RN, FAAN
Professor Emerita
Formerly Associate Dean for Academic Affairs
University of North Carolina – Charlotte
Charlotte, North Carolina

Peggy L. Chinn, RN, PhD, FAAN
Professor of Nursing
University of Connecticut
Storrs, Connecticut

Sheila Corcoran-Perry, PhD, RN, FAAN
Professor Emerita
University of Minnesota School of Nursing
Minneapolis, Minnesota

William Richard Cowling III, RN, PhD, CS
Associate Professor
School of Nursing
Virginia Commonwealth University
Richmond, Virginia

*Dorothy M. Crowley, PhD, RN
Formerly Professor
University of Washington
School of Nursing
Seattle, Washington

*(deceased)

Holly A. DeGroot, PhD, RN, FAAN
Chief Executive Officer of Catalyst Systems, LLC
Novato, California

Freda DeKeyser, RN, PhD
Lecturer and Coordinator
Nursing Research and Masters Program
Hadassah-Hebrew University School of Nursing
Jerusalem, Israel

Christine Sorrell Dinkins, PhD
Assistant Professor of Philosophy
Wofford College
Spartanburg, South Carolina

Sue Karen Donaldson, PhD, RN, FAAN
Professor of Physiology
School of Medicine
Professor of Nursing
School of Nursing
Johns Hopkins University
Baltimore, Maryland

*Rosemary Ellis, PhD, RN
Formerly Professor
Frances Payne Bolton School of Nursing
Case Western Reserve University
Cleveland, Ohio

Joan C. Engebretson, DrPH, HNC, RN
Associate Professor
School of Nursing and School of Public Health
University of Texas Health Science Center at Houston
Houston, Texas

Jacqueline Fawcett, PhD, FAAN
Professor
College of Nursing and Health Sciences
University of Massachusetts-Boston
Professor Emerita
University of Pennsylvania
Philadelphia, Pennsylvania

Anastasia A. Fisher, RN, DNSc
Director of Clinical Education, Programming, Quality Outcomes,
    and Research for Mental Health Services
Alta Bates Medical Center
Principal Investigator, Public Health Institute
Berkeley, CA

Joyce J. Fitzpatrick, PhD, MBA, RN, FAAN, FNAP
Elizabeth Brooks Ford Professor of Nursing
Case Western Reserve University
Frances Payne Bolton School of Nursing
Cleveland, Ohio

Sally Gadow, PhD, RN
Professor
School of Nursing
University of Colorado Health Sciences Center
Denver, Colorado

Denise Gastaldo, BScN, MSc, PhD
Assistant Professor
University of Toronto
    Faculty of Nursing and Centre for
    International Health
Toronto, Ontario, Canada

Susan Reichert Gortner, MN, PhD, FAAN
Orvis Endowed Chair in Nursing (.50)
University of Nevada Reno
Reno, Nevada

Margaret E. Hardy, PhD, RN, FAAN
Professor of Nursing, Retired
University of Rhode Island College of Nursing
Kingston, Rhode Island
Independent Scholar
Holliston, Massachusetts

Frank D. Hicks, PhD, RN
Associate Professor,
Adult Health Nursing
Rush University College of Nursing
Chicago, Illinois

Patricia A. Higgins, RN, PhD
Assistant Professor of Nursing
Case Western Reserve University
Cleveland, Ohio

Colin Adrian Holmes, BA(hons), TCert, MPhil, PhD
Professor of Nursing
James Cook University
Townsville, Queensland, Australia
Honorary Visiting Professor
University of Central Lancashire
England

*(deceased)

Dave Holmes, RN, BScN, MSc, PhD
Assistant Professor
University of Ottawa, Faculty of Health Sciences, School of Nursing
Ottawa, Ontario, Canada

June F. Kikuchi, RN (Retired), BScN, MN, PhD
Professor Emerita
Faculty of Nursing
University of Alberta
Edmonton, Alberta, Canada

Hesook Suzie Kim, PhD, RN
Professor
College of Nursing
University of Rhode Island
Kingston, Rhode Island

Susan K. Leddy, RN, PhD
Professor
School of Nursing
Widener University
Chester, Pennsylvania

Jeanne J. LeVasseur, PhD, FNP, RN
Associate Professor
Director, Graduate Nursing Program
Quinnipiac University
Hamden, Connecticut

Joan Liaschenko, RN, PhD
Associate Professor
Center for Bioethics
School of Nursing
University of Minnesota
Minneapolis, Minnesota

Patricia Liehr, PhD, RN
Professor
Department of Nursing Systems and Technology
University of Texas
Health Science Center at Houston
School of Nursing
Houston, Texas

Barbara Medoff-Cooper, RN, PhD, FAAN
Helen M. Shearer Professor in Nutrition
Director for the Center for Nursing Research
School of Nursing
University of Pennsylvania
Philadelphia, Pennsylvania

Afaf I. Meleis, PhD, DrPS(hon), FAAN
Margaret Bond Simon Dean of Nursing and
Professor
University of Pennsylvania School of Nursing
Philadelphia, Pennsylvania

Shirley M. Moore, RN, PhD, FAAN
Associate Dean for Research and Associate Professor of Nursing
Case Western Reserve University
Cleveland, Ohio

Patricia L. Munhall, EdD, ARNP, NCPsyA, FAAN
Clinical Director of Advanced Psychotherapy
Columbia, South Carolina
President and Phenomenological Psychoanalyst
International Institute for Human Understanding
Miami, Florida

Betty M. Neuman, PhD, RN, FAAN
Independent International Consultant
Watertown, Ohio

Margaret A. Newman, RN, PhD, FAAN
Professor Emerita
University of Minnesota
Minneapolis, Minnesota

John R. Phillips, RN, PhD
Retired, Division of Nursing
Steinhardt School of Education
New York University
New York, New York

Pamela G. Reed, PhD, MSN, FAAN
Professor
University of Arizona
College of Nursing
Tucson, Arizona

*Martha E. Rogers, RN, ScD, FAAN
Formerly Professor
New York University
New York, New York

Daniel Rothbart, PhD
Associate Professor
Department of Philosophy and Religious Studies
George Mason University
Fairfax, Virginia

*(deceased)

Barbara Sarter, PhD, RN, FNP
Associate Professor
University of Southern California
Department of Nursing
Los Angeles, California

Carole A. Schroeder, RN, PhD
Associate Professor
Psychosocial and Community Health
School of Nursing
University of Washington
Seattle, Washington

John R. Scudder, Jr., EdD
Professor of Philosophy, Emeritus
Lynchburg College
Lynchburg, Virginia

Phyllis R. Schultz, PhD, FAAN
Associate Professor Emerita
School of Nursing
University of Washington
Seattle, Washington

Mary Cipriano Silva, PhD
Professor and Director
Office of Healthcare Ethics
Center for Health Policy, Research, and Ethics
George Mason University
Fairfax, Virginia

A. Marilyn Sime, PhD
Professor Emerita
University of Minnesota
Minneapolis, Minnesota

Helen Simmons, BA, MA, PhD
Retired

Marlaine C. Smith, RN, PhD, HNC
Associate Professor and Associate Dean for Academic Affairs
Director of the Center for Integrative Caring Practice
University of Colorado Health Sciences Center School of Nursing
Denver, Colorado

Mary Jane Smith, PhD, RN
Professor and Associate Dean for Graduate Academic Affairs
School of Nursing
West Virginia University
Morgantown, West Virginia

Jeanne M. Sorrell, PhD, RN, FAAN
Professor and Associate Dean
Academic Programs and Research
College of Nursing and Health Science
George Mason University
Fairfax, Virginia

Chris Stevenson, RMN, BA(Hons), MSc(Dist), PhD
Reader
Nursing University of Teesside
United Kingdom

Mindy B. Tinkle, PhD, RNC, WHCNP
Intramural Program Director for Research & Training
National Institute of Nursing Research (NINR)
National Institutes of Health
Bethesda, Maryland

Paul Wainwright, SRN, DipN, DANS, MSc, PhD
Senior Lecturer
Centre for Philosophy and Health Care
School of Health Science
University of Wales Swansea
Wales, United Kingdom

Patricia Hinton Walker, PhD, RN, FAAN
Dean and Professor
Graduate School of Nursing
Uniformed Services University of the Health Sciences
Bethesda, Maryland

Philip John Warelow, RN, RPN, BN, MN, PhDc
Lecturer in Nursing
Deakin University
Geelong, Victoria, Australia

Catherine A. Warms, PhD, RN
Biobehavioral Nursing and Health Care Systems
School of Nursing
University of Washington
Seattle, Washington

Jean Watson, RN, PhD, FAAN, HNC
Distinguished Professor and Murchinson-Scolville Chair in Caring
    Science
University of Colorado Health Sciences Center School of Nursing
Denver, Colorado

Ann L. Whall, PhD, RN, FAAN
Professor
School of Nursing
Associate Director of Geriatrics Center
University of Michigan
Ann Arbor, Michigan

Jill White, RN, CM, BEd, MEd, FCN (NSW), FRCNA
Dean
Faculty of Nursing, Midwifery and Health
University of Technology
Sydney, Australia

Michael Yeo, PhD
Visiting Professor
Department of Philosophy
Carleton University
Ottawa, Canada

Reviewers

Geertje Boschma, RN, PhD
Assistant Professor
University of Calgary
Calgary, Alberta, Canada

Mary Jane Hamilton, PhD, MS, BSN
Professor of Nursing
Texas A & M University at Corpus Christi
Corpus Christi, Texas

Mary C. Kavoosi, PhD, RN
Associate Professor and Chair of Nursing
Clarion University of Pennsylvania
Oil City, Pennsylvania

Florence Myrick, PhD, RN
Associate Professor
University of Calgary
Calgary, Alberta, Canada

Janet Secrest, PhD, RN
Assistant Professor
University of Tennessee at Chattanooga
School of Nursing
Chattanooga, Tennessee

Mary Silva, RN, MS, PhD
Professor
George Mason University
Fairfax, Virginia

Preface

The term "theory" holds special meanings across disciplines, from the humanities to the sciences. In nursing, the term may refer to one of several meanings: a well known conceptual model of nursing, a middle range theory newly proposed by a doctoral student, the unobserved and conceptual as distinguished from the observed in clinical practice, and the metatheoretical or philosophical dimensions of the discipline. It is this last meaning that defines the focus of this book.

Perspectives on Nursing Theory, 4th edition is an anthology of classic and contemporary nursing articles that address various theoretical and philosophical perspectives on the nature of theory and knowledge development. It is designed to provide a comprehensive overview of the important discussions taking place regarding the structures and processes of knowledge building in nursing. A sampling of the articles within this book may be considered prerequisite or co-requisite knowledge for graduate level nurses, students, and faculty who philosophize, theorize, and conduct research in nursing. Further, we expect the discipline to someday advance to a stage where this knowledge is also expected of nurses who are practitioners of nursing, who are developers as well as users of nursing theory.

As many know, *Perspectives on Nursing Theory* has an important history. It began in 1985 with Leslie Nicoll as the founding editor, and continued through two additional editions at 6-year intervals, in 1991 and 1997. Dr. Nicoll carefully and skillfully selected articles

that captured 40 years of significant theoretical thinking in nursing. She included biographical information and original commentary by the authors. Pertinent articles were added with each edition, with her 3rd edition comprising 80 articles. The 4th edition maintains those elements of the previous editions that reviewers found valuable, with the selection of relevant articles and inclusion of authors' biographical information and commentary. But, importantly, this most recent edition also marks somewhat of a departure from the previous three editions, and not only in terms of its new editors! The 6-year period since the 1997 edition evidenced considerable evolution of theoretical thinking in nursing. Old or classic ideas were transformed into new meanings for nursing theory. This necessitated the addition of many new articles and a reconceptualization of the framework for the book.

This newly revised 4th edition of *Perspectives on Nursing Theory* has been trimmed down to 62 articles, replacing redundancies with substantive additions of cutting-edge and sometimes controversial ideas on nursing theory that include international perspectives. The book features 41 new articles. These articles reflect the changes in theoretical thinking in nursing that have occurred since the 1997 edition and are occurring as we move deeper into the new millennium. The 21 articles retained from the 3rd edition are indisputable classics in nursing theory and its authors represent a who's who in theoretical nursing. Together, the 62 articles orient readers to 21st century thought while maintaining a vital connection to the history of nursing theory.

Another feature of *Perspectives on Nursing Theory, 4th edition* is the inclusion of biographical information and personal commentaries by each author for each article. The information was updated for the retained 3rd edition articles as well. This approach reflects the biographical turn in understanding philosophies of science, and extends readers' insight into authors' theoretical ideas.

The 62 articles comprise the chapters of the book. The chapters are organized topically into five broad units. The flow of the chapters also often reflects the chronology of nursing theory. The five units (and their subsections) represent the breadth of metatheory:

- Unit One: Structures of Nursing Knowledge (Philosophy and Science; Theory; Evaluation Criteria)
- Unit Two: Historical Perspectives on Nursing Theory (Philosophies and Worldviews; Nursing Theory and Theories; Trends and Issues)
- Unit Three: Philosophic Foundations of Science and Theory (Worldviews; Epistemology; Ontology; Ethics; Philosophies and Knowledge Development)

- Unit Four: Nursing Theory and Practice (Practice and Knowledge; Nursing Aesthetics; Practice, Pragmatism and Praxis)
- Unit Five: Future Directions for Nursing Theory

Each unit consists of new articles, which are or soon will be often-cited sources concerning development of the science and the practice of nursing. Unit Five is an entirely new section in this book. The unit ends at the beginning in a sense, imploring readers to revisit 20th century assumptions and conceptions of nursing science.

In closing, this new edition of *Perspectives on Nursing Theory* is intended to not only inform scholars and future scholars of nursing, but to be used as a catalyst to facilitate continued thought and discussion among students and teachers, nurses and researchers, about the development of nursing knowledge. A diversity of philosophic sources is presented, from Rogerian to Foucauldian, as relevant to nursing. The beauty of these articles is that, like good art, whether they are studied for the first or the fifth time, they can generate new dialogue and fresh enthusiasm about the progress of nursing and one's role in its evolution.

Acknowledgments

Many people have contributed to making this book a success. We first thank the contributors whose timeless ideas and insights about nursing are recorded between the covers of this book. Their articles comprise the substance of this book and, together, provide conceptual perspectives about our discipline that are relevant to nursing theorizing.

We thank our students—past, present, and future—who helped inspire the selection of these chapters. It is our hope that these chapters will further students' learning about the metatheoretical foundations of their discipline.

We thank Leslie Nicoll, whose original vision brought the first three very successful editions of this book into existence for use by students, faculty, and others who valued having the ideas of noted metatheoretical thinkers in nursing at their fingertips.

We thank Margaret Zuccarini, Senior Acquistions Editor at Lippincott Williams & Wilkins, for having keen foresight about the need for this book in our rapidly evolving discipline, and for supporting our ideas for the 4th edition. We also thank Helen Kogut, Associate Managing Editor, and her very helpful Editorial Assistant, Carol DeVault. Helen was our rock — consistent, supportive, warm, and always there for us. We appreciate everyone at Lippincott Williams & Wilkins for working so closely with us to transform our ideas about nursing metatheory into this portable package.

Contents

UNIT **THREE:**
Philosophic Foundations
of Science and Theory

UNIT FIVE
Future Directions for Nursing Theory

Structures of Nursing Knowledge

This section is designed to ease the reader into the realm of metatheory, with its new terminology and philosophic approach to inquiry. The articles are well-written classics and several convey familiar ideas. Others entice readers with new challenges for thinking. The unit provides an essential overview of key elements of nursing theory and knowledge development, along with the relationships among these elements and the structures that emerge from these relationships. The reader is introduced to important elements in the structure of nursing knowledge and the distinctions between philosophy and science. The articles broadly address such topics as philosophy and science; middle range theories and conceptual models; and critique of structures of theory.

CHAPTER 1

Philosophy, Science, Theory: Interrelationships and Implications for Nursing Research

Mary C. Silva

If nurse researchers are to study the structure of nursing knowledge, they must first understand the relationships among philosophy, science, and theory. Although many articles have spoken to the nature of theory or science in nursing (Andreoli & Thompson, 1977; Hardy, 1974; Jacox, 1974; Leininger, 1968; Walker, 1971), few have examined the links between them and fewer yet have examined the role of philosophy in the deriving of nursing knowledge. To bridge this gap, I would like to present an overview of the relationships among philosophy, science, and theory, and then describe some implications for the conduct of nursing research.

Relationships Between Philosophy and Science

Although in western civilization the precise origin of what we call pure knowledge is difficult to trace, most scholars agree that significant advancements occurred during the great Age of Greece (500 B.C. to 300 B.C.). During this time those ideals commonly associated with western civilization—freedom, optimism, secularism, rationalism, and high regard for the dignity and worth of the individual—were developed (Burns, 1955).

Greek learning formed a single entry called philosophy and, even into the nineteenth century, this term was

About the Author

MARY CIPRIANO SILVA was born and raised in the small town of Ravenna, OH. She earned a BSN and an MS from Ohio State University and a PhD from the University of Maryland. She also undertook post-doctoral study at Georgetown University in health care ethics. The focus of her scholarship and key contributions to nursing has been in philosophy, metatheory, and health care ethics. She is a Professor and Director, Office of Healthcare Ethics, Center for Health Policy, Research, and Ethics, at George Mason University, Fairfax, VA. When not working, she attends foreign films, the Shakespeare Theatre, and fine and performing arts events.

used to designate man's total knowledge. To designate all knowledge as philosophy was possible because our body of knowledge was relatively small and no real distinctions were made between different kinds of knowledge.

The Industrial Revolution, however, dramatically altered man's perception about the structuring of knowledge. The Darwinian hypothesis of natural selection, cell and germ theories, revolutionary discoveries about energy and matter, and the advent of psychoanalysis were but a few contributors to the knowledge explosion. No longer was philosophy considered adequate to answer questions about natural phenomena, and science divorced itself from it. New disciplines were formed—embryology, cytology, immunology, anesthesiology, to name a few—each asking their own questions and seeking their own answers.

This specialization, however, created a new problem: Although each discipline revealed unique and enlightening aspects of man, the ultimate questions about his nature and purpose went unanswered. Science had taken man apart but had not put him back together. Once again philosophy was sought out—this time to unify scientific findings so that man as a holistic being might emerge. This is in keeping with Kneller's (1971) view of the philosopher as one whose work begins before and after the scientist has done his job.

The philosopher is concerned with such matters as the purpose of human life, the nature of being and reality, and the theory and limits of knowledge. Questions the philosopher might ask are "Is man inherently good or evil?", "Is truth absolute or relative?", "What does 'knowing' mean?". His approach to understanding real-

ity is characterized by formulating sets of assumptions and beliefs derived from his own personal experience and his contemplation of it in relation to the studied experiences of others (Association for Supervision and Curriculum Development [ASCD] Commission on Instructional Theory, 1968). Intuition, introspection, and reasoning are some of his methodologies.

The scientist, on the other hand, is primarily concerned with causality. Cause and effect, in one way or another, are central to his goal of deriving scientific laws (Labovitz and Hagedorn, 1976). Questions the scientist might ask are "Does treatment X, and only treatment X, cause Y?", or "What is the relationship between X and Y?" His approach to understanding reality is characterized by tentativeness, verifiability, observation, and experience. Reality becomes interpretable to him through such mechanisms as hypothesis-testing, operational definitions, and experiments. The scientists' position is summarized by Kerlinger (1973): "If an explanation cannot be formulated in the form of a testable hypothesis, then it can be considered to be a metaphysical explanation and thus not amenable to scientific investigation. As such, it is dismissed by the scientist as being of no interest" (p. 25).

However, despite different focuses and methodologies, the philosopher and scientist share the common goal of increasing mankind's knowledge.

Relationships Between Science and Theory

Before analyzing the relationships between science and theory, let us first briefly review some characteristics of science as a system, based on principles of Van Laer (1963, pp. 8–19):

1. **Science must show a certain coherence.** Science must constitute a coherent whole of interrelated facts, principles, laws, and theories which are appropriately ordered. An explication of unrelated data, no matter how valuable, does not constitute a science.
2. **Science is concerned with definite fields of knowledge.** Man is no longer able to know all things. Consequently, he must specialize so that he might know one field, or an aspect of it, well.
3. **Science is preferably expressed in universal statements.** Science ultimately is concerned with commonalities of properties that transcend the specific; science seeks to discover the universal characteristics of phenomena under investigation. Its goal is to reduce data to their most fundamental common denominator.
4. **The statements of science must be true or probably true.** What constitutes truth is a vexing epistemological question. One may suggest, however, that scientific statements are true if they express the nature of things as they are. But man, being finite, frequently does not know the true nature of things. And so it is to the scientist we often turn to help us find reality in a systematic, scholarly, and trustworthy way. His job, according to Scheffler, is "not to judge the truth infallibly, but to estimate the truth responsibly" (Scheffler, 1965, p. 54).
5. **The statements of science must be logically ordered.** One does not draw conclusions before stating hypotheses. Science is usually best served through careful observance of scientific methods such as the deductive-inductive or analytic-synthetic method.
6. **Science must explain its investigations and arguments.** Scientists have a responsibility not only to report their research findings, but as importantly, to explain the arguments and demonstrations which led them to their conclusions.

The above six principles certainly are not the exclusive domain of science. Many of them apply equally as well to philosophy or theory, once again underscoring the ebb and flow of relationships among philosophy, science, and theory.

We again see these relationships when we ask the question, "What is the aim of science? "Typical responses are that science aims to describe, understand, predict, control, or explain phenomena. But Kerlinger offers a different perspective: "The basic aim of science is theory" (Kerlinger, 1973, p. 8).

But what are the components of theory and how do they relate to science? There is no easy answer, no one correct response. Basic philosophical differences exist among scientists regarding the constructional processes composing science and theory. These differences stem from varying philosophical orientations—realism, idealism, pragmatism, and others—each with its own interpretation of reality.

To complicate the situation further, the many terms used to define theory can be bewildering. For example, words such as propositions, assertions, axioms, postulates and maxims, to name a few, are sometimes used interchangeably, at other times with different meanings. When one looks carefully, however, some common denominators of theory emerge. They are set, postulates, definitions, and hypotheses. Let us now briefly examine how each contributes to theory, and consequently, to science.

1. **Set.** Set is a well-defined collection of objects or elements. Facts, principles, and laws do not, in and of themselves, constitute theory. However, when a scientist selects particular facts, principles and laws from the universal set (i.e., from the set of all elements under discussion) because of their interrelationships and relevance to the problem under investigation, he fulfills the requirements of set needed for theory development.
2. **Postulates.** The central core of a theory consists of its postulates. These are statements of general truth that serve as essential premises for whatever is being investigated. Postulates are usually stated as generalizations which are consistent with scientific evidence related to one's research problem. They form the es-

sential presuppositions from which hypotheses are deduced and tested. Rogers (1970), for example, in developing her theoretical basis of nursing, identified four essential postulates about man. These postulates speak to man's wholeness, fluidity, sense of pattern and organization, and sentence.

3. **Definitions.** Definitions of terms are important for communication among scholars. Terms can be defined as primitive, theoretical, and key (ASCD Commission on Instructional Theory, 1968). Primitive terms are those which cannot be defined by specifying operations or by referring to other operationally defined terms. They represent entities which one can only intuitively experience. Purpose and need are examples of primitive terms. Theoretical terms are those which cannot be defined by pointing to particular operations, but which can be defined by their relationship to other terms which are operationally defined. Motivation is an example of a theoretical term. Key terms are those which can and must be operationally defined so that hypotheses under study can be tested. Learning is an example of a key term when it is essential to a hypothesis and can be operationally defined by use of valid and reliable instruments. Key terms are essential for replication research and theory verification.

4. **Hypotheses.** Hypotheses are predictions which have been deduced from a set of postulates and which state the relationship between two or more variables. They imply that the relationship between these variables can be observed and tested. This is no small matter, but one that is crucial in bridging theory and science. For if we cannot observe what we study, we cannot measure it. If we cannot measure it, we do not know whether or not it contributes to theory. If we do not know its impact on theory, we cannot know its potential contribution to science. Nurses are becoming more aware of these relationships. In a study of priorities in clinical nursing research, the highest priority in regard to "impact upon patient welfare" was given to items concerned with determining reliable and valid indicators of quality nursing care (Lindeman, 1975).

Because well stated hypotheses are based on observation of fact which permit them to be "proven" or "disproven," they are powerful instruments of science. Through systematic and rigorous testing of hypotheses, phenomena are explained and, depending on the amount of verifiable evidence, these phenomena have predictive ability, first as theory, then principles and laws (Weinland, 1975). Through the power of hypotheses, mankind's knowledge is increased, or at the very least in the case of disproven hypotheses, his ignorance is reduced.

If we now synthesize the above four common denominators of theory, we arrive at a workable definition: Theory refers to a set of related statements (most commonly, **postulates** and **definitions**) which have been derived from scientific data and from which plausible **hypotheses** can be deduced, tested, and verified. If verified, theory becomes part of the body of science from which other sets of postulates can be derived. The process of theory building, therefore, involves the formulation and testing of hypotheses which have been deduced from a set of statements derived from scientific knowledge and philosophical beliefs.

Implications for Nursing Research

When the research process is examined by studying the relationships among philosophy, science, and theory, one arrives at perspectives different from traditional viewpoints about the derivation and significance of nursing knowledge. These perspectives are discussed below:

1. **Ultimately, all nursing theory and research is derived from or leads to philosophy.** Traditionally, one is led to believe that nursing research begins with theory. I believe it begins and ends with philosophy and this awareness enhances one's perspective about the research process.

   If one examines the four main branches of philosophy—logic, epistemology, metaphysics, and ethics—one begins to see the links between them and the process of nursing research. Through logic, researchers are able to establish the validity of various thoughts and the correctness of their reasoning. Germane to the research process is the ability to establish logical relationships between theory selection and problem identification, problem identification and hypothesis testing, hypothesis testing and derivation of valid conclusions.

Epistemology, the study of the theory of knowledge, is also crucial to the process of nursing research. For is not the aim of research to discover, expand, or reaffirm knowledge? Yet, what constitutes knowledge is no simple matter. Inherent in the concept of knowledge are conditions of truth, secure belief, and evidence (Scheffler, 1965). The truth condition claims that if one "knows" something to be true, he must be judged not to be in error. The belief condition stipulates if one "knows" something to be true, he also believes it to be true. The evidence condition states that one evaluates knowledge against all adequate standards of evidence at a particular time. Although nurse researchers have recognized the evidence condition of knowledge, they seemingly have paid less attention to the truth and belief conditions. By identifying and applying the contributions of epistemology to nursing, nurse researchers can gain further insights into the research process.

Metaphysics studies the most general concepts used in ordinary life and science by examining the internal structure of the language used in various disciplines (Harré, 1972). Of particular interest to the nurse researcher is an examination of the concept of causality. Questions the researcher might ask include: Is causality a necessary condition of objective experience? Can causality be demonstrated empirically? What are acceptable scientific criteria for the establishment of causality?

Finally, the study of ethics comes to grips with moral principles and values. Although all researchers are, I hope, familiar with the ethical requirements of informed consent and protection of the rights of human subjects, some, perhaps, have not considered other pertinent concepts. For example, what are ethical implications inherent in the nature of the research problem? What ethical consider-

ations do advancements in science and technology present? What are the ethics involved in collaborative research and the reporting of research? To whom are researchers ultimately accountable? Although the "pure" scientist may argue that the use to which knowledge is put is not his business, I believe research cannot be conceived apart from its moral implications.

2. **Philosophical introspection and intuition are legitimate methods of scientific inquiry.** Historically and traditionally, nurses have been indoctrinated into a singular approach to the derivation of nursing knowledge—the scientific method. As early as the 1930s, scientific criteria were used to evaluate procedural demonstrations (Gortner & Nahm, 1977). In the 1960s, McCain (1965) stressed nursing by assessment, not intuition. This stress on the scientific method continues strongly today. For example, Riehl and Roy (1974), among others, express disapproval about nursing actions based on intuition. Gortner (1974) suggests that the logic of science is closed to intuition. In addition, many graduate nursing students have been indoctrinated into a methodology of nursing research which excludes anything but strict adherence to the scientific method.

The time has come to question this singular approach to the study of nursing knowledge. The time has come to value truths arrived at by intuition and introspection as much as those arrived at by scientific experimentation. For, in fact, the scientist has no greater claim to truth than does the theoretician or the philosopher. Yet, nurse scholars seem hesitant to acknowledge intuition and introspection as valid methods of acquiring knowledge.

However, what we scorn, others praise. Burner (1977), for example, tells us that the development of intuitive thinking is an objective of many highly regarded teachers and is considered to be a valuable asset in science. Intuition is not knowledge arrived at out of nothing; rather, it is knowledge arrived at by a deep grasp of a subject, although one may not be able to articulate the process by which a conclusion is reached. The derived knowledge may not always be correct, but neither is knowledge arrived at with all the advantages of the scientific method. The large numbers of unsubstantiated hypotheses support this assertion.

In addition, knowledge gained through introspection cannot be overlooked as it constitutes one of the major approaches to the derivation of knowledge—rationalism. The prime example, of course, is mathematics where truth is deduced from reasoning and not contingent on observation or experience. According to Scheffler, mathematicians conduct no experiments, surveys, or statistics, yet "they arrive at the firmest of all truths, incapable of being overthrown by experience" (Scheffler, 1965, p. 3).

The point to be made here is that we must keep our minds open to all potential avenues which lead to advancement of nursing knowledge. We must be careful not to impose our value judgments about the research process on others if, in the end, we narrow their thinking and undermine their creativity. For example, during the conduct of my dissertation, although never explicitly stated, it was inferred time and again that the experimental research design with its emphasis on causality is superior to all other types of research. Descriptive, historical, and other valuable types of research were quietly but steadfastly refuted.

3. **Nursing knowledge arrived at by the scientific method too often sacrifices meaningfulness for rigor.** Although rigorous research designs are praiseworthy, if not used judiciously, they can impede rather than enhance the research process. Too much rigor can (and often does) lead to trivial research problems with the logical outcome of trivial research results. The same is true of definition of terms and statistics. One can meticulously operationally define the independent and dependent variables in one's hypotheses, but if these definitions are so narrow that they have little or no meaning for nursing practice, what is the point? In terms of statistics, one can find statistically significant differences among groups (if they exist) if a large enough sample is used. However, for practical purposes, the differences may be so small as to be negligible. Such statistics can be impeccably and rigorously

applied, yet offer little to the advancement of nursing knowledge and, at best, be misleading.

Although one expects sufficient rigorism of design so that there is confidence in the results, the pursuit and worship of rigorism and experimentation for their own sake—as at times seems the case—needs questioning. Cook and LaFleur (1975) maintain that experimentation (with its implications for rigorism) as an exclusive method of obtaining knowledge is becoming a dead end as too little meaningful behavior can be understood by this method alone.

How can this situation be improved? As previously noted, researchers can begin to examine other ways to derive nursing knowledge. This does not necessarily mean that we give up a method we believe in, only that we open our minds to other approaches. Most of us, for example, have traditionally considered probability theory as the basis for accepting or rejecting hypotheses. Yet, Frank (1957) discusses another option: logical probability. Instead of reducing probability statements to statements about relative frequencies, one uses inductive logic to arrive at the probable truth or falsity of the data. The statements of inductive logic are purely logical and say nothing about physical facts; that is, they are not statements that are derived from observations. The basic premise is as follows: The inductive probability of a hypothesis h on the basis of a certain evidence e is high; or stated in another way, the evidence e confirms to a high degree the hypothesis h. Although the precise logical formulations derived to arrive at the above premise are beyond the scope of this paper, the possibilities of validating hypotheses in nontraditional ways are interesting to ponder.

In summary, when nurse researchers examine the total philosophy-science-theory triad, they develop a more holistic and less traditional approach to the possibilities of deriving nursing knowledge. They are more open to contributions of other disciplines and less likely to see the research process as though through a glass darkly.

REFERENCES

Andreoli, K. G., & Thompson, C. E. (1977). The nature of science in nursing. *Image, 9,* 32–37.

Association for Supervision and Curriculum Development Commission on Instructional Theory (ASCD). (1968). *Criteria for theories of instruction.* Washington, DC: National Education Association.

Bruner, J. (1977). *The process of education.* London: Harvard University Press (Originally published 1960).

Burns, E. M. (1955). *Western civilization: Their history and their culture* (4th ed.). New York: W. W. Norton.

Cook, D. R., & LaFleur, N. K. (1975). *A guide to educational research* (2nd ed.). Boston: Allyn and Bacon.

Frank, P. (1957). *Philosophy of science: The link between science and philosophy.* Englewood Cliffs, NJ: Prentice-Hall.

Gortner, S. R. (1974). Scientific accountability in nursing. *Nursing Outlook, 22,* 764–768.

Gortner, S. R., & Nahm, H. (1977). An overview of nursing research in the United States. *Nursing Research, 26,* 10–33.

Hardy, M. E. (1974). Theories: Components, development, evaluation. *Nursing Research, 23,* 100–107.

Harré, R. (1972). *The philosophies of science: An introductory survey.* London: Oxford University Press.

Jacox, A. (1974). Theory construction in nursing: An overview. *Nursing Research, 23,* 4–13.

Kerlinger, F. N. (1973). *Foundations of behavioral research* (2nd ed.). New York: Holt, Rinehart, and Winston.

Kneller, G. F. (1971). *Introduction to the philosophy of education* (2nd ed.). New York: John Wiley & Sons.

Labovitz, S., & Hagedorn, R. (1976). *Introduction to social research* (2nd ed.). New York: McGraw-Hill.

Leininger, M. (1968). Conference on the nature of science and nursing: Introductory comments. *Nursing Research, 17,* 484–486.

Lindeman, C. A. (1975). Delphi survey of priorities in clinical nursing research. *Nursing Research, 24,* 434–441.

McCain, R. F. (1965). Nursing by assessment—not intuition. *American Journal of Nursing, 65,* 82–84.

Riehl, J. P., & Roy, C. (1974). *Conceptual models for nursing practice.* New York: Appleton-Century-Crofts.

Rogers, M. E. (1970). *An introduction to the theoretical basis of nursing.* Philadelphia: F. A. Davis.

Scheffler, I. (1965). *Conditions of knowledge: An introduction to epistemology and education.* Glenview, IL: Scott, Foresman.

Van Laer, P. H. (1963). *Philosophy of science: An introduction to some general aspects of science* (2nd ed.). Pittsburgh: Duquesne University Press.

Walker, L. O. (1971). Toward a clearer understanding of the concept of nursing theory. *Nursing Research, 20,* 428–435.

Weinland, J. D. (1975). *How to think straight.* Totowa, NJ: Littlefield, Adams (Originally published 1963).

The Author Comments

Philosophy, Science, Theory: Interrelationships and Implications for Nursing Research

My inspiration for this article came from a long-standing interest in philosophy and the need I saw to bridge the gap between philosophy, science, and theory. In addition, when this article was written, the strong emphasis on empirical research offended my integrative and intuitive nature. The three implications for nursing research contained in this article continue to be important to the development, testing, and evaluation of nursing theory in the 21st century.

—MARY CIPRIANO SILVA

The Relationship Between Theory and Research: A Double Helix

Jacqueline Fawcett

Both theory development and research, when isolated endeavors, are excursions into the trivial. What could be less important than a theory about sweet peas or research that involved mating the peas? Yet Mendel combined these seemingly trivial activities and formulated classic genetic theory (Gardner, 1968). And what could be less meaningful than trying to interpret x-rays of sugars and proteins, drawing pictures of protein pairs and tinkering with cardboard and tin replicas of the substances? Yet from these activities emerged an understanding of the double helix structure of DNA (Watson, 1968). Thus only when theory and research are integrated do both become non-trivial; and only then can they contribute to the advancement of science.

The relationship between theory and research may be thought of as a double helix, much like DNA. Theory is one helix from the conception of an idea through modifications and extensions to eventual confirmation or refutation. Research is the second helix, spiralling from identification of research questions through data collection and analysis to interpretation of findings and recommendations for further study. The core of the double helix is the pairing of theory development with the research process. In the core, theory directs research and research findings shape the development of theory. It is this core that avoids the potential triviality of the separate helices.

The Theory Helix

The primary function of the theory helix is the development of theory. It is also concerned with such philo-

From Advances in Nursing Science, *October 1978, 1(1), 49-62.*
Copyright © 1978. Reproduced with permission of Lippincott Williams & Wilkins.

About the Author

JACQUELINE FAWCETT received her Bachelor of Science degree from Boston University in 1964, her master's degree in parent-child nursing from New York University in 1970, and her PhD in nursing from New York University in 1976. Dr. Fawcett is currently Professor, College of Nursing and Health Sciences, University of Massachusetts-Boston. She is Professor Emerita at the University of Pennsylvania. Starting with her dissertation, Dr. Fawcett conducted a program of research dealing with wives' and husbands' pregnancy-related experiences that was derived from Martha Rogers' conceptual system. Subsequently, she undertook a program of research dealing with responses to cesarean birth derived from the Roy Adaptation Model of Nursing. A third program of research, also derived from the Roy Adaptation Model, focuses on function during normal life transitions and serious illness. Dr. Fawcett is perhaps best known for her metatheoretical work, including many journal articles and several books. Since 1996, Dr. Fawcett has lived in the midcoast region of Maine with her husband John; two Maine Coon cats, Matinicus and Acadia; and a now-tame feral cat, Lydia Dasher. She and her husband own Fawcett's Art, Antiques, and Toy Museum. She swims laps and walks on a treadmill at a fitness center for exercise and relaxation and sails on a windjammer off the Maine coast during the summer.

sophic issues as "truth, the nature of reality, the processes of knowing, and the logic of meaning statements" (Dubin, 1978, p. 17).

A theory is defined as "a set of interrelated [concepts], definitions, and propositions that present a systematic view of phenomena by specifying relations among variables" (Kerlinger, 1973, p. 9). An empirically testable theory is composed of concepts that are narrowly bounded, specific and explicitly interrelated.

Content and Structure of Theory

As noted, a theory comprises concepts, definitions and propositions. A concept is an abstract idea expressed in words, a generalization from observed events which may range from a single word to several sentences to entire paragraphs. Concepts enable scientists to categorize, interpret and structure events and objects, helping them to make some sense of their world. Concepts refer to properties of things, not to the things themselves. Usually, they represent phenomena that vary in some manner and are thus referred to as variables (Burr, 1973; Dubin, 1978).

Concepts are the basic building blocks of theories and must therefore be precisely and explicitly defined to enable scientists to distinguish between the meanings of one concept and another. Concepts are defined constitutively and operationally. The constitutive definition, also referred to as the rational approach or the nominal definition, provides meaning for a concept by defining it in terms of the other concepts; it is a circular definition. The operational definition, in contrast, gives concepts empirical utility by linking them with the real world. These definitions, also called real definitions, rules of correspondence or rules of interpretation, define concepts in terms of observable data; i.e., the activities necessary to measure the concept or manipulate it.

Constitutive definitions facilitate communication about the meaning of concepts. Without them, as circular and imprecise as they are, it would not be possible to construct meaningful, logical theories. A theory composed of undefined concepts would be unintelligible, while one composed of only operationally defined concepts would probably be so complex that it too would be unintelligible. While all concepts in a theory should be defined constitutively, such a theory can be evaluated only on logical grounds and cannot be considered scientific. Therefore, for a theory to be empirically testable, operational definitions are required of at least some of its concepts. The operationally defined terms are called empirical indicators. Each is fully specified in terms of its measurement and is therefore clearly differentiated from others. It is important to point out that while constitutive definitions are a distinct part of a theory, operational definitions may be thought of as standing just outside the theory, serving as a link between it and research (Burr, 1973; Hempel, 1952; Torgerson, 1958).

Concepts are connected in a theory by verbal or mathematical statements called propositions. Propositions described the theoretical linkages between concepts. Two types of propositions are generally found in a theory. Axioms, or initial propositions, are the starting points for derivations; they are not to be tested, but rather are taken as givens in the theory. In contrast, postulates, also called deduced propositions or theorems, are statements of supposition regarding the type of relation between the concepts of the theory. A theory's explanatory power is found in its postulates (Burr, 1973; Skidmore, 1975).

The hypothesis is a postulate containing operationally defined terms. It is a descriptive, predictive or prescriptive statement about the presumed relations between the values of two or more empirical indicators. Like the operational definitions they contain, hypotheses are not part of a theory, but are derived from it. The theory is the explanation of relations between concepts; this explanation is tested through the tests of hypotheses (Dubin, 1978).

Theory-Building Strategies

Knowing what the elements of theory are does not, by itself, ensure adequate theory construction. For theory does not emerge out of a random selection and combination of concepts, definitions and propositions; it must be carefully constructed according to a defensible plan. Burr (1973) identified a taxonomy of theory building which includes strategies to assist the scientist to create, extend, integrate or modify theories.

Inductive strategies of theory building use relatively specific, concrete ideas to generate more general, abstract ideas. One such strategy is Glaser and Strauss's (1967) grounded theory, which requires scientists to immerse themselves, without preconceived ideas, in the data (preferably qualitative) of a research project in an attempt to generate new theoretical notions.

Merton (1957) describes another inductive strategy, codification; this is the process of systematizing apparently different empirical generalizations and using them as the basis for inducing new propositions. A third inductive approach is Zetterberg's (1965) definitional reduction in which several variables are redefined, or "collapsed," into a single variable. Thus a new theoretical formulation, more general than the original notions, is suggested.

A fourth theory-building strategy is Zetterberg's (1965) propositional reduction. This approach requires the scientist to select some of the original propositions as general axioms and then to derive other statements of relationships in a logical manner. This strategy qualifies as an inductive one because some propositions are taken to be more general than others.

Deductive strategies of theory building involve starting with relatively abstract, general propositions as the basis for logically deducing new theories that are more specific. One such strategy involves borrowing propositions from one discipline and applying them in another. However, this approach is appropriate only when the initial propositions are rather general and logically congruent with other knowledge in the discipline (Aldous, 1970; Jacox, 1969).

Another deductive strategy is the process of constructing a new theory by deductively extending an already established one. Zetterberg (1965) alludes to this approach, but it is not fully described in the literature.

Other theory-building strategies are not clearly classifiable as either inductive or deductive. The retroductive strategy, described by Hanson (1958), combines the two methods for the purpose of expanding theory. This approach requires the scientist to identify many specific propositions and then induce a more general proposition from which new, specific ones are deduced. Gibson's (1960) factor strategy is similar to induction and generates new theories by examining the interactions and contingencies of various independent variables and their influence on one or more dependent variables.

The final strategy in Burr's taxonomy is theory reworking, or the modification of a theory in light of new methodological tools, new conceptualization, new insights or new empirical data. Burr commented that while this strategy may not increase the amount of theory, "it can build theory in the sense of improving such things as the clarity, testability, communicability, parsimony, and heuristic value" (Burr, 1973, p. 281).

Burr (1973) also identified other activities that are indispensable to theory building. These include development of conceptual models; gathering of empirical data to generate, test of modify theory; improvement of data retrieval systems; and improvement of measurement instruments. However, the discussion of these techniques is beyond the scope of this article.

The ultimate purpose of theory is to order and systematize empirical observations. The scientist desires theory that is highly predictive and thus narrowly bounded; at the same time, he seeks theory that is highly explanatory and thus broad in scope. Since it is not possible to have both at once, decisions must be made as to which type of theory is most needed at any given time in the evolution of a science.

Merton's is perhaps the most popular solution for this paradox. He urged construction of "theories of the middle range" (Merton, 1957, p. 9)—that is, theories that focus on and are applicable to somewhat limited ranges of data. Such theories have some explanatory power and some predictive precision. Moreover, they are more readily testable than either grand theories that are initially too abstract for empirical testing, or partial theories that lack sufficient specification for empirical testing.

If scientists follow the procedures outlined above, they will produce theories that will probably have a de-gree of esthetic appeal. However, such theories could still be trivial. The theory helix becomes nontrivial only when theory is tested in the real world and modified accordingly.

The Research Helix

The primary function of the research helix is the development of prescriptions for empirical investigations. Its foci are measurement issues, translation of propositions into testable hypotheses and reliability of empirical indicators (Dubin, 1978).

Kerlinger defined scientific research as the "systematic, controlled, empirical, and critical investigation of hypothetical propositions about the presumed relations among natural phenomena" (Kerlinger, 1973, p. 11). Scientific research is systematic and controlled in that observations are sufficiently disciplined so that the investigator has confidence in the research outcomes. Systematization and control come from application of the "max-con-min principle" by which the investigator maximizes the variance of the variables of the research hypothesis, controls the variance of extraneous variables, and minimizes the error variance (Kerlinger, 1973, p. 306).

The empirical and critical nature of scientific research requires scientists to compare subjective belief against objective reality. They must continually subject their ideas to empirical inquiry and view their own and others' findings hypercritically.

Scientific research is a multiphase process which proceeds through several well-known stages: (a) formulation of a research issue, (b) identification of a specific research problem, (c) development of an appropriate research design, (d) selection of research instruments, (e) sampling of units of interest, (f) collection and analysis of data, (g) interpretation of findings and (8) dissemination of results.

Formulating Research Issues and Problems

The choice of research issues is typically based on scientists' current interests and their perceptions of what the crucial questions are in their discipline. Webb (1961) pointed out that scientists commonly base studies on: (a) their interest in the issues, (b) their belief that the answers to the problems inherent in the issues are available, (c) their compassion for society, (d) their belief that these issues will lead to expensive (and therefore important) studies, (e) their belief that the research will yield substantial personal rewards, (f) and their knowledge that everyone else is doing similar work. He noted that while each of these reasons may result in investigations of significant issues in the discipline, more often they result in delineation of pedestrian problems and trivial results.

Research Design and Instruments

The empirical expressions of research issues are the specific research problems, which state the relation between two or more variables. These statements should clearly indicate the scope of the research and should imply possibilities of empirical testing. Research design is the translation of research issues and derived problems into action. As noted above, scientific research attempts to deal with all sources of variance. The "max-con-min principle" is the basis of Campbell and Stanley's classic monograph comparing various research designs with regard to their likelihood of yielding valid inferences. Their work provides specific guidelines for research free from threats to internal and external validity (Campbell & Stanley, 1963).

The instruments selected for a particular study obviously should measure the variables identified in the problem statements. A major concern at this stage of the research process is the evaluation of instrument validity and reliability—their sensitivity in detecting significant differences or relations; their applicability to and appropriateness for the population of interest; and their objectivity. (Fox, 1976).

Sampling

Sampling techniques allow scientists to select for study groups of subjects that permit generalizations to the population of interest. While random samples are tradi-tionally the most valued, they are not the ones that are most precise and they cannot be used under some circumstances. It is therefore not surprising to find an increased interest in sampling methods that are more generally applicable and which yield more precise estimates of the population (Kish, 1965). Sample size must also be considered. Various techniques exist for the determination of optimum sample size and are documented in the literature (Cohen, 1969).

Data Collection and Analysis

Data collection, of course, directly depends on the research problems and instruments. However, it is not unusual in the course of a study for the scientist to collect data that are only indirectly related to specific study problems. As will be seen later, often these additional data ultimately prove more valuable in terms of the overall research issue.

Data analysis is a focal point of contemporary research. As more sophisticated and complex analyses are facilitated by the use of computers, it becomes increasingly possible for scientists to examine more sources of variance among study variables. However, it is important that they not be so seduced by advanced analytical methods as to lose sight of the original study issues and problems.

Interpretation and Dissemination of Findings

Interpretation of research findings follows the rules of logic explicit in the statistical procedures used in the investigation. Objectivity is a key component of this stage of the research process. While statistical significance of findings is almost always reported, few scientists consider the strength of association between variables, despite repeated urging by experts to do so (Dunnette, 1966).

The scientist has not completed the research helix until findings are reported to peers. The purpose of the research report is to communicate as precisely, concisely and clearly as possible "what was done, why it was done, the outcome of the doing, and the investigator's conclusions" (Kerlinger, 1973, p. 694). The readers must then make their own judgments regarding the adequacy and validity of the study.

Relating Research to Theory

If scientists apply the research process carefully, it is likely they will conduct sophisticated investigations free from methodological flaws. However, it is quite possible the studies will be irrelevant, for, just as the theory helix is trivial in isolation, so is the research helix. Knowledge of research methodology, no matter how extensive, is meaningless unless it can be utilized in the design and conduct of investigations that are grounded in theory.

The ultimate purpose of a research study, according to Popper (1965), is to refute the theory on which the study is based. The Popperian stance focuses on improving rather than proving a theory. This approach allows all data collected during an investigation to be used, giving "particular attention to deviant cases and nonfitting data that feed back immediately into the theory-building process by resulting in theory modifications" (Dubin, 1978, p. 232). From this perspective, it is impossible to discuss research without discussing theory.

The Core of the Double Helix

The double helix has as its core the interrelation between theory and research. As in DNA, the core is essential for structure and function. Merton emphasized this point by noting, "It is commonplace that continuity, rather than dispersion, can be achieved only if empirical studies are theory-oriented and if theory is empirically confirmable" (Merton, 1957, p. 100). Thus the body of knowledge of a science must rely on the repeated investigation of theoretically based problems that are redefined as research results accumulate. Theory should guide all phases of the research process, from choice of research issue to dissemination of results. All research, in turn, should be directed to one of two goals—theory building or theory testing.

Types of Theory-Related Research

Theory-building research has as its primary purpose the discovery of relations between variables on the basis of empirical observations. Once observations are made, they are analyzed and examined for generalizations that might lead to formulation of concepts and propositions. Traditionally, these activities have been labeled theoretical, descriptive, inductive or hypothesis-generating research. This type of research stems mainly from and relies heavily on inductive strategies of theory building to create new theories or to modify existing ones.

Theory-testing research, on the other hand, seeks to confirm or refute previously postulated relations between variables. Its major function is to determine the degree of correspondence between predicted and observed relations. These activities are usually labeled empirical, deductive or hypothesis-testing research. Predominantly through deductive theory-building strategies, hypotheses are formulated and tested in the real world (Dubin, 1978).

It should be clear that the two types of research are inextricably bound to theory and are differentiated only by the direction of movement between observation and theory within the double helix. It should also be obvious that all phases of the research process should be based on theory. Of course, research can be conducted without an explicit theoretical base. However, according to Popper (1965), even the most creative induction is based on observations made within some theoretical frame of reference.

Designing and Implementing Theory-Related Research

Since there is some evidence that scientists are not highly successful in uniting theory and research in their work, and since few research or theory construction texts consider this in any detail, the content of the double helix core needs to be examined.

The formulation of a research issue may justifiably stem from either theoretical or pragmatic concerns of the scientist. If theoretical interest is the point of departure, the research may lead to theory building or theory testing, depending on the state of theory in the discipline. Pragmatic concern, on the other hand, often leads initially to theory-building research, since frequently there is no prior theory bearing on this issue available for testing.

Many failures to integrate theory and research occur when the research impetus is pragmatic and the scientist "does not bother" to develop a theory to explain results. Such research may be very important in practical terms, but it is likely to be sterile and not advance the discipline. However, a theoretical interest can also get in the way of integration when scientists put all their energies into constructing elegant theoretical edifices which they do not trouble to test, or which, even worse, may be untestable.

Once the research issue has been identified, specific research problems must be outlined. The relation between theory and research is perhaps more clearly illustrated at this point than at any other in the double helix core. The specific problems ultimately derive from theory and prior research. Scientists should take care at this stage to explicitly relate the present study to the larger body of knowledge in the discipline. Furthermore, they should take care to either state the propositions of the theory being tested and to clearly derive hypotheses from them, or to identify specific observations expected to lead to propositions of the theory being built. The expression of the research problem is the culmination of the theoretical process, "the final step in the unfolding of the logic that provides the foundation for the empirical phase of research" (Batey, 1977, p. 329).

The specific research problems will suggest the research design to be used in conducting the investigation. The level of knowledge from which the research problem is derived is even more influential in selecting the design. For instance, if a review of the literature reveals no previous study of the relations between variables of interest, an exploratory theory-building study might be undertaken. Such a study enables the investigator to collect preliminary data which can then be used to formulate specific concepts and propositions using inductive theory-building strategies. However, if the literature indicates a well-developed body of theory, the research might focus on derivation of hypotheses using deductive strategies and empirical testing of hypothesized relations.

The choice of research instruments should also be guided by the study's theoretical base. Extreme care must be taken to select tools that are valid and reliable empirical indicators of the relevant concepts. It is important to recognize that the tools of a research project are the links between "a theoretically formulated research problem and the data to be gathered from observations" (Lin, 1976, p. 10).

Sampling, too, is based on the theory underlying the investigation. The majority of theories should be limited to certain populations. The scientist who wishes to build or test a theory must therefore be explicit about its boundaries. Furthermore, if the research is designed to extend a theory, the scientist must be certain it has been confirmed in one population before testing it in another.

The data analysis stage links research problem and the raw data. The form of analysis is also dictated by the theoretical base of the study. The statistics used in the analysis should come as no surprise to the reader, since the hypotheses should reveal these, at least in the broad categories of analysis of relations or of difference. Once data analysis is completed, the task is to interpret the findings. Theory serves to order the findings and to place them in context. Research findings should be clearly and explicitly related to the theory being built or tested.

Interpreting Theory-Related Research

The results of research lead directly to confirmation or rejection of hypotheses. If they are confirmed, the scientist should plan even more stringent tests of the theory or studies which will continue to build it. If, on the other hand, the hypotheses are rejected and the scientist is convinced the study was a legitimate test of the theory, it is probable the theory requires modification and subsequent rigorous testing.

Regardless of the outcomes of the study and of the care taken to integrate theory and research, several additional should be considered at this point in the research process. Those relating mainly to the theory include reexamination of the causal structure and of variables identified as causes and effects. (Although the scientist may not have considered his theory as causal, these factors require examination because causal thinking and theory cannot be separated.) Factors relating primarily to reexamination of the data include scale of measurement assumed, coding procedures used and validity of the data as empirical indicators of the concepts (Smelser & Warner, 1976). The conclusions which may be reached from such a critical review include: (a) the data are faulty and cannot be relied on; (b) the theory is faulty and should be discarded; (c) the data are accurate and the theory requires modification; and (d) the data are accurate but have no relevance to the theory (Downs, 1973).

Ultimately, a theory can never be confirmed or refuted. Since hypotheses are tested in a probabilistic manner, and since the probability of error in inference is normally never zero or one, it is always possible that replications of a study will yield different results. Moreover, there is always the possibility of other logical explanations why the data of one study provided or failed to provide support for the hypotheses. Any theory can therefore be considered no more than an approximation of the real world or a plausible explanation of events. As Selltiz and her associates commented:

> . . . the most plausible theory is the one for which we have the strongest evidential support. And it is this theory that is to be provisionally "believed" or "accepted" until another theory gains superior evidential support. Scientific knowledge is knowledge under conditions of uncertainty (Selltiz, Wrightsman, & Cook, 1976, pp. 47-48).

Theory and Research in Nursing Science

Nursing Theory

Nursing theory is not trivial; it is practically nonexistent. The nursing literature yield little evidence of formulations that might be considered nursing theory, that is, "a set of interrelated propositions and definitions which present a systematic view of one or more of the essential [concepts] of nursing—person, environment, health, nursing—by specifying relations among relevant variables" (Fawcett, 1978, p. 26).

Currently, nursing science has not progressed much beyond a knowledge base composed of conceptual models. A conceptual model is a highly abstract umbrella of related multidimensional concepts that provide a broad perspective for scientists, telling them what to look at (Reilly, 1975). The conceptual models of nursing certainly are not trivial, since they have a demonstrated usefulness in guiding nursing practice, research and education (Riehl & Roy, 1974). However, they cannot be empirically tested because of the abstract nature of their concepts. Nursing science thus remains essentially devoid of any substantive nursing theories that could be related to nursing research.

Nursing's theory helix has received considerable attention over the past several years. Nurse scholars have offered definitions of nursing theories and urged their construction; they have described techniques of theory formalization and construction; and they have cited the advantages and disadvantages of theory-building strategies using borrowed theories (Cleland, 1967; Hardy, 1974; Jacox, 1974; Silva, 1977). More recently, it has been advocated that nursing theories be derived from the conceptual models of nursing and that theory construction follow the master plan offered by Dickoff and James' (1968) four levels of theory (Fawcett, 1978; Menke, 1978).

Nursing scholars are essentially in agreement on the need for nursing theory and the strategies for its construction. They even seem to agree that nursing knowledge may be a synthesis of theory borrowed from other disciplines. What, then, has been the payoff for the theory helix of nursing science? Apparently, it has been almost nil. As Menke stated:

> Thus far there has been a dearth of theory developed for nursing. Efforts have not been organized in any specific manner. The theory that has been developed has followed a laissez-faire route or has not necessarily been focused in any specific direction (Menke, 1978, p. 218).

It may be concluded then that while knowledge of the content of the theory helix exists in nursing science, the application of that knowledge is not evident.

Nursing Research

The content of the research helix of nursing science is better developed. Even a cursory review of nursing research publications and presentations reveals increasing attention to the cornerstones of scientific research, i.e., systematization, control, empiricism and critical review. Despite this, given the preceding discussion, it should be clear that most nursing research must be trivial, since it is not connected to theory in any discernible way. This assertion is supported by Batey's (1977) review of 25 years of research published in *Nursing Research,* which discovered few explicit theoretical bases for the research. Batey's findings suggest that while nurse researchers may know that theory and research should be interrelated, they apparently do not comprehend this, or do not accept it, or do not know how to apply this knowledge.

The Theory-Research Core

It should by now be apparent that the double helix core is essentially nonexistent in nursing science. While this situation is not unique to nursing, as pointed out earlier, it is important that some rapid progress be made if nursing is to retain and increase its respectability as a science.

The underdevelopment of the theory helix of nursing science is obviously the main factor impeding the development of the double helix core. For without nursing theory, it is rather difficult, if not impossible, to design theoretically based nursing research. A review of the literature has identified several other factors retarding the development of the double helix core of nursing science.

First, nursing has no scientific heritage. There is no comprehensive body of knowledge or research tradition on which to construct a core of unified theory and research (Johnson, 1974). Second, although the derivation of research problems from the conceptual frameworks of nursing has been advocated (Schlotfeldt, 1975), here is little evidence that nurse researchers

have adopted this strategy, perhaps because of the effort required to deduce a theory and relevant empirically testable problems from these highly abstract models.

Third, the favoring of experimental research as the best way to test theories and of research with direct clinical practice implications has led away from basic descriptive studies that might provide the baseline data crucial for theory building. These research biases have, unfortunately, encouraged nurses to conduct "more sophisticated" studies that lack a firm theoretical foundation.

Fourth, the value placed on creativity, together with a "do your own thing" orientation in nursing, has inhibited study replication research that might provide empirical data needed for modification, extension or refutation of theories.

Fifth, since nurses are oriented to doing, it is evidently difficult for them to value "the time-consuming analysis and testing demanded by research before action is initiated" (Martinson, 1978, p. 159).

Sixth, as long as editorial reviews of research reports are less rigorous regarding theory helix content than for research helix content, it is doubtful that nurse researchers will be motivated to carefully delineate the type of research (theory building or theory testing) they are conducting or to explicitly integrate theory with research (Batey, 1977).

Finally, as long as published research is not related to theory, an implicit message of "why bother" is given to those who might otherwise attempt to relate theory to research and research to theory. Or, even worse, the effective message may be that this is not necessary.

Many other sciences have gone through a similar phase before the double helix core has come into being. For instance, only in the past decade has the literature of many of the behavioral sciences revealed integration of theory and research. It should not be surprising then that such integration has not yet occurred in the embryonic science of nursing. And it is probable that nursing's current preoccupation with this lack is the result of its quest for recognition as a distinct science, particularly in academe, but also in hallways of practice settings.

REFERENCES

Aldous, J. (1970). Strategies for developing family theory. *Marriage and the Family, 32*(2), 250–257.

Batey, M. V. (1971). Conceptualization: Knowledge and logic guiding empirical research. *Nursing Research, 26*(5), 324–329.

Burr, W. R. (1973). *Theory construction and the sociology of the family.* New York: John Wiley & Sons.

Campbell, D. T., & Stanley, J. C. (1963). *Experimental and quasi-experimental designs for research.* Chicago: Rand McNally.

Cleland, V. S. (1967). The use of existing theories. *Nursing Research, 16*(2), 118–121.

Cohen, J. (1969). *Statistical power analysis for the behavioral sciences.* New York: Academic Press.

Dickoff, J., & James P. (1968). A theory of theories: A position paper. *Nursing Research, 17,* 197–203.

Downs, F. S. (1973). Elements of a research critique. In F. S. Downs & M. A. Newman (Eds.), *A source book of nursing research.* Philadelphia: F. A. Davis.

Dubin, R. (1978). *Theory building* (rev. ed.). New York: Free Press.

Dunnette, M. D. (1966). Fads, fashions, and folderol in psychology. *American Psychologist, 21*(4), 343–352.

Fawcett, J. (1978). The 'what' of theory development. In *Theory development: What, why, how?* New York: National League for Nursing.

Fox, D. J. (1976). *Fundamentals of research in nursing* (3rd ed.). New York: Appleton-Century-Crofts.

Gardner, E. J. (1968). *Principles of genetics* (3rd ed.). New York: John Wiley & Sons.

Gibson, Q. (1970). *The logic of social enquiry.* New York: Humanities Press.

Glaser, B. G., & Strauss, A. L. (1967). *The discovery of grounded theory: Strategies for qualitative research.* Chicago: Aldine.

Hanson, N. R. (1958). *Patterns of discovery.* New York: Cambridge University Press.

Hardy, M. (1974). Theories: Components, development, evaluation. *Nursing Research, 23*(2), 100–107.

Hempel, C. G. (1952). *Fundamentals of concept formation in empirical science.* Chicago: University of Chicago Press.

Jacox, A. (1969). Issues in construction of nursing theory. In C. M. Norris (Ed.), *Proceedings, First Nursing Theory Conference.* Kansas City: University of Kansas Medical Center Department of Nursing Education.

Jacox, A. (1974). Theory construction in nursing. An overview. *Nursing Research, 23*(1), 4–13.

Johnson, D. E. (1974). Development of theory: A requisite for nursing as a primary health profession. *Nursing Research, 23*(5), 372–377.

Kerlinger, F. N. (1973). *Foundations of behavioral research* (2nd ed.). New York: Holt, Rinehart and Winston.

Kish, L. (1965). *Survey sampling.* New York: John Wiley & Sons.

Lin, N. (1976). *Foundations of social research.* New York: McGraw-Hill.

Martinson, I. (1978). Why research in nursing? In N. L. Chaska (Ed.), *The nursing profession: Views through the mist.* New York: McGraw-Hill.

Menke, E. M. (1978). Theory development: A challenge for nursing. In N. L. Chaska (Ed.), *The nursing profession: Views through the mist.* New York: McGraw-Hill.

Merton, R. F. (1957). *Social theory and social structure* (rev. ed.). New York: Free Press.

Popper, K. R. (1965). *Conjectures and refutations: The growth of scientific knowledge.* New York: Harper and Row.

Reilly, D. E. (1975). Why a conceptual framework? *Nursing Outlook, 23*(8), 566–569.

Riehl, J. P., & Roy, C. *Conceptual models for nursing practice.* New York: Appleton-Century-Crofts.

Schlotfeldt, R. M. (1975). The need for a conceptual framework. In P. J. Verhonick (Ed.), *Nursing Research, Vol 1.* (pp. 3–24). Boston: Little, Brown.

Selltiz, C., Wrightsman, L. S., & Cook, S. W. (1976). *Research methods in social relations* (3rd ed.). New York: Holt, Rinehart and Winston.

Silva, M. C. (1977). Philosophy, science, theory: Interrelationships and implications for nursing research. *Image, 9*(3), 59–63.

Skidmore, W. (1975). *Theoretical thinking in sociology.* New York: Cambridge University Press.

Smelser, N. J., & Warner, R. S. (1976): *Sociological theory: Historical and formal.* Morristown, NJ: General Learning Press.

Torgerson, W. S. (1958). *Theory and methods of scaling.* New York: John Wiley & Sons.

Watson, J. D. (1968). *The double helix.* New York: New American library.

Webb, W. B. (1961). The choice of the problem. *American Psychologist, 16,* 223–227.

Zetterberg, H. L. (1965). *On theory and verification in sociology* (3rd ed.). Totowa, NJ: Bedminster Press.

Reactions

Advances in Nursing Science, April 1979, *1*(3), viii.

. . . [In] "Theory and Research: A Double Helix," Jacqueline Fawcett noted that Marge Batey's review of 25 years of research published in *Nursing Research* discovered few explicit theoretical bases for research. Hopefully, members of editorial review teams in nursing journals will heed Dr. Fawcett's admonishments, namely factors six and seven listed as retarding nursing. Journals reporting nursing research must act to allow the researcher to delineate relevant theory as explanation of relations between concepts in presenting empirical tests of these relationships.

BETTY D. PEARSON, RN, PhD
Associate Dean
Graduate Program in Nursing
School of Nursing
University of Wisconsin
Milwaukee, Wisconsin

On the "Relationship Between Theory and Research," *Advances in Nursing Science,* April 1979, *1*(3), x-xi.

To the Editor:

"The Relationship Between Theory and Research: A Double Helix" by Jacqueline Fawcett clearly identifies many important issues and concerns regarding relationships between theoretical and research components and the need for unification of these elements.

I would agree with the author that integration of theory development and research is paramount to a highly productive approach toward scientific advancement, this being particularly true for nursing in its embryonic theoretical state. However, while the integration of the two is highly desirable, lack of such integration need not deem such research to be trivial if by trivial one means of little importance or worth. While benefits of such research are greatly minimized, no valid scientific effort is without some significant value.

As was noted by the author, other sciences have experienced a process analogous to nursing's prior to integration of theory with research. Those sciences were also initially concerned with development of a knowledge base and survival as a profession much as nursing is. Perhaps this evolutionary process is indispensable to emerging sciences . . . is in fact a necessary part of that science's evolution. All previous nursing research, for example, with or without implications for practice, has significance in that it has increased skills of nurse investigators and has broadened the scope of nursing research. Both theory and research are valuable in and of themselves for the new avenues, ideas and implications for further research they may afford, and we should not be demoralized by the slow progress to date.

The various parts comprising the whole may lead to vistas unrecognized at earlier stages, as Dr. Fawcett noted when she described Mendel's combination of seemingly trivial activities which led to formulation of classical genetic theory. The pulling together of pieces of accumulated knowledge led ultimately to significant theory. Perhaps nursing has not yet recognized possible theoretical bases within its own accumulating body of knowledge; perhaps there are unidentified links or connections in research already done. While forging ahead we would do well to systematically evaluate connections in research which has already been documented. One wonders what contributions to theory building might be made out of existing empirical data, whether in fact we have not connected possible existing theoretical concepts.

The greater is not triviality so much as the need for nursing to decide whether it will take the position of firmly specifying directions for nursing research in the future. On the one hand we can continue the evolutionary course we have followed in the past, progressing at a snail's pace towards substantive theory, as it will take an inordinate amount of time to connect isolated research findings to theory development. On the other hand, we can purposely choose the fastest, most productive route towards theory building.

Nursing does not have the luxury of unlimited time; there is need to survive as a viable scientific discipline. Therefore the tremendous need for theory development behooves us to choose the most productive of the two approaches. Empirical research which tests theories and allows us to confirm, refute or modify those theories is of greatest value for steady, cumulative progress in nursing science. Isolated endeavors may indeed prevent us from "seeing the forest for the trees." Yet each tree is an integral, viable part of the forest, and in that sense nontrivial to its growth and development. Isolated theory and research indeed contribute to the advancement of science by providing new answers to questions. The larger issue is whether nursing, in developing its theoretical base, feels it is more valuable to speed this evolutionary process by consciously and consistently integrating the two.

CAROLYN ERICKSON D'AVANZO, MS, RN
Bolton, Connecticut
Student, Doctor of Nursing Science Program
Boston University
Boston, Massachusetts

The Author Comments

The Relationship Between Theory and Research: A Double Helix

Doctoral coursework with Florence S. Downs at New York University sensitized me to the need for a strong and explicit theoretical base for empirical research and to the implications of research findings for theory development. No publications of the time included more than a cursory explanation of the close connection between theory and research. An invitation from Peggy L. Chinn to submit an article for the first issue of *Advances in Nursing Science* provided the opportunity to share my ideas about the relationship between theory and research. Further development of those ideas has been catalyzed by students' and colleagues' questions and appear in my book, *The Relationship of Theory and Research* (3rd ed., Philadelphia: F. A. Davis, 1999; the first two editions were coauthored with Florence S. Downs). I believe that understanding the relationship between theory and research is crucial for the advancement of theory-guided nursing practice throughout the 21st century.

—JACQUELINE FAWCETT

CHAPTER 3

Nursing Questions
That Science Cannot Answer

June F. Kikuchi

Science—what nursing questions can it answer? What nursing questions can it *not* answer? Indeed, are there *any* nursing questions that science, as a mode of inquiry, cannot answer? Certainly, given the tremendous success of science to date and the omnipresence of science, it is easy to be lured into thinking that we not only can, but must, turn to science for answers to all of our questions. That we have been so lured is clear: Science reigns supreme in the world of nursing research.

That science dominates nursing research is not problematic—in fact, because nursing as a discipline is a science, it is to be expected. What *is* of concern is that nurses are erroneously subjecting to scientific study nursing questions that are nonscientific—beyond the scope of science to answer. This misuse of science is clearly evident in the scientific studies being conducted

using the grounded theory method (à la Glaser and Strauss) to answer philosophical nursing questions such as "What is the nature of nursing?" and "What is the nature of the nurse-client relationship?" Adequate answers to such questions will not be forthcoming until they are recognized as philosophical in nature and are pursued philosophically, not scientifically.

It is my contention that the present misuse of science by nurses, and its attendant consequences, will persist unless and until philosophy, as a mode of inquiry, is allowed to take its rightful place in the nurse's world, for it is only by philosophizing that we can ascertain the kind of nursing question that is (and those that are not) amenable to scientific study. In this essay, with the hope of goading us into philosophizing about those nursing questions that science cannot answer, I present

About the Author

JUNE F. KIKUCHI was born on the west coast of Canada in 1939 and, being of Japanese ancestry, she spent some of her early years in an internment camp in the interior of British Columbia during World War II. She received her BScN degree in 1962 from the University of Toronto and her MN and PhD degrees in the nursing care of children in 1969 and 1979, respectively, from the University of Pittsburgh. Postdoctorally, she studied philosophy at the University of Toronto. She has held various nursing positions, including staff nurse, instructor, head nurse, clinical nurse specialist, clinical nurse researcher, and, most recently, professor. With Dr. Helen Simmons, she cofounded the Institute for Philosophical Nursing Research at the University of Alberta in 1988 and served as its director until 1997, when she retired early to engage leisurely in philosophic nursing inquiry, gardening, and volunteer work with hospitalized children. The aim of her scholarly work continues to be raising nurses' awareness of the need to think philosophically about their world.

a position that is grounded in the *moderate realist* view of reality—a view that in my estimation is the most tenable and that nurses must adopt if nursing is to have a future as a learned profession (i.e., as a societal institution with an organized body of knowledge and with activities of its own, which exists to serve a practical end, a "particular human good" (Maritain, 1930, p. 111). I say this because in this view the existence of reality independent of the mind is supposed: objective reality with natural forms, boundaries, and orders, against which the truth of propositions can be tested, making possible the attainment of knowledge (in the form of probable truth) of reality. The importance of this supposition becomes evident as this essay unfolds.

In putting forward my position, given the time constraint and the theme of the conference, I have decided to focus on only one kind of nursing question that science cannot answer: the philosophical. Let me begin by defining three key terms: nursing question, science, and philosophy. Other key terms will be defined as they arise.

What is a nursing question? An answer to this philosophical nursing question presupposes an answer to another philosophical nursing question: What is the nature of nursing? As we all know, in searching for an adequate definition of nursing, we have hit dangerous potholes and landmines. Given that we are without adequate answers to both of these questions and that in this

essay I do not intend to seek such answers, in order that I might proceed, permit the term *nursing question* to be incompletely defined as follows: questions that are controlled by the end or goal of nursing practice. To define it in terms of the end or goal of nursing practice seems proper because, as Wallace (1977) correctly states, "That which is final in the place of action is the cause of all the activity leading to it" (p. 157). I acknowledge that for many purposes this definition would not be useful, in that it includes the undefined term *nursing;* however, it is adequate to the task at hand.

Because of the various ways in which the terms *science* and *philosophy* are used, it is problematic, especially in epistemological treatises, if these terms are left undefined. Unless otherwise specified, in speaking of science and philosophy, I am referring to specific modes of inquiry, the aim of which is to attain knowledge, in the form of probable truth, about reality—a world of real existences that exists outside and independent of our minds (Adler, 1965). As a mode of inquiry, science inquires into the phenomenal aspects of reality, philosophy into those aspects that transcend the phenomenal (Maritain, 1930). An elaboration of this distinction follows in the next section.

In agreement with Adler (1965), I am taking probable truths to be truths that are "(1) testable by reference to evidence, (2) subject to rational criticism, and either (3) corrigible and rectifiable or (4) falsifiable"

(p. 28). Such truths are distinctively different from necessary truths, which are characterized by certainty and finality, such as self-evident truths; and from statements we make from time to time about our own subjective experiences, such as "I feel ill," which unless we are prevaricating also have certitude and finality for us when we make them (p. 26). Furthermore, probable truths are not to be confused with mere opinion, which is "irresponsible, unreliable, unfounded, unreasonable" (p. 29).

Having defined some key terms, let me now present my position. I will proceed by first establishing the essential distinction between scientific and philosophical questions. Then I will consider the kinds of questions that constitute the realm of philosophical nursing questions—a realm beyond science's investigative power.

Scientific and Philosophical Questions

Why is it that science cannot answer philosophical questions? Is it merely that science does not yet have the means to do so? What if we devised additional scientific methods? It is my contention that no scientific method would help us here. Philosophical questions are questions regarding aspects of reality that are not amenable to scientific study in that they transcend the material. Being metaphysical, they lie outside science's realm—the realm of the phenomenal (Maritain, 1930). Scientific questions, then, are questions regarding the phenomenal (material) aspects of reality. Let me try to make this distinction between philosophical and scientific questions clear, by calling upon the work of Aristotle (as interpreted by Wallace, 1977) concerning the matter of change.

In grappling with the perplexing philosophical problem of change (how it is that things change and yet remain the same), Aristotle reasoned that two coexisting intrinsic principles were operative in every change: (a) *form,* the principle that actuates matter (i.e., that makes a thing be what it is); and (b) *matter,* the principle that receives the actuation (i.e., that of which a

thing is made). Now, there are (a) two kinds of form: substantial and accidental, and (b) two kinds of matter: primary and secondary. *Substantial form* actuates *primary matter* (or what may be thought of as undifferentiated protomatter) making it *be* a thing of a specific kind or essence (such as "a dog" or "a human"), or what is called *secondary matter.* Operating on this secondary matter (i.e., the actuated primary matter), *accidental forms* qualify it to be this way or that in certain respects (such as its color and size), resulting in, for example, "a large, brown dog."

According to Aristotle, *substantial change* entails a change of substantial form; in such a change, a thing wholly becomes a thing of another kind, such as takes place at death. *Accidental change* entails a change of accidental form(s); in this kind of change, a thing changes in one or more respects while retaining its substantial form, such as takes place when a baby grows. To illustrate, as a baby grows, it changes only in an accidental way. For example, it becomes larger in size, and its hair color and tone of voice may change; however, throughout such changes, the baby does not change substantially—it retains the human form or essence that it had at conception (albeit in potency) and will retain until death.

Now—relating Aristotle's work to the matter at hand—science concerns itself with the accidental or phenomenal; philosophy with the substantial or non-phenomenal. Science has the power to answer questions regarding the accidental aspects of things (e.g., questions about how babies change as they grow); however, it has no power to answer questions regarding the substantial aspect of things (the essence of things, such as the babies' humanness). Questions about essences or forms per se, the metaphysical aspects of things, lie in the metaphysical realm, a realm addressed by philosophy.

When we are faced with philosophical questions (speculative questions regarding metaphysical aspects of reality and the normative questions grounded in them), science's investigative observational and measurement tools are useless. We have no recourse but to use that wonderful power that we possess—reason—

which, unfortunately, seems to be taking a backseat to feelings lately. Moderate realism, a common-sense philosophy, holds that by reflecting on and discursively analyzing our common-sense knowledge (that which we know, not through investigation, but by common sense in light of common experience available to all of us by virtue of being awake), answers to philosophical questions can be attained that are empirically grounded and, furthermore, do not conflict with our common-sense knowledge (Adler, 1965). If you will recall, I have grounded my position on the matter of nursing questions that science cannot answer in moderate realist thought. Therefore, all of its tenets are presupposed, the most important being that philosophy can attain probable truths about reality through the use of reason.

Having made the essential distinction between philosophical and scientific questions, let us turn to the nurse's world and consider the structure of the realm of philosophical nursing questions: philosophical questions controlled by the end or goal of nursing practice.

Philosophical Nursing Questions

An examination of the contemporary nursing literature (apart from an examination of the reported methods used by nurse researchers) might lead one to conclude that philosophical nursing questions are of two kinds: ethical and epistemological. Would we be correct in so concluding? To answer this question, it may be fruitful to look first at ethical nursing questions: There seems to be little dispute within nursing that these questions are philosophical in nature.

Ethical Nursing Questions

In the last decade, numerous publications have appeared in which the term *nursing ethics* has been used, leading one to conclude that the realm of philosophical nursing questions includes, at minimum, ethical nursing questions. In point of fact, ethical nursing knowledge is the only kind of philosophical nursing knowledge identified by Carper (1975), Jacobs-Kramer and Chinn (1988), Schlotfeldt (1988), and Walker (1971) in their conceptualizations of nursing knowledge. Furthermore, it is equated by the latter two authors with "nursing philosophy" and "philosophy of nursing," respectively. However, as a recent issue of *Advances in Nursing Science* devoted to ethical issues (Chinn, 1989) indicates, a point yet to be resolved is whether or not there are, indeed, ethical nursing questions—whether or not the ethical principles that guide nursing activities are attained by nursing ethics or by ethics proper.

It would seem that because ethics proper addresses questions about what is good to do and to seek, specifically as human, in order to attain a good human life, nursing ethics would be required to address questions about what is good to do and to seek, specifically as nurses, in order to attain the end or goal of nursing practice—in short, to answer ethical nursing questions. It would also seem that given the nature of ethics proper and of nursing ethics, the latter derives ethical nursing principles from principles that the former has worked out. If so, nursing ethics, as knowledge, would not (as the previously mentioned nurse scholars claim) consist of ethical theories or professional codes of behavior: the former would be presupposed and the latter derived from nursing ethics (ethical nursing principles).

Let me hasten to add that nursing politics would also be required to address questions about what nursing, as a political institution, ought to do and to seek in order to meet its social mission—to answer political nursing questions. As is the case for nursing ethics, answers to political nursing questions, it would seem, are derived from principles that politics proper (i.e., political philosophy) has worked out.

Moving along to epistemological questions, let us consider the existence of epistemological nursing questions.

Epistemological Nursing Questions

As is the case for nursing ethics, it would seem that because epistemology proper addresses questions regarding human knowledge in general (its nature, scope, and object), nursing epistemology would be required to address questions regarding nursing knowledge (its nature, scope, and object)—epistemological nursing questions. That these questions do exist and have been addressed by nurse scholars with increasing frequency is evident, for example, in the compilation of papers published in *Perspectives on Nursing Theory* by Nicoll (1986).

Again, it would seem that, as is the case for nursing ethics and nursing politics, answers to epistemological nursing questions are derived from principles that epistemology proper has worked out. It is important to note that this would only be the case if epistemology were conceived as giving us new knowledge. It would not be the case if the position taken up by some contemporary philosophers, such as Adler (1965), were adopted: the position that epistemology "gives us no new knowledge, it serves only to clarify what we already know . . . [it gives us] only a better understanding of the facts already known by other disciplines" (Adler, 1965, p. 47).[1]

In adhering to the positive position—that epistemology proper and nursing epistemology give us new knowledge—it then becomes possible to raise epistemological nursing questions with a future, the asking and answering of which will bring us ever closer to identifying and developing the body of nursing knowledge required for attaining the end of nursing practice. What are these questions? Because the focus of the conference is epistemological in nature, it may be helpful to identify some of these questions and also concerns related to them.

Some critical questions come immediately to mind: Is there such an entity as nursing knowledge? If so, what is its nature? What are its parameters? What is its object? There are those who have dismissed these questions, saying that it is pointless to ask them because there are no genuine boundaries to knowledge of any sort. Others who have tried to answer them, but without success, have dismissed them, saying that it is a waste of time and energy to continue to struggle with them because the answers are too elusive. Still others, myself included, contend that these questions are not so easily dismissed. They continually crop up in our interactions with other disciplines, funding agencies, the public, the media, health care institutions, and so

forth. I submit that we must *not* try to escape asking and answering these questions but rather face them squarely. Only by so doing can we attain the knowledge that will ensure that the research endeavors of nurses directly and essentially serve the end or goal of nursing.

In addressing the aforementioned epistemological nursing questions, three epistemological distinctions must be made. It is of concern that these distinctions are not being made in the nursing literature. If made, the confusion that currently pervades our thinking stands to be replaced by clarity.

First, a distinction must be made between (a) the knowledge nurses use in order to nurse, and (b) the knowledge that comprises the body of nursing knowledge. Are these synonymous? Some nurses certainly seem to be treating them as such. I contend that they are not synonymous and that the latter is part of the former—the knowledge that comprises the body of nursing knowledge is only one kind of knowledge that nurses use in order to nurse. Furthermore, it is only the body of nursing knowledge that nursing is responsible for developing. Nursing is not responsible for developing the other kinds of knowledge nurses use, such as the preclinical and personal knowledge nurses use to do their work. By *preclinical knowledge* I mean that knowledge that nurses use or take on as assumption, which lies outside their discipline; by *personal knowledge* I mean that knowledge described by Carper (1975) as subjective, incommunicable, publicly unverifiable, and therefore not possessed by anyone other than the one whose direct knowledge it is. Indeed, how could nursing be held responsible for developing such private knowledge?

Another distinction requiring our attention is the difference between (a) private ways of knowing, such as intuiting, that may contribute to the development of nursing's body of knowledge but *only* indirectly; and (b) public ways of knowing, such as scientizing and philosophizing, that stand to contribute directly. Private ways of knowing serve only as possible means to public ways of knowing—ways that possess the power to make available, for public examination and testing, their methods and resultant evidence and, thereby, directly serve the development of knowledge. How can intuition be other than an indirect contributor, given that it is a private experience?

The failure to make these two distinctions may be a result, in part, of the failure to make a third distinction: the difference between (a) that which is private, and (b) that which is public. According to Adler (1985), that which is private "belongs to one individual alone and cannot possibly be shared directly by anyone else" (p. 10); and that which is public is "common to two or more individuals" (p. 10). Private ways of knowing and knowledge, then, are subjective: "differ[ent] from one person to another and . . . exclusively the possession of one individual and no one else" (p. 9). They are incommunicable and publicly unverifiable. Public ways of knowing and knowledge, on the other hand, are objective: "the same for me, for you, and for anyone else" (p. 9). They are communicable and publicly verifiable.

Of late, nurses (e.g., Carper, 1975; Jacobs-Kramer & Chinn, 1988; Kidd & Morrison, 1988; Schultz & Meleis, 1988) seem not to be paying heed to these three distinctions in setting down their conceptualizations of nursing knowledge. Consequently, when a reference is made to nursing knowledge, at times it is impossible to determine if the referent is (a) the knowledge that nurses possess and/or use, or (b) the knowledge that lies within the body of nursing knowledge. Perhaps the failure to make these distinctions is intentional in that it is being presupposed that there are no differences in kind (i.e., no natural forms and boundaries) in reality, only differences in degree. Such a presupposition would explain nurses' growing reluctance to differentiate between (a) nursing's body of knowledge and (b) those of other disciplines; and between (a) ways of knowing and knowledge that are public and objective and (b) those that are private and subjective. It seems likely that this presupposition may be operative, because questions about whether or not nursing knowledge is borrowed or unique seem to have disappeared from the nursing literature and to have been replaced with questions about the knowledge that nurses possess and use.

Let me move on now to another kind of philosophical nursing question, a kind that is, unfortunately, neglected in the nursing epistemological literature: the ontological.

Ontological Nursing Questions

It is problematic that in contemporary conceptualizations of nursing knowledge, for the most part, no reference is made to ontological nursing knowledge: knowledge about nursing as a *being*. Are we to take, from this absence, that it is being presupposed, as identified earlier, that there are no differences of kind in reality, only differences of degree? I suspect this may be so because, if such were the case, no ontological nursing questions regarding the nature, scope, and object of nursing would be asked. However, we do ask such questions. How would those who deny the existence of ontological and ontological nursing questions account for the occurrence of such questions? I suspect that they would identify them as scientific, in which case they would also claim that answers to such questions would be found in the science of nursing, both of which are errors.

I submit that if ontological nursing questions are treated as scientific and "answered" scientifically, then we will attain merely knowledge of nursing as it exists phenomenally or accidentally and as it appears to us. But then, if it is being presupposed that there are no natural forms and boundaries in reality, this is the end of the line. To acknowledge the existence of ontological nursing questions and the possibility of attaining philosophical knowledge of nursing as it exists substantially, as a being, would require our holding the presupposition that natural forms and boundaries, differences of kind, do exist in reality. In my estimation, to do otherwise is suicidal. If only differences of degree exist, then we are left with no universal natural truths or order and with having to impose meaning and order on the world. This bodes ill in terms of knowledge development, because all we can possibly attain in that case is a plurality of mere opinions, which may be upheld by consensus or by what can be referred to as "might makes right."

As is the case for nursing ethics, nursing politics, and nursing epistemology, it would seem that answers to ontological nursing questions are derived from principles that ontology proper has worked out. It would also seem that because ontology proper addresses questions about being *qua* being, nursing ontology would be required to address questions about nursing as a being—in short, to answer ontological nursing questions, questions about the substantial nature, scope, and object of nursing. It is imperative that we identify these aspects of nursing, because without doing so it is impossible to identify the substantial nature, scope, and object of nursing knowledge. Furthermore, it would be impossible to establish the end of nursing practice, because the object in nursing thought is the end in nursing action. Without knowledge of the object of nursing, we would be left with no proper end to direct our actions in nursing practice and, furthermore, to direct them in an ethical manner. Without the direction provided by ontological nursing knowledge, the end result of our efforts at inquiry would be chaos and, to use an apt phrase of Maritain's (1930), "a formless agglomeration" (p. 116).

Are there other kinds of philosophical nursing questions? I do not think so. I do not see a place for a derived nursing philosophy of man or of nature but instead hold that the principles of philosophy of man proper and of the philosophy of nature proper are taken on as assumption by nursing.

Concluding Remarks

During the last 2 decades, we have devoted much of our time and energy to the development of what has been called "the science of nursing." This devotion is misguided in that science cannot answer all of our questions. It is only by allowing philosophical inquiry to take its rightful place in nursing knowledge development that nurses stand a chance of not unknowingly violating the nursing profession, but rather of letting it be and become the powerful force that potentially lies in its nature to benefit humankind.

Note

1. This quote reflects the position taken by Adler (1965) with regard to the role of epistemology. However, it should be noted that when Adler made this statement, he was arguing that there is more to philosophy than epistemology—that philosophy addresses both first-order questions (i.e., "questions about that which is and happens or about what men should do and seek" [p. 44]) and second-order questions (i.e., "questions about our first-order knowledge, questions about the content of our thinking, when we try to answer first-order questions, or questions about the ways in which we express such thought in language" [p. 44]).

REFERENCES

Adler, M. J. (1965). *The conditions of philosophy*. New York: Atheneum.

Adler, M. J. (1985). *Ten philosophical mistakes*. New York: Macmillan.

Carper, B. (1975). *Fundamental patterns of knowing in nursing*. Unpublished doctoral dissertation, Columbia University, New York.

Chinn, P. L. (Ed.). (1989). Ethical issues [Special issue]. *Advances in Nursing Science, 11*(3).

Jacobs-Kramer, M. K., & Chinn, P. L. (1988). Perspectives on knowing: A model of nursing knowledge. *Scholarly Inquiry for Nursing Practice: An International Journal, 2*(2), 129–139.

Kidd, P., & Morrison, E. F. (1988). The progression of knowledge in nursing: A search for meaning. *Image, 20*(4). 222–224.

Maritain, J. (1930). *An introduction to philosophy* (E. I. Watkin, Trans.). London: Sheed & Ward.

Nicoll, L. H. (Ed.). (1986). *Perspectives on nursing theory*. Boston: Little, Brown.

Schlotfeldt, R. M. (1988). Structuring nursing knowledge: A priority for creating nursing's future. *Nursing Science Quarterly, 1*(1), 35–38.

Schultz, P. R., & Meleis, A. I. (1988). Nursing epistemology: Traditions, insights, questions. *Image, 20*(4), 217–221.

Walker, L. (1971). *Nursing as a discipline*. Unpublished doctoral dissertation, Indiana University, Indiana.

Wallace, W. A. (1977). *The elements of philosophy*. New York: Alba House.

The Author Comments

Nursing Questions That Science Cannot Answer

My doctoral nursing studies in the 1970s focused only on the scientific mode of inquiry, and I graduated thinking that science was the only road to knowledge. A few years later, I discovered to my amazement that the question "What is nursing?" is a philosophic question to be answered philosophically. I then realized that I was ignorant about philosophic inquiry, and, as they say, the rest is history. Nursing Questions That Science Cannot Answer is one of the first papers I wrote after my life-changing discovery. The sound development of nursing theory in the 21st century depends, in part, on our seeking answers to the types of philosophic nursing questions identified in that paper, particularly those of an ontologic nature about the nature, scope, and object of nursing.

—JUNE F. KIKUCHI

CHAPTER 4

Scientific Inquiry in Nursing: A Model for a New Age

Holly A. DeGroot

Despite the acknowledged need for widespread and rapid scientific advancement in nursing, little systematic attention has been paid to the progenitor of research, the individual investigator. The nature of scientific problem solving as the fundamental process of research practice is explored, and a model of scientific inquiry is proposed. Variables in the model are discussed in relation to their potential effect on the inquiry process, and strategies that facilitate the practice of research are identified.

Concern with the growth of nursing science has received full attention from nursing scholars over the past decade. The need for nursing as a foundation for nursing science and professional growth has been repeatedly acknowledged by contemporary nursing authors (Donaldson & Crowley, 1978; Hardy, 1983). Roy (1983) considers theory development as the number one priority for this decade. Current economic pressures have added unprecedented urgency to this scientific quest as health care policy makers and administra-

tors demand research verification of nursing's disciplinary contribution.

Theory development literature in nursing has largely focused on theory construction (Dickoff, James, & Weidenbach, 1968; Jacox, 1984; Meleis, 1985), the nature of nursing's scientific advancement (Hardy, 1983; Newman, 1983), and the identification of conceptual and methodological deficiencies (Batey, 1977; Gortner, 1977; Jacobsen & Meininger, 1985). Despite agreement that creative strategies are required to re-

About the Author

HOLLY A. DEGROOT is currently Chief Executive Officer of Catalyst Systems, LLC, Novato, CA, a nurse-owned and nurse-operated firm dedicated to evidence-based staffing decisions in health care. As founder of Catalyst 15 years ago, Dr. DeGroot has developed the largest objective database of its type on nursing workload and staff utilization patterns. In addition, she has created a family of patient classification measures and staffing methodologies for virtually every inpatient and outpatient clinical area where patient care is provided. She has been closely involved in regulatory and legislative issues involving nurse staffing throughout the United States, frequently providing expert testimony and advice on related topics. Dr. DeGroot has worked in several administrative, faculty, and research positions throughout her career and also serves as faculty in the graduate program in Nursing Administration and Informatics at the University of California, San Francisco. Born in Pittsburgh, PA, Dr. DeGroot has spent the majority of her life in northern California, where she enjoys swimming, reading, traveling, and writing.

solve these theoretical inadequacies (Caper, 1978; Oiler, 1982), surprisingly little attention has been paid to the process and practice of scientific inquiry with the individual investigator as the unit of analysis. An understanding of the nature of scientific activity and the factors that influence individual inquiry and research practice is essential if nursing is to exercise its fullest intellectual power for theory development.

The Nature of Scientific Activity

Science has been characterized as a "creative and imaginative human activity" (Goldstein & Goldstein, 1978, p. 4) and as a form of contemplative wisdom (Weiskopf, 1973). Bronowski observes that "all science is the search for unity and hidden likenesses" (Bronowski, 1965, p. 14). As the method of inquiry employed in this quest, the research process is virtually indistinguishable from what Bigge (1982) calls reflective thinking. This is "a reflective process within which persons either develop new or change existing tested generalized insights or understanding. So construed, reflective thinking combines both inductive—fact gathering—and deductive processes in such a way as to find, elaborate and test hypotheses" (Bigge, 1982, p. 105).

It is clear that the research process and the reflective thinking process constitute parallel attempts di-

rected toward problem solving. Polanyi (1962) distinguishes between two phases of problem solving: an initial stage of perplexity and a subsequent stage of taking action directed toward dispelling the perplexity. Polanyi summarizes the four well-known stages of discovery in problem solving: (a) stage of preparation, during which a problem is initially recognized; (b) stage of incubation, which is an unconscious preoccupation with the problem; (c) stage of illumination, characterized by the tentative discovery of a possible solution; and (d) stage of verification, during which the solution withstands tests of practical reality. Implicit in this notion of scientific activity as a process of reflective thinking and of problem solving is the fundamental relationship of both to creativity. Bronowski (1965) asserts that while science is involved in a search for hidden likenesses, creativity is the discovery of hidden likeness.

Creativity can be viewed as a five-step process that is triggered by identifying or sensing a problem (Mackinnon, 1979). The first stage is called the period of preparation, during which experience, cognitive skills, and problem-solving techniques are acquired. The second stage, or period of concentrated effort, is often accompanied by frustration that results from unsuccessful attempts to solve the problem. Next comes a period of withdrawal, which is akin to the incubation stage of problem solving. In this stage the problem and its possible solutions are considered on a conscious as well as subconscious level. This stage is characterized by what Worthy (1975) has termed "fruitful obsession." The fourth stage, or moment of insight, is accompanied by a feeling of exhilaration that comes from the sudden discovery of a solution to the problem. Worthy calls this "aha thinking," which results in intuitive leaps and sudden insights related to problem solution. The last step in the creative process, the period of verification, is characterized by the elaboration of the newly created insight or solution and its subsequent testing, refinement, extension, and evaluation. The attainment of this fifth and final step in the creative process forms the foundation and the starting point for further creative activities. That this creative process bears a striking resemblance to the problem-solving and reflective thinking processes of scientific activity, as outlined earlier, is central to the discussion of scientific inquiry.

Since scientific problem solving necessarily involves an individual's contribution to the creative process, characteristics of creative persons and their work are also important to consider. Creativity in individuals has been associated with divergent thinking, intelligence, commitment or involvement, and a preference for complexity from which simplicity and order may be derived (Nicholls, 1983). The willingness to take risks (Albert, 1983) and to use imagination and intuition (Yukawa, 1973) are other fundamental characteristics of creative individuals. Introversion, playfulness, and a well-developed sense of humor also figure heavily with these individuals (Worthy, 1975).

Characteristics of the outcomes or products of creative problem solving (e.g., research findings and theories) have also been identified (MacKinnon, 1979). Originality and the ability of the solution to actually solve an existing problem are key characteristics. In addition, the solution must be "produced," which implies development, refinement, and communication of the problem solution. Additional criteria have relevance if nursing theory is considered to be the creative "product." These criteria are that the creative outcome or theory contains truth and beauty and that it contributes to the quality of human existence. It has also been observed that creativity can be generated as much by the nature of the problem as by the person attempting to solve it (Albert, 1983;

Yukawa, 1973). Creative problem solving has beneficial psychological effects on others who are exposed to the process by encouraging and engaging them in more imaginative and creative activity. Although creativity alone does not ensure successful problem solving, it is a vital ingredient for the theoretical complexity of knowledge generation in human sciences. It should be remembered that less than successful problem solving can be equally rich in stimulating creative scientific problem solving because it forces the consideration of alternative possibilities (Yukawa, 1973).

Phases of Inquiry

It is clear from this discussion that the quintessence of scientific inquiry is creative problem solving conducted through the research process. Scientific inquiry thus comprises at least four interrelated phases: (a) formulation of the research problem, (b) method selection, (c) method implementation, and (d) communication of findings. Each of these phases shares common characteristics that have implications for a model of scientific inquiry. Although these phases are typically presented as the orderly and normative approach to inquiry, it has been pointed out that the actual research process has little resemblance to such a rational model (Martin, 1982). The inquiry process has been aptly described as a series of dilemmas that can be neither solved nor avoided (McGrath, 1982).

Problem Formulation

The pivotal point for a system of scientific inquiry is the research problem, question, or hypothesis, for it reflects all that came before and directs all research activity that will follow. Kerlinger goes a step further, calling the research problem or hypothesis the "working instrument of theory" (Kerlinger, 1973, p. 20). The research problem (a term to be used alternatively with "research question" or "research hypothesis," denoting the same or similar entity) is a highly subjective construction. As such, it is an intensely personal and intimate creation because of its contextual and historical proximity to the very essence of its creator. Not surprisingly, Polanyi calls research problems "intellectual desires" (Polanyi, 1962, p. 152), noting that in any scientific controversy personal attacks rather than scientific arguments are the norm because intellectual passions, not reason, are truly at odds.

Since the formulation of a research question is a creative effort based on imagination, ingenuity, and insight (Polit & Hungler, 1983), the research results stemming from it ultimately reflect the intellectual power of the question and, undeniably, the researcher. Research problem selection is closely related to personal values (Kaplan, 1964; Tucker, 1979) and actually discloses the direction of human will and intuition (Noddings & Shore, 1984). Runkel and McGrath observe that as a researcher attempts to formulate the research problem, "he begins with his own previous way of thinking about things; he seeks help in organizing his complexities from literature and colleagues; finally, he is inevitably affected by his own personal experience as he interacts with the world" (Runkel & McGrath, 1972, p. 13). Not surprisingly, this characteristic of subjectivity is inherent in the other phases of inquiry as well.

Selection of Methods

Although Kaplan (1964) acknowledges at least four distinct usages of the term "methodology," only the fourth is inclusive enough for a discussion of the process of scientific inquiry. This definition incorporates specific techniques and procedures as well as abstract philosophical imperatives. Kaplan asserts that the use of this expanded meaning allows for the inclusion of a wide range of activities, including concept delineation, hypothesis formation, observation and measurement, and model and theory construction, as well as explanation and prediction. The advantage of such a definition is that it treats all tools that a researcher has at his or her disposal (including the conceptual and the concrete) and the research implementation phases, such as data collection and analysis, as interrelated components of inquiry. Conceived in this way, factors influencing problem formulation directly or indirectly influence all phases of inquiry.

The implications of this expanded and integrated view of research methodology are not universally appreciated. At the very least, authors agree that the methods are dictated by the research question (Kerlinger, 1973; Kaplan, 1964; Runkel & McGrath, 1972; Wilson, 1985). However, there seems to be tacit endorsement of a greater rationality and objectively of method selection than actually exists. For example, some authors (Polit & Hungler, 1983) subscribe to a design selection hierarchy, usually with experimental designs at the top and nonexperimental approaches clearly at the bottom. This view implies that the selection of design methodology is based primarily on whether the research can meet the three requirements for a true experiment, namely, the ability for manipulation, control, and randomization. If these requirements can be met by the proposed study, the choice of methods is clear. If researchers are somehow unable to meet these requirements for experimentation, they are at once relegated to the realm of nonexperimental methodology. Kerlinger (1973) goes as far as to categorize nonexperimental methods as "compromise designs," consigning them rather casually to the bottom of the design hierarchy. Unfortunately this stance serves to create a methodological double bind: Methods are purportedly dictated by the question, but it is less desirable to ask questions that must be answered by "lower-order" designs and methods.

Brink and Wood (1983) propose a similarly straightforward and deductive approach to method selection based on the level of the research question. These levels are a function of existing amounts of knowledge related to the phenomena of interest. These authors also suggest that selection of methods may be based primarily on the existence of valid and reliable measures. Little attention is given to other factors that may influence the selection of research methods.

Method Implementation and Communication of Findings

How methods are implemented through the use of data collection techniques and analytical strategies is affected by the same subjective considerations inherent in problem formulation and method selection phases of inquiry. There is a wide range of methodological possibilities open to experimental and non-experimental approaches, with choices to be made at each juncture. Whether one decides to use open-ended interview *v* standardized questionnaire, grounded theory *v* hermeneutic interpretation, analysis of covariance (ANCOVA) techniques *v* multiple regression correlation (MRC), or a convenience *v* a stratified random sample is influenced by a combination of interrelated factors. Even the communication of research findings is similarly influenced as choices are made about which journal to submit the results to, what information should be included in the report, how conservative or liberal the interpretations will be, and what the theoretical implications of the findings are.

Despite the rigorous assertions that method selection and implementation are primarily rational processes, some authors concede the influence of subjective factors on these phases of inquiry (Martin, 1982; Kuhn, 1970; Luria, 1973; Polkinghorne, 1983). These include factors such as disciplinary norms, personal research style, fund-

ing realities, and other value-laden considerations. Tucker (1979) points out that scientific activity is essentially a process involving a series of value decisions to be made by the researcher and that perhaps the largest number of these decisions is made in relation to methodological issues. Polkinghorne goes one step further, asserting that "particular methods do not operate independently of a system of inquiry" and in fact "the use of a method changes only as a researcher uses it in different systems of inquiry" (Polkinghorne, 1983, p. 6). This perhaps is the most important point of all, for it posits the inextricable relationship between each phase of inquiry and the subjective factors that necessarily influence each phase.

A Model of Scientific Inquiry

The model proposed here is fundamentally a systems/process model applied to a human system of inquiry (see Figure 4-1). As such, the system comprises

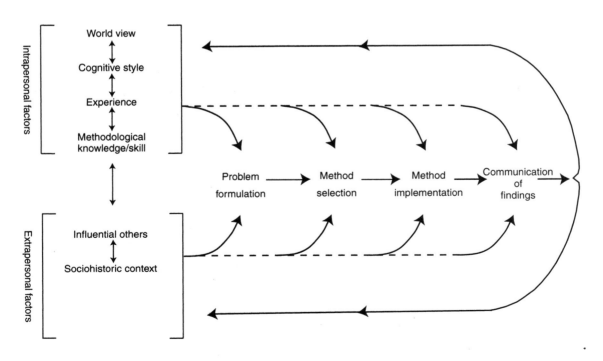

Figure 4-1 *A model of scientific inquiry.*

Table 4-1
Major Factors Influencing Scientific Inquiry in Nursing

Intrapersonal factors

World view
   Nature of human beings
   Nature of knowledge and truth
   Nature of nursing science
Cognitive style
Experience
   Life experience
   Professional nursing experience
   Research experience
   Theoretical experience
Methodological knowledge and skill

Extrapersonal factors

Influential others
   Individual
   Institutional
Sociohistorical context

---

six interrelated influencing variables, subdivided into four intrapersonal factors and two extrapersonal factors (Table 4-1). The six factors are assumed to be in constant and mutual interaction, and when there is a change in one variable the other variables are affected. There are four basic phases to the inquiry process, and each phase is influenced by the six variables. Accordingly, the cumulative effect of the variables on the system as a whole is greater than the sum of the influence of the individual variables.

The system is characterized by continual change and is directed toward growth and increasing sophistication. In addition, it operates according to the principal of equifinality (Von Bertalanffy, 1968), which asserts that the same final or end state can be achieved from different beginnings and by different paths or routes. Even though there is never a final state in the research process for the researcher, this proposed inquiry system accepts and encourages individual differences throughout the practice of research, since each path chosen can get equally close to the "truth." The six factors or influencing variables are not intended to represent all intrapersonal or extraper-

sonal possibilities. Rather they should be viewed as a major class of variables that operate in addition to other factors such as personality, intelligence, or other values and beliefs. In addition, individual investigators vary in their awareness of the existence and nature of these variables as well as in the relative degree of influence any one factor may exert on the inquiry process.

Intrapersonal Factors

World View

The first personal variable that influences the process of inquiry is called world view, which consists of the researcher's general philosophical orientation, or world view, of the nature of human beings, the nature of knowledge and truth, and the nature of nursing science. Beliefs about human nature are fundamental to the development of the researcher's theoretical learnings, to the delineation of appropriate research questions, and, ultimately to the selection of research methodology. Relevant beliefs about human nature include such considerations as whether human beings are considered to be rational or irrational, whether human behavior is predetermined, and what the basis is for motivation of behavior. For example, are human motivations primarily conscious or unconscious? Is human behavior dictated by the need for growth or by the deprivation humans feel? Research questions generated will differ sharply, depending on whether human beings are viewed as highly self-directed individuals constantly striving for self-actualization v individuals who are at the mercy of their subconscious and who are constantly suppressing the primal urges the subconscious seeks to satisfy. Tucker points out that these latter beliefs as espoused by Freud and others, for example, have very specific implications for research methodology as well. He reminds us that the belief that one cannot ask a person directly about his or her thoughts and feelings provided the primary impetus for the development of popular psychological methods that employ unobtrusive and often deceptive testing techniques (Tucker, 1978).

Other beliefs related to a researcher's world view include how human beings are perceived in relation to their environment. For example, are people viewed as primarily passive reactors to events that impinge on them, or are they seen as proactive or mutually interactive with the environment? Does the human boundary end at the skin, or does the human field extend, as Rogers (1970) insists, beyond the skin to actually merge with the environmental field? Other perceptions that contribute to a researcher's world view relate to the multidimensionality of human beings. Are people seen as the popularized "biopsychosocial" beings, or are they seen as "biopsychosocial-spiritual-cultural" being? The very nature of the research questions would be altered by these two alternative views in that they would contain a very different constellation of variables and possible methodological implications.

These beliefs form the basis for establishing theoretical congruence, or the degree to which prevailing theories comfortably conform to one's world view. For example, if one believed that human beings were passive reactors to their environment and that behavior is motivated by the desire to avoid discomfort, it is unlikely that a systems perspective or symbolic interaction-based method would be very appealing. In this way beliefs about human nature delimit the realm of theoretical possibility in the practice of research.

Beliefs about the *nature of knowledge and truth* also affect a researcher's world view and thus the process of inquiry. Two major competing schools of thought best illustrate the diversity of these beliefs. Logical positivism, later known as the received view, asserts that objective, axiomatic truth exists that is discoverable and able to be verified by hypotheticodeductive methods (Suppe, 1977). Only certain methods that are objective and produce sense data can appropriately demonstrate this truth with any certainty, and only that knowledge derived in this manner counts as true scientific knowledge. The received view, as the dominant contemporary conception of science, conflicts sharply with what Polkinghorne (1983) calls the postpositivist view. A postpositivist conception of scientific knowledge and truth has evolved in reaction to the rather obvious limitations of the received view, especially for the human sciences. This view holds that the pursuit of knowledge and truth is necessarily historical, contextual, and theory laden. It claims no access to certain truth or knowledge but rather accepts certain knowledge to be "true" if it withstands practical tests of reason and utility. In this way, although knowledge may be useful, it is still fallible. Postpositivism does not cling to any one method of science and in fact encourages the use of the most appropriate method for the particular research question. Polkinghorne notes that "those methods are acceptable which produce results that convince the community that the new understanding is deeper, fuller, and more useful than the previous understanding" (Polkinghorne, 1983, p. 3).

The received view, or logical positivist approach to science, conforms closely to the correspondence norms of truth (Kaplan, 1964). What constitutes truth is the degree of correspondence between facts and their related theories and the degree to which propositions can be verified or shown to be false. Truth can be achieved only when it is shown that a proposition cannot be falsified. The received view also relies, in part, on the coherence theory of truth and its appreciation of theoretical aesthetics and logical simplicity in content and form. The postpositivist view, on the other hand, aligns itself with the pragmatic theory of truth, which emphasizes practical utility in problem solving and the degree of community consensus about that utility.

In the conduct of research positivism lends itself to reductionistic observables that must be quantified and verified, while postpositive concerns can be deductive or inductive in nature and can use either quantitative or qualitative strategies. It is clear that whether a researcher has positivist or postpositivist leanings and consciously or unconsciously subscribes to one theory of truth over another, these beliefs have a major effect on the formulation of the research question and the methodological strategy chosen. Thus it is unlikely that a researcher steeped in positivistic principles would ever ask a research question requiring the existential research methods of hermeneutic analysis.

A researcher's world view is also shaped by his or her beliefs about the *nature of nursing science.*

Whether or not one believes that nursing is a "science of human health and behavior across the life span" (Gortner, 1983, p. 5) and is specifically concerned with "the diagnosis and treatment of human responses to actual or potential health problems" (American Nurses' Association, 1980, p. 9) has ultimate implications for the types of events, states, and situations perceived to be problematic. Although client, nursing, environment, and health have all been considered phenomena central to nursing (Fawcett, 1978), one might disagree as to the emphasis that one component has in relation to another or on whether some or all of these concepts must be included in a theoretical formulation for nursing. For example, Stevens (1979) deemphasizes the environmental aspects, while Fawcett (1978) states that at least one or more of the four concepts must be present if the theory is to be called a nursing theory. Flaskerud and Halloran (1980) insist that the concept of nursing must always be included in any theoretical formulation for it to be considered nursing theory, while Conway (1985) believes the inclusion of nursing is inappropriate.

Whether nursing science is believed to conform more to a human science model (postpositivist) or to a natural science model (positivist) also has implications for the formulation of research problems. As a human science nursing must take into account various characteristics of the human realm. For example, the systemic character of human phenomena and the unclear nature of their boundaries are important to consider (Polkinghorne, 1983). The former necessitates investigating the whole rather than its individual parts, while the latter implies acceptance of indistinct conceptual boundaries. The process nature of the human realm must also be taken into consideration, as it signifies continual growth and repatterning over time. This implies the use of longitudinal or time series designs to fully explicate our phenomena of interest (Metzger & Schultz, 1982).

Fundamental to human sciences is the additional awareness that our perceptions about human phenomena are limited by our perceptions as human being. Total objectivity is an unattainable ideal because "there is no absolute point outside phenomena from which to investigate. Moreover, the knowledge gained in the investigation changes the character of what has been investigated" (Polkinghorne, 1983, p. 263). It also is not possible to directly access the human realm by direct observation. Rather, it must be observed indirectly through our interpretation of human behavioral expressions. This is an important point, since one of the major forms of human expression is through language. This implies that access to human phenomena is rightly obtained from written or oral expressions, for example. Credibility is thus established for subjective data collection methods that include interviews and questionnaires. A natural science mode, however, dictates a hypotheticodeductive approach to research with reliance on objective quantitative methods.

This notion of nursing as a human science—one modeled after a natural science—also has implications for expectations regarding nursing's scientific advancement. Some authors (Hardy, 1983; Newman, 1983) propose carte blanche acceptance of Kuhn's model for scientific growth, even though Kuhn clearly indicates that the model was developed for natural sciences (Kuhn, 1970). Expecting periods of normal science that will be periodically interrupted by scientific revolutions is perhaps unrealistic for nursing as a human science (Meleis, 1985). It may, in fact, lead to erroneous conclusions about scientific progress and, worse yet, hopelessly distort nursing's future direction. Kuhn points out that the rigid pattern of education for normal activity in the natural sciences "is not well designed to produce the man who will easily discover a fresh approach" (Kuhn, 1970, p. 166). It might well be that alleged patterns of revolution in natural science exist only because there is no other way for creative change to occur or for discoveries to be incorporated in such severely structured disciplines. It is clear that an investigator's fundamental beliefs about the nature of human beings, the nature of knowledge and truth, and the nature of nursing science contribute mightily to the definition of a research problem and ultimately to its solution.

Cognitive Style

It has long been observed that individuals have a preferred style of problem solving (Bloom & Broder, 1950) and that this style is a major factor in successful problem solving (Shouksmith, 1970). These cognitive styles "represent a person's typical modes of perceiving, remembering, thinking and problem solving" (Messick, 1970, p. 188). As such, cognitive styles exert a major influence on both the identification of a research problem and the ultimate approach to a solution.

In his theory of experiential learning, Kolb (1981) conceives of learning as a fourstage cycle that includes observations and reflections, formation of abstract concepts and generalizations, testing of implications of concepts and new situations, and concrete experience. Four kinds of abilities are required if this process is to be effective. Concrete experience (CE) is characterized by open, unbiased involvement, while the second ability, reflective observation (RO) involves considering experiences from many perspectives. Abstract conceptualization (AC) involves formulation and integration of concepts into logical and sound theories, and active experimentation (AE) reflects the ability to apply these theories in decision making and problem solving. These abilities can be considered polar opposites on two bisecting dimensions with CE and AC on either end of one continuum and AE and RO as opposites on the other. Kolb points out that the most sophisticated and highly evolved ability, that of creative insight, actually involves synthetic interaction between these abstract and concrete dimensions. In addition, individuals appear to develop cognitive styles that generally emphasize some abilities over others, and those abilities remain remarkably stable over time. It can be demonstrated, however, that styles tend to become somewhat more reflective and analytical as an individual gets older.

Through his research Kolb identifies four cognitive styles. *Convergers* operate predominantly between abstract conceptualization and active experimentation, with an aptitude toward practical application of ideas. These persons approach problems in a hypotheticodeductive way, focusing on a single solution to a problem, often preferring to deal with nonhuman entities. The opposite of convergers are *divergers,* whose abilities lie in concrete experience and reflective observation. These people are "idea generators" who have strong

and active imaginations and who are able to connect many unrelated but specific instances into a meaningful whole. Divergers are social and aesthetic in orientation and are often drawn to the humanities and the liberal arts. *Assimilators* operate predominantly in the abstract conceptualization and reflective observation modes and thus show great strength in inductive reasoning and theory formulation. These people are drawn to the logical and the abstract, with little attention to the need for practical application. *Accommodators,* operating on the opposite dimension from assimilators, are adept at concrete experience and active experimentation. These are action-oriented, risk-taking individuals who are often involved in implementation of an idea or a study. Accommodators are highly adaptive to changing situations and use the trial and error approach to problem solving.

These cognitive styles provide a useful way to conceive of general learning and problem-solving styles in individuals. Kolb (1981) warns against strict stereotyping, however, noting that research on cognitive style has consistently demonstrated how diverse and complex these processes actually are in real life. For example, cognitive function will vary in an individual according to the cognitive domain or situational demand.

The four cognitive styles described by Kolb (1981) can be related to inquiry norms in an academic discipline as well. Natural sciences and mathematics generally fall into the abstract-reflective quadrant; science-based professions are abstract-active; and social professions are more concrete-active. The concrete-reflective quadrant is characteristic of humanities and social sciences. Interestingly, in one study of a single university setting described by Kolb (1981), nursing fell into the abstract-active quadrant (converger), while in a much larger study nursing students and faculty fell into the concrete-reflective (diverger) category.

Kolb also proposes a typology of knowledge structures and inquiry processes in academic disciplines, suggesting that "forms of knowledge in different fields can be differentially attractive and meaningful to individuals with different learning styles" (Kolb, 1981, p. 245). That convergers would be drawn to or flourish in science-based empirical disciplines devoted to discrete analysis and conformance to correspondence norms is not surprising, nor is the attraction that the humanities and social science hold for divergers who profess to humanism, norms of coherence, and the conduct of research by historical analysis, field study, or clinical observation. That individuals with various cognitive styles would be attracted to nursing is also not surprising given the acknowledged complex and multifaceted nature of nursing's domain of interest. Certain cognitive styles are undoubtedly drawn to some scientific inquiry strategies more than others. For instance, the assimilator style might prefer theory generation using grounded theory methodology (Glaser & Strauss, 1967), while the accommodator style might choose involvement in clinical trials or intervention studies. A researcher whose predominant style is that of a converger might choose to be involved in theory-testing physiological research with animal subjects, while divergers might be drawn to phenomenological studies. Cognitive style appears to be a variable with major influence in a model of scientific inquiry.

Experience

The role of personal experience in scientific inquiry should not be underestimated. Both *life experience and professional nursing experience* provide fertile ground for problem awareness to grow. Problem identification and formulation of the research question become the fruit of that experience. Evidence of the verification or refutation of theories in the real world is also provided by this experience. Theories that work well are easily identified, while theories that fall short can be revised, extended, or discarded. Anomalous cases become readily apparent, as do continuing perplexities that remain unexplained by existing theories. One's sense of substantive significance stems from this experience, and intuition serves as a guide to the problems that have the most personal and professional meaning.

Prior *research experience* is also an important aspect of this variable, for it is through this experience that investigators learn which questions are able to be answered by current methods, which research ap-

proaches have worked in the past, and which ones have not. Experience also teaches what research needs to be conducted in the future and how it might best be accomplished. It also tells researchers whether prior research endeavors fit well enough with what Luria (1973) calls their research style. If prior research experience has been satisfactory and successful, an attempt will be made to replicate aspects contributing to that success, whether substantive or methodological in nature. While research success teaches investigators to utilize similar problem-solving strategies in the future, less than successful research is often as instructive because of the demand for increasingly novel and creative approaches in subsequent studies.

Theoretical experience is another type of experience that affects the process of inquiry. One aspect of this experience relies upon the existing knowledge base in a substantive area and the researcher's individual perception of that knowledge base. Theoretical experience allows the researcher to identify the existing gaps in knowledge and the significant areas that remain unexplored or unexplained. Individual researcher perception is important in this type of experience, for it is that perception that drives interest in unexplored domains. Scientific advancement depends on theoretical experience over time because of the necessarily progressive nature of research questions based on prior studies. Insight gained from longstanding familiarity with theoretical issues is of inestimable value and contributes to the overall level of understanding about the phenomenon of interest. This level of understanding in turn affects the content and level of subsequent research questions.

A second aspect of theoretical experience relates to the degree to which the researcher has been open to various theoretical approaches and intellectual strategies related to the exploration of the research problem area. If the researcher remains intellectually open to diverging and opposing views, the quality of theoretical understanding will be affected even though initial theoretical orientation may be maintained. Obviously the greater the clarity of understanding of the problem area the greater the possibility of significant answers. This type of intellectual exploration also allows for greater problem tension to exist, which in turn results in greater efforts to resolve the problems (Polyani, 1962). Bruner (1966) points out that it is precisely this dialectical tension between the concrete and the abstract that allows for creativity in problem solving.

Methodological Knowledge and Skill

The level and type of methodological knowledge and skill possessed by a researcher have a major influence on the process and product of scientific inquiry. Since the seeds of the answer lie in every research question (Mackinnon, 1979) and it is asserted that researchers have a preferred style of problem solving (Kolb, 1981), it is natural that researchers pose research questions that they will be able to answer. Kaplan calls this the "law of the instrument" and observes that "it comes as no particular surprise to discover that a scientist formulates problems in a way which requires for their solution just those techniques in which he himself is especially skilled" (Kaplan, 1964, p. 28). He also points out that the cost of becoming an expert in any one research area results in what can be called a "trained incapacity." That is, the more expert one becomes in something the harder it is to solve a problem any other way. Maslow agrees, asserting that "it is tempting, if the only tool you have is a hammer, to treat everything as if it were a nail" (Maslow, 1966, pp. 15-16).

It would seem that the relationship of methodological skills to the formulation of the research question and the process of inquiry for a single investigator study is closer than is often admitted. This limitation may be easier to overcome in larger studies with more than one investigator or over many studies, each conducted by different investigators. Capitalizing on the methodological strengths of multiple investigators to study complex nursing phenomena allows for greater theoretical possibilities through the use of multiple research methods. Polkinghorne points out that multiple methods allow more to be learned about a research problem than could be discovered from any one procedure or method alone (Polkinghorne, 1983).

Extrapersonal Factors

Two classes of extrapersonal variables are proposed to relate to the process and practice of scientific inquiry: influential others and the sociohistoric context.

Influential Others

Two major types of influence on scientific inquiry are inherent in the variable of influential others: individual and institutional. Individual influences are initially conveyed primarily by mentors and other professors in graduate school, the primary wellspring of research values and training for the budding nursing scientist (Tinkle & Beaton, 1983). Here, individual faculty methodological preferences and research values are made known implicitly or explicitly, and disciplinary norms are passed on (Kuhn, 1970). Expectations regarding appropriate methods of scientific inquiry are embedded in each experience and are reinforced at every juncture. It is the prevailing "faculty view" that determines the ultimate breadth and depth of curricular exposure to various research strategies, and it is faculty expertise that delimits actual research opportunities for students. It is here in graduate research training that a nursing scientist's individual research style is born (Luria, 1973).

While the acquisition of disciplinary norms is unquestionably important, the notion implies existing disciplinary consensus on what those norms actually are. Nursing has not quite come to such a conscious consensus, although there is no evidence of the consistent use of diverse research methods to study nursing's complex phenomena (Jacobsen & Meininger, 1985). When disciplinary research norms are not collectively shared, Toulmin points out that "theoretical debate in the field becomes largely— and unintentionally—methodological and philosophical; it is directed less at interpreting particular empirical findings than at debating the general acceptability (or unacceptability) of rival approaches, patterns of explanation and standards of judgment." (Toulmin, 1972, p. 380). The result is, of course, adamant assertions about one method over another, and the student scientist may be forced early on to align with one camp or another. Thus the norms that are acquired become not disciplinary but methodological and evaluative in nature. Kaplan calls this the "myth of methodology" and warns that "by pressing methodological norms too far, we may inhibit bold and imaginative adventure of ideas. The irony is that methodology itself may make for conformism—conforming to its own favored reconstructions" (Kaplan, 1964, p. 25). Polkinghorne (1983) points out that overall conceptual capacity, or what he calls "conceptual instruments," is also acquired by researchers in their graduate research training. However, he also notes that the unfortunate tendency is for these conceptual abilities to remain relatively unimproved throughout one's research career, even though the scientist may be exposed to diverse inquiry strategies throughout his or her research life. This notion lends support to the considerable influence of faculty norms on student scientists and to the relative strength of the other variables in the model of scientific inquiry as well.

Institutional influences, whether local, regional, or national in origin, also affect the process of scientific inquiry in a similar manner. Institutional norms function as operational imperatives for disciplinary activity in a given setting. Faculty researchers are thus expected, to some degree, to conform to these institutional norms, thus ensuring personal and professional prestige and survival. For example, on a large health science campus where the received view dominates the general conception of science, the faculty and student research in a school of nursing must reflect quasi conformance to these norms to exist at all. In the absence of such conformity university and extramural funding for the school and its research-related activities would be virtually impossible to secure. However, serious scientific repercussions can result when methodological conformity becomes the unquestioned status quo. Thompson (1985) warns that nurse researchers may not even be aware of the extent to which their research questions are prejudiced by the prevailing view. Martin (1982) notes the related influence of resource availability on the selection of the research problem, choice of methodology, and, less commonly, the interpretation of research findings. It is essential to recognize these theoretical and methodological prejudices and the extent to which they enable or disable nursing's scientific progress.

Luria reminds us that "research in a university is free to the extent that the university itself is free" (Luria, 1973, p. 82). The same can be said for research in a school of nursing. Diverse faculty research expertise and activity are characteristic of research climates that are intellectually free. It has also been observed that "the progress of science, good science, depends on novel ideas and intellectual freedom" (Feyerabend, 1981, p. 165). Innovative inquiry and methodological diversity among faculty beget similar opportunity and ability in student scientists. It is upon this foundation of scientific inquiry that the most important advancements in nursing science will be made.

Sociohistorical Context

Sociohistorical influences also affect the process of scientific inquiry in two significant ways. First, significant research problems are often sociohistorically defined and prioritized, thus affecting health policy decisions and funding levels. One obvious example is the current and intense research interest in the causes, cure, and treatment for acquired immune deficiency syndrome (AIDS). This disease has existed in less virulent forms throughout the world for a long time. However, it was the sudden and virulent occurrence of AIDS in western urban population centers, predominantly in otherwise healthy young males, that prompted research interest and subsequent funding by virtue of its threat to public health. Other examples of sociohistorically defined research problem areas include the current focus on quality of life issues, such as stress and coping, as well as the management of chronic illness. These current research concerns are a natural focus in a society that has conquered communicable disease and has extended the human life span. As the aging population grows, so also grows involvement in gerontological health concerns and research problems ultimately related to controlling or decreasing health care expenditures for the elderly.

The second way that the sociohistorical context affects the conduct of inquiry is a function of the idiosyncratic relationship of research style to disciplinary fashion (Luria, 1973). Kaplan wryly observes that "the pressures of fad and fashion are as great in science, for all its logic, as in other areas of culture" (Kaplan, 1964, p. 28). Contemporary scientific fashion alone has the power to dictate substantive focus, theoretical perspective, and methodological approach. For individuals and disciplines in search of academic prestige or research funding, the pressures and priorities of fashion often prove too great to resist. These influences may have the intended effect of stimulating creativity and the solution of significant problems, or they may serve to stultify research activity and to make it less creative than usual.

It is clear from this discussion that the intrapersonal factors of world view, cognitive style, experience, and methodological knowledge and skill as well as the extrapersonal factors of influential others and sociohistorical context together exert a major influence on the progress of scientific inquiry. In the proposed model the process of scientific inquiry is thus depicted as evolutionary emergent, fueled by continual feedback and ultimately directed toward growth and self-actualization. In this way individual research programs develop and progress throughout a scientific career.

Implications for Nursing Science

Several assumptions are fundamental to a discussion of the implications of the model of scientific inquiry for nursing. It will be helpful to state them explicitly:

- The model of scientific inquiry is a reasonable representation of reality.
- As such, the model can be considered to be an existing disciplinary norm for research problem solving in nursing.
- The demand for methodological diversity is implicit in this model or norm because of the complex and multifaceted nature of nursing phenomena and the nature of the individual inquiry process.
- The progress or success of nursing science must be judged by the degree to which the most significant disciplinary problems are actually solved.

These assumptions carry certain implications for nursing science. For example, that this model can be viewed as a norm of nursing science implies ultimate respect for the individual researcher's personal process of problem formulation and resolution. Actions that enhance this personal process ultimately will positively affect the development of nursing theory and science, while actions that interfere or interrupt this process will adversely affect the developing science.

Creativity

The assumption of methodological diversity implies certain mandates for student scientists, their graduate school professors and mentors, and for schools of nursing and other institutions. It has been established that science, at its best, demands the highest degree of creativity in problem solving. Nursing science, in its quest for rapid scientific advancement, is bound even closer than usual to this "constraint of creativity." Creativity coupled with sound methodological expertise is the rightful key to scientific progress. It is hypothesized that a creative scientist using a creative process and operating in a creative situation or climate is more likely to produce research results or theories that answer significant disciplinary questions. Fortunately there are several ways to enhance this creativity, beginning (for the purposes of this article) in doctoral study.

Creativity flourishes in a climate of intellectual freedom and open exploration. Creative problem solving must begin with self-exploration and self-knowledge. Student scientists should be provided with planned opportunities or activities designed for systematic, philosophical self-exploration so that one's world view can be explored and made known. This would contribute to more conscious decision making related to theoretical alignment, research methods, and the like. Opportunities to share and to discuss one's world view with peers and professors are also fundamental to scientific self-acceptance and acceptance of others. This obviously contributes to an academic atmosphere of openness and intellectual freedom.

Intuition

Intuition is ultimately associated with creativity and must be actively encouraged through the use of intuition-acknowledging and enhancing techniques. Students' exploration of their own pattern of receptivity and creativity should be part of every doctoral curriculum, as well as exposure to the processes of other creative thinkers. Faculty should share their own intuitive and creative processes freely, acknowledging the starts, stops, and detours inherent in the process. Other intuition-enhancing techniques can be employed throughout the educational experience as well. These include providing initial problem contexts or situations and encouraging students to explore the research problem, reformulating it in a manner appropriate to their experience and insight. Involvement in heuristic arguments, exercises in induction, and reasoning by analogy or metaphor all are activities directed toward increasing intuitive and receptive ability (Noddings & Shore, 1984). Ignoring the relationship of intuition to creativity or stifling its natural inclination exacts a terrible price from nursing theory development. To avoid the widespread underuse of such an obvious personal and professional resource implies ultimate acceptance of intuition as a legitimate partner to scholarly creativity and successful scientific enterprise. That intuition and creativity have "female" connotations should not worry those seeking scientific status, for it is relevant only to the observation that female scientists may be superior scientific problem solvers.

Cognitive Style

Assessment of personal cognitive style is also a highly useful strategy for beginning scientists so that existing abilities can be strengthened and weaker ones identified for possible intervention. Although there are obvious advantages and disadvantages to matching cognitive style of students and faculty, it has been proposed that the benefits of matching might be more related to the purpose of the student-faculty relationship (Rogers, 1970). If the relationship is instrumental, or for the purpose of learning particular skills, as in a research residency or mentor relationship, matching cognitive styles may be productive. If the purpose of the relationship is developmental and aimed at developing critical thinking skills, for example, then a mismatch of cognitive style might be more productive because of the exposure to diversity in thinking. Cognitive style assessment would provide useful baseline information upon which later decisions about course work, mentor relationships, research strategies, and the like might be made. The important point is that the assessment process should be a purposive activity within the doctoral curriculum.

Another important consideration related to cognitive style is the degree to which reflective thinking processes are enhanced or encouraged. Although creative and intuitive processes are important to scientific problem solving, critical thinking and analytical ability are equally important (Bigge, 1982). Inherent in reflective thinking is the ultimate balance between the cognitive and affective domains, the rational or analytical intuitive modes, the abstract and concrete levels of thinking, and, finally, the deductive and inductive approaches. Ideally these abilities would exist in exquisite balance in each researcher, but a more realistic focus would be to develop these abilities in each individual as much as possible. Fortunately many of the strategies directed toward enhancing intuition, creativity, and scientific problem solving also serve to improve reflective thinking abilities. Obviously if student scientists are to have adequate opportunity to refine these thinking skills in doctoral study, a faculty similarly skilled must be available to model and engage the students in appropriate exercise. If students are afforded the chance to increase skill in both analytical and intuitive modes, the gaps and flaws in existing theoretical conceptualizations will be easier to see and to overcome. Encouraging such creative yet critical thinking skills is the obvious antidote for nursing education's "long history of squelching curiosity and replacing it with conformity and a nonquestioning attitude" (Meleis, 1985, p. 37).

Methodological Diversity

Because the demand for methodological diversity is based as much on researcher characteristics as on the phenomenon of interest, opportunities for exposure to all types of research methods are essential. Thus a faculty must be carefully constructed so that quantitative and qualitative expertise exist side by side. This does not imply that a university cannot develop a research reputation for excellence in certain methodological strategies or theoretical orientation, merely that it should not gain it at the expense of other approaches. If faculty with varied philosophical orientation, cognitive styles, and methodological expertise are not available, then students are forced to match their process of inquiry to that of the available faculty. This can result in rather dire and sometimes dramatic consequences if a gross mismatch exists. At the outset the basic assumptions of the model of scientific inquiry are violated. Since the research problem that is formulated may not be a product of that intensely personal interactive process, there may be less investment in the research problem (Bigge, 1982). With decreased personal investment there may be diminished intellectual desire to solve the problem. When this natural obsession with one's problem is lost, so is what Polanyi calls "the mainspring of all inventive power" (Polanyi, 1962, p. 127). Once this power is lost, the research problem is essentially relegated to the routine, and it becomes a chore instead of an exciting process of discovery. One wonders if the plethora of one-shot studies in nursing is in part a function of the lack of investment in the research problem.

When prevailing scientific attitudes and norms directly conflict with the intellectual-intuitive orientations of the researcher or student scientist and no safe haven for one's methodological learnings exists, interest is lost and so is another opportunity for scientific advancement. Jacox warns that "we have to be careful not to catch students and others who express these alternative views of science in our own somewhat narrower interpretations of science and theory. We must be cognizant that students may be in some jeopardy from faculty not knowledgeable or not accepting of emerging alternative views of science" (Jacox, 1981, p. 20). When it comes to the degree of faculty influence on a student scientist's process of inquiry, it is wise to take heed of Feyer-abend's advice: "The hardest task needs the lightest hand or else its completion will not lead to freedom but to a tyranny much worse than the one it replaces" (Feyerabend, 1981, p. 167).

Nursing scientists are a scarce national resource and as such their scholarly productivity must be promoted whenever possible. The ultimate success of nursing science depends wholly on the ability to answer significant disciplinary questions. A creative research effort at all levels of theory building is required to accomplish this formidable task. This demands the existence of an intellectual climate most conducive to creative scientific problem solving and must allow a full array of cognitive and methodological possibilities for use by nursing's budding scientists. This climate should be responsive to individual differences in cognitive style, methodological preference, and the like but should simultaneously foster a fundamental appreciation for divergent approaches and styles.

Admittedly the costs of creating such a climate might appear to be high initially. In the extreme, widespread and epistemological anarchy and methodological revolution might result. At the very least it will require renouncement of scientific conformism, a return to individualism, and acceptance of methodological relativism. In either case the investment will yield a critical mass of highly committed and creative nursing scientists who are intrigued by nursing's scientific complexities and who are fully engaged in finding their solutions. In addition, an increasingly diverse pool of applicants will be attracted to doctoral study in nursing because of the increasing disciplinary consonance with a wide range of philosophical and intellectual possibilities. This can only further enhance the ability to address all levels of theory development.

Once the tremendous force of nursing's unclaimed creative potential is unleashed, a new age of inquiry in nursing science will be born. This new age of inquiry will be characterized by the generation of sophisticated methodological strategies suited to the complexities of a human science, the existence of sound theoretical formulations, and the general societal acknowledgement of nursing's sizable contribution to human welfare. A renewed sense of professional pride will prevail and nursing's scientific competence will be rightly judged by the ability to solve the discipline's most significant problems.

REFERENCES

Albert, R. S. (Ed.). (1983). *Genius and eminence: The social psychology of creativity and exceptional achievement.* Oxford, England: Pergamon Press.

American Nurses' Association (1980). *Nursing: A social policy statement.* Kansas City: Author.

Batey, M. V. (1977). Conceptualization: Knowledge and logic guiding empirical research. *Nursing Research, 26*(5), 324–329.

Bigge, M. (1982). *Learning theories for teachers* (4th ed.). New York: Harper & Row.

Bloom, B., & Broder, C. (1950). *The problem solving process of college students.* Chicago: University of Chicago Press.

Brink, P., & Wood, M. (1983). *Basic steps in planning nursing research, from question to proposal* (2nd ed.). Monterey, CA: Wadsworth.

Bronowski, J. (1965). *Science and human values.* New York: Harper & Row.

Bruner, J. (1966). *The process of education.* New York: Atheneum.

Carper, B. A. (1978). Fundamental patterns of knowing in nursing. *Advances in Nursing Science, 1*(1), 13–23.

Claxton, C., & Ralston, Y. (1978). *Learning styles: Their impact on teaching and administration.* Washington, DC: The American Association for Higher Education.

Conway, M. (1985). Toward greater specificity in defining nursing's metaparadigm. *Advances in Nursing Science, 7*(4), 73–81.

Dickoff, J., James, P., & Weidenbach, E. (1968). Theory in a practice discipline: Part I—practice oriented theory. *Nursing Research, 17*(5), 415–435.

Donaldson, S. K., & Crowley, D. M. (1978). The discipline of nursing. *Nursing Outlook, 26*(2), 113–120.

Fawcett, J. (1978). The relationship between theory and research: A double helix. *Advances in Nursing Science, 1*(1), 49–62.

Feyerabend, P. (1981). How to defend society against science. In I. Hacking (Ed.), *Scientific revolutions.* London: Oxford University Press.

Flaskerud, J. H., & Halloran, E. J. (1980). Areas of agreement in nursing theory development. *Advances in Nursing Science, 3*(1), 1–7.

Glaser, B., & Strauss, A. (1967). *The discovery of grounded theory: Strategies of qualitative research.* New York: Aldine.

Goldstein, M., & Goldstein, I. (1978). *How we know: An exploration of the scientific process.* New York: Plenum Press.

Gortner, S., & Nahm, H. (1977). An overview of nursing research in the United States. *Nursing Research, 26,* 10–33.

Gortner, S. (1983). The history and philosophy of nursing science and research. *Advances in Nursing Science, 5*(2), 1–8.

Hardy, M. (1983). Metaparadigms and theory development. In N. L. Chaska (Ed.), *The nursing profession: A time to speak* (pp. 427–435). New York: McGraw-Hill.

Jacobsen, B., & Meininger, J. (1985). The design and methods of published nursing research: 1956–1983. *Nursing Research, 34,* 306–311.

Jacox, A. (1974). Theory construction in nursing: An overview. *Nursing Research, 23*(1), 4–13.

Jacox, A. (1981, June). *Competing theories of science.* Paper presented at the 1981 Forum on Doctoral Education in Nursing, Seattle, WA, June 1981.

Kaplan, A. (1964). *The conduct of inquiry.* New York: Harper & Row.

Kerlinger, F. (1973). *Foundations of behavioral research* (2nd ed.). New York: Holt, Rinehart & Winston.

Kolb, D. (1981). Learning styles and disciplinary differences. In A. Chickering (Ed.), *The modern American college* (pp. 232–255). San Francisco: Jossey-Bass.

Kuhn, T. S. (1970). *The structure of scientific revolutions* (2nd ed.). Chicago: University of Chicago Press.

Luria, S. E. (1973). On research styles and allied matters. *Daedalus, 102*(2), 75–84.

Mackinnon, D. (1979). Creativity: A multifaceted phenomenon. In J. D. Roslansky (Ed.), *Creativity* (pp. 19–32). Amsterdam: North-Holland.

Martin, J. (1982). A garbage can model of the research process. In J. McGrath, J. Martin, & R. Kulka (Eds.), *Judgment calls in research* (pp. 17–39). Beverly Hills, CA: Sage.

Maslow, A. H. (1966). *The psychology of science: A reconnaissance.* South Bend, IN: Gateway Editions.

McGrath, J. E. (1982). Dilemmatics: The study of research choices and dilemmas. In J. McGrath, J. Martin, & R. Kulka (Eds.), *Judgement calls in research* (pp. 69–102). Beverly Hills, CA: Sage.

Meleis, A. I. (1985). *Theoretical nursing: Development and progress.* Philadelphia: J.B. Lippincott.

Messick, S. (1970). The criterion problem in the evaluation of instruction: Assessing possible, not just intended extremes. In M. Wittrock & D. Riley (Eds.), *Evaluation of instruction: Issues and problems.* New York: Holt, Rinehart & Winston.

Metzger, B., & Schultz, S. (1982). Time series analysis: An alternative for nursing. *Nursing Research, 31*(6), 375–378.

Newman, M. A. (1983). The continuing revolution: A history of nursing science. In N. L. Chaska (Ed.), *The nursing profession: A time to speak* (pp. 385–393). New York: McGraw-Hill.

Nicholls, J. G. (1983). Creativity in the person who will never produce anything original or useful. In R. S. Albert (Ed.), *Genius and eminence: The social psychology of creativ-*

ity and exceptional achievement (pp. 265–279). Oxford, England: Pergamon Press.

Noddings, N., & Shore, P. (1984). *Awakening the inner eye intuition in education.* New York: Teachers College Press.

Oiler, C. (1982). The phenomenological approach in nursing research. *Nursing Research, 31*(3), 178–181.

Polanyi, M. (1962). *Personal knowledge.* Chicago: University of Chicago Press.

Polit, D., & Hungler, B. (1983). *Nursing research: Principles and methods* (2nd ed.). Philadelphia, J.B. Lippincott.

Polkinghorne, D. (1983). *Methodology for the human science systems of inquiry.* Albany, NY: State University of New York Press.

Rogers, M. E. (1970). *A theoretical basis for nursing.* Philadelphia: F.A. Davis.

Roy, S. C. (1983). Theory development in nursing: Proposal for direction. In N. L. Chaska (Ed.), *The nursing profession: A time to speak* (pp. 453–465). New York: McGraw-Hill.

Runkel, P., & McGrath, J. (1972). *Research on human behavior: A systematic guide to method.* New York: Holt, Rinehart & Winston.

Shouksmith, G. (1970). *Intelligence, creativity and cognitive style.* New York: Wiley Interscience.

Stevens, B. (1979). *Nursing theory: Analysis, application, evaluation.* Boston: Little, Brown.

Suppe, F. (1977). *The structure of scientific theories* (2nd ed.). Chicago: University of Illinois Press.

Thompson, J. (1985). Practical discourse in nursing: Going beyond empiricism and historicism. *Advances in Nursing Science, 7*(4), 59–71.

Tinkle, M. B., & Beaton, J. L. (1983). Toward a new view of science: Implications for nursing research. *Advances in Nursing Science, 5*(2), 27–36.

Tucker, R. (1979). The value decisions we know as science. *Advances in Nursing Science, 1*(2), 1–12.

Toulmin, S. (1972). *Human understanding* (Vol. 1). Oxford, England: Clarendon Press.

Von Bertalanffy, L. (1968). *General system theory.* New York: George Braziller.

Weiskopf, V. (1973). Introduction. In H. Yukawa (Ed.), *Creativity and intuition: A physicist looks east and west* (J. Bester, trans.). Tokyo: Kodansha International.

Wilson, H. S. (1985). *Research in nursing.* Menlo Park, CA: Addison-Wesley.

Worthy, M. (1975). *Aha! A puzzle approach to creative thinking.* Chicago: Nelson Hall.

Yukawa, H. (1973). *Creativity and intuition: A physicist looks at east and west* (J. Bester, trans.). Tokyo: Kodansha International.

The Author Comments

Scientific Inquiry in Nursing: A Model for a New Age

This work arose from an intensely passionate intellectual process that kept me in its grips for the first 2 years of doctoral study at the University of California, San Francisco. Coursework in theory development, the philosophy of science, and research methods challenged my assumptions about the research process, forcing a reflective process unlike any I had ever experienced. To understand my role as a budding nurse scientist and how I might best contribute to nursing's knowledge base, I struggled with the question, "How does science really happen?" and, more to the point, "What factors truly affect the conduct of research?" It seemed reasonable that insight into the many influences and pressures I was facing in defining my own research interests would be crucial to the resolution of these issues in my career. Fortunately, the new understanding I gained led to the creation of the model for scientific inquiry in nursing and a sense of peace about my career decisions.

—HOLLY A. DEGROOT

CHAPTER 5

Nursing Systems and Nursing Models

John R. Phillips

Since the primary goal of nursing theory is the generation of knowledge specific to nursing, the process of theory building must be couched in a nursing frame of reference. Otherwise, the obtained knowledge will not be nursing knowledge which can be used to build or expand nursing science or be used for nursing education, practice, or research.

The evolution of nursing science as any young science is dependent upon knowledge borrowed from other disciplines. There will always be a core of knowledge which will be used by all the sciences. However, the process of borrowing theories and models from other disciplines has hampered nurses in learning how to ask questions which are of specific concern to nursing or in conceptualizing how the borrowed knowledge is to be used to generate theory to expand nursing science.

The creation of nurse scientist programs was an attempt to avoid the pitfalls of borrowing knowledge from other disciplines. One would wonder how effective these programs have been in the testing of theory to obtain knowledge to advance nursing science. Newman (1972), in reference to nurse scientist programs, points out that the testing of theory in another discipline's framework relates the data more to that discipline than to nursing. Nurse scientists may contribute to the general knowledge of order in man, but it will continue to be borrowed knowledge (Johnson, 1968). As long as nurses continue to borrow theories and models and test theory in other disciplines and not relate the data to nursing, the evolution of nursing science will be slow. Borrowed knowledge from other disciplines must be synthesized into conceptual systems and models of

About the Author

JOHN R. PHILLIPS left the hills of Virginia, his birthplace, by enlisting in the U.S. Air Force. After discharge from the military, he went to New York City to attend the Bellevue and Mills Schools of Nursing. While in staff and administrative positions at the Bellevue Hospital Medical Center, he received his bachelor degree from Hunter College and his master's degree from New York University (NYU). John's contributions to nursing science and theory, particularly Rogerian science, began when he was a doctoral student at NYU under the tutelage of Martha E. Rogers and Margaret Newman. While a doctoral student at NYU and a faculty member at Hunter College, he created and taught the first core nursing theory course in the master's program at Hunter College. Since his recent retirement from NYU after 25 years on the faculty, he devotes more time to the collection of art, art glass, and pottery, as well as first-edition books. His interest in all dimensions of humanity is enriched by his participation in the arts and leisure activities of New York City.

nursing; otherwise, the focus of nursing will remain within the conceptual systems and models of other disciplines.

Nursing practice is another method nursing uses to discover theory (Wald & Leonard, 1964). The lack of success of this method in building nursing knowledge is related to nurses practicing within borrowed conceptual models and theoretical frameworks of other disciplines. In other words, the gestalt for practice is not uniquely nursing because of inadequate synthesis of theories and models from other disciplines into nursing systems and models. The advancement of nursing science will occur only when nursing systems and models are created which nurses can use to construct theories from practice and from which principles and theories can be evolved to explain, describe, and predict phenomena of man. When this inductive and deductive approach to nursing theory becomes more a reality, nursing will have a "ground" for education, practice, and research.

The method of borrowing theories and models from other disciplines has been of benefit, but the point in the evolution of nursing has arrived where nursing must be more productive in the creation of conceptual systems and models of nursing. One needs only to analyze some of the models borrowed from other disciplines to understand why the advancement of nursing science has been stymied. The analysis will help to clarify why nursing has had difficulty in differentiating itself from other disciplines and in identifying the boundaries which are unique to nursing.

The Medical (Disease) Model

The most pervasive model borrowed by nursing is the medical model. The medical model forces nursing to view health-illness manifestations as organic phenomena where emphasis is upon disorders in the structure and function of the body. With this disease-oriented approach to clients, the nurse is concerned with underlying defects or structural aberrations—changes in organs, tissues, and cells—which "must be identified, prevented, removed, counteracted, neutralized, or corrected" (Wu, 1973). The medical model framework of signs and symptoms, cause, pathology, course and prognoses, and treatment is used by the nurse to plan care. The utilization of the medical model compels a person to view disease as the failure of the body as a physiochemical machine, and patients are helped by interventions in bodily processes (Engel, 1970). As long as nurses use the medical model, chronic illnesses will present a difficult problem. To treat a person as sick rather than impaired gives rise to discouragement of normal behavior (Shagass, 1975).

The process of nursing education within the medical model has its theoretical base derived primarily from the biological sciences. A look at nursing textbooks which are medically oriented reveals principles directed toward minimization or elimination of disease processes. Nursing interventions are directed toward causal factors or pathology. The medical model purports also that mental disorders are illnesses like any other illness. Nursing educators who held this view taught this belief to students under the assumption that there is an underlying cause for the individual's behavior. Thus, the educational process focused on the causes of abnormal or maladaptive behaviors rather than the behaviors themselves. Nursing is not medicine but nursing!

The medical model posits a dichotomy between mind and body which is not congruent with the philosophy of nursing in its concern with the whole person. Not only is nursing concerned with the structure and function of the body but also with human experience, behavior, feelings, and the influence of social forces upon the body—manifestations of the man-environment interaction, whether they be termed normal or abnormal. As nurses became dissatisfied with the medical model with its focus upon the body, the psychologic model was borrowed to look at the health-illness of man.

The Psychologic Model

The psychologic model concerns itself with normal human growth and development and deficits which occur with the maturation process. Emphasis is placed upon disruptions in the individual's development and the undesirability of certain states of mind, feeling, or conduct (Leifer, 1970-1971). Using the psychologic model nursing added theories of psychodynamics, interpersonal relations, crisis intervention, and ego development and defense mechanisms to its repertory of borrowed knowledge. The use of the word "added" can be understood after an examination of nursing texts is carried out. The importance of understanding the psychological component of man is stressed; yet, the content of the texts deals with alterations in physical structure and function of the body. Here, specific reference is made to the medical-surgical nursing texts where interest is shown in the mind and behavior of man for the purpose of understanding and altering bodily mechanisms.

When one looks at the psychiatric texts, there is still mention of alterations in physical structure and function. But, when mention is made of physical and structural disruptions, it is for the purpose of understanding their effect on mind and behavior. However, the borrowing of the psychologic model enabled the nurse to begin to move away from a disease orientation to one whereby the psychologic meaning of events, feelings, and behaviors could be explored and incorporated into nursing interventions. The psychologic model gave nurses an opportunity to teach patients how to experience their feelings. The model also gave nurses the opportunity to explore with clients how to bear feelings which appeared to be beyond bearing.

The medical and psychologic models place a dichotomy between mind and body which is built into nursing curricula where separate courses in medical-surgical nursing, parent-child nursing, psychiatric nursing, psychosocial aspects of nursing, and interpersonal relations in nursing are presented. Fortunately, the inadequacy of such curricula has been recognized, and integrated curricula have been and are being developed. The proposed success of these curricula will remain a myth, however, as long as they remain under the aegis of models borrowed from other disciplines. To be successful, the borrowed knowledge must be synthesized into nursing systems from which conceptual models for curricula can be created.

The medical and psychologic models are oriented toward individuals, but man does not exist as an entity unto himself but interacts with his environment. The medical and psychologic models do not deal with the relationship of man to his environment. The borrowing of the ecologic model was one attempt by nursing to gain a better understanding of the interaction of man with his environment.

The Ecologic (Public Health) Model

The ecologic model is an extension of the medical model (Pasewark & Rardin, 1971). Disease in this model is postulated as not being caused by disruptions in the structure and function of the body but by multiple factors both within the outside man. In other words, an ecological relationship between the host (man) and the environment where illness is a function of genetic man and the total effects of his environment (E. S. Rogers, 1960).

The effects of the ecologic model upon nursing can be seen with the addition of public health nursing and epidemiology into nursing curricula. The ecologic model gave rise to the concept of prevention which is one of the prime foci of nursing today. There is movement away from tertiary and secondary prevention (medical model) to primary prevention. Even though the ecologic model is an extension of the medical model, it helped to open paths for nurses such as primary care and independent nurse practitioners in their attempt to move away from the constraints of the medical model. The passage of new Nurse Practice Acts was a tremendous impetus toward independent practice in nursing.

Nursing's rejection of the medical model and movement toward more autonomy has the medical profession in an uproar about the role and function of nursing. The physician still "tries to legislate out of existence those who would cure human ills" (Nemiah, 1970-1971), even nursing. As long as the physician can enforce the medical model, only he will be able to confer the sick role through his diagnoses (Shagass, 1975). As long as nurses continue to function within the medical model, only the physician will be allowed to make diagnoses and prescribe treatment for manifestations of illness.

The Social Model

The social model explicates further the influence of the environment upon man since the primary assumption of the model is that the manifestations of an individual are essentially the consequence of cultural variables that impinge upon him. These forces upon the individual come directly from the culture or from such cultural groups as the family, social institutions, and agencies (Pasework & Rardin, 1971).

The social model enables the nurse to have concern for individuals as they exist in a group of meaningful others and to have better understanding of how groups of individuals influence each other. However, the social model is not a specific frame of reference for nursing. Manifestations of illness in the social model are viewed as "an impairment of capacity to perform one's social roles and/or valued tasks relative to his status in society" (Parsons, 1958). Within this frame of reference, illness is defined in terms of the social position or role a person is expected to occupy or play (Wu, 1973).

Nursing borrowed from the social model theories of group dynamics and group socialization and theories concerning the development of various role patterns. The borrowed knowledge helped the nurse to focus on the ways individuals function in social systems. But, the frame of reference for nursing still remained within another discipline. Theories constructed within this frame of reference are tainted by another discipline's views of the health needs of people.

The analysis of the models borrowed by nursing in its attempt to expand nursing knowledge elucidates two major questions with which nursing is concerned. Will the process of borrowing knowledge make nursing unique from the other disciplines? What are the boundaries of nursing? It is hoped that the present conceptual systems and models of nursing will provide answers to these questions. However, the use of some of the models cannot be successful in providing the answers. Some nursing theorists have simply taken theories and models from other disciplines and transposed them into what is called a "nursing" model. The dangers of this method of model construction are that the theories and models borrowed may not have been supported in the other disciplines, and the theories and models may not be generalizable to nursing. If the borrowing method is to be used by nursing, the theories and models must be supported from a nursing frame of reference before being synthesized into conceptual systems and models for nursing. Other nursing models have great potential in providing answers to the questions. Theories and models from other disciplines were not borrowed; instead, concepts were used to construct the nursing model. With the nursing models constructed from concepts, it is possible to build theories to generate knowledge unique to nursing. This knowledge in turn might be borrowed by other disciplines to expand their knowledge!

The discussion of the models which nursing has borrowed to advance nursing science makes clear the fact that not one of the models views man in his totality in his interaction with the environment. Some of the nursing models constructed from borrowed theories and models perpetuate this dichotomy of man and environment. The more abstract nursing models constructed from concepts and not from borrowed theories and models look at the complementarity of the man-environment interaction. Two examples of the more abstract nursing models are the *Rogers Life Process Model* (M. E. Rogers, 1970) and the *Johnson Behavioral System Model* (Auger, 1976; Riehl & Roy, 1974). These models can be used as a framework for theory construction which can generate nursing knowledge—knowledge which can be used for nursing education, practice, and research. Nursing must continue to construct systems and models which are truly nursing so theory can be developed to generate nursing knowledge. Nursing can no longer afford to have its frame of reference couched in the systems and models of other disciplines.

REFERENCES

Auger, J. R. (1976). *Behavioral systems and nursing.* Englewood Cliffs, NJ: Prentice-Hall.

Engel, G. L. (1970). Sudden death and the 'Medical Model' in psychiatry. *Canadian Psychiatric Association Journal, 15,* 527–37.

Johnson, D. E. (1968). Theory in nursing: Borrowed and unique. *Nursing Research, 17,* 206–209.

Leifer, R. (1970–71). The medical model as ideology. *International Journal of Psychiatry, 9,* 13–21.

Nemiah, J. C. (1970–71). The myth of mental illness. *International Journal of Psychiatry, 9,* 26–29.

Newman, M. A. (1972). Nursing's theoretical evolution. *Nursing Outlook, 20,* 449–453.

Parsons, T. (1958). Definitions of health and illness in light of American values and social structures. In E. G. Jaco (Ed.), *Patients, physicians, and illness.* New York: Free Press.

Pasewark, R. A., & Rardin, M. W. (1971). Theoretical models in community mental health. *Mental Hygiene, 55,* 358–364.

Riehl, J. P., & Roy, C. (1974). *Conceptual models for nursing practice.* New York: Appleton-Century-Crofts.

Rogers, E. S. (1960). *Human ecology and health, Part III.* New York: Macmillan.

Rogers, M. E. (1970). *An introduction to the theoretical basis of nursing.* Philadelphia: F. A. Davis.

Shagass, C. (1975). The medical model in psychiatry. *Comprehensive Psychiatry, 16,* 405–413.

Wald, F. S., & Leonard, R. C. (1964). Towards development of nursing practice theory. *Nursing Research, 13,* 309–313.

Wu, R. (1973). *Behavior and illness.* Englewood Cliffs, NJ: Prentice-Hall.

The Author Comments

Nursing Systems and Nursing Models

In the preparation of the theory course, I was surprised to find how sparse the nursing theoretic underpinnings were. A survey of nursing texts indicated that much of what was being taught in nursing schools was based on knowledge from other sciences. Also, there was little substantive nursing research that indicated this knowledge was appropriate for nursing. Thus, I felt a need to write about the evolution of the theoretic base for nursing and to postulate how nursing science should be developed through the use of nursing systems and models. More important, I believed that nursing students had to be taught theory and theory development from a nursing perspective if nursing science were to develop at a more rapid pace. During the past 25 years, nurse scholars have developed a sophisticated nursing science through the use of nursing models and theories. However, recently, some fraudulent nurse scholars are emphasizing the use of models and theories from other disciplines to advance nursing science. I am making a plea to all nurses to heed the suggestions in the article so that nursing, as a science, will survive in the 21st century and beyond.

—JOHN R. PHILLIPS

CHAPTER 6

Levels of Theoretical Thinking in Nursing

Patricia A. Higgins
Shirley M. Moore

Development of a knowledge base is an iterative and ongoing process that requires periodic analysis and synthesis of an entire body of work. This article examines 4 related levels of theoretical thinking that are currently used in developing knowledge for nursing practice, education, and science: meta-theory, grand theory, middle-range theory, and micro-range theory. Each level of theory is discussed according to typology, scope, and generalizability, level of abstraction, and role. Suggestions are made for clarification of terminology, and examples are provided for each level of theoretical thinking. Evidence associated with the 4 levels of theoretical thinking is discussed, and applications for use of the levels of theoretical thinking to meet future challenges in nursing's knowledge development are offered.

In an effort to build a knowledge base for the clinical, educational, and scientific endeavors of the discipline, nursing theory has undergone several phases of development. In the earliest period, scholars focused their attention on building grand theory and debating the structure and methods for developing nursing theory. More recently, there has been a call for the development of middle-range theory. Thus theory in nursing has been conceptualized as existing on several levels although there are wide differences in the definitions and terminology associated with the levels of theoretical thinking and the classification of theoretical products. This lack of clarity impedes our use of theoretical thinking to extend and communicate our nursing knowledge. Therefore, the purpose of this article is to present an examination of levels of theoretical thinking in nursing and

Reprinted from Nursing Outlook, *Levels of theoretical thinking, 48(4),179-183,*
Copyright © 2000, Mosby, Inc., with permission from Elsevier Science.

About the Authors

PATRICIA HIGGINS is an Assistant Professor of Nursing, Case Western Reserve University (CWRU). Her first nursing diploma was from Henry Ford Hospital (1970) and her second from Akron University (BSN, 1986). These were followed by graduate degrees from CWRU (MSN, 1989; PhD, 1996). Her teaching concentrates on theory and philosophy of science, and her program of research focuses on understanding and improving the health of adults who live with chronic conditions. In her time off, Dr. Higgins enjoys her family, gardening, and reading.

SHIRLEY MOORE is an Associate Dean for Research and Associate Professor of Nursing at Case Western Reserve University (CWRU), Cleveland, OH. Born at the beginning of the baby boom, she began her nursing career during a shift in nursing education from hospital training programs to more academic-focused programs, and she considers herself a product of both. Dr. Moore received her diploma of nursing from the Youngstown Hospital Association School of Nursing (1969) and her bachelor's degree in nursing from Kent State University (1974). At CWRU, she earned a master's degree in nursing-psychiatric mental health nursing (1990) and a PhD in nursing science (1993). Dr. Moore has taught nursing theory and nursing science to all levels of nursing students and has a program of research and theory development that addresses recovery after acute cardiac events. Her hobbies include traveling with her family, reading, and music.

provide examples of how several existing nursing theories can be classified within the theoretical levels. Applications of levels of theoretical thinking to meet challenges in knowledge development in nursing are suggested.

A theory in its simplest view is the creation of relationships among two or more concepts to form a specific view of a phenomenon. As constructions of our mind, theories provide explanations about our experiences of phenomena in the world.[1] The understanding provided by theories is of two types: explanatory (describing concepts and understanding interactions among concepts) or predictive (anticipating a particular set of outcomes).[2] Theories consist of the following components: (1) concepts that are identified and defined, (2) assumptions that clarify the basic underlying truths from which and within which theoretical reasoning proceeds, (3) context within which the theory is placed, and (4) identified relationships between and among the concepts.[3]

The terms theory, theoretical (or conceptual) model, theoretical framework, and theoretical system are often used to distinguish different types of theory.

This practice has created confusion among scholars and practitioners, and we believe a more useful approach to understanding theory is to consider all of the aforementioned terms as parallel synonyms. Each can be used interchangeably, but each term also requires further specification through an adjective modifier, such as "grand" or "middle range," that describes its fit with other theoretical work. Thus the notion of different levels of theoretical thinking can be a more useful way to develop, disseminate, and use knowledge in nursing. We use the word "level" to imply a relative degree of relationship rather than a ranking or a distinct advantage. Each level of theoretical thinking has defining characteristics and purposes that are specific to that level. The scope or breadth of the concepts and goals of a theoretical system determine its use for research and practice. Therefore, theoretical thinking in nursing uses concepts and their relationships to organize and critique existing knowledge and guide new discoveries to advance practice. Its development and use is not limited to particular venues, time frames, or formats, and although *all* nurses may not use theoretical thinking *at all times*, its actual use is more frequent than some nurses may acknowledge. For instance, theoretical thinking regarding a family's psychologic well being can be briefly and automatically accessed as part of the gestalt of clinical practice or formally developed into a more permanent, written framework. Both types of theoretical thinking are crucial for practice, and either may be critiqued, modified, and tested.

Linkages between the theoretical world and the empirical world to which it applies are made through the formulation and testing of hypotheses. Both scientists and practitioners use this process to make the empirical world and the theoretical world as congruent as possible. It is important to distinguish an empirical system from a theoretical system. An empirical system is what we apprehend, through senses, in the environment. A theoretical system is what we construct in our mind's eye to model the empirical system.[1] Nurse scientists and practitioners focus on understanding the variables of a particular practice situation. To better understand a specific event, they formulate working definitions and associations among variables (hypotheses) and either develop a new theoretical system or link them to existing organizing frameworks. The theoretical system then serves as guidance about how to proceed, and as long as the abstraction of a theory can be represented with empiric indicators, hypotheses can be generated and empirically tested.[2]

Levels of Theoretical Thinking

Theory in the human sciences has been used to delineate and legitimate the emerging disciplines and substantiate knowledge development.[4] There are 4 levels of theoretical thinking in nursing: meta-theory, grand theory, middle-range theory, and micro-range theory.[5] Each level of theory will be discussed according to level of abstraction and scope, generalizability, typology, and role. Figure 6-1 describes the relationships among the 4 levels and provides examples of theoretical thinking for each level.

Meta-theory

Meta-theory, the most abstract and universal of the 4 levels of theoretical thinking, addresses issues related to the conduct of inquiry. Therefore, it is the theory of inquiry. Meta-theory or philosophic inquiry uses logic and analytic reasoning to examine the direction, methods, and standards of inquiry and thus it differs from the other levels of theory as its product is primarily knowledge-about-knowledge (second-order knowledge), rather than specific theoretical frameworks that explain the empirical world (first-order knowledge). Meta-theoretical inquiry related to scientific issues is known as philosophy of science, and it focuses on a critical examination of science, its processes, and products. Used by both scientists and practitioners, meta-theoretical inquiry also addresses questions that science cannot answer. For example, in the study of death and dying, scientific inquiry seeks to answer questions about the physiologic changes leading to death. However, philosophic inquiry is needed to address the question, "Is death best understood as a process or a product?" Therefore, an understanding of meta-theoretical thinking is central to both the research and practice of nursing.

As the most well established of the 4 levels, the significance and role of meta-theoretical knowledge in nursing is revealed through a partial list of issues addressed through this mode of inquiry: (1) clarification of the relationship between nursing science and practice, (2) definition, development, and testing of nursing theory, (3) establishment of the academic discipline of nursing, and (4) examination and interpretation of fundamental philosophic perspectives and their connection to nursing science. The long list of exemplary scholarship that represents these 4 categories of philosophic inquiry in nursing is well represented in anthologies such as the one by Nicoll,[6] but one example also illustrates the value of the discipline's meta-theoretical thinking. In 1978 when Carper[7] published her influential article on the fundamental patterns of knowing in nursing, she initiated a spirited dialogue that continues to this day—in print, classrooms, and practice arenas throughout the world.

Grand Theory

Nursing grand theories are the global paradigms of nursing science.[8] They are formal, highly abstract theoretical systems that frame our disciplinary knowledge

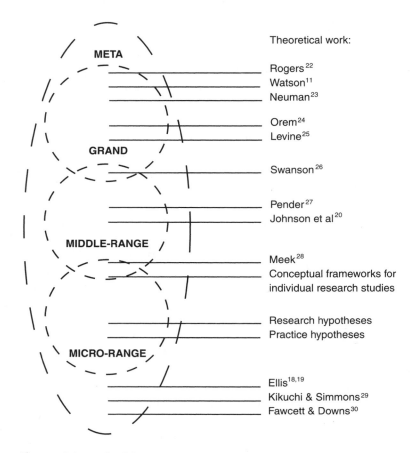

Theoretical work:

Rogers[22]
Watson[11]
Neuman[23]

Orem[24]
Levine[25]

Swanson[26]

Pender[27]
Johnson et al[20]

Meek[28]
Conceptual frameworks for individual research studies

Research hypotheses
Practice hypotheses

Ellis[18,19]
Kikuchi & Simmons[29]
Fawcett & Downs[30]

Figure 6-1 *Levels of theoretical thinking.*

within the principles of nursing, and their concepts and propositions transcend specific events and patient populations. The substantial body of analytic and philosophic reasoning that has emerged from grand theory provides evidence of scholarship that distinguishes nursing from other closely related disciplines and legitimizes its existence among academic disciplines.[9] Thus grand theory's most significant contribution to nursing is the establishment and substantiation of the discipline's identity and boundaries.

Given their abstract nature, grand theories provide universal explanations and an understanding of nursing, but not the particulars that are necessary for empirical testing. As a result, they have little predictive capability. Some grand theories also use language that is difficult for the beginning student and unfamiliar to many potential users. Nevertheless, they have significantly influenced knowledge development within the discipline and there are numerous examples of their use in guiding nursing research, practice, and education. Grand theories also contribute to the historical perspective of nursing, reflecting the time and context in which the authors developed their theories, as well as their philosophic underpinnings and their educational and practice perspectives. In charting the growth of the discipline, Nightingale[10] can be considered the first grand theorist and *Notes on Nursing,* the original paradigm of contemporary nursing.

There is debate about what constitutes a grand theory and thus, which nursing scholars' work should be classified as grand theory. For example, is Jean Watson's[11] *Philosophy and Science of Caring* more accurately categorized as a "philosophy" or "grand theory" of nursing? Further, should Madeleine Leininger's[12] conceptual model, *Culture Care: Diversity and Universality Theory,* be classified as a grand or middle-range theory? Our view is that this type of debate reflects the growth of nursing's disciplinary knowledge. Although we may never have a consensus of answers for such questions, it also indicates that we have sufficiently established our external boundaries, and we can now redirect our energy to further distinguish the internal substance and structure of our knowledge through the construction of middle-range theories.

Middle-range Theory

In terms of historical development, middle-range theory is the relative newcomer to nursing science. Similar to grand theory, middle-range theory explains the empirical world of nursing, but it is more specific and less formal. For example, the philosophic underpinnings and assumptions of the middle-range theorist may be more implicit than explicit. As indicated by its name, any explanation of middle-range theory requires discussing "what it is" and "what comes before and after in its range." Suppe[4] was one of the first to clarify and define middle-range theory for nursing science. By using Merton's examination of sociologic theory,[13] Suppe[4] provided 3 criteria for delimiting middle-range theory from grand theory and the next lower level, micro-range theory. These 3 criteria, scope, level of abstraction, and testability are widely accepted.[14,15]

In terms of scope and level of abstraction, Lenz et al[15] stated that "middle-range theories (are those) that are sufficiently specific to guide research and practice, yet sufficiently general to cross multiple clinical populations and to encompass similar phenomena." In the quote from Lenz et al,[15] the guidance for research and practice is much more direct than is that offered by grand theory; therefore, middle-range theory can be tested in the empirical world. The concepts or phenomena of interest can be coded objectively (by using either qualitative or quantitative methods) and it has the potential to postulate measurable relationships between the phenomena; thus it has a "time-relativistic distinction."[4] The generalizability of middle-range theory is further defined by boundaries that limit measurement of the person-environment interaction. Although testable across several different patient populations and environments, a particular middle-range theory does *not* address *all* patients in *all* environments. For example, Good and Moore's[14] theory on pain management applies only to adults who experience acute surgical pain and is appropriately tested only during the immediate postoperative period. Because of the aforementioned characteristics, middle-range theory is not as limited as grand theory in its typology and can be classified as either explanatory or predictive. A major role of middle-range theory is to define or refine the substantive content of nursing science and practice, and it should be an important focus of both nurse scholars and practitioners as we continue to build knowledge for the discipline.

Micro-range Theory

Micro-range theory is the least formal and most tentative of the theoretical levels discussed in this article. It also is the most restrictive in terms of time and scope or application. However, its particularistic approach is invaluable for scientists and practitioners as they work to describe, organize, and test their ideas. We propose 2 levels of micro-range theory. At the higher level, micro-range theory is closely related to middle-range theory but is comprised of 1 or 2 major concepts, and its application frequently is limited to a particular event; for example, theories related to decubitus or catheter care.[16]

At the lower level, micro-range theory is defined as a set of working hypotheses or propositions.[17] Scientists and practitioners use these working propositions to tentatively categorize, explain, or test health-related person-environment interactions. As such, they are not coded and entered into a formal theoretical system, but two examples serve to illustrate their invaluable contribution to science and practice. In the first example, scientists interested in developing and testing larger theoretical frameworks isolate and organize proposed conceptual relationships into propositions. The scientific literature is then used to investigate the relationships of the propositions and, if there is evidence for the truth of the relationships, to determine conceptual-empirical correspondence. In the second example, the clinician also uses propositions to identify, describe, and organize the working conceptual relationships in practice. The investigation, although identical in process to the scientist's, differs in terms of its scope and its generalizability; that is, the practitioner investigates more particular and immediate relationships in a smaller group of persons; or frequently, a single person. For instance, a nurse working on a general medical unit is assigned to admit an elderly patient with the medical diagnosis of chronic obstructive pulmonary disease. Before meeting the patient, and in attempt to organize knowledge, the nurse hypothesizes several possible conceptual relationships; for example, the patient's age and medical diagnosis limit the patient's functional status. The nurse then tests the working hypothesis through assessment and works to directly change the concepts' relationships through manipulation of the person-environment interaction.

Any discussion of micro-range theory must consider the term "practice theory." We jump into the debate on what constitutes practice theory with the realization that numerous definitions exist and many authors consider micro-theory, as the most concrete and applicable of all theoretical levels, to be an equivalent term for practice theory.[5,16] We believe this categorization limits the understanding of theoretical thinking in nursing and a broader definition of practice theory is more useful. Based on Ellis,[18,19] who stated that *all* nursing knowledge ultimately is developed for practice, we maintain that all nursing theory, regardless of level, is practice theory.

Evidence and Levels of Theoretical Thinking

Regardless of the method used to create the theory or whether the theory is explanatory or predictive, the amount of evidence accrued to support it promotes confidence in its use by practitioners and scientists. In addition to the previously cited examples, varying degrees of evidence exist among the different types and levels of theoretical thinking.

On the meta-theoretical level, the accrual of bodies of research findings (evidence) demonstrates our ability to produce and critique our knowledge. Our progress is measured by the usefulness of the knowledge that is accrued, the explanatory and predictive theories that are created and tested, and the articulation of philosophic perspectives that are connected to nursing science and practice.

At the grand theory level, evidence is represented by practitioners' and scientists' use of the philosophic approaches presented in the theories. As we have sought to build an academic discipline, grand theories have assisted in legitimizing the emerging discipline by providing broad guidelines about the focus of the discipline. There are varying degrees of evidence about the usefulness of existing nursing grand theories. Their frequent use by schools of nursing, care institutions, and practitioners, and their use in guiding research initiatives are examples of their value.

Middle-range theories often have evidence that is acquired by using many repetitions under controlled conditions (scientific method). An example is Johnson's[20,21] self-regulation theory that addresses the use of preparatory information to assist persons in coping with threatening illness situations. Middle-range theoretical frameworks provide some evidence to support the relationships posed. However, to date no nursing theories have sufficient evidence to be considered "laws," which is not unexpected, given that nursing is a newly established discipline and our phenomena of interest are highly complex.

In micro-range theory, relationships exist among a limited number of concepts that characterize a specific situation. The working hypothesis (of either the practitioner or the scientist) has the least amount of evidence behind it. The evidence behind this kind of theoretical thinking is not usually accrued by planned repetitions under controlled situations, but instead it is built from a limited number of repetitions and observations. For example, the best way to approach first-time ambulation for surgical patients may be hypothesized by a nurse as the result of providing postoperative care to a series of patients. The theoretical-empirical congruence of this hypothesis is then tested in subsequent surgical patients.

Use of Levels of Theoretical Thinking to Enhance Knowledge Development in Nursing

Several challenges prevail in the development of nursing knowledge. Conceptualizing theory at different levels of theory may assist us to address some of these challenges. For example, one challenge is to determine how different levels of theory relate to each other. How can one level of theory be used to develop related theories at another level? As we analyze and generate theory, we often use traditional methods of theory construction and substruction. The appropriate use of inductive and deductive approaches to develop nursing knowledge may be improved by the consideration of the relationships among levels of theories. Conceptualizing levels of theories also provides a beginning tool to assess whether the philosophic roots of our grand theories are reflected in our middle-range and micro-range theories. Such analyses can potentially enhance the consistency and logic in our decision making about care issues and the theoretical design of future research.

As a discipline, we also are looking for ways to integrate related theories that have arisen from the multiple ways of building knowledge. For instance, how does the theory about stages of behavior change, developed from grounded theory methods, relate to theories of self-efficacy for health behaviors that were developed by using hypothesis-testing methods? Similarly, we are searching for ways to integrate related theories from different disciplines. For example, how do middle-range theories of health promotion in psychology relate to those in sociology and nursing? The analysis and integration of related theories may be facilitated by comparison of related theories at the same theoretical level across disciplines and arising from multiple methodologic approaches.

Another challenge in the discipline's knowledge development is understanding the mechanisms needed to enhance articulation of the knowledge produced by practitioners and researchers. Regardless of whether the methods used to develop theory are inductive or deductive, and originate from a philosophic, practice, or research perspective, multiple levels of theoretical thinking exist. Although practitioners and researchers may use divergent methods, each uses theoretical thinking for the generation of knowledge. Recognition and discussion about the levels of theoretical thinking can serve as a vehicle for increased communication between practitioners and scientists about the knowledge each is developing.

Conclusion

Knowledge development in any discipline is a dynamic process that pursues probable truths about reality. It begins with creative approaches from multiple perspectives and continues by testing the knowledge according to appropriate truth criteria. In nursing, our "reality" is clinical practice, and we construct theories about probable truths related to the experience of health in the person-environment interaction. Development of a knowledge base is an iterative and ongoing process that requires periodic analysis and synthesis of an entire body of work. In an attempt to further the understanding of the current status of nursing theory, we provided an examination of the different levels of theory currently being used to develop nursing knowledge. This meta-theoretical discussion of theory is not meant to create artificial domains; rather, it is an attempt to understand the current status of nursing theory through clarification of the terminology and a discussion of the related categories of theoretical thinking. Perhaps more important, the final purpose of this article is to recognize the strength of our disciplinary knowledge base and generate public discussion about the future of theory development and testing.

REFERENCES

1. Stevens BJ. Nursing theory, analysis, application, evaluation. 2nd ed. Boston: Little Brown & Co Inc; 1984.
2. Dubin R. Theory building. 2nd ed. New York: Free Press; 1978.
3. Chinn PL, Kramer MK. Theory and nursing. 5th ed. St. Louis: Mosby; 1999.
4. Suppe F. Middle range theories: what they are and why nursing science needs them. Proceedings of the ANA/Council of Nurse Researchers Symposium; 1993 Nov 15.
5. Walker LO, Avant KC. Strategies for theory construction in nursing. 3rd ed. Norwalk (CT): Appleton & Lange; 1995.
6. Nicoll LH. Perspectives on nursing theory. 3rd ed. Philadelphia (PA): Lippincott-Raven; 1997.
7. Carper BA. Fundamental patterns of knowing in nursing. Adv Nurs Sci 1978;1:13–23.
8. Whall AL. Current debates and issues critical to the discipline of nursing. In: Fitzpatrick JJ, Whall AL. Conceptual modes of nursing. 3rd ed. Stamford (CT): Appleton & Lange; 1996. p. 1–12.
9. Fawcett J. Analysis and evaluation of conceptual models of nursing. 3rd ed. Philadelphia (PA): FA Davis Co; 1995.
10. Nightingale F. Notes on nursing. New York: Churchill Livingstone; 1859.
11. Watson J. Nursing: the philosophy and science of caring. Boston: Little Brown & Co Inc; 1979.
12. Leininger M. Transcultural nursing: concepts, theories, and practices. New York: Wiley; 1978.
13. Merton RK. On sociological theories of the middle range. In: Merton RK. Social theory and social structure. New York: Free Press; 1968. p. 39–72.
14. Good M, Moore SM. Clinical Practice guidelines as a new source of middle-range theory: focus on acute pain. Nurs Outlook 1996;44:74–9.
15. Lenz ER, Suppe F, Gift AG, Pugh LC, Milligan RA. Collaborative development of middle-range nursing theories: toward a theory of unpleasant symptoms. Adv Nurs Sci 1995;17(3): 1–13.
16. Whall AL. The structure of nursing knowledge: analysis and evaluation of practice, middle-range, and grand theory. In: Fitzpatrick JJ, Whall AL. Conceptual modes of nursing. 3rd ed. Stamford (CT): Appleton & Lange; 1996. p. 13–25.
17. Kim HS. The nature of theoretical thinking in nursing. East Norwalk (CT): Appleton-Century-Crofts; 1983.
18. Ellis R. The practitioner as theorist. Am J Nurs 1969;69:428–35.
19. Ellis R. Values and vicissitudes of the scientist nurse. Nurs Res 1970;19:440–5.
20. Johnson JE, Fieler VK, Jones LS, Wlasowicz GS, Mitchell ML. Self-regulation theory: applying theory to your practice. Pittsburgh (PA): Oncology Nursing Press; 1997.
21. Leventhal H, Johnson JE. Laboratory and field experimentation: development of a theory of self-regulation. In: Wooldridge PJ, Schmitt MH, Skipper JK, Leonard RC, editors. Behavioral science and nursing theory. St Louis: Mosby; 1983, p. 189–262.
22. Rogers ME. An introduction to the theoretical basis of nursing. Philadelphia (PA): F. A. Davis Company; 1970.
23. Neuman B. The Neuman systems model: application to nursing education and practice. New York: Appleton-Century-Crofts; 1982.
24. Orem DE. Nursing: concepts of practice. New York: McGraw Hill; 1971.
25. Levine ME. The four conservation principles of nursing. Nurs Forum 1967;6:45–59.
26. Swanson KM. Empirical development of a middle range theory of caring. Nurs Res 1991;40(3): 161–6.
27. Pender NJ. Health Promotion in nursing practice. New York: Appleton-Century-Crofts; 1982.
28. Meek SS. Effects of slow stroke back massage on relaxation in hospice clients. IMAGE J Nurs Sch 1993;25:17–20.
29. Kikuchi JF, Simmons H, editors. Philosophic inquiry in nursing. Newbury Park (CA): Sage Publications; 1992.
30. Fawcett J, Downs FS. The relationship of theory and research. 2nd ed. Philadelphia (PA): FA Davis Co; 1992.

The Authors Comment

Levels of Theoretical Thinking in Nursing

We wrote this article in response to our need to understand and explain middle-range theory to our students. As the discipline's understanding of theoretic thinking evolved, we were asked for detailed definitions of theory and how to distinguish the meaning and application of the different types. Because we both also have programs of research, we're pragmatists when it comes to theoretic thinking. Therefore, using "levels" of theory was a natural approach for categorizing and explaining the range of theoretic thinking used by all nurse theorists, from practitioners to scientists to philosophers. The article is dedicated to all our students. Thank you for your questions, skepticism, and willingness to take on the adventure of understanding human health and illness.

—Patricia Higgins
—Shirley Moore

CHAPTER 7

Theoretical Thinking in Nursing: Problems and Prospects

Hesook Suzie Kim

The development of nursing's knowledge-base for its practice has exercised the minds of nursing scholars in recent years as evidenced in the literature. Many of the nursing theories and conceptual frameworks initially proposed in the 1970s have gone through several revisions and testing by nursing scientists. There are some evidences that nursing's theoretical frameworks are producing an array of explanatory knowledge and some predictive or prescriptive notions about human phenomena and nursing practice. Many doctoral programs in nursing which have been implemented during the past 5 years to a total of more than 40 in the United States have also been instrumental in forcing nursing scientists to seek theoretical bases of their own research and of their students within the nursing perspective.

However, such culmination has received very little systematic scrutiny in the literature as to how far and to what extent the nursing's theoretical development has progressed. Nursing scientists in general are either interested in or pressured into 'testing' theories empirically rather than 'evaluating' or 'reflecting' on what theories are being produced or how they are being produced. Of course this is not to say that there have not been any critical analyses of nursing theories. Summaries and critiques of nursing theories and conceptual frameworks have been published in recent years as evidenced in such books as Chinn and Jacobs (1983), Fitzpatrick and Whall (1983), Fawcett (1984), and Meleis (1985). However, much of these analyses were limited to evaluation of the contents of theories and conceptual frameworks which I consider to be only one level of analysis.

About the Author

HESOOK SUZIE KIM was born in Korea and came to the United States as an undergraduate student at Indiana University. She received a BS in nursing and an MS in nursing education from Indiana University and an MA and a PhD in sociology from Brown University. She has been in Rhode Island since 1964 and has been a faculty member at the University of Rhode Island College of Nursing since 1973, having taught mostly in the graduate programs. Her scholarly work has focused on metatheoretical questions in nursing, and she considers her two books, *The Nature of Theoretical Thinking in Nursing* (2nd edition published in 2000) and *Nursing Theories: Conceptual and Philosophical Foundations* (edited with Ingrid Kollak, published in 1999), to be her major contributions to the discipline. Her empirical research has been on nursing practice issues from the cross-national perspective, including research on collaboration, pain assessment, clinical decision making, and the nature of nursing practice carried out in Finland, Japan, Korea, Norway, the United States, and Sweden. She reads (Günter Grass is her favorite author), listens to jazz, plays golf, and skis for sheer enjoyment and relaxation.

Inherent in this state of affairs is a lack of systematic framework upon which various levels of questions related to knowledge generation can be posed for the discipline of nursing. In general, questions related to how theories should be developed and what theories should be like are left to scholars in the philosophy of science to grapple with while very little systematic attention is paid to such questions by nursing scholars. In nursing, the products of theoretical work are evaluated only with respect to their contents and forms. My view is that this approach is limiting. A comprehensive system of theory evaluation that poses questions beyond those related to theory's content and form is needed to assess the broader questions of epistemological orientations as well as content adequacy.

This paper attempts to integrate several levels of analysis to examine the nature of theoretical thinking in nursing, beginning with the questions at the level of the philosophy of science and moving to the examination of the contents of theories being developed in nursing. The major assumption underlying this form of analysis is in the belief that the nature of scientific products is influenced by the scientists' views regarding the methods of knowledge generation, the definitions of knowledge structure, and the aims of disciplines as well as the focus of scientific attention.

A Framework for Examining the Nature of Theoretical Thinking

Whether or not a scientist is aware of the connections among his/her theory or research piece and the beliefs about what a theory should be like or what the content of a theory should be and the contributions of the work on the discipline is irrelevant. This is because the articulation between what Popper (1972) calls World 2, a 'subjective' world, and World 3, 'an objective' world occurs in scientific activities regardless of such awareness. What cannot be ignored is the idea that a scientist who is working within the frame of his/her own World 2 (a personal data system) is engaged in creating and adding to a World 3, the objective world of ideas, knowledge, and understanding which becomes interwoven with that particular scientist's perspectives about the world and science.

While it is apparent that most scientists go about with their work, i.e. their scientific activities, paying very little attention to fundamental questions related to the nature of science and scientific methodologies, cumulatively their work results in forming prevailing patterns and forms in the discipline's scientific development. Hence the nature of theoretical thinking or theorizing in nursing has to be examined by looking not only into the contents of theories·being developed or the products of theory testing but more importantly into the various levels of philosophical and perspective based orientations from which the scientist's work is being developed. From this assumption, I propose a five-level analysis framework for reviewing and evaluating theoretical work in nursing, articulating the following questions. These questions are similar to the ones discussed by Turner (1986) for sociological theorizing.

• What is the kind of knowledge possible for nursing? And, what kinds of theories are possible for nursing?
• What procedures are appropriate for developing this knowledge for nursing? And, what are the appropriate ways to develop nursing theories?
• What is it that nursing should try to develop knowledge about?
• What should nursing theories be concerned with? And, how can we decide what are important questions for nursing science?

• What are the ultimate goals of nursing knowledge being generated?
• What qualifies a given nursing theory to be scientifically sound?

These questions within the five-level framework are shown within the Figure 7-1, indicating the increasing specificity with which descending level influences theorizing and theoretical products in nursing. The five levels are thus specified as (1) the philosophy of science level, (2) the metaparadigm level, (3) the nursing philosophy level, (4) the paradigm level, and (5) the theory level.

The philosophy of science level is concerned with questions related to a scientist's positions regarding the nature of nursing as a science and the nature of scientific theory and theorizing. Analyses at this level will reveal the foundations upon which theories take their form and theorizing progresses. The second level focuses on a scientist's definitions regarding the essential phenomena of nursing requiring scientific attention and

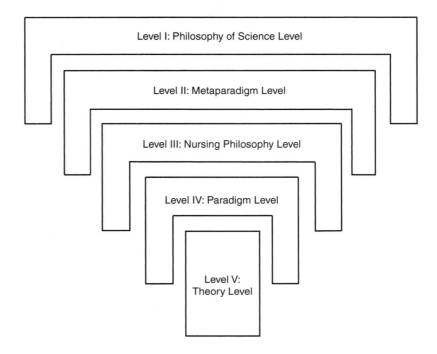

Figure 7-1 *Framework for analysis of theoretical thinking in nursing.*

the selection of subject matters with which a given nursing theory is concerned. This level of analysis can be examined within a metaparadigmatic structure for nursing science as developed by Kim (1983, 1987). What the analysis at this level can reveal is the boundary within which nursing theories are being developed and how such a boundary changes over time within the discipline's revisions regarding the 'critical problems' for scientific attention. While the first level (the philosophy of science level) is concerned with the fundamental positions regarding scientific methodologies for theory development and theory testing, the second level (the metaparadigm level) allows examinations of the 'content' choices which are made for the science.

The third level concerned with nursing philosophy is essential to the extent that a given nursing philosophy directs the development of nursing theories in their orientations for understanding, explanation, prediction, and prescription. Therefore, this level articulates closely with the philosophy of science level by directing the nature of nursing theory being developed in a methodological sense.

The fourth level is concerned with paradigmatic orientations and perspectives from which the actual theorizing is carried out. The term paradigms is used to mean general scientific perspectives and traditions in this discussion, not used in the strict sense with which Kuhn (1962, 1970) described paradigms for the natural sciences. The concept of paradigm for this level is appropriate for our analysis because nursing science is being developed from various scientific traditions, maybe because it is paradigmatic as Kuhn might argue, and furthermore because the critical scientific problems of the discipline seem to require various perspectives for understanding.

The fifth level is concerned with theories themselves. Analyses at this level will reveal the content of a theory with respect to its scope, logic and preciseness (i.e. form) of theoretical statements, testability and use. While there have been many nursing theoreticians who proposed different criteria for theory analysis and evaluation, for example, Stevens (1984), Hardy (1974) and Meleis (1985) among many, these four criteria have been adopted to be critical

for the analysis of the contents of theory for nursing within this proposed framework. These four criteria have linkages to the preceding four levels of analysis, in that the questions of scope and use have direct relevance to the metaparadigm and nursing philosophy levels while the questions of form and testability are related to the philosophy of science and paradigm levels.

For the present exposition, this framework is used to scan the status of nursing's theoretical development and point up the areas in which gaps and deficiencies are apparent with respect to our efforts in nursing science. However, many fundamental questions related to the nature of nursing knowledge and scientising of nursing vis-à-vis nursing practice are lurking unresolved behind the scene of fervour with which scientific knowledge is being produced within nursing. Such questions are most troublesome, for example, as we encounter a nurse at a patient's bedside who is grappling with a decision to apply or not to apply a bed restraint.

Theoretical Development in Nursing: Status, Problems and Prospects

Level I: Philosophy of Science Questions

Nursing within the last three decades in its attempt to be treated as a legitimate knowledge discipline has embraced the belief that its knowledge has to be scientific and that scientific theories are the foundations upon which knowledge about nursing phenomena may be accumulated. There are three basic questions which have constantly been circumvented by nursing scientists in their quests for nursing knowledge:

1. Is the primary goal of nursing science in understanding or in control?
2. What kinds of knowledge are appropriate for nursing discipline and nursing science?
3. What is (are) the appropriate form(s) of theorizing in nursing?

While it appears that modern nursing is comfortable with the notion that the best way to accumulate knowledge relevant to nursing and nursing practice is through scientific methods, we continue to argue regarding the extent to which the science of nursing should control nursing practice. In addition, dichotomising the science and art of nursing as separate entities requiring some form of integration has been one of the major struggles articulated by many nursing scholars including Florence Nightingale, Henderson, and more recently Carper (1978) and Watson (1981). On the one hand is the belief that nursing practice encompassing the art of nursing goes beyond the scope of nursing science, while the counter argument goes with the belief that nursing practice has to be based on scientific knowledge and the science of nursing. This argument, in a sense, is more fundamentally embedded in the question regarding the nature of nursing science rather than the seeming dichotomy of the science and art. The fundamental question therefore is whether the nursing science is concerned with 'what is' or 'what should be.'

Since all prescriptive theories must be based on the notion of what is the right thing to do, they are based on value premises. The proposal for situation-producing theories as the ultimate goal of nursing in the early years of nursing theory development (Dickoff, James & Wiedenbach, 1968a) had set the stage for nursing science to be normative science for many nursing theorists. Donaldson and Crowley (1978) also argue for the development of prescriptive theories which can govern the clinical practice of nursing. They view 'the syntax of nursing as value systems (both of science and professional ethics) . . . '(p 119), and suggest that this syntax influences theory generation in nursing by providing a context from which judgments regarding the appropriateness, reliability and validity of knowledge being developed are made.

Suppe and Jacox (1985) also argue that since situation-producing theories presume goal states as the starting points, they are normative although satisfying as a species of teleological theory within the semantic concept of theories, and indicate that goal selection or the justification of selection are based on nonscientific normative or ethical assumptions requiring extra scientific procedures for analysis.

To the extent that prescriptive theories presume to differentiate what should be desired or preferred from what should not be, they are ideological and normative in nature. However, the procedures followed by developing prescriptive theories in nursing have not incorporated the procedures which are necessary in developing ideological knowledge. One form of argument has been advanced by Beckstrand (1978a, 1978b, 1980) in arguing against practice theories and by proposing that 'the goal of modern 'scientific' practice is to bring about changes in entities through scientific and moral means so that a good is acknowledged and defined within the ethical theory of value is realized or becomes increasingly capable of being realized' (Beckstrand 1978a, p 136). Beckstrand thus believes that scientific theory as value-forming knowledge may be developed separately, requiring juxtapositioning of two bodies of knowledge at the instances of practice.

It appears then that there are at least two schools of thought regarding the nursing science as value-free or value laden. Nursing scientists who believe in the notion that science is 'value-free' will have to be interested in understanding the nature of nursing phenomena as the basic goal of nursing's scientific enterprise, while prescriptive theorists' goal of nursing science is in controlling nursing phenomena in selected contexts of goal attainment. This differentiation certainly will result in different types of nursing theories advanced and different methodologies used to develop such theories. Whether or not nursing scientists in general are aware of this differentiation in orientation is highly questionable in the light of the paucity of literature available on the subject.

Somewhat related to the above problem but related to the maturing of nursing as a scientific discipline is the current awareness among the nursing scholars of the role that various philosophies of science have played in influencing the kinds of nursing knowledge being developed. It appears that the debates in the philosophy of science have finally filtered onto nursing scientists, raising sensitivities and questions about the nursing's scientific enterprise as well as their own work in terms of methodologies and contents. This awareness may have been stimulated in recent years by the necessity to delve into the developments in philosophy of science by faculty members in the many newly created doctoral programs in nursing. Hence, we are recently engaged in debating about the nature of nursing science in terms of form and procedures of development (Watson, 1981; Webster, Jacox, & Baldwin, 1981; Hardy, 1983; Gortner, 1983). Uys (1987) even suggests that many of the so-called nursing theories are pretheoretical and may be considered as foundational studies that try to answer such questions as foundationalism, development of language system, and philosophical analysis regarding the discipline of nursing science.

Nevertheless, the literature indicates that during the past 30 years many nursing scientists who had been trained in the tradition of the received view of science, with or without realizing their commitment to it, led the development of nursing science to the path that emphasized essentialism (Silva, 1977; Jacox, 1974), deductive theory building and formalization (Hardy, 1974; Chinn & Jacobs, 1983; Walker & Avant, 1983), operationalization and empirical testing (Fawcett & Downs, 1986) and the rules of confirmation and verification (Silva, 1977; Gortner, 1980).

However, sensitizing to the new developments in the philosophy of science with the exposures to and assimilation of the works by Hanson (1958), Popper (1968), Kuhn (1962, 1970), Lakatos and Musgrave (1970), Suppe (1977), Laundan (1978), and Feyreabend (1978) has created a great deal of confusion and uncertainties among nursing scientists in recent years (see Silva & Rothbart, 1984; Suppe & Jacox, 1985). Thus, many theoretical writings by metatheorists and theorists in nursing (e.g., Fawcett, 1980; Stevens, 1984; Meleis, 1985; Rogers, 1983; King, 1981) seem to have embraced selected views regarding the nature and form of nursing science. Some are holdovers from the Received View tradition, while others are encompassing of the new ideas suggestive of the perspective view of Hanson, the semantic conception of theories espoused by Suppe, and the historicism of Kuhn, Laudan, and Shapere, henceforth creating muddiness in the position taken by them regarding the nature and form of nursing theories and theory development. Whether or not this is only transitional and should eventually fall into distinct positions and schools of thought regarding the nature of nursing science has to be borne out by the history, it seems.

Attempts deviating from the earlier efforts in nursing theory development and methodologies for theory testing have become more varied and aggressive in recent years. Phenomenological theories (Parse, 1981; Paterson & Zderad, 1976), inductive theorizing (Benoliel, 1977, 1983; Norris, 1982), use of qualitative methodologies (Munhall, 1982; Watson, 1985), and hermeneutics (Benner, 1983) have been proposed as appropriate or better ways of developing nursing knowledge.

Level II: Metaparadigm Questions

A metaparadigm refers to a boundary structure which consists of items or phenomena for investigation for a given disciplinary perspective. Thus a nursing metaparadigm provides a structure from which the subject matters for nursing may be described and/or selected for scientific attention. Fawcett (1980) uses four essential concepts: person, environment, health, and nursing (Yura & Torres, 1975) as those encompassing the phenomena of interest to nursing science, and suggests these concepts as the components of a metaparadigm for nursing. Meleis (1985) expands this list in what she terms 'domain concepts' for a metaparadigm of nursing theories, and includes nursing client, transitions, interaction, nursing process, environment, nursing therapeutics, and health. Both authors use these metaparadigm concepts to indicate the extensiveness of a given nursing theory in its scope, and suggest that theories describing or dealing with any one of the major concepts are nursing theories—although Fawcett (1984) considers that the most sophisticated nursing theory would encompass all four of the essential concepts. With a view that these metaparadigms are limited in the specification for the purpose of subject matter selection and of considering what would constitute critical scientific problems, a more comprehensive metaparadigm was proposed for consideration (Kim, 1983, 1987).

A metaparadigm topology of four subdomains for structuring nursing knowledge proposed in my earlier work (Kim, 1987) provides a freedom with which nursing theorists and scientists can select out phenomena of concern for theoretical or empirical attention within the nursing perspective at various levels of scope. This metaparadigm containing four subdomains (the client domain, the client-nurse domain, the practice domain, and the environmental domain) is based on the assumption that the goal of nursing science is to gain knowledge about the nature of human phenomena in the context of nursing practice. With such knowledge, it is possible to understand, explain, or predict human phenomena requiring nursing attention with respect to other human phenomena, environment, client-nurse interaction, or practice. Further, it is also possible to understand the nature of nursing therapeutics and interpret or predict outcomes of nursing practice. Table 7-1 shows a matrix based on this metaparadigm useful in examining the concept selections within nursing theories. It can be used to analyze theories in terms of in what domain the concepts requiring explanation reside and from what domain or domains the concepts providing explanation are selected.

Obviously, the domain of environment does not qualify to be the major domain of interest for explanation in the nursing perspective and is only appropriate in providing the focus of explanation. The matrix therefore can point up within-domain theories and across-domain theories at various degree of scope.

What has been found in our analyses of nursing theories so far is that the general theoretical frameworks, such as Rogers's unitary man model, Orem's self-care model, Roy's adaptation model, and Parse's man-health-living model deal with the client domain concepts in either nonselective or holistic manners, in the form of what Turner (1986) calls 'analytical schemes' rather than as theories containing a network of well developed propositions. Hence, these models may be considered theoretical to the extent that they try to order human phenomena in specific schemata with given orientations for the client domain.

In contrast, many middle range theories being developed and tested in nursing are more specific in the selection of metaparadigm concepts. For example, Johnson's theoretical and empirical work on a theory of self-regulation (1983) is concerned with the concept of identity development, both of them with the metaparadigm orientation in the client domain.

Interests in concepts of the client-nurse domain among nursing scholars are longstanding. Peplau (1962), Orlando (1961), Wiedenbach (1963), and King (1981) have taken concepts from the client-nurse domain for explanation of client phenomena or nursing practice. As it is true of the client domain theories, nursing theories dealing with the client-nurse domain tend to focus on global concepts of interaction and communication rather than on delineated aspects of client-nurse phenomena such as conflict, collaboration, competition, frequency, or quality of interaction.

Table 7-1
Nursing Domain in Matrix for Identification of Metaparadigm Focus of Theories

Domain of Focus Providing Explanation	Domain of Focus for Theory		
	Client Domain	Client-Nurse Domain	Practice Domain
Client domain	*		
Client-nurse domain		*	
Practice domain			*
Environment domain			

*Within domain theories.

What is important at this level of analysis is the identification of metaparadigmatic focus with the ultimate purpose of assessing whether or not nursing's theoretical work is adequately and sufficiently dealing with critical problems of the discipline. As one fills the matrix with nursing theories in the process of analysis, it is possible to identify the gaps in theoretical development in nursing. We have thus far limited theoretical advances in making specific connections between concepts from the client domain and the environment domain and between those from the client domain and the practice domain. Hence, the metaparadigm level questions permit us to examine to what extent a given theory or a collection of theoretical work handle the critical problems or subject matters of interest to the discipline of nursing.

Level III: Nursing Philosophy Questions

As debated by Walker (1971), the term "philosophy of nursing" has been used in several senses in the literature. The specific sense it is adopted for this level of analysis refers to one's beliefs about the nature of humanity and what nursing "should" do about this humanity. These are preparadigmatic choices one has to be committed to in order to streamline one's theoretical thinking, and are closely related to the kinds of philosophic choices one makes in terms of the nature of science and scientific theories. This notion of choice in philosophies of nursing is not universally accepted. Munhall (1982) treats as given that there is an adherence to "a basic philosophy" of individuality and advocacy in nursing. Sarter (1988) points out common philosophical views as well as some divergent ones in her analysis of four nursing theorists' work, and suggests dangerously that the commonly shared philosophical views among the four theories may form "an appropriate philosophical foundation for the discipline." Sarter's conclusion thus is derived with the assumption that nursing science requires a single metaparadigm based on an appropriate philosophical foundation. Sarter therefore equates a common metaparadigm of nursing with a world view, a philosophical foundation for the discipline of nursing. This no-

tion is contrary to the position expressed in this paper, calling for multiple philosophies of nursing as appropriate.

While it is possible that there can be a prevailing philosophy of nursing at a given time, it does not mean that multiplicity in philosophies of nursing is impossible or inappropriate insisting on a unified philosophy of nursing is pigeon-holing the development of theoretical thinking in nursing to only one direction and one paradigm. Certainly for an essentialist who believes in one and only one truth, this view would be appropriate. However, philosophy is an intellectual choice and commitment one makes regarding metaphysics which becomes integrated into the lower level theoretical thinking.

My review, contrary to Sarter's analysis, indicates divergent nursing philosophies with orientations in such positions as rationalism, existentialism, causal determinism, instrumentalism, humanism, and pragmatism. As stated by Bernstein (1986), intellectual currents of a given period may have common philosophical concerns, but philosophical positions culminate into diverse idea systems according to the way the problems of humanity are analyzed. For nursing, this diversity in philosophical orientations will eventually influence the types of praxiology (theories of practice) that get developed.

What is usually portrayed in the nursing literature is a separate treatment of nursing philosophy without integrating it into theoretical positions. Hence, it is often that we encounter a theorist who advocates free will and individualism but whose theory is based on the assumption of normative determinism or behaviouristic holism. It appears that nursing scholars in general take the position that there is a unified nursing philosophy upheld by the nursing community, national or international, and that its significance to theory development is rudimentary at best. My view is contrary to this in that nursing philosophy having a close linkage to the philosophy of science has to be articulated into theory so that the whole network of theoretical thinking that goes into theory building maintains internal consistency and is based on a compatible thread of idea-system.

Level IV: Paradigm Choices

Paradigm choices in theory development refer to choices related to theoretical tradition and perspective as discussed earlier. A given theoretical tradition for nursing holds specific assumptions about the nature of human phenomena or nursing. A theoretical perspective also advocates specific ideas about theory building and theory testing, thus guides theoretical activities in dealing with selected metaparadigm concepts. The most prevailing paradigm choices which seem to have guided and continue to guide the theoretical work in nursing are:

1. General systems perspective in the tradition of von Bertalanffy's work
2. Behavioral perspective inclusive of all varieties of stimulus-response and adaptation/coping frameworks
3. Phenomenological perspective
4. Functional perspective
5. Sensory/cognitive perspective
6. Interaction perspective.

Although these seem to be the major paradigms, theories are more often based not on a single perspective but on two or more perspectives combined to guide the work.

At the same time, nursing scholars are beginning to pay attention to nontraditional theoretical perspectives such as Habermas' critical theory (Holter, 1988) and hermeneutics and interpretive perspective (Benner, 1984). It appears that as we become increasingly sophisticated and diversified in asking questions about the nature of critical nursing problems, we seek out alternative explanations based on different theoretical perspectives rather than holding onto those which have offered unsatisfactory answers in the past. This diverse approach to theory building in nursing may eventually fall into major paradigms for the three domains of nursing, as theorists and researchers working independently with concepts from different domains but from similar theoretical perspective begin to realize integration into major theoretical themes.

Level V: Aspects of Theory

This level of analysis is concerned with the content of a theory in terms of key concepts and propositions. Questions of "form" and "testability" refer to the internal structure of a theory, while the questions of "scope" and "use" refer to the degree with which a theory contributes to the development of nursing science. These four are considered to be the elementary, fundamental criteria to evaluate the content of a theory partly in line with Reynolds (1971), Hardy (1978), Stevens (1984), and Meleis (1985).

Form as the criterion of evaluation deals with:

1. The clarity, abstractness and consistency with which key concepts in a theory are specified and derived, and
2. Identification of the types, network and internal structure of propositions and theoretical statements contained within a theory.

An evaluation of a theory with respect to form will reveal the degree of completeness in the development of conceptual system in terms of logic, clarity, and abstractness. On the other hand, testability as the criterion of evaluation deals with the degree with which a theory can be translated for empirical testing. Hence, the more abstract a theory is the more deductive or interpretive steps it would require for empirical testing.

The questions of scope and use have been well articulated by Stevens (1984), and refer to degrees with which a given theory provides explanations for various subject matters in nursing and suggests usefulness in providing the types of knowledge for application. While middle range theories tend to be narrower in scope but are more useful in providing both explanatory and predictive knowledge, grand theories of nursing tend to be broader in scope but very troublesome in terms of utility.

Summary

The foregoing exposition suggests a global approach to evaluate theoretical thinking in nursing. Several issues have come to light in examining the current status of nursing's theoretical work within the proposed framework.

In most of the theoretical pieces of work in nursing, major threads of theoretical thinking are difficult to identify. It seems that even if it were to be an afterthought, any major theoretical work should be committed to certain positions at the four higher levels so that it becomes obvious for the kind of theory that gets developed.

As has been stated by many nursing scholars, the so-called grand nursing theories or conceptual frameworks require further specification to be called theories. There seems to be two ways these frameworks could be developed further:

1. They may be developed into paradigms of nursing by specifying advocated assumptions about the nature of human beings and nursing, theory-building strategy or strategies assumed to be appropriate for the perspective, an image of nursing practice the perspective holds, and types of theoretical statements that are possible within the perspective; or
2. They may be developed as bona-fide theories by rigorously following the criteria at the fifth level.

It seems that the time is ripe for nursing scholars working within similar theoretical perspective to come together in order to formulate integrative nursing theories covering concepts from different domains of nursing.

For example, much work in nursing within the symbolic interactionist tradition may be ready to be assimilated into a nursing theory of "self-identity."

Similarly, much of the theoretical and empirical work dealing with how people develop competence in living with chronic illness (for example, cancer) can also be integrated into one nursing theory for further testing.

The community of nursing scholars at large has not dealt with the meaning of prescriptive theories for nursing science and nursing practice. There should be more rigorous debates regarding the normative nature of prescriptive theories and their effects on the development of nursing science and application to nursing practice in the context of scientific philosophy, nursing philosophy, and praxiology. The beliefs that praxiology follows

naturally from prescriptive theories and that prescriptive theories are naturally the goal of nursing science are both naive and dangerous.

Certainly, we are becoming increasingly sensitive and competent to carve out those requiring scientific explanation in the nursing perspective. And in doing so, we have created world views of nursing that seem both socially and epistemologically relevant to pursue. However, theoretical thinking in nursing will require a greater degree of specificity in terms of process and products if we are to move away from the intellectual infancy on which we have been comfortably resting. This attempt will require not only a greater degree of specificity, but also a more rigorous self-criticism.

REFERENCES

Beckstrand, J. (1978a). The notion of a practice theory and the relationship of scientific and ethical knowledge to practice. *Research in Nursing and Health, 1,* 131–136.

Beckstrand, J. (1978b). The need for a practice theory as indicated by the knowledge used in the conduct of practice. *Research in Nursing and Health, 1,* 175–179.

Beckstrand, J. (1980). A critique of several conceptions of practice theory in nursing. *Research in Nursing and Health, 3,* 69–79.

Benner, P. (1983). Uncovering the knowledge embedded in clinical practice. *Image, 15,* 41.

Benner, P. (1984). *From novice to expert: Excellence and power in clinical nursing practice.* Menlo Park, CA: Addison-Wesley.

Benoliel, J. (1977). The role of the family in managing the young diabetic. *The Diabetic Educator, 3,* 5–8.

Benoliel, J. (1983). Grounded theory and qualitative data: The socializing influences of life threatening disease on identity development. In P. J. Wooldridge, M. H. Schmitt, J. K. Skipper Jr., & R. C. Leonard (Eds.). *Behavioral science and nursing theory* (pp. 141–187). St. Louis: C. V. Mosby.

Bernstein, R. J. (1986). *Philosophical profiles: Essays in a pragmatic mode.* Cambridge: Polity Press.

Carper, B. A. (1978). Fundamental patterns of knowing in nursing. *Advances in Nursing Science, 1,* 12–23.

Dickoff, J., James, P., & Wiedenbach, E. (1968a). Theory in a practice discipline: Part I, Practice-oriented theory. *Nursing Research, 17,* 415–435.

Dickoff, J., James, P., & Wiedenbach, E. (1968b). Theory in a practice discipline: Part II, Practice-oriented theory. *Nursing Research, 17,* 545–554.

Donaldson, S. K., & Crowley, D. M. (1978). The discipline of nursing. *Nursing Outlook, 26,* 113–120.

Fawcett, J. (1980). A framework for analysis and evaluation of conceptual models of nursing. *Nurse Educator, 5,* 10–14.

Fawcett, J. (1984). *Analysis and evaluation of conceptual models in nursing.* Philadelphia: F. A. Davis.

Fawcett, J., & Downs, F. S. (1986). *The relationship of theory and research.* Norwalk, CT: Appleton-Century-Crofts.

Feyerabend, P. (1978). *Against method.* London: Verso.

Fitzpatrick, J. J., & Whall, A. L. (1983). *Conceptual models of nursing: Analysis and application.* Bowie, MD: Brady.

Gortner, S. R. (1980). Nursing science in transition. *Nursing Research, 29,* 180–183.

Gortner, S. R. (1983). The history and philosophy of nursing science and research. *Advances in Nursing Science, 5,* 1–8.

Hanson, N. R. (1958). *Patterns of discovery.* Cambridge, England: Cambridge University Press.

Hardy, M. E. (1974). Theories: Components, development, evaluation. *Nursing Research, 23,* 100–107.

Hardy, M. E. (1978). Perspectives on nursing theory. *Advances in Nursing Science, 1,* 27–48.

Hardy, M. E. (1983). Metaparadigms and theory development. In N. L. Chaska (Ed.). *The nursing profession: A time to speak* (pp. 427–437). New York: McGraw-Hill.

Holter, I. M. (1988). Critical theory: A foundation for the development of nursing theories. *Scholarly Inquiry for Nursing Practice, 2,* 223–232.

Jacox, A. (1974). Theory construction in nursing: An overview. *Nursing Research, 23,* 4–13.

Kim, H. S. (1983). *The nature of theoretical thinking in nursing.* Norwalk, CT: Appleton-Century-Crofts.

Kim, H. S. (1987). Structuring the nursing knowledge system: A topology of four domains. *Scholarly Inquiry for Nursing Practice, 1,* 99–110.

King, I. M. (1981). *A theory for nursing: Systems, concepts, process.* New York: John Wiley & Sons.

Kuhn, T. S. (1962). *The structure of scientific revolutions.* Chicago: University of Chicago Press.

Kuhn, T. S. (1970). *The structure of scientific revolutions* (2nd ed.). Chicago: University of Chicago Press.

Lakatos, I., & Musgrave, A. (Eds.) (1970). *Criticism and the growth of scientific knowledge.* Cambridge, England: Cambridge University Press.

Laudan, L. (1978). *Progress and its problems: Toward a theory of scientific growth.* Berkeley, CA: University of California Press.

Leventhal, H., & Johnson, J. E. (1983). Laboratory and field experimentation: Development of a theory of self-regulation. In P. J. Wooldridge, M. H. Schmitt, J. K. Skipper Jr., & R. C. Leonard (Eds.). *Behavioral science and nursing theory* (p. 262). St. Louis: C. V. Mosby.

Meleis, A. I. (1985). *Theoretical nursing: Development and progress.* Philadelphia: J. B. Lippincott.

Munhall, P. L. (1982). Nursing philosophy and nursing research: In apposition or opposition? *Nursing Research, 31,* 176–181.

Norris, C. M. (1982). *Concept clarification in nursing.* Rockville, MD: Aspen.

Orlando, I. (1961). *The dynamic nurse-patient relationship.* New York: J. P. Putnam's Sons.

Parse, R. R. (1981). *Man-living health: A theory of nursing.* New York: John Wiley & Sons.

Paterson, J. G., & Zderad, L. T. (1976). *Humanistic nursing.* New York: John Wiley & Sons.

Peplau, H. (1962). Interpersonal techniques: The crux of psychiatric nursing. *The American Journal of Nursing, 62,* 50–54.

Popper, K. R. (1972). *Objective knowledge.* Oxford, England: Clarendon Press.

Reynolds, P. D. (1971). *A primer in theory construction.* Indianapolis, IN: Bobbs-Merrill.

Rogers, M. E. (1983). Science of unitary human being: A paradigm for nursing. In I. W. Clements & F. B. Roberts (Eds.). *Family health: A theoretical approach to nursing.* New York: John Wiley & Sons.

Sarter, B. (1988). Philosophical sources of nursing theory. *Nursing Science Quarterly, 1,* 52–59.

Silva, M. C. (1977). Philosophy, science, theory: Interrelationships and implications for nursing research. *Image, 9,* 59–63.

Silva, M., & Rothbart, D. (1984). An analysis of changing trends in philosophy of science on nursing theory development and testing. *Advances in Nursing Science, 6,* 1–13.

Stevens, B. J. (1984). *Nursing theory: Analysis, application, evaluation* (2nd ed.) Boston: Little, Brown.

Suppe, F. (Ed.) (1977). *The structure of scientific theories* (2nd ed.). Urbana, IL: University of Illinois Press.

Suppe, F., & Jacox, A. K. (1985). Philosophy of science and the development of nursing theory. In H. H. Werley & J. J. Fitzpatrick (Eds.). *Annual review of nursing research: Vol. 3* (p. 267). New York: Springer.

Turner, J. H. (1986). *The structure of sociological theory* (4th ed.). Chicago: Dorsey Press.

Uys, L. R. (1987). Foundational studies in nursing. *Journal of Advanced Nursing, 12,* 275–280.

Walker, L. O. (1971). Toward a clearer understanding of the concept of nursing theory. *Nursing Research, 20,* 428–435.

Walker, L. O., & Avant, K. C. (1983). *Strategies for theory construction in nursing.* Norwalk, CT: Appleton-Century-Crofts.

Watson, J. (1981). Nursing's scientific quest. *Nursing Outlook, 29,* 413–416.

Watson, J. (1985). *Nursing: Human science and human care.* Norwalk, CT: Appleton-Century-Crofts.

Webster, G., Jacox, A., & Baldwin, B. (1981). Nursing theory and the ghost of the received view. In J. C. McCloskey & H. K. Grace (Eds.). *Current issues in nursing* (pp. 26–35). Boston: Blackwell.

Wiedenbach, E. (1963). The helping art of nursing. *American Journal of Nursing, 63,* 54–57.

Yura, H., & Torres, G. (1975). Today's conceptual frameworks within baccalaureate nursing programs. In National League for Nursing. *Faculty, curriculum development. Part 3: Conceptual framework: its meaning and function* (pp. 17–25). New York: Author.

The Author Comments

Theoretical Thinking in Nursing: Problems and Prospects

This article was written to address my concerns regarding the one-dimensional approach to analysis and evaluation of nursing theories espoused by many authors who are mostly concerned with the structure and meaning of theories rather than with the fundamental epistemologic roots from which nursing theories emerged. I found that when master's and doctoral students relied on such sources to understand nursing theories, they often became dogmatic, procedural, and superficial. I believe that nursing theories, as any other theories, emerge from and are rooted in various sorts of epistemologic assumptions. To understand theories more comprehensively, it is necessary to engage in analyzing and evaluating their epistemologic foundations before addressing theory structure and contents. My doctoral students have been engaged in the framework I proposed in this article to study nursing theories, as well as other theories they encounter, and their work has shown this approach to be valuable and enriching. My hope is that any nursing scholar who engages in theory building would consider the epistemologic questions I address in this article as the starting points for theory development.

—Hesook Suzie Kim

EVALUATION CRITERIA

CHAPTER 8

Theories: Components, Development, Evaluation

Margaret E. Hardy

The roles of concepts, statements of relationship, and models in theory development are examined. Criteria for evaluating theories are outlined, and the tentative nature of theories is discussed.

Although nurses in their everyday work are expected to evaluate health conditions of persons under their care, usually little thought is given to evaluating the soundness of the theory and knowledge which guides their action. If the theory is poorly suspended by evidence (i.e., the theory is not "true"), the health of the persons for which nurses are responsible may be severely jeopardized. As health professionals, nurses need to be able to make sound judgments about the rationale for various treatments, therapies, and care. It is often assumed that because an idea is in print (particularly if in a textbook or professional journal), it must be true. Many of the theories on which health professionals base their activities, however, are open to severe criticisms. With the speed with which new ideas are published, nurses now more than ever need to keep abreast of the development of relevant knowledge and be able to evaluate that knowledge in order to make informed judgments.

Unless nurses can assess the knowledge generated in such diverse areas as stress, systems, decision making, leadership, self-concept, body image, family, groups, body systems, they cannot use that knowledge wisely and constructively. Failure or inability to assess knowledge relevant to her area of work means the

About the Author

MARGARET E. HARDY was born in Edmonton, Alberta, Canada, in 1938. She received her BSN in 1960 from the University of British Columbia in Vancouver, Canada; her MA in 1965 from the University of Washington School of Nursing, with a major in community mental health; and her PhD in sociology in 1971 from the University of Washington. Her employment includes a faculty position at Boston University from 1971 to 1985, where she held a joint appointment in the School of Nursing and the Department of Sociology. From 1985 to her early retirement in 1993, she was Professor at the University of Rhode Island School of Nursing. Her major contribution to nursing evolved serendipitously as a result of her teaching assignment at Boston University; development of courses for the graduate program led to the publication of her award-winning books *Theoretical Foundations for Nursing* and *Role Theory*, as well as a book *Research Readings*. Through her publications and teaching hundreds of graduate students throughout New England during the 1970s and 1980s, Dr. Hardy provided foundational knowledge on metatheory and inspired many to initiate theory development for nursing. Dr. Hardy enjoys watercolor painting, reading, walking, hiking, traveling, and camping in the mountains with her husband and two dogs.

nurse must function as a technician, depending on others to interpret the knowledge-base which guides her actions. If nurses intend to direct their own actions in a responsible manner, they must become well informed on developing knowledge, they must be able to evaluate critically the knowledge developed, and they must make informed judgments based on this knowledge. They also must learn to function optimally as generalists. A competent practitioner really does not have the luxury of concentrating her efforts in a restricted area (psychiatry is currently under attack for the narrowness of its activities), but must take into account a wide variety of phenomena which have bearing on her clients.

Our comprehension of the world around us is based on the use of concepts, hypotheses, and theories. Nurses, as practitioners in the health field, apply and use knowledge generated from theories. In spite of the pervasiveness of theories in guiding and controlling our everyday life, the literature on theory development is diverse and confusing, and it generally is little related to the activities of practitioners. This article attempts to identify the structure of theory, to differentiate between different types of theoretical statements, and to identify criteria for evaluating theories.

Concepts

Concepts are labels, categories, or selected properties of objects to be studied; they are the bricks from which theories are constructed. Concepts are the dimensions, aspects, or attributes of reality which interest the scientist. Patients, illness, cardiovascular diseases, nurses, or physicians are examples of concepts used in health-related fields on which research may be based. The scientist constructs theories in his domain of interest by linking concepts of one class or attribute to concepts of other classes or attributes. When he has a set of interrelated statements or hypotheses concerning the relationships between concepts (i.e., when he has filled between the bricks with mortar), he has a theory. Concepts are the basic elements of theory. A major part of the evaluation of a theory is the identification and assessment of the concepts.

Components and Structure of Theory

A theory may be viewed from a variety of perspectives. For the purpose of exploring the structure of a theory, one may view theory as a language (Rudner, 1966). Like any language, theory consists of elements, formulations, and a set of definitions, i.e., it is comprised of syntax and semantics. When an investigator studies a scientific theory, he is interested in the logical structure or the relation between the elements (concepts) of the theory (the syntax) and the meaning given to the elements (the semantics). Syntax, then, is concerned with the occurrence of concepts in the axioms, postulates, or hypotheses of a theory and the relationship between the concepts and between the hypotheses of a theory, while semantics is concerned with the specific meaning attributed to the concepts. When a theory is made explicit or is formalized, one can examine the syntax and determine if the structure of the theory is consistent with the rules of logic.

The Semantics of Theory

Theories consist of two types of elements or terms. One set, the *derived* terms, are specifically introduced through definition whereas the other set, the *primitive* terms, remain undefined (Hempel, 1952). The primitive terms (or concepts) are the primary building blocks of theories from which new terms are derived. Both primitive and derived terms appear in a theory's axioms and postulates and give meaning to an otherwise uninterpreted or formalized system.

Concepts are defined and their meanings are understood only within the framework of the theory of which they are a part. Much conceptual confusion exists in theoretical areas upon which nurses draw. Concepts are often vaguely defined; the same concept may be defined and described many different ways (each writer providing his own definition). For example, within the area of role theory the concepts of role, status, and role behavior overlap and are often used interchangeably. Concepts develop as part of theory and are altered and refined as a body of knowledge grows. The concern for clarifying concepts involves a dilemma of trying to achieve consistency in meaning without premature closure of theories. Conceptual confusion and vagueness in theories appear to be a necessary and an important condition for creativity in science as elsewhere. Persons in the more applied professions often find this state of confusion difficult to cope with.

The refinement of concepts (improving the bricks) is a continuous process which involves not only sharpening of theoretical and operational definitions, but also modification of existing theory. Theories and concepts are reformulated by relating the theoretical world to the empirical, by organizing a great many concrete items into a small number of classes (regrouping the bricks), and by relating diverse concepts within a more general system of concepts.

General or Abstract

Concepts may be ordered on the basis of their level of abstractness. A specific occurrence, such as a patient's chest pain, is treated as a special case of a more general condition, such as heart disease. Heart disease, in turn, is a special condition of the more general area, the circulatory system.

Concepts are also appraised for their degree of generality; they are assessed according to the extent they change or vary. Concepts which refer to classes or categories of phenomena may be called *nonvariable* (Hage, 1972). Such concepts are found in typologies in which classes are clearly defined; an observation either fits or does not fit into a given category, depending upon the presence or absence of the property of interest, e.g., male, female. Concepts which are used to order phenomena according to some property or concepts which refer to dimensions of phenomena are called *variables* (Hage, 1972). When the results of observations fall on a continuum, the property being observed is a variable concept, e.g., 27 years, 82 years. It has been argued (Hage, 1972) that concepts that have a continuum should be utilized more frequently in conceptualizing and theory construction because such concepts facilitate theory development, are not restricted to time and place, and are more subtle for description and classification. The following illustrates the difference between nonvariable and variable concepts: Schizophrenia, manic depression, phobic reactions, and passive-aggressive traits are nonvariable concepts; they are bound by culture. The following general variable concepts are not so bound: anxiety, the degree of depression, intensity of affect, extent of contact with reality, frequency of phobic reactions. These general variable concepts may be utilized to describe the specific mental disorders listed above as well as other normal and abnormal mental states, whereas the nonvariable concepts (disease entities) are specifically either-or types of abnormal phenomena. By using both abstract and variable concepts, the scientist is able to develop laws and theories which have a wide range of applicability.

Theoretical or Operational

Concepts, whether nonvariable or variable, may have both a theoretical definition and an operational definition. The theoretical definition gives meaning to the terms in context of the theory and permits any reader to assess the validity of that definition. The operational definition tells how the concept is linked to concrete situations. An operational definition, which is used in the process of giving experiential meaning to the concept of a theory, describes a set of physical procedures which must be carried out in order to assign to every case a value for the concept. For example, the concept of level of aggression may be operationally defined as the number of times a child hits another child during an hour of play. How adequately the operational definition reflects the theoretical concept is another matter for consideration. That is, not only do concepts need operational definitions but the operational definition must be a valid reflection of the theoretical meaning of the concept. In this example, the operational definition certainly permits an observer to assign a level of "aggression" to each child observed. The level of aggression score for a child, however, may not reflect the theoretical meaning of the concept. The operational definition does not take into account the intent of the child, aggressive acts other than hitting, or the intensity of the act. The dilemma encountered in trying to link observable events to theoretical constructs is that the more concretely concepts are defined, the more restricted is the scope of the theory and the less useful is the theory. In spite of the difficulty in developing operational definitions, it is necessary to define theoretical terms in a way that the concepts can be measured. Only

through developing measurements of concepts can hypotheses and, in turn, theories be tested.

Operational definitions are a necessary part of theory construction. Operational definitions permit the validity of concepts to be assessed. They permit hypotheses to be tested and the empirical relevance of a theory to be assessed. They also permit other scientists to replicate the study. Operational definitions, which form the bridge between the theory and the empirical world, are modified over time as both theoretical and technological knowledge grow.

Theoretical concepts only make sense when considered within the framework of the theories of which they are a part. Such concepts may be examined on the basis of the degree of observability of their referent. Observable concepts (concepts that refer directly to observable objects) are likely to be found in derived theorems which are to be tested, whereas nonobservable concepts are found in axioms. Nonobservable concepts—intervening variables or hypothetical constructs—are derived on the basis of inferences from observable referents. Intervening variables are concepts that are based on inferences from observations. To illustrate this point, consider the following: A state of anxiety is often inferred on the basis of observations of increased heart rate, sweaty palms, and nausea. Anxiety per se is not observable.

Hypothetical concepts are more abstract than intervening variables. Belief in their existence is based primarily on theoretical support, and only indirectly on supporting empirical data. The id and the unconscious are examples of hypothetical constructs. The distinctions between intervening variables and hypothetical constructs are not at all clear. In one theory, a concept may be a hypothetical construct; in another theory, the same concept may be an intervening variable.

Attributes of Concepts
Utilized for Evaluation

Concepts are abstractions from concrete events; concepts themselves can have a varying degree of abstraction. As one moves up the level of abstraction in order to develop systematic explanations of general phenomena, one is faced with the problem of relating back from the symbolic concepts to concrete phenomena. Part of the difficulty in doing this is dependent on the adequacy of the rules of correspondence (or the links one is able to make) between the theoretical concepts and their empirical referents. The generality (abstraction) of concepts and the relationship between the concepts and the empirical referent (testability) are criteria used to evaluate a theory. Examination of the semantics of a theory provides another means for evaluation. This may, in part, be examined by assessing the intersubjectivity of meaning. The intersubjectivity of the meaning of concepts refers to whether the concepts are given a meaning similar to the meaning used by other scientists in related areas (Reynolds, 1971).

Statements of Relationships Between Concepts

Syntax of Theory

If a theory is formalized or made explicit, the syntax, or relationship, between concepts can be examined and the logical adequacy of the theory can be assessed. In assessing a theory's logical structure, the meanings of the concepts themselves are not taken into consideration. That is, symbols may be used to represent the concepts. This facilitates the examination of the logical structure without confusing the issue by considering the explicit meaning of the concepts. For example, the statement that social stress "results in" heart disease can be expressed symbolically. If social stress is represented by X, heart disease by Y, and results in by → then the statement social stress results in heart disease can be expressed by X→Y. A formalization of statements like this and other interrelated statements in a theory facilitate the examination of the structure of a theory.

Types of Relationships

To analyze the structure of a theory it is necessary to identify the relationships between concepts. Some types of relationships and their meanings are summarized in Figure 8-1. Relationships listed are not mutu-

Nature of Relation[1]	Meaning
Symmetrical	If A, then B; if B, then A
Asymmetrical	If A, then B; but if no A, no conclusion about B
Causal	If A, always B
Probabilistic	If A, probably B
Time order	If A, later B
Concurrent	If A, also B
Sufficient	If A, then B, regardless of anything else
Conditional	If A, then B, but only if C
Necessary	If A and only if A, then B

[1]The relations are not all mutually exclusive

Figure 8–1 *Relationships between concepts*

ally exclusive. Some of the relationships between concepts may be illustrated by using Selye's (1956) theory of stress. This stress formulation indicates that stressors result in a physiological syndrome identified as General Adaptive Syndrome (GAS). If in this formulation the relationship between stressors and GAS is determinate, then this implies that the concepts are *time-ordered* (stressors occur prior to the development of GAS), *sufficient* (if stressors occur, then GAS occurs regardless of anything else), and *necessary* (if stressors and only if stressors occur, then GAS occurs). The determinate relationship between stressors and GAS is asymmetrical (if stressors occur, then GAS occurs; if no stressors occur, then no conclusions may be reached about the occurrence of GAS) rather than symmetrical (if stressors occur, GAS occurs; if GAS occurs, then stressors occur). It is possible, however, that the relationship between stressors and GAS is not determinate but probabilistic (if stressors occur, there exists a 90 percent chance that GAS will occur) or conditional (if stressors occur, then GAS occurs, but only if specific physiological condition W exists). For clarity in theoretical formulations, it is necessary to specify the type of relationships between concepts. Although the identification of causal relationships in the health sciences is the reason for considerable success in disease prevention, relationships which are stochastic and relationships which are conditional are valuable in the prediction and control of disease-related events and hence should be identified rather than ignored.

Sign of the Relationship

An additional characteristic of the relationship between concepts is the sign (+/-) of the relationship. Concepts may be either positively (+/-) or inversely (-) related. The sign of relationships, though being discussed here in the context of theory development, really relates to the concept of measures of association or correlation. Thus, in the postulates—the greater X, the greater Y, and the greater Y, the greater Z—a positive relationship is implied between concepts as measured by some measure of association. Knowing that Y increases with X and Z increases with Y, it can be logically deduced that Z increases with X. The sign of the relationship between X and Z depends upon the sign of the relationships between the concepts X and Y, and Y and Z in the postulates. The sign rule has been summarized from work by Zetterberg (1963); Costner and Leik (1964) stated that the sign of the deduced relationship is the algebraic product of the signs of the postulated relationships. If Y is positively correlated with X and Z is positively correlated with Y, then it can be concluded by deduction and the sign rule that Z is positively correlated with X. This process of deduction may be expressed as:

$$\begin{array}{ll} \text{If} & X \overset{+}{\rightarrow} Y \\ \text{and} & Y \overset{+}{\rightarrow} Z \\ \hline \text{then} & X \overset{+}{\rightarrow} Z \end{array}$$

It is still an empirical question as to whether this logically deduced relationship actually exists. A relationship which is true according to logic is not necessarily true empirically.

Formalizing and Examining a Set of Statements

This discussion has emphasized that the evaluation of a theory's structure is facilitated if the concepts and the relationships between the concepts are formalized. The following stress formulation will be utilized to illustrate ways of assessing the syntax of theory: Social stress results in emotional tension whereas cognitive dissonance and social stress are inversely related; emotional tension results in somatic dysfunctioning. These statements may be formalized and displayed di-

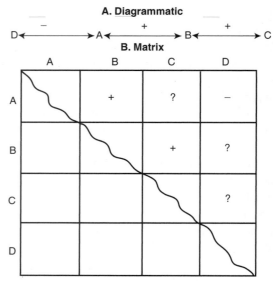

A. Diagrammatic

B. Matrix

[1]Concepts: Social stress, A; emotional tension, B; somatic dysfunctioning, C; cognitive dissonance, D. Sign of the relationship: Positive, +; inverse, −; unspecified, ? Relationships between concepts: Symmetrical, ↔; asymmetrical, →.

Figure 8-2 *Diagrammatic (A) and matrix (B) representation of stress formulation: concepts and their relationships.*[1]

agrammatically or in a matrix (Figure 8-2). The matrix used here is an adaptation of a data correlation matrix. The visual representation of the formalized model makes it relatively simple to examine the theory's structure. The diagram shows the relationship between the concepts while the matrix readily displays the completeness and logical consistency of the formulation. Discontinuities in the stress formulation are evident in both the diagram (lack of connections between the concepts) and the matrix (empty cells). Deductions can be made from the postulates stated. Using the sign rule and the deduced relationship, we may conclude that A and C are positively associated. That is, an increase in social stress is associated with an increase in somatic dysfunctioning. From this deduction the formulation is made more complete; no logical inconsistencies exist. The formalization of a theory to facilitate an evaluation of it will be discussed later.

Types of Statements

Although "postulates," "proposition," "hypothesis," "axiom," "laws," "principles," and "empirical generalizations" refer to different types of statements, they have a common characteristic in that they link together two or more concepts. A theory is made up of a set of interrelated propositions, theorems, or hypotheses derived from axioms, initial hypotheses, or postulates. Hypotheses refer to facts that are as yet unexperienced; they are corrigible in view of fresh knowledge. Principles and empirical generalizations are statements about data and are generally believed to be true. The distinguishing characteristic between empirical generalizations and hypotheses is that a hypothesis may be formulated in the absence of data, while an empirical generalization summarizes empirical evidence. Statements differ in their degree of generality and degree of empirical support. Empirical generalizations, since they summarize data, are closer to reality than are hypotheses. However, hypotheses, because they are at a higher level of generalization, are invaluable in aiding our understanding of events which have not yet been systematically tested.

Scientific hypotheses are more or less *grounded* on previous knowledge, i.e., they are partially supported (or at least not refuted) by empirical evidence and by theory. Hypotheses are developed from a rationale; they are not wild, groundless guesses. They should show reasonable conjecture—not fly in the face of existing knowledge.

Laws are well grounded; they have strong empirical support. They state a constant relation among two or more variables, each representing (at least partly and indirectly) a property of concrete systems. An example of a law is $E = Mc^2$. In the psychosocial area few, if any, laws exist. Laws are propositions that assert universal connections between properties.

Statements on the highest level of generality are laws and axioms. Statements on a lower level of generality (propositions, theorems, hypotheses) can be deduced from laws. The purpose of deduction is to test the general statements. In a deductive system, high-level statements can be falsified by the falsification of lower-level (deduced) statements. In any hypotheticodeduc-

tive theory, the less universal statements or lower-level statements are themselves still, strictly speaking, universal statements; they are empirical generalizations and must have the character of hypotheses. Postulates, axioms, and laws are primitive statements about an infinite universe, whereas hypotheses and empirical generalizations are statements about a finite universe.

The following examples may illustrate the difference between laws and hypotheses: A law in physiology is: Cardiac output = heart rate × stroke volume. This statement is true under all conditions (i.e., for all human hearts regardless of time or culture and also for nonhuman hearts). An hypothesis in physiology is: Resting potentials in nerve and muscle cells depend only on the difference in potassium ion concentration across the cell membrane. The statement has not reached the status of a law. Although there is reasonable evidence to support this statement, experimental evidence suggests that other ions may affect resting potentials. The generalization holds true for most muscle and nerve cells rather than for all cells. An hypothesis in social psychology is: In any task-oriented group, inequality in task activity among group members occurs and results in role differentiation. This generalization has mixed empirical support. Some experimental studies corroborate this hypothesis, while other experimental studies identify conditions under which role differentiation in task-oriented groups does not occur. The generalization may only apply under specific conditions and only in the American culture.

Models

Although a scientific theory is considered to be a deductive system, the relationship between variables may best be expressed in terms of a model. That is, an investigator may formalize a theory, identify its postulates, identify or derive the remaining propositions, and then decide that the problem of relationships is best represented by a model. A model is a simplified representation of a theory or of certain complex events, structures, or systems. Constructing a model forces the theorists to specify the precise relationship between components.

Models, like theories, are isomorphic systems; they are selective representations of the empirical world with which the scientist is concerned; crucial aspects of the phenomena are identified and aspects not considered important are ignored. Models are descriptive; they simplify the area of concern and can help the scientist grasp key elements and the relationships between these elements. The distinction between theories and models is not always clear. For example, what is considered a well-established theory in one academic area may be used as a model to represent phenomena in another area. Modeling is a technique used to describe and explain as well as to generate ideas and predictions.

Types

One type of model is an *analog* model, or an analogy. This model directs attention to resemblances between theoretical entities and familiar subject matter (Kaplan, 1964). For example, a nurse may use the analogy of a mechanical pump to explain to a patient the workings of his heart. In doing this, the nurse is using properties of the pump (an entity with which the patient is familiar) to explain characteristics about the heart (an entity with which the patient is unfamiliar). A problem which is difficult to understand may be made more comprehensible by the use of an analogy. The study of social organizations has been based on an organic model, e.g., Parsons' (1951) description of social systems, and social interactions have been described in terms of economic exchanges (Blau, 1964). Because the model is "true" in one area of science, however, does not mean that it will be true or hold up on another area. The model must be tested for its validity in each area of application. Although many characteristics of the organic model are inappropriate for describing social systems, the organic model has been a useful starting point for the study of social phenomena.

Iconic models are used if a direct representation of the subject is wanted (DiRenzo, 1966). The model may vary as to the number of properties represented and the level of abstraction. A kidney machine, for example, although it does not resemble the kidney in appearance, does represent relatively accurately some of the kidney processes. A model of the heart (built to scale), a scaled model of a DNA molecule, an organizational chart of a hospital, and a miniature social system depicting the hierarchical structure and communication processes in an organization are examples of iconic models. These models represent the original phenomena but in another form. Such models are useful to the extent that they increase our sense of understanding of the entity. This type of modeling has been utilized more perhaps in the physical sciences than in the social sciences. The usefulness of iconic models for understanding social phenomena may be directly related to our ability to identify key variables and to abstract these characteristics. For many persons it is easier to accept a plastic model of the heart as a useful model than it is to accept a three-person decision-making network as a useful model of a social organization. The value of models is dependent upon the extent to which they increase understanding, explain phenomena, or give us a sense of what is going on and why.

Another type of model is the *symbolic* model which represents phenomena figuratively (DiRenzo, 1966). A set of connected symbols, objects, or concepts may be used to represent a problem of interest. The relationship between concepts may be represented diagrammatically to facilitate conceptualization and understanding.

Use

Although models have proved to be extremely helpful in theory construction, they should be used carefully. Models have no truth value themselves. There is no guarantee that a model that has been successfully used in one area of study will be useful in another area. A major question to consider is the extent to which the model faithfully represents the phenomena of interest. There may be a tendency to overlook the differences between the phenomena of interest and the model since the scientist is more interested in the similarities. The differences, however, may completely negate the usefulness of the model. Models are tools for understanding reality which should be used judiciously and be replaced or modified when outmoded or inappropriate.

Criteria for Evaluating Theories

Theories are sets of interrelated hypotheses which are subject to reformulation and refinement. The development of adequate theories to describe, explain, predict, and control phenomena is a slow process and requires the cooperative effort of many persons. Knowledge is not acquired by one person in isolation but results from the cumulative efforts of many persons over a long period of time. Various writers, primarily philosophers, have suggested criteria to assist in the evaluation of theory. A theory may be evaluated in terms of its logical adequacy, abstractness, testability, empirical adequacy, and pragmatic adequacy (Schrag, 1967). These criteria are not meant to hinder the development of theories but to provide guidelines.

Theories are developed to help describe, explain, predict, and control phenomena in the world around us whether the theory is concerned with the area of astronomy, genetics, physics, chemistry, psychology, sociology, physiology, or biology. Implicit in the discussion of theories is the assumption that a theory can be evaluated according to certain universal standards. Regardless of the content of the theory, an investigator examines the underlying assumptions, the validity of the concepts and of the general perspective, the degree of generality of the theory, the soundness of the reasoning, the testability of the hypotheses, the empirical support for the hypotheses, the ability to control and manipulate the phenomena, and the degree of accuracy with which predictions can be made.

Meaning and Logical Adequacy

That few theories successfully meet all these criteria does not mean that theories should not be evaluated. A first step in evaluating theory is to identify basic assumptions (these may not be stated), the concepts, and the relationships between the concepts and to consider the validity of the assumptions, the validity of the meaning attributed to the concepts (are the concepts defined in a manner similar to that used by other scientists in the area?), and the logic of the theoretical system.

When an investigator has reached a conclusion about the validity of the concepts and proposed theory, he can assess the logic of the argument. In doing this, the scientist is concerned with the reasonableness of the argument. The logical adequacy of a theory can be evaluated by formalizing the theory and examining it for discontinuities, discrepancies, and contradictions. In the example cited earlier (Figure 8-2a and b), discontinuities in the theory were evident. When the theory was formalized, it was apparent that nothing was said about the relationship between social stress and somatic dysfunctioning or about the relationship between cognitive dissonance and emotional tension and cognitive dissonance and somatic dysfunctioning. From the postulates and using the sign rule, it was deduced that A and C are positively associated. Since D is related (inversely) only to A, nothing can be said about its relationship to B or C. Because the relationships between A and B and B and C are asymmetrical (A B, B C), the conclusion that A is positively correlated with and results in C is logical. Had the relationship between the variables been symmetrical (A = B, B C), then the conclusion that A is related to C might not hold up. The relationship between A and B, for example, says that A and B vary together; the relationship is not necessarily causal. A and B may be related because of their common relationship to another variable, i.e., the relationship could be spurious.

Likewise, the symmetrical relationship between B and C might be spurious. If either or both of the relationships in these postulates are spurious, then the relationship between the concepts in the deduced proposition is open to question. No contradictions were evident in the stress formulation. Formalizing a theory increases the probability that discontinuities and contradictions will be identified.

Operational and Empirical Adequacy

Next, the theory can be assessed for its testability. To be testable, a theory must have operationally defined concepts. Since Bridgman's (1927) introduction of the phrase, "operational definition," scientists in all areas have been concerned with identifying adequate operational definitions for their concepts. When operational definitions for theoretical concepts have been established, the theory can be tested. Assessing the operational adequacy of a theory requires consideration of (a) whether the concepts can be measured and (b) how accurately the operational definitions reflect the theoretical concepts.

In testing a theory, it can be subjected to falsification (be found false) rather than to confirmation (Popper, 1959). If a sincere attempt is made to refute a theory and the theory stands up, the theory is considered supported or tentatively confirmed. Terms such as "confirmation," "verification," "support," "corroboration," "disconfirmation," "falsification," "failure to support," relate to the empirical base for a theory. Hypotheses may not be proved true, verified, or falsified by limited evidence, but evidence gathered over time from a variety of sources may tend to support, bear out, corroborate, or be in accord with an hypothesis, and thus be confirming evidence. If the evidence does not support the hypothesis, the evidence may be viewed as disconfirming rather than falsifying; the hypothesis is not "proved false." The use of the term "evidence" and the terms "disconfirming," "supporting," and "corroborating" suggests that one recognizes the status of the hypothesis as tentative—awaiting further testing. An hypothesis is not an absolute statement or a truth statement; it should be stated in a way that it can be tested and refuted. For data from any one study and for cumulative evidence from numerous studies, the question of the empirical adequacy of the theory is raised, i.e., how well does the evidence support the theory?

Over time, evidence that both supports and fails to support a theory accumulates. When the relative strengths of the evidence are evaluated, some conclusion about the empirical adequacy of a theory may be reached. Assessing the empirical adequacy of a theory requires the determination of the degree of congruence between the theoretical claims and the empirical evidence.

Generality

Another criterion used to evaluate a theory is the degree of generality or the degree of abstractness which characterizes it. The more general a theory, the more useful it is. A theory of the grieving process which can be applied to persons of all ages, to persons in any culture, and to losses of any object is more useful than a theory of grieving which can be applied only to middle-aged persons who lose a spouse.

Contribution to Understanding

A theory may be assessed as to how much it increases understanding. Does it describe the phenomena and give a sense of insight? Does it suggest new ideas and a new way of looking at the phenomena? The scientist constantly looks for theories that will increase his understanding of phenomena, which are relatively simple explanations, and which suggest new lines of reasoning and new avenues of exploration.

Predictability

Another criterion used to assess theory is the extent to which predictions can be made. A theory may describe a process, may increase the understanding of the process, but it may not assist in making any predictions about the outcomes of that process. A theory, for example may permit a description and explanation of a process after it has occurred; i.e., it is possible to look at a family which has suffered a "loss" and describe the family behavior in terms of adjustment to a crisis, but it may not be possible to predict accurately the behavior of family members in response to this crisis before the crisis occurs.

Pragmatic Adequacy

Since the purpose of a theory is to explain, predict, and control, the ability to control phenomena of interest is one means for assessing a theory. This criterion is pragmatic adequacy (Schrag, 1967). A theory may permit explanation and accurate prediction, but the theory may not permit the scientist to control the phenomena of interest.

The business of the applied professions (nursing, engineering, social work, medicine, architecture, political science) is to make *use* of existing theory to predict certain processes or outcomes and to control "events" in such a way that desired outcomes are achieved. The usefulness of a theory (pragmatic adequacy) for changing conditions is of major importance to the health professions. In the biological sciences many theories enable scientists or professionals to control outcomes; e.g., disease control, (prevention) of degenerative process in the body, and control or replacement of defective body parts. Although it is recognized that science has as its goal the production of knowledge for predicting and controlling phenomena, the ethics of using this knowledge is only now being examined in detail. Some of the decisions as to whether man should use the knowledge he had generated to control and alter the forces around him are being questioned more in some areas than in others, i.e., few question the use of vaccines to prevent disease, but the use of abortions to prevent overpopulation has been severely attacked by some segments of the population. Although there are relatively few theories (particularly in the area of social behavior) which permit the scientist to control phenomena, the development of such theories is likely to increase. The problems associated with the use of these theories by the applied professions will also increase.

Tentative Nature of Theories

Although rules and guidelines can be postulated to aid in the development and evaluations of theories, theories are tentative. With new knowledge, old facts are subject to different interpretations, and different data are brought to light. The development of theory is man's attempt to establish structure and meaning in his world. In assessing existing knowledge, one needs to take into account the culture of the scientific community as well as the values of society in general. The values of both communities come into play in many aspects of the process of establishing knowledge. The selection of problem areas and the development and use of concepts involve arbitrary choices. The theories that develop reflect the interests of the scientific community and of society and do not necessarily represent the areas that are in most need of examination.

REFERENCES

Blau, P. M. (1964). *Exchange and power in social life.* New York: John Wiley & Sons.

Bridgman, P. W. (1927). *The logic of modern physics.* New York: Macmillan.

Costner, H. L., & Leik, R. K. (1964). Deductions from axiomatic theory. *American Sociological Review, 29,* 819–835.

Di Renzo, G. J. (Ed.). (1966). *Concepts, theory and explanation in the behavioral sciences.* New York: Random House.

Hage, J. (1972). *Techniques and problems of theory construction in sociology.* New York: John Wiley & Sons.

Hempel, C. G. (1952). Fundamentals of concept formation in empirical science. In *International encyclopedia of unified sciences.* Chicago: The University of Chicago Press.

Kaplan, A. (1964). *The conduct of inquiry.* San Francisco: Chandler.

Parsons, T. (1951). *The social system.* Glencoe, IL: Free Press.

Popper, K. (1959). *The logic of scientific discovery.* New York: Basic Books.

Reynolds, P. D. (1971). *A primer in theory construction.* Indianapolis: Bobbs-Merrill.

Rudner, R. S. (1966). *Philosophy of social science.* Englewood Cliffs, N.J.: Prentice-Hall.

Schrag, C. (1967). Elements of theoretical analysis in sociology. In L. Gross (Ed.), *Sociological theory: Inquiries and paradigms* (pp. 220–253). New York: Harper & Row.

Selye, H. (1956). *The stress of life.* New York: McGraw-Hill.

Zetterberg, H. (1963). *On theory and verification in sociology (A much revised edition).* Totowa, NJ: Bedmeister Press.

The Author Comments

Theories: Components, Development, Evaluation

The motivation for writing this article was the need for students to have an organizing framework for selecting one theory over another when faced with a clinical situation, regardless of clinical specialty or unit of study, from the physiologic to the organizational. Students also needed to link theoretic areas, which, at the time, often included the concepts of stress, crisis, and adaptation. To do this, students had to know the characteristics and components of a theory and the criteria for selecting and evaluating theory. This metatheoretic knowledge was and still remains a necessary prerequisite for comparing and selecting theories for nursing practice, as well as for evaluating one's own theories. At the time this article was written, there was no literature published on this topic. This article, along with the book publications, forged new and important territory in knowledge development for nursing.

—Margaret E. Hardy

CHAPTER 9

Framework for Analysis and Evaluation of Conceptual Models of Nursing

Jacqueline Fawcett

Conceptual models are important in guiding the development of the discipline of nursing. Yet the difference between these abstract schemes and substantive theory is often confused. This article defines and describes both types of knowledge and offers a framework for analysis and evaluation appropriate for nursing models.

Nursing knowledge is rapidly organizing around and developing from several abstract conceptual models. Among the best known are the Roy Adaptation Model (Roy, 1976), Orem's (1971) Self-Care Model, the Johnson Behavioral Systems Model (Grubbs, 1974), M. E. Rogers's (1970) Life Process Model, and King's (1971) Social Systems Model. If nursing is to continue to emerge as a distinct discipline, nursing educators must define and explore semantic and substance issues surrounding these models and their relation to other forms of knowledge. Even if we can't agree on major points, we should clarify language usage and terminology.

This article seeks to provide a clear definition of conceptual models, to delineate the particularly confused distinction between conceptual models and theories, and to develop an appropriate framework for analysis and evaluation of conceptual models. Educators must understand this material before they can effectively incorporate conceptual models into nursing program curricula. The framework presented here will permit educators and students to fully examine several models before adopting the one most congruent with their philosophy. It will also help those who prefer a more eclectic approach to choose those bits and pieces from several models that

About the Author

JACQUELINE FAWCETT received her Bachelor of Science degree from Boston University in 1964, her master's degree in parent-child nursing from New York University in 1970, and her PhD in nursing from New York University in 1976. Dr. Fawcett is currently Professor, College of Nursing and Health Sciences, University of Massachusetts-Boston. She is Professor Emerita at the University of Pennsylvania. Starting with her dissertation, Dr. Fawcett conducted a program of research dealing with wives' and husbands' pregnancy-related experiences that was derived from Martha Rogers' conceptual system. Subsequently, she undertook a program of research dealing with responses to cesarean birth derived from the Roy Adaptation Model of Nursing. A third program of research, also derived from the Roy Adaptation Model, focuses on function during normal life transitions and serious illness. Dr. Fawcett is perhaps best known for her metatheoretical work, including many journal articles and several books. Since 1996, Dr. Fawcett has lived in the midcoast region of Maine with her husband John; two Maine Coon cats, Matinicus and Acadia; and a now-tame feral cat, Lydia Dasher. She and her husband own Fawcett's Art, Antiques, and Toy Museum. She swims laps and walks on a treadmill at a fitness center for exercise and relaxation and sails on a windjammer off the Maine coast during the summer.

can be combined into a meaningful and logical whole. Moreover this material may be used as an organizing structure for courses focused on conceptual models.

Definition of Conceptual Model

The term conceptual model, and synonymous terms such as conceptual framework, system, or scheme, refer to global ideas about the individuals, groups, situations and events of interest to a science. These phenomena are classified into concepts, which are words bringing forth mental images of the properties of things. Concepts may be abstract ideas, such as adaptation and equilibrium, or concrete ones, such as table and chair.

Concepts are linked to form propositions stating their interrelationships. These statements constitute the basic assumptions of the science. An example of this kind of relational statement is: "People and their environments are open systems."

A conceptual model may therefore be defined as a set of concepts and those assumptions that integrate them into a meaningful configuration (Nye & Berardo, 1966). Each model, then, specifies certain phenomena by identifying relevant concepts and by describing the connections among them. Thus, a conceptual model might outline the environmental forces or stressors acting on a person to create adaptive change, as well as the resources available to help the person maintain equilibrium while coping with these stressors.

The concepts in a conceptual model are highly abstract and usually not directly observed in the real world. Similarly, the assumptions linking the concepts are abstract generalizations that are not immediately testable. By identifying relevant phenomena, a conceptual model provides a perspective for scientists, telling them what to look at and speculate about. By describing these phenomena and their interrelationships in general and abstract terms, *the model represents the first step in developing the theoretical formulations* needed for scientific activities.[1]

It is not unusual to find that more than one discipline or school of thought is interested in the same concepts. What distinguishes these fields of inquiry are different definitions and measures of the concepts, and different assumptions tying them together. For while sociologists

---

[1]Theoretical Formulations, as used here, refers to ideas ranging from loosely constructed conjectures to fully developed, widely accepted theories. The substantive knowledge of a discipline is made up of these untested or partially validated speculations, as well as of established principles and laws.

explore social origins of language, psychologists may examine genetic influences on the ability to communicate.

Conceptual models usually evolve from the intuitive insights of scientists often initially within the frame of reference of a related discipline. The synthesis that occurs in the development of a new conceptual scheme, however, results in a product unique to the field. Conceptual models may also represent deductive systems that creatively combine propositions from several areas.

Conceptual models can clearly specify the phenomena of interest to nursing science, encompassed by four essential concepts: person, environment, health, and nursing (Yura & Torres, 1975). Existing nursing models define and describe person and environment and their interrelations. Most conceptualizations view the person as a biopsychosocial being who interacts with family members, the community, and other groups, as well as with the physical environment. However, each scheme presents these essential concepts in such unique ways as adaptive systems, behavioral subsystems, or complementary four-dimensional energy fields. The models further provide a definition of health, often describing both the well and ill person and environments conducive or detrimental to health. They also identify the goals of nursing, which usually derive directly from the definition of health. For example, a nursing goal might be to assist the person to attain, maintain, or regain health as defined by that conceptual scheme. Finally, each model spells out its version of the nursing process, frequently in great detail.

The several conceptual models of nursing represent various schools of thought within the discipline of nursing. As such it is not surprising that each operationalizes the four essential concepts differently and links these concepts with diverse assumptions.

Distinctions Between Conceptual Model and Theory

A conceptual model is *not* a theory. A theory is formally defined as "a set of interrelated constructs (concepts), definitions, and propositions that present a systematic view of phenomena by specifying relations among variables" (Kerlinger, 1973, p. 9). It postulates specific relations among concepts and takes the form of a description, an explanation, a prediction, or a prescription for action. Any theory presupposes a more general abstract conceptual system; the concepts, definitions, and propositions of the theory are derived from the concepts and assumptions of the model.

The literature contains many different routes from model to theory, but there is little agreement as to which path is the best. A discussion of these diverse theory-building strategies, using inductive, deductive, or retroductive thought is beyond the scope of this article (Burr, 1973). Two points, however, may be made here. First, whichever path is chosen, reaching its end requires imagination, knowledge of the subject matter, and logical thinking. And second, this road must be a rocky one, since so few conceptual models ever lead to theories.

The crucial distinction, then, between a conceptual model and a theory is the level of abstraction. As noted earlier, a conceptual model is a highly abstract system of related global concepts. A theory, in contrast, contains more concrete concepts, along with their definitions and the propositions linking them. A theory also provides greater specification of phenomena and more detailed explanations of postulated relationships than does a conceptual model. A conceptual model embodies the "world view," the paradigm, of a discipline or school of thought. Each theory derived from the model explains some or all of the paradigm's phenomena but only within a limited range. A theory is both more precise and more limited in scope than its parent conceptual scheme. For example, a nursing model might suggest that the individual's health status is a function of total environmental influences. A theory of mental health nursing might then postulate that certain patterns of family interaction foster psychological dysfunction in a given family member and explain the reasons for this outcome.

Although some people consider conceptual models to be what Merton called "grand theories"—global orientations that attempt to explain a totality of events—the position taken here is that conceptual schemes are too abstract to be considered any type of theory. As used here, theory refers to Merton's "theory of the middle range"—speculations concerned with relatively narrow ranges of data (Merton, 1957, pp. 5-6).

With these distinctions in mind, we can define a nursing theory. Nursing theories are most appropriately derived from the conceptualizations of nursing. They are characterized as sets of interrelated propositions and definitions that present systematic views of the essential concepts of nursing—person, environment, health, nursing—by specifying relations among variables derived from these ideals (Fawcett, 1978a).

Theoretical model, theoretical framework, and theoretical rationale are essentially synonymous terms frequently seen in the nursing literature. These terms refer to networks of theoretical ideas and research results from which we can deduce empirically testable hypotheses. In some articles, two or more specific theories may be connected to form a more general theory that is still sufficiently concrete to permit testing. In other articles, the rationale may rest upon generalizations from a series of observations and descriptive research findings that do not comprise a formal theory.

By now we can see that conceptual models are not specific enough to provide more than general guidelines for scientists' endeavors. Therefore, theoretical formulations must accompany the model if definitive directions for action are needed. The function served by a model determines the type of speculations required to further explain events. In nursing, conceptual frameworks act as general guides for practice, research, curricula, and administrative systems. The particular practice situation, research problem, educational program, or management setting will dictate the explanations needed to flesh out the skeleton provided by the model. To date, we have borrowed most of these theoretical ideas from other disciplines, including psychology, sociology, biology, physics, and chemistry. Nursing theories probably will amplify or replace this borrowed knowledge as scholars succeed in their efforts to establish a body of nursing knowledge.

Some examples will help to clarify this point. Conceptual models and related theories are beginning to be used in clinical practice. For instance, Roy's assessment scheme has been applied by a family nurse in her clinical practice. Intervention strategies for this nurse's clients were guided by the model and by knowledge of physiology. In this case, we expect that the nurse's accrued observations will eventually lead to nursing theories (Roy & Obloy, 1978).

Similarly, models are now being used in development of nursing research projects. A study of body image changes of pregnant women and their husbands was derived from Rogers's conceptualization of person-environment complementarity. Since this model is highly abstract, it was necessary to base the research hypotheses on the more concrete tenets of body image theory. The study findings of similar alterations in spouses' body images during and after pregnancy lent support to both specific aspects of body image theory and global assumptions about person-environment interactions. The next step in this research program will be to develop a unique nursing theory to explain these and other aspects of the experience of pregnancy as shared by family members (Fawcett, 1977, 1978b).

Educational programs have employed conceptual frameworks to organize content for several years. Indeed, so many articles have documented this process that further elaboration is hardly required here.

Finally, conceptual models are also useful in administrative situations. For example, a hospital or community health agency could arrange nursing care plans according to the categories of a particular model's nursing process. Or, as one author suggested (C. G. Rogers, 1973), areas of clinical specialization could be developed from categories outlined in a model. In each case, additional detail would follow from relevant theories now borrowed from other sciences. However, as we accumulate observations in each category, the building blocks of nursing theories will emerge.

Analysis and Evaluation of Conceptual Models

Clearly, the distinctions between conceptual models and theories are sufficiently great to warrant different frameworks for analysis and evaluation. The nursing literature contains such excellent presentations of criteria for theories that further effort in that direction seems unnecessary (Ellis, 1968; Hardy, 1978; Torres & Yura, 1975).

The literature also includes evaluative schemas that reflect the confusion between conceptual models and theories. The one proposed by Riehl and Roy (1974) used the Dickoff and James (1968) survey list for situation-producing theory, and therefore, from our position, is too concrete for abstract conceptualizations.

Conversely, two other review systems claimed to be designated for theory evaluation but were applied to conceptual models. Both the Duffey and Muhlenkamp (1974) and the Stevens (1979) plans include some questions appropriate to model's level of abstraction, but like the Riehl and Roy schema, offer other items more germane to a concrete theories.

Two additional schemas are appropriate for conceptual model evaluation but seem too limited for comprehensive reviews. Johnson's (1974) criteria are focused solely on social decisions while Peterson's (1977) questions lack necessary scope and detail. However, taken together, these several plans provided some building blocks for construction of the analytic and evaluative framework presented in Figure 45-1.

This framework separates questions dealing with analysis from those more appropriate to evaluation. The former queries permit nonjudgmental, detailed examination of the conceptual model, including its philosophical base, content, and scope. In contrast, evaluation questions allow one to draw judgmental conclusions by focusing on internal validity of a model, although not on external comparisons among various conceptualizations. This important distinction implies "that any conceptual model is valid insofar as it is reasonably sound with regard to the particular anthropology employed (i.e., man as developing, adapting, interacting)" (Zbilut, 1978, p. 128). Indeed, it is imperative that the reader understands on what level conceptual models may be compared. Since models explain the phenomena of district disciplines or schools of thought, we can make direct comparisons. Reese and Overton cautioned that "because of basic lack of communication, the par-

tial overlap in subject matter and the difference in truth criteria, (each model) must be evaluated separately, and in obedience to its own ground rules" (Overton, 1970, p. 122). Thus, judgments must be limited to the adequacy of each conceptual scheme as it stands alone.

In sum, the framework for analysis and evaluation leads to a decision to retain, modify, or discard the model, and also provides an answer to the pragmatic question of whether I can use the conceptual model for *my* nursing activities.

Questions for Analysis

A conceptual model is derived from an author's personal philosophy and scientific orientation. This philosophic base and the method of model development (usually inductive but sometimes deductive) are often revealed in the author's earlier writing and in preliminary versions of the conceptual system. The first aspect of analysis, then, asks the questions:

- What is the historical evolution of the conceptual model?
- What approach to development of nursing knowledge does the model exemplify?

Earlier we established that a conceptual model comprises a set of concepts and linking assumptions, and that the essential concepts of any nursing model are person, environment, health, and nursing. These components lead to the second aspect of analysis. The questions are:

- How are the four essential concepts of nursing explicated in the model?
- How is person defined and described?
- How is environment defined and described?
- How is health defined? How are wellness and illness differentiated?
- How is nursing defined? What is the goal of nursing?
- How is the nursing process described?
- What statements are made about the relationships among the four concepts?

The final aspect of analysis derives from the fact that any model must be limited in scope; it cannot deal with *all* things in the universe. Although most authors start with the same view of the general purpose of nursing, in final form nursing models reflect different perspectives of the essential concepts and hence lead to considerations of different problems in the person-environment interactions related to health. Moreover, the source of these problems may vary from, for example, dysfunctional internal factors to hostile environmental factors. Borrowing from Duffey and Muhlenkamp, the questions to be raised are:

• With what problems is the conceptual model concerned?
• What is the source of these problems?

Questions for Evaluation

The first aspect of evaluation concerns the philosophic underpinnings of the model. The question is:

• Are the biases and values underlying the conceptual model made explicit?

The next aspect of evaluation deals with content of the model and relates back to the answers supplied by the second aspect of analysis.

Here the questions to be posed are:

• Does the conceptual model provide complete descriptions of all four essential concepts of nursing?
• Do the basic assumptions completely link the four concepts?

This portion of the evaluation must also consider the logic of the model; its internal structure must be evaluated for congruity. Internal consistency also takes the classification of models into account. Nursing models have been categorized according to the discipline or anthropology from which they were derived and are most often labeled development, interaction, or systems models. Each of these "world views" has distinct characteristics that shape organization of knowledge and methodologies for application.

Internal consistency is especially important if the model incorporates more than one view of any of the essential concepts, since each has different criteria for

determining the truth of statements. A synthesis that mixes perspectives also mixes truth criteria.

However, we can translate viewpoints by redefining them in a consistent manner. Translation represents the construction of a brand-new, unmixed model that is logical (Reese & Overton, 1970). The questions to be raised, then, are:

• Is the internal structure of the conceptual model logically consistent?
• Does the conceptual model reflect the characteristics of its category type?
• Do the components of the model reflect logical translation of diverse perspectives?

Johnson's evaluation criteria represent another aspect for consideration. She maintained that conceptual models are validated by social decisions. The first is *social congruence,* and the question is:

• Does the conceptual model lead to nursing activities that meet social expectations or do the expectations created by the conceptual model require societal changes?

The second decision is *social significance,* and here the question is:

• Does the conceptual model lead to nursing actions that make important differences in the client's health status?

The third decision is *social utility,* and the question to be raised is:

• Is the conceptual model comprehensive enough to provide general guides for practice, research, education, and administration?

The next part of evaluation reflects the relation between models and theories. As was noted earlier, theories are derived from models; thus, the theory generating contributions of the model should be judged, as well as the result of empirical tests of any theories derived from the model. The questions to be posed are:

• Does the conceptual model generate empirically testable theories?

- Do tests of derived theories yield evidence in support of the model?

The final aspect of evaluation is as general as the models themselves. This question judges the contribution of the model to nursing knowledge, asking:

- What is the overall contribution of this conceptual model to the body of nursing knowledge?

Questions for Analysis

- What is the historical evolution of the conceptual model?
- What approach to development of nursing knowledge does the model exemplify?
- How are the four essential concepts of nursing explicated in the model?
- How is person defined and described?
- How is environment defined and described?
- How is health defined? How are wellness and illness differentiated?
- How is nursing defined? What is the goal of nursing?
- How is the nursing process described?
- What statements are made about the relationships among the four concepts?
- With what problems is the conceptual model concerned?
- What is the source of these problems?

Questions for Evaluation

- Are the biases and values underlying the conceptual model made explicit?
- Does the conceptual model provide complete descriptions of all four essential concepts of nursing?
- Do the basic assumptions completely link the four concepts?
- Is the internal structure of the conceptual model logically consistent?
- Does the conceptual model reflect the characteristics of its category type?
- Do the components of the model reflect logical translation of diverse perspectives?
- Is the conceptual model socially congruent? Does the model lead to nursing activities that meet social ex-

pectations or do the expectations created by the model require societal changes?

- Is the conceptual model socially significant? Does the model lead to nursing actions that make important differences in the client's health status?
- Is the conceptual model socially useful? Is the model comprehensive enough to provide general guides for practice, research, education, and administration?
- Does the conceptual model generate empirically testable theories?
- Do tests of derived theories yield evidence in support of the model?
- What is the overall contribution of this conceptual model to the body of nursing knowledge?

Conclusion

This article sought to distinguish between two forms of knowledge—general conceptualizations and specific theoretical formulations. Further, in light of the current expansion and elaboration of nursing models, a framework for analysis and evaluation appropriate to their level of abstraction was developed. This plan can assist nurses in comparing various methods before choosing one to guide their activities. My own work in applying these questions to individual conceptual schemes indicates that gaps and logical inconsistencies are identifiable and readily corrected. Moreover, my experience in teaching nursing science courses shows that the framework greatly facilitates students' comprehension and fuller use of the models as bases for nursing practice, research, education, and administration.

REFERENCES

Burr, W. R. (1973). *Theory construction and the sociology of the family.* New York: John Wiley & Sons.

Dickoff, J., & James, P. (1986). A theory of theories: A position paper. *Nursing Research, 17,* 197–203.

Duffey, M., & Muhlenkamp, A. F. (1974). A framework for theory analysis. *Nursing Outlook, 22,* 570–574.

Ellis, R. (1968). Characteristics of significant theories. *Nursing Research, 17,* 217–222.

Fawcett, J. (1977). The relationship between identification and patterns of change in spouses' body images during and after pregnancy. *International Journal of Nursing Studies 14,* 199–213.

Fawcett, J. (1978a). The 'what' of theory development. In *Theory development: What, why, how?* (NLN Pub. No. 15–1708). New York: National League for Nursing.

Fawcett, J. (1978b). Body image and the pregnant couple. *The American Journal of Maternal Child Nursing, 3,* 227–233.

Grubbs, J. (1974). An interpretation of the Johnson behavioral system model. In J. P. Riehl & C. Roy (Eds.), *Conceptual models for nursing practice* (pp. 160–197). New York: Appleton-Century-Crofts.

Hardy, M. E. (1978). Evaluating nursing theory. In *Theory development: What, why, how?* (pp. 82–86) (NLN Pub. No. 15–1708). New York: National League for Nursing.

Johnson, D. E. (1974). Development of theory: A requisite for nursing as a primary health profession. *Nursing Research, 23,* 376–377.

Kerlinger, F. N. (1973). *Foundations of behavioral research* (2nd ed.). New York: Holt, Rinehart and Winston.

King, I. M. (1971). *Toward a theory of nursing.* New York: John Wiley & Sons.

Merton, R. F. (1957). *Social theory and social structure* (Rev. ed.). New York: Free Press.

Nye, F. I., & Berardo, F. M. (1966). *Emerging conceptual frameworks in family analysis.* New York: Macmillan.

Orem, D. E. (1971). *Nursing: Concepts of practice.* New York: McGraw-Hill.

Peterson, C. J. (1977). Questions frequently asked about the development of a conceptual framework. *Journal of Nursing Education, 16,* 22–32.

Reese, H. W., & Overton, W. F. (1970). Models of development and theories of development. In L. R. Goulet & P. B. Baltes (Eds.), *Life-span development psychology* (p. 122). New York: Academic Press.

Riehl, J. P. & Roy, C. (Eds.) (1974). *Conceptual models for nursing practice.* New York: Appleton-Century-Crofts.

Rogers, C. G. (1973). Conceptual models as guides to clinical nursing specialization. *Journal of Nursing Education, 12,* 2–6.

Rogers, M. E. (1970). *An introduction to the theoretical basis of nursing.* Philadelphia: F. A. Davis.

Roy, C. (1976). *Introduction to nursing: An adaptation model.* Englewood Cliffs, NJ: Prentice-Hall.

Roy, C. & Obloy, M. (1978). The practitioner movement—Toward a science of nursing. *American Journal of Nursing, 78,* 1698–1702.

Stevens, B. J. (1979). *Nursing theory: Analysis, application, evaluation.* Boston: Little, Brown.

Torres, G., & Yura, H. (1975). The meaning and functions of concepts and theories within education and nursing. In *Faculty-curriculum development, Part III: Conceptual framework—Its meaning and function* (NLN Pub. No. 15–1558) (pp. 5–6). New York: National League for Nursing.

Yura, H., & Torres, G. (1975). Today's conceptual frameworks within baccalaureate nursing programs. In *Faculty-curriculum development, Part III: Conceptual framework—Its meaning and function* (NLN Pub. No. 15–1558) (pp. 17–25). New York: National League for Nursing.

Zbilut, J. P. (1978). Epistemologic constraints to the development of a theory of nursing [Letter to the Editor]. *Nursing Research, 27,* 128.

The Author Comments

Framework for Analysis and Evaluation of Conceptual Models of Nursing

Doctoral course work with Martha Rogers at New York University sensitized me to the differences between conceptual models and theories. I began developing the framework for analysis and evaluation of conceptual models of nursing in a graduate seminar I conducted at the University of Connecticut School of Nursing during the fall 1976 semester, because I was dissatisfied with evaluative schemata found in the literature, which either reflected the confusion between conceptual models and theories or were too limited for a comprehensive analysis and evaluation. I have revised and refined the framework since the publication of this article in *Nurse Educator.* The most recent revision appears in chapter 3 of my book, *Analysis and Evaluation of Contemporary Nursing Knowledge: Nursing Models and Theories* (Philadelphia: F. A. Davis, 2000). A framework for analysis and evaluation of nursing theories appears in chapter 11 of that book. I believe that the development of nursing knowledge will truly progress during the 21st century only if nurses understand the differences between and content of nursing conceptual models and theories.

—JACQUELINE FAWCETT

Historical Perspectives on Nursing Theory

The articles in this unit provide an overview of the history and trends in theory development, nursing's theoretical evolution, and the state of the science. The articles span 4 decades of ideas about worldviews, philosophies, and theories in nursing, and conclude with a call for a nursing reformation. The critical distinction between borrowed and unique theories in nursing as first put forth by Dorothy Johnson in the 1960s re-emerges as an issue of the 1990s. Authors propose other positions and issues that have become integral to understanding the history and possible future of nursing theory.

CHAPTER 10

Nursing's Scientific Quest

Jean Watson

Nursing seems to be suffering in its quest for a scientific foundation for its practice. Like the mythological Danaids who kept filling their jars with water only to have it leak through holes, nursing finds its search for scientific underpinnings as elusive as the liquid. Its quest has been influenced by a traditional philosophy of science that is outdated and inappropriate for nursing as are newer concepts from the behavioral sciences. The result has been confusion with nursing and concern about its scientific progress.

In spite of Florence Nightingale's foresight and progressive views on nursing and nursing research, the profession has perpetuated a practice-oriented "doing" culture, almost to the exclusion of its intellectual and scientific development. The term nursing science was rarely used in the nursing literature until the 1950s. Ab-

dellah cites an incident in 1949, whereby a researcher sent a report of a study to a leading nursing journal only to have it returned because "nurses do not do research; they are not interested in research and that furthermore, research has no place in nursing" (Abdellah, 1969, p. 390). However, as nursing education became more associated with higher education in general, nursing norms and expectations began to change. Educators realized that baccalaureate, graduate nursing, and nurse scientist programs required a theoretical-research orientation to prepare students, improve practice, and further nursing's scientific base. Charges were then made that nursing was becoming too removed from practice, too theoretical: Knowing was separated from doing. As recently as the 1960s, there was debate as to whether it was appropriate for nurses to do re-

About the Author

JEAN WATSON is Distinguished Professor of Nursing and holds the Murchinson-Scolville Chair in Caring Science at the University of Colorado Health Sciences Center (HSC). She is founder of the original Center for Human Caring and previously served as Dean of the University of Colorado HSC School of Nursing. She is a Past President of the National League for Nursing. Born in West Virginia, July 21, 1940, Dr. Watson earned undergraduate and graduate degrees in nursing and psychiatric-mental health nursing and holds her PhD in educational psychology and counseling. Dr. Watson is known for her theoretical work on the art and science of human caring. Her latest books and articles address empirical measurements of caring and new postmodern philosophies of caring and healing that bridge paradigms and point toward transformative models for the 21st century. Dr. Watson is the recipient of many awards and honors, including an international Kellogg Fellowship in Australia, a Fulbright Research Award in Sweden, five honorary doctoral degrees, the National League for Nursing's Martha E. Rogers Award, New York University's Distinguished Nurse Scholar Award, and the Fetzer Institute's Norman Cousin's Award. Her hobbies include international travel, skiing, hiking, biking, and writing.

search, and nursing theory development was questioned or had to be justified (Norris, 1969).

Nursing has indeed received contradictory messages regarding its legitimacy in pursuing research, theory, and scientific advancement both within and outside the profession. Even now nurses have to justify and rationalize a theory-research goal far more often than those in other professional or academic disciplines. The reasons are many. In some important ways nursing has been subjected to different social, political, and scientific forces than those in other disciplines.

Historically, medical and male norms influenced nursing's earlier professional practice and educational development and more recently norms from the fields of science and behavioral science have influenced nursing's scientific development. Nursing's established ties and control by doctors and hospitals and society's male-female role expectations played an important part in nursing's emphasis on "doing," its status, problems with authority, self-denial, and lack of esteem. Its recent attempts in scientific development have often been guided by other fields that are inappropriate models for nursing and have resulted in nurses becoming sociologists, biologists, and psychologists, without their directly addressing nursing problems and issues.

Somewhere in the midst of these strong opposing external forces nursing lost sight of its nursing leaders' call for research aimed fundamentally at the solution of human health problems. Such leaders as Nightingale (1860), Henderson (1964), Krueter (1957), and Hall (1964) were advocates of an integrated approach to scientific study that would capitalize on nursing's richness and complexity and not separate practice from research, the art from the science, the "doing" of nursing from the "knowing," the psychological from the physical, and theory from clinical care.

Nursing needs to take a fresh look at its scientific progress, particularly in light of the insights of these earlier leaders. Perhaps then we can unravel and explain some of the obstacles and find direction in which nursing can move forward as a science in its own right, without apologies or excuses, and with confidence and zeal.

Changes in the Philosophy of Science

During the past three or four decades, the philosophy of science influencing nursing has undergone review and change. Theory concerning the nature of science has largely been the product of philosophers who were either Vienna Circle Logical Positivists, the dominant group in the early 1930s, or others who shared similar views (Webster, Jacox, & Baldwin, 1981). Their orientation to science and its progress consisted of a set of assumptions that became dogma. These assumptions had to do with standards of logic, formalization, objectivity, falsity, truth, observational and operational terms, laws, predictions, and reductionism. Their research was based on a single scientific methodology that was neutral with respect to human values. This set of assumptions has been called the "Received View" of the nature of science, scientific theory, and scientific methodology (Laudan, 1977; Suppe, 1977).

The assumptions of the Received View concerning the nature of science have since been overthrown by those scientists and philosophers who were original proponents of Logical Positivism. During the years that these scientific assumptions were being revised and rejected within the science community, other developing disciplines such as psychology, sociology, education, and later nursing were trying to adhere to some of the Received View principles. Many of these disciplines still adhere to these principles even though these views have long since been abandoned by others in the science community and are clearly incompatible with the scientific problems and aims of the disciplines in question, especially nursing.

The changing, and at the same time unchanging, views of the history and philosophy of science have contributed to the confusion and ambivalence surrounding nursing's scientific development. The results are that once nursing began its scientific quest, it seemingly accepted uncritically the Received View as the truth about science. Consequently, when scientific advancement became a legitimate pursuit for nursing theorists and researchers began to translate their understanding of the nature of nursing into Received View notions and attempted to promote nursing research according to its scientific methodology—such as reductionism, quantifiability, objectivity, and operationalization. In the meantime, some of the rich, nonquantifiable, qualitative, subjective, emotional "wholes of nursing" that have

long been proposed by nursing's leaders became submerged. Why? Because they weren't scientific or researchable or testable. Some of the components of nursing may never be scientific by the criteria of the Received View, but does that make nursing phenomena bad science?

Dichotomies Within Nursing

Many physicists, philosophers, and mathematicians have been aware of the fundamental problems associated with the Received View of Science. Bronowski emphasized that no scientific theory is a collection of facts, that no theory is true or false. He reports, "Science is nothing else than the search to discover unity in the wild variety of nature or...in the variety of our experiences. Poetry, painting, the arts are the same search..." (Bronowski, 1965, p. 16). He pointed out that the discoveries of science are the act of creation—the same act in original science as well as in original art. Unfortunately, only now are some of the "younger" disciplines—education, psychology, nursing, sociology—seeing the light. As a result, nursing has created a host of false dichotomies as to what is nursing and what is credible and legitimate for the development of nursing science. We are all familiar with the confusions and dichotomies evident in such schisms as:

Nursing art vs Nursing sciences
Nursing profession vs Nursing discipline
Doing vs Knowing
Caring vs Curing
Nursing practice vs Nursing Theory
Subjective vs Objective
Mind vs Body
Psychosocial vs Psychobiological

At the same time, nursing is replete with conflicting methodologies for practice, research, and theory development. Nursing possesses a set of rights and wrongs that are still largely guided by outdated Received View notions. Criteria from psychology, education, sociology, physiology, and formal philosophy still influence nursing research development. The scientific method is considered the one and only process for scientific discovery, experimental quantitative research methodology, and design. Philosophy, in particular, has guided nursing theory development with hierarchical notions of prescriptive theory, predictive theory, descriptive theory, factor-isolating theory, factor-relating theory, as well as created some nurse researchers' preoccupation with syntax, correspondence rules, formalization, and axiomatization. But, clearly nursing's history is full of other notions associated with intuitionism, subjectivism, wholism, traditionalism, utilitarianism, and humanism. The results are sets of conflicting research traditions, leading nursing into a double bind.

If nursing's scientific progress is viewed from a Received View perspective, it may be considered out of step with the mainstream of science because it is largely impressionistic, nonscientific and not readily quantifiable, objective, or formalized. However, in the view of recent scientific influences, largely from the social sciences and education, nursing may be considered more in step with that notion of scientific progress because it has tried to conform to Received View standards. On the other hand, if nursing is viewed from a non-Received View perspective, it is still considered out of step because it has been adhering too closely to the reductionist, logical, positivist view of science. A set of false dichotomies has been established that makes many facets of nursing incompatible. But the situation may change; revisions in nursing's views about research are emerging.

Nursing's Changing Research Tradition

Upon reflection, it appears that early nursing leaders were attempting to create a research tradition for nursing. That is, they tried to establish a set of general assumptions about entities and processes in the domain of study and the appropriate methods to be used for investigating problems and constructing theories (Laudan, 1977). For example, Nightingale talked of a "new art and a new science" and presented nursing as an art that required organized and scientific training. She did not create a false dichotomy between science and art. Later leaders—Virginia Henderson, Lydia Hall, Frances Krueter—promoted concepts of nursing that were consistent with Nightingale. For example, Henderson defined the nurse's role as very subjective and qualitative. She believed the nurse should, "...get inside the skin of each of [her] patients in order to know what [he] needs" (Henderson, 1964, p. 63). In describing the richness of this role, she said the nurse is "temporarily the consciousness of the unconscious, the love of life for the suicidal, the leg of the amputee, the eyes of the newly blind, a means of locomotion for the infant, knowledge and confidence for the young mother, the mouthpiece for those too weak or withdrawn to speak and so on" (Henderson, 1964, p. 63). At the same time, she emphasized the necessity of clinical nursing research. Hall believed the uniqueness of nursing was its nurturing aspect of care; she emphasized feelings as well as knowledge. Krueter discussed nursing care as "more related to 'pathos' in that the feelings are touched" (Kreuter, 1957, pp. 302, 304).

While these leaders have strongly influenced the development of nursing and more or less succeeded in promoting a nursing research tradition, nursing has still not actualized what these leaders have described as the essence of nursing or that aspect that is self-directed. One reason is the impact of the later competing and compelling research traditions from other fields, along with the Received View prejudices about the nature of science. It may be more than a coincidence that this transaction and break from the early research tradition, including the generation of a new research tradition, roughly corresponds to the development of nurse scientist programs in which nurses were doctorally prepared in a field outside of nursing. However, as nursing has advanced with its own doctoral programs, it has been subjected to the same processes of scientific development as other sciences—that is, first adopting Received Views ideas and then undergoing its own processes of rejection. For example, consider the following quotes from nurse scientists in the late 1960s and even late

1970s, most of whom were doctorally prepared outside of nursing:

> Definitions...are operationally defined...whenever possible, they should be expressed in observable and quantifiable terms.
>
> The testing of hypotheses either serves to confirm the validity of the theory or leads to a modification of the postulate upon which the theory was based.
>
> All concepts must be subjected to rigorous testing...
>
> The art of nursing must not be confused with the science of nursing.
>
> The former concerns itself with intuitive and technical skills and also the more important supportive aspects of nursing; the latter concerns itself with scientific truths...(Abdellah, 1969, pp. 391-392)
>
> Our contention is that any practice-minded nursing theory must be a theory of the situation-producing level. (Dickoff & James, 1968, p. 201)
>
> What is significant for nursing...is that which pertains to practice. Generation of knowledge for the sake of knowledge is not the raison d'être for the profession. (Ellis, 1968, p. 222)
>
> Theories must be rigorously tested by empirical studies before they can be accepted and then utilized in the real world of nursing practice, clinical research, and education. (Fawcett, 1978, p. 27)
>
> In science, the term theory refers to a set of verified interrelated concepts and theoretical statements. (Hardy, 1978, p. 77)
>
> The clinical of nursing requires the development of prescriptive theories. (Donaldson & Crowley, 1977, p. 14)

What a dilemma for nursing's scientific advancement. On one hand, nursing has been told, and we all know in a priori Kantian sense, it is rich, sensitive, complex, caring, subjective, artistic, practice-directed, focused on doing, feelings, and so on. On the other hand, it is presented with insistence on being scientific in the

traditional objective Received View sense of science—clearly a double bind. However, more recent authors are suggesting alternative views consistent with Laudan's context for understanding the evolution of the nature of science. The following examples illustrate the change in view during the 1970s and early 1980s that perhaps will generate a new research tradition for nursing.

> Nurse scientists must...tolerate loosely constructed theoretical notions. (Hardy, 1989, p. 77)
>
> Theorizing is a form of dialogue with reality, an attempt to find meaning in the world one lives in. (Zderad, 1978, p. 39)
>
> Like the nurse scientists, the nurse poets, the nurse artists also share an articulated vision of experience. (Zderad, 1978, p. 48)
>
> Nursing is moving from actions based on facts, or limited units of knowledge (such as nursing procedures), to actions based on theories or broad units of knowledge with wide applicability...We are a practice discipline, but we must not be exclusively practice-oriented. (Rinehart, 1978, p. 74)
>
> One of the reasons I have been pursuing cross-cultural studies on caring behaviors and processes is that scientific knowledge of care is limited; and yet, I hold it is the central concept and essence of nursing. (Leininger, 1979, p. xii)
>
> The way to understand nursing is to identify, describe, and research those central humanistic-scientific factors that are essential to effecting positive health change...The science of caring combines sciences with the humanities. The science of caring cannot be completely neutral with respect to human values. (Leininger, 1979, p. xii)
>
> The current discussion of the role of the observer in physics (quantum mechanics and relative theory) challenges the traditional view of the scientist as purely objective...The observer, therefore, cannot be a neutral point in the study...In the future, it will probably be more important to state the observer's position, values and beliefs, or whatever

else is pertinent, as part of the research protocol. (Winstead-Fry, 1980, p. 6)

In recent years, nursing has become disenchanted with traditional approaches to health and illness care. This disenchantment has lead to a re-examination of the concept of health and the role of the nurse...(Naravan & Joslin, 1980, p. 27)

These views suggest a new research tradition that can provide nursing with the scientific and social freedom and openness to solve both conceptual and empirical problems. It is an alternative to the Received View and permits nursing to return to the richness and complexities inherent in its social and scientific roots and goals. It may not be totally explanatory, predictive, or directly testable. Its success will be judged as to whether it can provide nursing with some adequate solution to an ever increasing range of empirical conceptual problems (Laudan, 1977).

Nursing is subject to all the problems of an emerging discipline that wishes to make itself credible and respectable. It has been burdened not only by the Received View of the nature of science, but by similar, rigid views associated with women in society, and by traditional ties to a male-dominated medical care system. Nursing now has both the scientific and sexual-social freedom to integrate and synthesize the false dichotomies and explore a whole range of scientific and methodological options. These options are consistent with past visions of nursing as well as the changing views of scientific growth. New alternatives found in nursing doctoral programs rather than in other disciplines may free nursing to recover and restore what it rightfully owns.

REFERENCES

Abdellah, F. G. (1969). The nature of nursing science. *Nursing Research, 18,* 390–393.

Bronowski, J. (1965). *Science and human values* (ref. ed.). New York: Harper & Row.

Dickoff, J., & James, P. (1968). A theory of theories: a position paper. *Nursing Research, 17,* 197–203.

Donaldson, S. K., & Crowley, D. M. (1977). Discipline of nursing: Structure and relationship to practice. In M. V. Batey (Ed.). *Optimizing environments for health: Nursing's unique perspective.* Communicating Nursing Research, Vol. 10 (pp. 1–22). Boulder, CO. WICHE.

Ellis, R. (1968). Characteristics of significant theories. *Nursing Research, 17,* 217–222.

Fawcett, J. (1978). The 'what' of theory development. In *Theory development: What, why, how?* (NLN Pub. 15–1708, pp. 75–86). New York: National League for Nursing.

Hall, L. E. (1964). Nursing—what is it? *Canadian Nurse, 60,* 150–154.

Hardy, M. E. (1978). Evaluating nursing theory. In *Theory development: What, why, how?* (NLN Pub. 15–1708, pp. 75–86). New York: National League for Nursing.

Henderson, V. (1964). The nature of nursing. *American Journal of Nursing, 64,* 62–68.

Kreuter, F. R. (1957). What is good nursing care? *Nursing Outlook, 5,* 302–304.

Laudan, L. (1977). *Progress and its problems: Towards a theory of scientific growth.* Berkeley, CA: University of California Press.

Leininger, M. (1979). Foreword. In J. Watson (Ed.). *Nursing: The philosophy and science of caring* (p. xii). Boston: Little, Brown.

Narava, S. M. & Joslin, D. J. (1980). Crisis theory and intervention: A critique of the medical model and proposal of a holistic nursing model. *Advances in Nursing Science, 2*(4), 27–39.

Nightingale, F. (1860). *Notes on nursing: What it is and what it is not.* New York: Appleton.

Norris, C. M. (Ed.). (1969). *Proceedings, First Nursing Theory Conference.* Kansas City: Department of Nursing Education, University of Kansas Medical Center.

Rinehart, J. M. (1978). The 'how' of theory development in nursing. In *Theory development: What, why, how?* (NLN Pub. 15–1708, pp. 75–86). New York: National League for Nursing.

Suppe, F. (Ed.). (1977). *The structure of scientific theories* (2nd ed.). Champaign: University of Illinois Press.

Webster, G., Jacox, A., & Baldwin, B. (1981). Nursing theory and the ghost of the received view. In H. Grace & J. McCloskey (Eds.). *Current issues in nursing* (pp. 26–35). Boston: Blackwell Scientific.

Winstead-Fry, P. (1980). The scientific method and its impact on holistic health. *Advances in Nursing Science, 2*(4), 1–8.

Zderad, L. T. (1978). From here-and-now to theory: Reflexations on 'how.' In *Theory development: what, why, how?* (NLN Pub. 15–1708, pp. 75–86). New York: National League for Nursing.

The Author Comments

Nursing's Scientific Quest

The ideas for this article evolved from my concern with nursing's human dimensions and the conflict between traditional science and the view of nursing as a human science. This article was also influenced by my work with PhD nursing students. Together we explored the basis of nursing science in relation to medical science. Hopefully the article will continue to raise questions about the nature of nursing science and its evolution.

—JEAN WATSON

CHAPTER 11

The History and Philosophy of Nursing Science and Research

Susan R. Gortner

The research tradition is so young in nursing that only in the past few years has there been comment about the philosophical orientations that might guide research, including methods; discovery in contrast to justification or proof; and ethics and politics. These topics of philosophy of science are now beginning to intrigue many who have been involved with developments in nursing science. For example, one can ask if nursing practice should continue to be the major source of research ideas (as historically it has). One can posit, as has Munhall (1982), that experimental or scientific methods are incompatible with a humanistic, holistic philosophy. Munhall's solution is to discard quantifications. For many of these issues that intrigue us and others, a review of the history of science is illuminating.

Practice as the Source of Knowledge

Early Years

Concepts of nursing practice have influenced the subject matter of research since the beginning of our history. The concerns of the times have varied over the past 150 years, with some early concerns remaining prominent even today. From the Nightingale era onward, the poor quality of care for the sick in hospitals and in the home called attention to the need for qualified caregivers and thus prompted the development of formal programs of nursing education. For over 100 years, education was viewed as the means to the improvement of practice.

From Advances in Nursing Science, *January 1983, 5(2), 1-8. Copyright © 1983 by Aspen Systems Corporation. Reprinted with permission from Lippincott Williams & Wilkins.*

About the Author

After graduating from Stanford University in 1953 with an AB degree in social sciences, SUSAN REICHERT GORTNER enrolled in the generic master's program at Frances Payne Bolton School of Nursing, Case Western Reserve University, graduating with honors in 1957. She completed a PhD in higher education from the University of California, Berkeley, in 1964, which coincided with the births of her children. She relocated with her scientist husband to Maryland and joined the Division of Nursing as a health scientist administrator, first to evaluate the 1964 Nurse Training Act and later to serve as Branch Chief for Research and Research Training. She was the first Associate Dean for Research (Nursing) at the University of California, San Francisco (UCSF). Dr. Gortner's many honors and recognitions include Frances Payne Bolton School of Nursing Distinguished Alumna, UCSF Helen Nahm Research Lecturer, Fulbright Association Lecturer/Research Scholar in Norway (Oslo University), and, most recently, the American Academy of Nursing "Living Legend" award in 2001. Internationally known for her views on nursing science and research, she developed a collaborative program of research on cardiac surgery recovery, examining patient and family treatment choices and outcomes and recovery processes. Dr. Gortner was honored for this work by the National Center for Nursing Research (now NINR) and the American Heart Association. She lives full-time in the High Sierras in California, enjoys summer and winter sports with her Border collies, and recently joined the Orvis School of Nursing as Endowed Chair (.50) to help faculty development in research.

At the turn of the century, the concern was for improvement of the public's health. Mortality rates were high due to the major communicable diseases of childhood and adulthood. Maternal and infant health had yet to profit from prenatal care and improved obstetrical practices. Most surgery was done in the home. The literature in professional journals addressed problems associated with tuberculosis, meningitis, scarlet fever, and other communicable diseases. By the early 1920s, case studies began to appear in the literature, as did care plans based around specific groups of patients and procedures. A review of the literature for the period 1930-1960 (Gortner & Nahm, 1977), as well as interviews with such leaders as Lucile Petry Leone, suggest that the need for systematic evaluation of nursing techniques had its origins in the post-depression years. In part, this was because the graduate nurse had returned both to the hospital and to the graduate nursing programs that had begun to develop. Case study presentations also occurred in the field of medicine, in which usual symptomatology was presented, followed by a discussion of medical and nursing therapies.

Nationwide Development

World War II prompted the collection of national data on nursing needs and resources, which heightened the concerns of this period toward identification of professional practice. The Division of Nursing Resources of the United States Public Health Service was formed in 1948. Its staff developed and published guides for institutions on techniques for studying nursing activities (U.S. Public Health Service, 1964). As a result of these guides, a number of "activity" studies were carried out (Roberts, 1964). In 1950, The American Nurses' Association announced plans for a 5-year study of nursing functions and activities. This resulted in the enumeration of functions, standards, and qualifications for practice, as well as the publication *Twenty Thousand Nurses Tell Their Story* (Hughes, Hughes, & Deutscher, 1958). Research in the organization and delivery of health services continued into the late 1950s, often attempting to link nursing staff and unit arrangements to improvement in patient care and patient satisfaction.

Twenty-five years ago, studies of nurses outnumbered studies of patient care 10 to 1. The need for research on problems encountered in patient care began to be addressed at this time. By the early 1960s, the literature was reflecting a shift in focus to the patient instead of the nurse as the object of research. Such a shift was forecast in the 1950 statement of the Chief Nurse Officer of the Public Health Service. Leone (1954) recommended generating a research base through new methods to use nursing skills, nursing care most essential to patient recovery, analysis of nursing techniques, conditions reducing turnover and promoting job satisfaction, use of management theories in the health care arena, and therapeutic effectiveness of interpersonal relationships. It was reemphasized in editorials in the fledgling organ, *Nursing Research*. Both the United States Public Health Service and the American Nurses' Association issued statements of priorities directed toward enlargement of the knowledge base and improvement of patient care.

Thus the efforts to generate a knowledge base for nursing through research have been concentrated in the past two decades. The work has been mainly experiential, not emanating from a solid conceptual or theoretical base until recently. Interest in the theoretical or scientific bases of practice and research was stimulated by the development of programs for training nurse scientists in a number of major universities, by research development activities in these settings, by a growing number of those trained in the scientific methods, and by a tremendous federal investment in the improvement of nursing education over a 15-year period.

Research Development

Early research approaches included the development of critical resources, documentation of need through surveys, use of the conference mechanism, studies of procedures (the technology), case analysis (the art and science), and alliance with other disciplines. Critical resources were identified in terms of numbers of personnel, facilities, and finances.

The survey mechanism was a successful technique for documenting need for personnel and has resulted in a number of classics: the Goldmark report of 1923 (Committee on Nursing and Nursing Education in the United States, 1923), the Committee for the Grading of Nursing Schools reports of 1928 and 1934, and Brown's (1948) *Nursing for the Future*, to name a few. The conference mechanism also has been a successful strategy. Many of these studies were commissioned by conference groups, e.g., the Committee on the Grading of Nursing Schools, the National Nursing Council of the War Years, and the Surgeon General's Consultant Group. This mechanism employed expert panels to convene and deliberate on nursing needs and resources. Other early techniques included the study of procedures and the use of case analysis.

Alliance with other disciplines originated with medicine and education and, as the research base enlarged, also with the social sciences. This alliance has had important implications for the disciplinary technology and modes of inquiry in nursing. The profession has rapidly gained a health-oriented perspective with behavioral, social, and cultural components. Reliance on sociological and anthropological research techniques has provided good capability for description, but perhaps less ability to draw associations and causation.

Current Resources for Research

Current research strategies include:

- enlargement of critical resources with increasing numbers of earned doctorates, increasing postdoctoral activities, and improving the quality of doctoral training
- public support
- colleagueship
- communication
- design and methods, including sampling, instrumentation, multivariate analysis, reproducibility, and generalizability.

Critical resources have an impact on education and practice. Today the research doctorate pool stands at its greatest size since count has been kept. There has been a steady growth in nursing as the major disciplinary field for predoctoral training. Postdoctoral opportunities are being sought by young as well as senior doctor-ate holders. Public support of research is measured by the size of the private gift and the public tax dollar. The latter has averaged $5 million annually since 1976. There are sufficient numbers of nurse scientists prepared now that some colleagueship within and among institutions is possible in areas of mutual interest. Communication is at an all time high, with two new refereed research journals started within the past 3 years and the number of research symposia growing rapidly. Such media are important sources of contact and comment on scientific work. They should provide an opportunity for those beginning to enjoy the meaning of communality.

To assume that the choice of research methods used in nursing was influenced by a particular philosophy of science, e.g., logical positivism, is to attribute too much deliberation or rationality to what was the result of social, political, and economic events. By virtue of their doctoral training in fields other than nursing, nurse scientists brought to the study of nursing those problems and techniques that had served them well in their own doctoral disciplines of sociology, anthropology, biology, psychology, and epidemiology. Socialization into these sciences included the expectation of funding for one's research program. Granting agencies prefer controlled studies in which variables are well specified and instrumentation is precise. What had worked for one science was expected to work for another. Advanced techniques from biostatistics, psychometrics, and computer science were incorporated in the resolution of nursing research problems. Attention is now paid to sampling plans so that enough cases are reported on with sufficient controls to attain some credibility. Design elements are sophisticated enough to allow reproduction and confirmation of findings and to provide some comprehensive treatment of multiple variables under study. A growing body of instruments was evidenced by the recent compilations of research tools. Finally, generalizability has become a critical factor in nursing research efforts. The capacity to affect practice depends heavily on this factor.

Conceptualizations of Nursing and Nursing Science

Nursing has been depicted at various times as a series of tasks and technology (a subset of medicine); as a broad, compassionate, and supportive human service; and, most recently, as a science of human health and behavior across the life span. This current conceptualization includes understanding of biological, behavioral, social, and cultural factors in health and illness and the definition of health outcomes and indicators of health status. These features are reflected in Donaldson and Crowley's (1978) well-publicized themes of inquiry: (a) the principles and laws that govern life processes, well-being, and optimum functioning of human beings; (b) the patterning of human behavior in interaction with the environment in critical life situations; and (c) processes by which positive changes in health status are effected.

Nursing science has been defined as the body of codified understanding of human biology and behavior in health and illness, with particular attention to response states (Barnard, 1980; Gortner, 1980b). There appears to be a growing consensus on the nature of the research paradigms as representing human responses in health and illness. Fawcett (1981) has described person, environment, health, and nursing as elements of a metaparadigm. But while consensus grows among theorists on the subject matter of the discipline and its science, the philosophical orientation of the science is mainly empirical and naturalistic. The orientation involves exploration, description, and classification of phenomena by direct observation and inspection.

It now attempts to incorporate theoretical propositions, however tentative, and seeks to discover relationships. Carper (1978) has described the philosophical base (explanatory base) for many of the present conceptualizations of nursing as teleological, or consequential and functional. The concept of adaptation, an excellent illustration of such an orientation, is represented in the conceptualizations offered by Roy (1970), Neal (1976), and others. With some exceptions, nursing's current theory is rationally or deductively arrived at, with few empirical verifications. Eventually, the interface will come between the two major modes of inquiry, observation and experimentation, and between the observed phenomena and their logical explanations.

The Philosophy of Science Emerges

The movement from empiricism to rationalism (to theory-laden observations) is heartening—a gain in the level of sophistication of nursing research. There appears to be a move in some settings toward greater specificity of theoretical frameworks and of their concepts and propositions for purposes of empirical testing.

How the empirical testing will be carried out is a matter of debate. Scientific approaches to the study of human health and illness need not eliminate the features of design and methods that have served other sciences well. The logic inherent in the scientific method and the discipline of the method can aid in the identification of correlates of healthy behavior and illness (Winstead-Fry, 1980). Science (empirics), art (aesthetics), morality (ethics), and intuition (personal or subjective) all represent sources of knowledge, but nursing research activity has largely concerned itself with the empirics (Carper, 1978). It has been hoped that nursing could maintain its humanistic value orientation as it became more involved in scientific work and thus not repeat the loss of humanism evident in medicine's evolution as a scientific discipline (Gortner, 1974). The profession would be unwise to reject scientific techniques now because of fear of dehumanization or concerns about the validity of analytical approaches. The hypothetico-deductive methods of science can be as much a part of the nursing research repertoire as are the descriptive, inductive, and theory-generating forms. The profession surely can accommodate multiple paradigms (analytic, humanistic) and modes of inquiry (naturalistic, experimental, historical).

Formation of Research Questions

Concepts are ideas or abstractions that form part of our rational perspective and guide the formulation of research questions. Examples of concepts that are frequently in the research literature in nursing include social support, attachment, self-image, pain or discomfort, chronicity, and parenting. Examples of recently completed and ongoing research dealing with these topics may be found in the published proceedings of the 1980 and 1981 meetings of the Western Society for Research in Nursing. Symposia on parenting and nursing, papers on parental assessment, family wellness, and family illness, and instrumentation to measure social support illustrate current scientific interests in only one region of the country.

At another level of abstraction are the following concepts or constructs: health, illness, function and dysfunction, affiliation, adaptation, development, prevention, and promotion. It can be expected that inquiry will be directed toward these constructs and concepts and that the work will be of a more fundamental nature in the future than was true of the past (Gortner, 1980a). The profession is clarifying the sources of its knowledge. It is generally agreed that nursing practice should not be the exclusive source. Accordingly, fundamental knowledge derived from related disciplines and from investigations carried out today in nursing and made relevant to existing theory will be the basic scientific foundation for research.

Areas of Inquiry

Such fundamental questions are generally considered to hold no immediate hope for clinical utility or application in their undifferentiated or basic form. Rather, they contribute a general understanding of events across a wide variety of disciplines. Examples of general areas of fundamental inquiry essential to human health, illness, and recovery include genetic endowment, organ system integrity, psychological well-being, life styles, and culture. Examples of phenomena that have particular relevance for nursing include compliance, chronicity, self-care, social support, parenting, family functioning, and stress.

Besides these areas of fundamental inquiry, there is another area that is concerned with clinical therapeutics. This area has been defined by a number of writers as representing that set of studies of interpersonal and physical techniques that assist patients and families in coping with the effects of illness and in promoting health. The focus is on both the characteristics and outcomes of the interventions, the psychobiological circumstances under which they take place, and the effect they have on modifying psychological and pathophysiological processes (Gortner, Bloch, & Phillips, 1976).

A final area of inquiry that represents a domain of scientific work is investigation of environments. These are viewed as complex multidimensional sets of forces and elements affecting the development and maintenance of healthy and unhealthy states in human beings (Barnard, 1980). Nursing research gives attention to the characteristics of internal and external environments that promote, maintain, and support states of health.

Future Contributions

Nursing science will make a major contribution, as science, in the interface of the biological and social sciences concerned with illness and health. Examples of research questions dealing with the phenomena of chronicity, parenting, and family functioning are as follows:

- How does chronic illness modify self-image?
- What coping mechanisms are effective with chronic and acute pain?
- What factors influence maternal role attainment?
- What constitutes health-seeking behavior among adolescents?
- What is the relationship of family functioning to recovery from episodic illness?

These vital questions have the following features in common. The emphasis is on the psychosocial and biological dimensions of health and illness and on the whole organism. The work produces findings that can be verified and thus contribute to the general understanding of human behavior and response. The questions will ultimately have relevance for the practice field.

As is true of other fields, "good" science in nursing is known by the significance of the questions asked, by the presence of one or more reasonable propositions or hypotheses that can be tested in a verifiable manner, and by the characteristics of creativity, responsibility, and discipline. "Good" scientific work has developed in nursing in a short time. It appears to be well established in a number of areas and settings. The modern university has been a mainstay of important scientific activity in many fields. Will it also house and nurture the fledgling science of nursing, recognizing its potential and its contributions to date? The answer to that critical question may well accelerate or impede nursing's progress as an academic discipline in the next decade.

REFERENCES

Barnard, K. (1980). Knowledge for practice: Directions for the future. *Nursing Research, 29,* 208–212.

Brown, E. L. (1948). *Nursing for the future.* New York: Russell Sage Foundation.

Carper, B. A. (1978). Fundamental patterns of knowing in nursing. *Advances in Nursing Science, 1*(1), 13–23.

Committee on the Grading of Nursing Schools. (1928). *Nurses, patients and pocketbooks: A report of a study of the economics of nursing.* New York: Author.

Committee on the Grading of Nursing Schools. (1934). *Nursing schools today and tomorrow.* New York: Author.

Committee on Nursing and Nursing Education in the United States. (1923). *Nursing and nursing education in the United States: Report of the committee and report of the survey by Josephine Goldmark, secretary.* New York: Macmillan.

Donaldson, S., & Crowley, D. (1978). The discipline of nursing. *Nursing Outlook, 26,* 113–120.

Fawcett, J. (1981, November). Hallmarks of success in nursing theory development. Paper presented at Vanderbilt University, School of Nursing, Nashville, TN.

Gortner, S. R. (1974). Scientific accountability in nursing. *Nursing Outlook, 22,* 764–768.

Gortner, S. R. (1980a). Nursing research: Out of the past and into the future. *Nursing Research, 29,* 204–207.

Gortner, S. R. (1980b). Nursing science in transition. *Nursing Research, 29,* 180–183.

Gortner, S. R., Bloch, D., & Phillips, T. (1976). Contributions of nursing research to patient care. *Journal of Advanced Nursing, 1,* 507–517.

Gortner, S. R., & Nahm, H. (1977). An overview of nursing research in the United States. *Nursing Research, 26,* 10–33.

Hughes, E. C., Hughes, H. M., & Deutscher, I. (1958). *Twenty thousand nurses tell their story.* Philadelphia: J.B. Lippincott.

Leone, L. P. (1954). *Comments of the need for studies and researchers in nursing.*

Munhall, P. L. (1982). Nursing philosophy and nursing research: In apposition or opposition? *Nursing Research, 31,* 176–177, 181.

Neal, M. V. (Ed.). (1976, March). *A conceptual basis for maternal child health nursing practice.* Proceedings of a perinatal conference. Baltimore: University of Maryland School of Nursing.

Roberts, D. E., & Hudson, H. H. (1964). *How to study patient progress* (Public Health Service publication No. 1169).

Washington, DC: U.S. Department of Health, Education, and Welfare.

Roy, S. C. (1970). Adaptation: A conceptual framework. *Nursing Outlook, 18,* 42–45.

Unpublished staff paper, historical file. U.S. Public Health Service, Division of Nursing, Nursing Research Branch, Bethesda, MD.

U.S. Public Health Service. (1964). *Patients and personnel speak* (Public Health Service publication No. 527). Washington, DC: U.S. Department of Health, Education, and Welfare.

Winstead-Fry, P. (1980). The scientific method and its impact on holistic health. *Advances in Nursing Science, 2*(4), 1–7.

The Author Comments

The History and Philosophy of Nursing Science and Research

This essay was the culmination of several presentations, beginning with a distinguished scholar's presentation at the University of Pennsylvania and then at Vanderbilt, where Jacqueline Fawcett's *Hallmark of Success in Nursing Theory Development* (1983) also was presented. Here, I attempted to depict some of the major conceptualizations in the history of nursing science and research and to show how our empirical work (research studies) and our theoretical or rational work (theory development) have been carried out on parallel and nonintersecting planes. Fortunately, 20 years later, this disconnect is not apparent, because most research now is theory based. Because this essay was written during the heyday of debates over "proper" methodology, I argued against the position that research methods must be compatible with what was then called the philosophy of the discipline (no other profession placed such a requirement on its scientists at the time). Given the tremendous growth in nursing research activity in U.S. universities, nursing science is well grounded in its intellectual home, the university, with increasing collaborative and interdisciplinary features.

—Susan Reichert Gortner

CHAPTER 12

Nursing's Theoretical Evolution

Margaret A. Newman

The need for knowledge which is specific to nursing has been recognized since the beginning of modern nursing. Florence Nightingale wrote:

> I believe . . . that the very elements of nursing are all but unknown . . . are as little understood for the well as for the sick. The same laws of health or of nursing, for they are in reality the same, obtain among the well as among the sick. (Nightingale, 1859, p. 6)

The elements which Nightingale identified and attempted to explicate focused on the environment, nourishment, and observation of the patient and on the interpersonal relationship between the nurse and the patient. Even then, participants in nursing confused knowledge of the laws of health. In her attempt to clear up the confusion, Nightingale explained:

Pathology teaches the harm that disease has done. But it teaches nothing more. We know nothing of the principle of health, the positive of which pathology is the negative . . . .

It is often thought that medicine is the curative process. It is not such thing; medicine is the surgery of functions, as surgery proper is that of limbs and organs. Neither can do anything but remove obstructions . . . .Surgery removes the bullet out of the limb, which is an obstruction to cure, but nature heals the wound. So it is with medicine; the function of an organ becomes obstructed; medicine, so far as we know, assists nature to remove the obstruction, but does nothing more. And what nursing has to do, in ei-

About the Author

MARGARET A. NEWMAN was born in Memphis, TN, on October 10, 1933. She received her first degree (BSHE, 1954) in home economics at Baylor University. She entered nursing at the University of Tennessee, Memphis, in 1959 and received a BSN in 1962. Her graduate study included an emphasis on medical-surgical nursing at the University of California, San Francisco (MS, 1964) and a further emphasis on rehabilitation nursing and nursing science at New York University (PhD, 1971). Except for a short tenure as director of nursing for the clinical research center at the University of Tennessee, the emphasis of her work has been in education (at New York University, Penn State University, and the University of Minnesota). The focus of her scholarship has been on theory development in nursing. The books *Health as Expanding Consciousness* (1986, 1994) and *A Developing Discipline* (1995) represent her major contribution to nursing theory. She is an avid fan of live theater and music, with subscriptions to two local theater groups' offerings and the St. Paul Chamber Orchestra.

ther case, is to put the patient in the best condition for nature to act upon him. (Nightingale, 1859, p. 74)

Although over a hundred years ago our charge was clear, the direction we have taken in search for nursing knowledge has led us at times away from our responsibility. Only within the past decade have we begun to discover the kinds of information that will assist us in establishing optimal health for man, in sickness and in health.

Historical Development

Throughout most of the past century, the approach to nursing was based largely on medical knowledge. Nurses, taught by physicians, were instructed in what physicians thought they needed to know to carry out the medical regimen for the patient. Even the advent of university education for nurses did not change the approach, for curriculums were organized by medical specialty areas. To some extent, this organizational focus persists today.

Another approach to nursing knowledge has been pursuit of the educational process and method. The earliest opportunities for nurses to pursue graduate education were provided by schools of education. The nursing leaders who were prepared in this way thought that the key to improving the quality of nursing care was

in improving nursing education (McManus, 1961). Consequently, the research these nurses pursued related primarily to educational and, to some extent administrative problems in nursing.

Along with the increase in the number of collegiate programs in the early fifties came a growing awareness on the part of nursing faculty of the need for scientifically based knowledge specific to the nursing process. A major step in directing the attention of nurses to research was accomplished with the publication of the first issue of *Nursing Research* in 1952. One of the purposes of this journal, as stated in the first issue, has been to stimulate research in nursing.

An overview of the categories of research and concerns reported in *Nursing Research* during the past 20 years suggests the trends of nursing's theoretical evolution. (Frequencies reported are based on the major articles of the journal and the first-named author.) The magazine's expansion from an original three-times-a-year publication to its bimonthly status has been accompanied by change both in the quantity of research published and in its content and quality. For example, during the early period, the number of studies that emphasized the role and characteristics of nurses comprised approximately 32 percent of the articles. At the same time, studies relating to the nursing process and the behavior of man accounted for only about 12 percent. Since 1968, although the number of studies emphasizing the functions and characteristics of nurses continued at approximately 24 percent, the number relating to nursing process and the behavior of man has risen to approximately 36 percent.

The change in types of contributors to *Nursing Research* through the years is also indicative of the changes that have taken place in theory development. Whereas 36 percent of the contributors in the 1952-58 period were non-nurses and 26 percent were nurses with doctorates, only 16 percent of the contributors since 1968 have been non-nurses and the proportion of articles contributed by nurses with doctorates has risen to 49 percent.

The large proportion of non-nurse contributors during the early period may explain the bulk of studies on functions and characteristics of nurses. During those years nurses tended to turn to social scientists for help in studying nursing. This approach resulted in restatement of nursing problems as social science questions, with nurses studying nurses, rather than nursing. Wald and Leonard point out that the "pure" scientist was trained to pursue his own discipline and "it might have been expected that he would help nurses develop his discipline rather than nursing practice" (Wald & Leonard, 1964, p. 309).

Approaches to Nursing Theory

Concern about nursing theory, which began to become evident in the early sixties, has received considerable attention since 1968. During this period, three main approaches to the discovery of nursing theory emerged: (1) the "borrowing" of theory from other disciplines with an intent to integrate it into a science of nursing; (2) an analysis of nursing practice situations in search of the theoretical underpinnings; and (3) the creation of a conceptual system from which theories could be derived.

Theory From Other Disciplines

Since 1962, when the federal government started funding the nurse-scientist program to enable nurses to study in other disciplines for the purpose of relating their theory to nursing, the number of nurses who have received doctorates has increased considerably. In exercising the diligence necessary to attain competence in these other disciplines, however, nurses who pursed this type of research preparation have been confronted with a problem in maintaining an intimate relationship with nursing. Although many theories from other disciplines are relevant to nursing, the testing of these theories within the framework of another discipline relates the data more clearly to that discipline than to nursing.

Dorothy Johnson has said that knowledge from the basic sciences is relevant to nursing but that the knowledge needed for nursing practice is incomplete until "we learn to ask . . . nursing questions about events in nature of specific concern to us" (Johnson, 1968, p. 206). One of the purposes of encouraging nurses to obtain research preparation in related disciplines was to provide a means for enlarging the research potential of nursing faculties. Since this purpose has been accomplished to some extent, supporters of this approach to the development of nursing theory are now beginning to recommend the development of doctoral programs in nursing, with the accompanying emphasis on research of nursing questions (U.S. Health Manpower Education Bureau, 1971).

Practice Theory

The second approach, that of analyzing nursing practice in search of conceptual relationships, has gained support since 1968. Wald and Leonard (1964) exhorted nurses to direct their attention toward building knowledge directly from a systematic study of nursing experience. They asserted that nursing is a professional practice rather than an academic discipline and that the purpose of a practitioner-scientist is to study ways to achieve changes—changes in patients' responses to such experience as hospitalization or other health measures. They believed that theory of this type could best be derived from and tested in the actual nursing arena.

One of the problems inherent in an analysis of the nursing situation is the lack of agreement on answers to such questions as: What is nursing? What is the specialized role of the nurse? Only three years ago, at a conference organized for the purpose of synthesizing a theory of nursing, the participants, who were considered leaders in theory development, found these questions stumbling blocks to the advancement of theory basic to nursing (Norris, 1969).

Most recently, in a critique of current nursing theory, Walker begins her discussion with what she considers "the leading question in a science of nursing, that is, What is occurring in nursing?" (Walker, 1971, p. 428). After a century of asking ourselves that question, we are still not much closer to our goal of nursing theory.

A Conceptual System

Much of the confusion about what we should be studying was eliminated, in my opinion, when Rogers (1964) identified the phenomenon which is the center of nursing's purpose: *man.** It sounds simple, yet many a graduate student will attest to the difficulty of reorganizing one's thinking about man in order to consider him a unified being and not as a composite of organs and systems and various psycho-social components. The clear-cut delineation of man as the focus of nursing gave direction for the development of theory that is not just relevant to nursing, but basic to nursing.

Thus, a conceptual framework of nursing theory was born. Confident in her designation of man as the phenomenon which is the focus of nursing's purpose, Rogers reviewed the available literature in an effort to identify basic assumptions regarding man and determined that the following statements could be accepted as true:

- Man is a unified whole possessing his own integrity and manifesting characteristics more than and different from the sum of his parts (wholeness) (Rogers, 1970, 46-47).

---

*The author wishes to apologize for the sexist language of the late sixties and early seventies, and asks the reader to substitute "human being" or "person" wherever "man" is used.

- Man and environment are continuously exchanging matter and energy with one another (open system) (Rogers, 1970, p. 54).
- The life process evolves irreversibly and unidirectionally along the space-time continuum (unidirectionality) (Rogers, 1970, p. 59).
- Pattern and organization identify man and reflect his innovative wholeness (pattern and organization) (Rogers, 1970, p. 65).
- Man is characterized by the capacity for abstraction and imagery, language and thought, sensation and emotion (sentience) (Rogers, 1970, p. 73).

On the basis of these assumptions, she proceeded to synthesize a conceptual model of man and from there to formulate some general principles from which theories of man can be derived and tested. The relationship of Rogers' conceptual system to data is shown on Figure 12-1.

Hempel, in emphasizing the importance of developing a system of concepts from which general explanatory and predictive principles can be formulated, points out that "science is ultimately intended to systematize the data of our experience . . . ." (Hempel, 1952, p. 21). He perceives a scientific theory as simi-

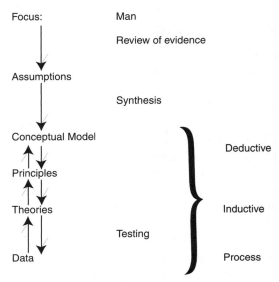

Figure 12-1 *Relationship of conceptual system to data.*

lar to a complex spatial network: the concepts represented by the knots and the unifying principles represented by the strings. Using this network, the scientist can proceed back and forth in the system to observable data and thereby expand the explanatory power of the system.

Other theorists in nursing have called for a conceptual system from which nursing theory can be derived (Batey, 1971; Brown, 1964). King (1971) has recently proposed four ideas as the conceptual base of the dimensions of nursing: social systems, health, perception, and interpersonal relations. She agrees that the basic abstraction of nursing is the phenomenon of man and his world. The selection of her conceptual base is rooted in her belief that "nurses, in the performance of their roles and responsibilities, assist individuals and groups in society to attain, maintain, and restore health." More specifically, "man functions in *social systems* through *interpersonal relationships* in terms of his *perceptions* which influence his life and *health*" (King, 1971, pp. 21-22). Although on the surface King's system may appear to be quite different from that proposed by Rogers, comparison of statements from the two positions reveals a certain amount of congruity (see Table 12-1).

The principles and postulates identified by Rogers and the premises formulated by King indicate that there is some agreement in the evolving theoretical framework from which hypotheses are being derived and tested and the data therefrom are fed back into the system. The comparisons are by no means complete, either for these two theorists or for other nursing theo-

Table 12-1
Comparison of Excerpts From Rogers' (1970) *An Introduction to the Theoretical Basis of Nursing,* and King's (1971) *Toward a Theory of Nursing*

Rogers	King
The principle of reciprocity: The human field and the environmental field are continuously interacting with one another. The relationship . . . is one of constant mutual interaction and mutual change (pp. 96–97).	The dynamic life process of man involves a constant restructuring of the real world. The transactions . . . that occur in human interactions are an exchange of energy and information within the persons involved (intrapersonal) and between the individual and the environmental (interpersonal) (pp. 87–88) . . . .thus action results from factors in the situation and in the individual at any point in time (p. 88).
Basic assumption: Man and environment are continuously exchanging matter and energy with one another (p. 54).	
The principle of synchrony: Change in the human field depends only upon the state of the human field and the simultaneous state of the environmental field at any given point in space-time (p. 98).	
Man is a unified whole possessing his own integrity and manifesting characteristics that are more than different from the sum of his parts (p. 47).	Man as a composite of mind and body reacts as a total organism to his experiences which are viewed as a flow of events in time (p. 88).
The human field possesses its own identifiable wholeness . . . it maintains identity in its everchanging but omnipresent patterning (pp. 90–91).	
Helicy: . . . the life process evolves unidirectionally in sequential stages . . . is a function of continuous innovative change growing out of the mutual interaction of man and environment along a spiraling longitudinal axis bound in space-time (pp. 99–101).	Time is an irreversible process in the life cycle . . . (p. 88).
Man is characterized by the capacity for abstraction and imagery, language and thought, sensation and emotion (p. 73).	Man is a social being. Through language man has found a symbolic way of communicating his thoughts, actions, customs, and beliefs over time (p. 88).

rists whose formulations may provide additional elaboration of the system. The examples are selected to illustrate that a conceptual system of nursing focused on man is evolving similarly in the minds of nursing theorists and does provide meaningful direction for research. As Rogers has said, "the science of nursing aims to provide a body of abstract knowledge growing out of scientific research and logical analysis and capable of being translated into nursing practice" (Rogers, 1970, p. 86).

The fruitfulness of this conceptual approach to theory development is borne out by the research which has been conceived from ideas based on the wholeness of man's constant interaction with his environment. A series of studies of the effect of the stimulation of total body movement on man have resulted in an evolving theory of movement or motion (Earle, 1969; Neal, 1968; Porter, 1971). Other studies are beginning to outline characteristics of man's spatial and temporal awareness and have implications for his continuous reciprocal interactions with his environment (Felton, 1970; Newman, 1972; Rodgers, 1971; Schlachter, 1971).

Continued exploration of patterns of stimulation are introducing evidence regarding man's capacity for maintaining his pattern in an ever-changing environment. Again, these examples are only a few of the rapidly growing number of studies designed to test the theory of man, with the ultimate purpose of identifying laws regulating this continuous interaction of man and his environment. Knowledge of such laws would then guide nursing practitioners in their goal which is, in essence, to help man achieve his maximum health potential.

Theory of Theories

Proponents of practice theory assert that theory for a profession must go beyond merely describing, explaining, and predicting a particular phenomenon. Dickoff and James (1968) have described four levels of theory: (1) factor-isolating theory (classification); (2) factor-relating theories (situation-depicting); (3) situation-relating theories (predictive); and (4) situation-producing theories (prescriptive). Theory, they assert, must provide conceptualization intended to guide the shaping of reality to a profession's purpose. Situation-producing theory, they believe, incorporates the other three levels of theory and, in addition, prescribes the desired outcome of a situation and the activities necessary to produce that outcome. Inherent in this approach is the assumption that the "desire" outcome can be identified.

Nursing is referred to, from time to time, as a learned profession, an applied science, and a practice discipline—somehow with the connotation that these terms have different meanings. Each of the terms, however, has two components: one which indicates the rigors of scientific inquiry, and another which implies a commitment to service. The development of theory for nursing, therefore, is likely to proceed at more than one level of generalization. At present, nursing theorists are working primarily at the descriptive and predictive levels, but the possibility of a prescriptive level exists.

There now appears to be consensus among nursing theorists that nursing is concerned with assisting man to maintain optimal health throughout his life process. There is also some agreement regarding the conceptual framework of nursing. Whether the theory evolves inductively from ideas conceived in clinical practice or deductively from broad generalizations within the theoretical framework does not seem particularly important. What is important is that the nursing investigator determine the relationship of her study question to the overall conceptual system in nursing and thus expand and elaborate the system by the testing of theories that have derived from it.

Validation of Theory

One of the problems we face in nursing is the need for more valid methods of measuring the variables of our research if we are to learn anything about the reality of the world in which we live. The rigidly controlled experimental studies necessary for baseline studies do not adequately explain the totality of man's interaction with his environment. Field work studies, on the other hand may be of equally questionable validity. If the phenomenon of man's interaction with his environment is to be described, explained, and predicted in such a way that it is applicable to man in his environment, we must continue to seek new methods of measurement.

On the Threshold

Nursing is coming of age. We have established a viable conceptual system—one that provides us with clear, relevant guidelines for theory-building and research. We are no longer overly concerned with ourselves as nurses. Concerned with the phenomenon of man, we are beginning to understand man. We no longer are completely dependent on other disciplines for the knowledge of our practice, but neither are we completely independent. We are beginning to realize our own potential for discovering a particular kind of knowledge that is relevant to other disciplines and essential to nursing. The problem of the past has been the dearth of nursing knowledge. The problem of the future will be the acceleration of that knowledge.

REFERENCES

Batey, M. V. (1971). Conceptualizing the research process. *Nursing Research, 20,* 296–301.

Brown, M. I. (1964). Research in the development of nursing theory. *Nursing Research, 13,* 109–112.

Dickoff, J., & James, P. (1968). A theory of theories: A position paper. *Nursing Research, 17,* 197–203.

Earle, A. (1969). *The effect of supplementary postnatal kinesthetic stimulation on the developmental behavior of the normal female newborn.* Unpublished doctoral dissertation, New York University, New York.

Felton, G. (1970). Effect of time cycle change on blood pressure and temperature in young women. *Nurse Research, 19,* 48–58.

Hempel, C. G. (1952). *Fundamentals of concept formation in empirical science.* Chicago: University of Chicago Press.

Johnson, D. E. (1968). Theory in nursing: Borrowed and unique. *Nursing Research, 17,* 206–209.

King, I. M. (1971). *Toward a theory of nursing.* New York: John Wiley & Sons.

McManus, R. L. (1961). Nursing research—its evolution. *American Journal of Nursing, 61,* 76–79.

Neal, M. V. (1968). Vestibular stimulation and the developmental behavior of the small premature infant. *Nursing Research Report 3,* 3–5.

Newman, M. A. (1972). Time estimation in relation to gait tempo. *Perceptual and Motor Skills, 34,* 354–366.

Nightingale, F. (1859). *Notes on nursing: What it is, and what it is not.* London: Harrison and Sons.

Norris, C. M. (Ed.) (1969). *Proceedings of the First Nursing Theory Conference.* Kansas City, KA: Department of Nursing Education, University of Kansas Medical Center.

Porter, L. S. (1971). Physical-physiological activity and infants growth and development. *American Nurses' Association Seventh Nursing Research Conference.* New York: American Nurses' Association.

Rodgers, J. A. (1971). *The relationship between sociability and personal space preference among college students in the morning and in the afternoon.* Unpublished doctoral dissertation, New York University, New York.

Rogers, M. E. (1964). *Reveille in nursing.* Philadelphia: F. A. Davis.

Rogers, M. E. (1970). *An introduction to the theoretical basis of nursing.* Philadelphia: F. A. Davis.

Schlachter, L. (1971). *The relation between anxiety, perceived body and personal space and actual body space among young female adults.* Unpublished doctoral dissertation, New York University, New York.

Wald, F. S., & Leonard, R. C. (1964). Towards development of nursing practice theory. *Nursing Research, 13,* 309–313.

Walker, L. O. (1971). Toward a clearer understanding of the concept of nursing theory. *Nursing Research, 20,* 428–435.

U.S. Health Manpower Education Bureau. (1971). *Future directions of doctoral education for nurses.* Report of conference held in Bethesda, Md. (DHEW Publication No. NIH 72–82) Washington, DC: U.S. Government Printing Office.

The Author Comments

Nursing's Theoretical Evolution

As suggested by the date of publication, this article represents my early attempt to make sense out of the "theories" and curricular foci of the day. It was an outgrowth of my first teaching experience at the doctoral level. I was convinced that the content of doctoral education should be based on the discipline of nursing, yet there was little in the literature to bring it all together. The reader will notice that we have come a long way since then.

—Margaret A. Newman

Reactions

"Theory Development," *Nursing Outlook, 20*(10), 630.

. . . Margaret A. Newman's article "Nursing's Theoretical Evolution" is excellent in that she has succinctly identified the highlights in the historical development of nursing theory. Her discussion of three main approaches to discovery of nursing theory should be helpful to graduate faculty and students.

I agree wholeheartedly that there is more "congruity between the King and the Rogers theoretical systems." It is my hope these and other theoretical systems in nursing are widely tested through research during the next decade.

IMOGENE M. KING
Professor,
School of Nursing
Ohio State University
Columbus, Ohio
1972

NURSING THEORY AND THEORIES

CHAPTER 13

Perspectives on Nursing Theory

Margaret E. Hardy

In recent years, the discipline of nursing has invested considerable time and effort in developing knowledge about theories, models and conceptual frameworks in order to direct nursing practice and establish the boundaries of its knowledge. Nursing conferences, journals and graduate curricula reflect this interest and concern. Nurses are now asking: What is nursing theory? What theory can nurses use? What is a theory as opposed to a conceptual framework? Although some of us may at times be dissatisfied and impatient at the speed with which these questions are being answered, we can perhaps gain a better understanding of theory development by looking at the total process objectively. Furthermore, the evaluation of nursing theory may be more appropriate and useful if the evaluator is aware of the stages of scientific development.

Stages of Scientific Development
Paradigms and Preparadigms

The dissent and confusion about "what is theory" and "what is nursing theory" may be typical of the early stages of scientific development in any discipline. Kuhn (1970), in *The Structure of Scientific Revolutions,* presents a fascinating thesis on the development of scientific knowledge; some of his points may shed considerable light on nursing's present concern with theory. Kuhn points out that the early stage of scientific development, the preparadigm stage, is characterized by divergent schools of thought which, although addressing the same range of phenomena, usually describe and in-

From Advances in Nursing Science, *October 1978, 1(1), 27-48. Copyright © 1978, by Aspen Systems Corporation.*
Reprinted with permission of Lippincott Williams & Wilkins.

About the Author

MARGARET E. HARDY was born in Edmonton, Alberta, Canada, in 1938. She received her BSN in 1960 from the University of British Columbia in Vancouver, Canada; her MA in 1965 from the University of Washington School of Nursing, with a major in community mental health; and her PhD in sociology in 1971 from the University of Washington. Her employment includes a faculty position at Boston University from 1971 to 1985, where she held a joint appointment in the School of Nursing and the Department of Sociology. From 1985 to her early retirement in 1993, she was Professor at the University of Rhode Island School of Nursing. Her major contribution to nursing evolved serendipitously as a result of her teaching assignment at Boston University; development of courses for the graduate program led to the publication of her award-winning books *Theoretical Foundations for Nursing* and *Role Theory*, as well as a book *Research Readings*. Through her publications and teaching hundreds of graduate students throughout New England during the 1970s and 1980s, Dr. Hardy provided foundational knowledge on metatheory and inspired many to initiate theory development for nursing. Dr. Hardy enjoys watercolor painting, reading, walking, hiking, traveling, and camping in the mountains with her husband and two dogs.

terpret these phenomena in different ways. Nursing appears to be now in this preparadigm stage.

Kuhn challenges the commonly held belief that scientific knowledge advances through slow and steady increments; he proposes that while accumulation of knowledge plays a major role in the advances of scientific knowledge, progress occurs as a result of scientific revolution. Kuhn's model of the development of scientific knowledge may be represented as given in Figure 13-1. In each revolution, a prevailing paradigm with its associated theories, concepts and research methods is overthrown when anomalies in the accumulating data cannot be accounted for. Then a new paradigm with its own theories, concepts and methods, which more fully accounts for the anomalies, replaces the prevailing paradigm. If a paradigm is to prevail in a discipline, it must attract an enduring group of adherents away from competing scientific orientations, and it must be sufficiently open-ended to leave all sorts of scientific problems to solve.

The paradigm of interest in this article is the *metaparadigm*. This is a gestalt or total world view within a discipline; it provides a map which guides the scientist through the vast, generally incomprehensible world. It gives focus to scientific endeavor which would not be present if scientists were to explore randomly.

The metaparadigm is the broadest consensus within a discipline. It provides the general parameters of the field and gives scientists a broad orientation from which to work. A more restricted type of paradigm is the *exemplar*. This paradigm is more concrete and specific than a metaparadigm. A discipline may have several exemplar paradigms which direct the activities of scientists. For example, in the field of social psychology scientists may group according to their agreement on the model of human nature: noble (Maslow), hedonist (Skinner) and cognator (Mead). This discussion of the metaparadigm and the exemplar paradigm will make the reader aware that the two types of paradigms exist, differentiated primarily on their level of abstraction; a

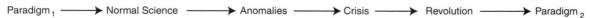

Paradigm$_1$ ⟶ Normal Science ⟶ Anomalies ⟶ Crisis ⟶ Revolution ⟶ Paradigm$_2$

Figure 13-1 *Process of scientific revolutions.*

metaparadigm may subsume several exemplar paradigms.

In summary, the metaparadigm or prevailing paradigm in a discipline presents a general orientation or total world view that holds the commitment and consensus of the scientists in a particular discipline. In general the paradigm: (1) is accepted by most members of the discipline, (2) serves as a way of organizing perceptions, (3) defines what entities are of interest, (4) tells the scientists where to find these entities, (5) tells them what to expect and (6) tells how to study them (i.e., the research methods available).

What do paradigms have to do with nursing theory? Kuhn's (1970) discussion of paradigms suggests that the metaparadigm and the exemplar paradigm are endorsed by a discipline and its subgroups because of their scientific-empirical support. The existence of a prevailing paradigm facilitates the normal work of science. Research is purposeful, orderly and raises few unanswerable questions.

When a dominant paradigm does not exist, a discipline may be in a crisis situation characterized by competing paradigms or it may be in a *preparadigm* stage with different, ill-defined perspectives that are heatedly argued and defended. In the preparadigm stage of a discipline, there is little agreement among its scientists as to what entities are of particular concern, where to locate these entities or how to study them. Such is the status of nursing today, with energy going into attempts to justify one of several embryonic paradigms rather than into purposeful, orderly research. Confusion prevails as to what exactly nursing should be studying; the research that is conducted is often poorly focused and unsystematic.

Kuhn's theory of paradigms and scientific revolution suggests that the development and evaluation of knowledge in nursing may proceed at a very slow pace, not because nurse-scientists lack the necessary ability to develop empirically-based scientific knowledge but because so much time is being devoted to justifying the various preparadigms. Until there is a prevailing paradigm and exemplar paradigms to give focus to the thinking and work of nurse-scientists, knowledge in nursing will develop slowly and somewhat haphazardly. This leaves the practicing nurse in a difficult position of deciding what knowledge is usable and how it should be evaluated for use.

Nursing as a Preparadigm Science

If Kuhn's conception of science is correct and if nursing is indeed in the preparadigm stage, then the time spent in defending one of the existing nursing conceptualizations (Riehl & Roy, 1974), the present concern with conceptual frameworks, models, theory construction and research methods are all part of an evolutionary process that other disciplines have either experienced already or have yet to face. Although this period of theory development in a discipline is characterized by ambiguity and uncertainty, nurse-scientists can help build the knowledge base that will help formulate an acceptable paradigm. They can do this by being well informed in a substantive area and participating actively in both theory construction and research. Nursing cannot decree that a specific paradigm will be adopted; the adoption of a paradigm will be based on its scientific credence and its potential for advancing scientific knowledge in nursing.

The preparadigm stage of science is one of confusion and frustration, with much dispute over theory, research and frequent factional power struggles. Nurse-scientists who realize this may be able to raise themselves above the battleground and focus their efforts and skills on developing sound nursing knowledge. Their work to solve very specific nursing-care problems may contribute significantly to developing exemplar paradigms and a predominant paradigm in nursing. The predominant nursing paradigm, when developed, will make it possible for other nurses to define more clearly their own "turf" or subject matter. While working on knowledge for practice, nurse-scientists must at present tolerate loosely constructed theoretical notions. This preparadigm stage of nursing science is difficult not only for those developing theory and research but also for those attempting to evaluate and use nursing knowledge.

The Development of Theory

The Nature of Theory

Before addressing the question of theory evaluation, the term theory must be defined. In common usage, the meaning of theory ranges from a hunch or a speculative explanation to a body of established knowledge. Kaplan (1964), in *The Conduct of Inquiry,* elaborates on the process of theorizing, suggesting that theory formation may well be the most important and distinctive attribute of human being. He does not perceive theorizing as a process removed from experience as opposed to brute fact.

In science, the term *theory* refers to a set of verified, interrelated concepts and statements that are testable. In his discussion of the human ability to develop scientific theory, Kaplan says:

> In the reconstructed logic,...theory will appear as the device for interpreting, criticizing, and unifying established laws, modifying them to fit data unanticipated in their formulation, and guiding the enterprise of discovering new and more powerful generalizations. To engage in theorizing means not just to learn by experience but to take thought about what is there to be learned. (Kaplan, 1964, p. 295)

Nurses will do well to remember the vital part that experience plays in theorizing.

Since a theory is a validated body of knowledge about some aspect of reality, it is appropriate that in developing theory nurses should concern themselves with identifying aspects of reality they wish to focus on, developing relevant theory and evaluating the soundness of the knowledge they develop. The scientist, in developing theory, looks for lawful relationships, patterns or regularities in the empirical world. Such relationships between concepts, sets facts or variables are carefully studied in order to identify conditions that modify or alter the original relationship.

Few "theories" in nursing or related disciplines are sufficiently well developed to permit specification of both lawful relationships and the condition under which these relationships vary. One possibility is behavior modification theory, which expresses a lawful relationship between specified behavior and reinforcement. Furthermore, this relationship may alter according to the type of reinforcement schedule employed.

Relationship Between Theory and Practice

Kaplan stresses the interrelatedness of theory and experience. In nursing, scientists and practicing nurses are frequently out of touch with one another. The nurse-scientist is a thinker unconcerned with the practice setting, while the practitioner is a provider of nursing care and is sometimes referred to as a technician. But it is from the practice setting that the nurse-scientist should derive ideas, and it is for the nurse in the clinical setting that ideas are developed. If the nurse-scientist is to be the major developer of theoretical knowledge, the practitioner must be in a position to provide the nurse-scientists with research-worthy problems and, at the same time, must be able to evaluate the knowledge generated for its soundness and applicability. A similar symbiosis has been highly successful in other fields. For instance, the theoretical physicist develops ideas and the engineer applies those ideas for the practical benefit of human beings.

Nursing has a mandate from society to use its specialized body of knowledge and skills for the betterment of humans. The mandate implies that knowledge and skills must grow in such a way as to keep up with the changing health goals of society. Furthermore, nursing must regulate its own practice, control the qualifications of its practitioners and implement *newly developed knowledge.*

The majority of nurses are clearly "doers" or practitioners. However, the discipline must also include scientists dedicated to generating knowledge. These scientists must be committed to finding things out, to obtaining an understanding and explanation of phenomena in their world and to identifying means for controlling significant phenomena. Nursing practice and nursing science, as pointed out earlier, are not antithetical; each depends on the other. It is important that theory be useful and encompass significant concepts and conditions that can be applied and favorably altered in the clinical setting.

Drawing on Work in Other Disciplines

Nursing draws on theories and knowledge from the disciplines of psychology, sociology and physiology. This is entirely legitimate; there is no reason for nurse-scientists to spend years of hard work duplicating knowledge that already exists but is housed in other disciplines. However, theory from another discipline must first be empirically validated to determine if its generalizations are applicable to nursing and its particular problems and needs. For example, generalizations from cognitive dissonance theory should be assessed to see if they can be used by nurses in practice settings; it is conceivable and, in fact likely, that modifications will first be necessary.

A large number of hours has been expended by social scientists in developing empirically based theoretical frameworks on role and social exchange. If nurses and nurse-scientists wish to employ these two sets of knowledge, they will need to determine how, when and where the concepts and empirical generalizations are applicable. In making this evaluation, they are likely to identify conditions unique to nursing practice which alter the social scientists' generalizations; they may also find they need to expand the original theory.

Types of Theory: Grand Versus Circumscribed

If the discipline of nursing is indeed in the preparadigm stage, consideration must be made for the level of theory development. Given a set of criteria for evaluating theory, the evaluator must make a decision as to what can be considered to be theory. A body of knowledge which is in the preparadigm stage cannot be evaluated as rigorously as a theory, nor can formulations which are "grand theories" or philosophies about nursing. They provide neither solid nor practical foundations for nursing practice; they are difficult to evaluate for their scientific value.

A theory in the early stage of development is characterized by discursive presentation and descriptive accounts of anecdotal reports to illustrate and support its claims. The theoretical terms are usually vague and ill defined, and their meaning may be close to everyday language. A paradigm at this embryonic stage is very readable and provides a perspective rather than a set of interrelated theoretical statements. This type of formulation *lacks empirical support;* the empirical illustrations accompanying it are not tests of the theoretical perspective.

This type of formulation, the "grand theory" or "general orientation," is aimed at explaining the totality of behavior (Merton, 1957). Grand theories tend to use vague terminology, leave the relationships between terms unclear and provide formulations that cannot be tested. Examples of grand theory might be Parsons's theory of Social Systems, Rogers's (1970) formulations of nursing theory, crisis theory, and some of the stress formulations. All present unique ways of looking at reality, but their ill-defined terms and questionable linkages between concepts make them impossible to put into operation and test empirically—and testability of a theory is one of the most important conditions a formulation must meet (Gibbs, 1972).

In addressing the problem of grand theories, Merton (1957) makes a plea for scientists to move into the study of partial theories. Since this plea, social scientists seem to have been successful in developing and testing partial or circumscribed theories. These circumscribed formulations may become exemplar paradigms; the move from grand formulations to circumscribed theory may take a discipline from a preparadigm stage to a paradigm stage with exemplar paradigms.

Circumscribed theories focus on selective aspects of behavior such as communication, social exchange, role behavior and self-consistency. In time, these formulations may lead to explication of theoretical terms and hypotheses which can be tested by carefully designed studies. The cumulative research and resulting theory is sound. Of the paradigms developed, one may eventually predominate, several may combine into a new paradigm which will address a larger part of reality, and several may coexist as exemplar paradigms.

The circumscribed theories on which scientists focus may seem irrelevant and unimportant when compared to the complex day-to-day problems confronted by nurses. Yet nurses must recognize that such complex problems cannot be solved quickly—as is evident in the enormous number of hours this country has spent trying to determine what cancer is and how it develops. Complicated scientific problems usually must be broken down into smaller, more manageable parts and tackled one by one. The scientific process for developing knowledge is slow, but it is the only sure one we have.

The norms that guide scientific activities seem to be universal; they are not specific to a discipline or country (Hardy, 1978). These norms include the need for public discourse on knowledge; the need for establishing the validity of scientific work; the need for critical assessment of both theory and research; and the need for empirical, objective work which can be replicated by others. It is in a milieu influenced by these norms that knowledge is generated and theory is developed; thus the outcome of the scientific process, the scientist's major goal, is achieved. If theory application is to contribute to the advancement of knowledge and to the professional code of ethics, nurse-scientists must adhere to these norms when developing knowledge.

Evaluation of Theory

Scientists have a variety of criteria for assessing knowledge. They examine their theories for explanatory and predictive power, for parsimony, generality, scope and abstractness (Hage, 1972; Hardy, 1978). For nurse-scientists, there is also a subset of criteria relating to the application of a particular theory in clinical practice. The following questions might be asked for such a theory: Is it internally consistent or *logically adequate?* How sound is its *empirical support?* Does the theory present concepts and conditions which the nurse can

actually *modify?* Can the theory be used in bringing about *major, favorable changes?*

Logical Adequacy (Diagramming)

Since a theory is a set of interrelated concepts and theoretical statements, its structure can be analyzed for internal consistency or logic (Hardy, 1978; Rudner, 1966). This involves examining the syntax of the theory rather than its content. If the structure is inconsistent or illogical, then empirical testing may not provide a test of the theory itself but only of unrelated or loosely related hypotheses.

One method for examining a theory's internal consistency involves identifying all the major theoretical terms. These may include constructs, concepts, operational definitions or referents. Once identified, each term can be represented by a symbol. Use of symbols serves to decrease the evaluator's bias and thus lessens the likelihood that substantive meaning will be attributed to the theory when it is not present.

The next step is to identify the relationships or linkages between terms. The linkages are usually expressed as follows: direction, type of relationship (positive or negative) and form of relationship (Hage, 1972). Symbols are used to signify the linkages; if the theory does not specify a linkage, this will become obvious as the structure of the theory is diagrammed.

To illustrate this process, consider the statement "high role conflict experienced by a person results in less communication with coworkers" and the statement "frequent communication with coworkers is associated with job satisfaction." The structure of these two statements would then be as shown in Figure 13-2. Diagramming these statements shows clearly that there are no contradictions in the specified linkages, and that there is no link specified between role conflict and satisfaction. This type of diagramming makes it possible to identify gaps, contradictions and overlaps. Linkages between constructs, concepts and operational definitions can also be diagrammed. (See Figure 13-3.) Diagramming a theoretical formulation will clearly show whether the hypothesis to be tested flows logically from the more abstract theoretical statements.

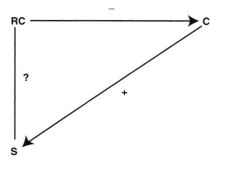

RC = role conflict
C = communication
S = satisfaction
+ = positive linkage
− = negative linkage
? = unspecified linkage

Figure 13-2 *Typical linkage diagram.*

Empirical Adequacy

Empirical validity is perhaps the single most important criterion for evaluating a theory which is to be applied in a practice setting. However, a theory cannot be empirically valid if it is logically inadequate. Many theories are

proposed but only a few are testable. Unfortunately, it is all too easy to select a theory which seems plausible or fits our own belief system and then use it in teaching students and working with patients. Among others, popular theories which have such questionable empirical support are psychoanalytic theory, crisis intervention theory and Erikson's theory of developmental crisis.

Assessment of Empirical Support

Assessing the empirical support for a theory is a rigorous but exciting puzzle-solving activity which involves several independent but closely related steps. Suppose an individual is planning to go to a major theoretical work and attempt to identify the key theoretical terms and the linkages between them. This process is identical to the processes used in determining the internal consistency of the theory, and a linkage diagram is used. When the individual has diagrammed the theory and identified predictions and hypotheses, it is necessary to examine the empirical support which actually exists. This requires going to the literature and identifying related studies.

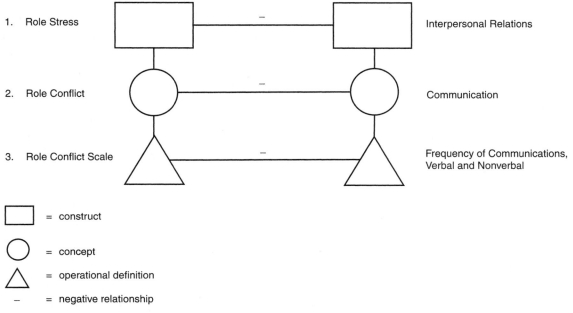

1. Role Stress — Interpersonal Relations
2. Role Conflict — Communication
3. Role Conflict Scale — Frequency of Communications, Verbal and Nonverbal

☐ = construct
○ = concept
△ = operational definition
− = negative relationship

Figure 13-3 *Linkage diagram showing relationships between terms.*

After the pertinent studies have been reviewed, they may be classified according to the strength of their research methodology and the empirical support given to the hypotheses tested. Care must be taken in judging which studies represent valid empirical tests of the theory. Case studies, anecdotal reports or descriptions of processes presented in discursive accounts of the theory do not constitute empirical tests. Such accounts are generally presented to give the reader the feeling that the theory is plausible and congruent with life events. This type of material may, however, be used to assess the theory's potential scope and generality.

It should not be forgotten that researchers usually have vested interests in their studies and may have introduced biases that alter the interpretation of the findings. During the critical reading, a study's hypotheses and their empirical referents may be diagrammed, as may the empirical relationship found between the concepts. The congruence between theoretical predictions and empirical outcomes can then be readily assessed in a relatively objective manner.

Factors to Consider

In evaluating research, possible changes in meaning of terms and concepts should be kept in mind. For example, in the literature of the 1950s on therapeutic communication theory, the concept of negative feedback may have been defined as derogatory (negative) communication, while in the 1970s, negative feedback has been redefined to mean any communication that alters (increases or decreases) the communication of the other person.

In analyzing a theory and its empirical support, it is necessary to determine that the hypotheses tested are clearly deduced from the theory. If they are not, the research is not testing that theory. In examining theoretical terms and their corresponding operational definitions, one's immediate concern is with the validity of the operational definitions. A theory may be logically sound—the hypotheses may follow clearly from it and be stated in a form that can be confirmed or rejected—but if the operational definitions do not reflect the meaning of the theoretical concepts, the research is not really addressing the theory and results will have limited or no bearing on it.

To complete the assessment, the entire body of relevant studies must be evaluated in terms of the extent to which it supports the theory, or some part of the theory. This assessment should result in a decision as to whether empirical support is sufficient to warrant the theory's application. The absolute necessity for determining the empirical adequacy of a theory cannot be overemphasized. If nurses are taught "theories" that have little or no empirical support, the nursing care interventions based on such "theories" may have deleterious effects on clients who believe in the nurse's skill, expertise and competence. And indeed there has been a tendency to base nursing actions on tradition, intuition and conceptual frameworks which seem sound but have not been empirically tested. Though they may be creative and may give nurses a sense of security in what they do, these sources of knowledge remain in the realm of myth and nonscientific knowledge.

For example, even if a conceptual framework for crisis intervention makes intuitive sense to a nurse, using it as a basis of action when it does not have sound empirical support is a serious error in judgment and one that has considerable ethical implications. There is a need to develop and use empirically sound scientific knowledge if nursing is to retain its reputation as a profession. And the process of evaluating a theory empirically should be shared with students since they, as practicing nurses, should carry out this same process for the remainder of their nursing careers.

Usefulness and Significance

Since nursing is an applied profession, it follows that relevant theories are those which nurses may use in the clinical setting. After a theory has been identified as having internal consistency and strong empirical support, can it actually be put to use by a nurse? The theory is *useful* to the degree that the practitioner is able to control, alter or manipulate the major variables and conditions specified by the theory to realize some desired outcome. Knowing multiple sclerosis is caused by a virus that lies dormant in a person for 30 years does not provide nurses with a basis for immediate intervention. On the other hand, the awareness of the empirical association between smoking and both lung cancer and heart disease allows the nurse to manipulate variables that can decrease the occurrence and severity of these diseases. Here theoretical knowledge is useful. Inhaling carcinogens from cigarettes is an activity over which the nurse can exert some influence, either through persuading individual patients not to smoke or by assisting in more general public education efforts.

Related to the usefulness of a theory is its *significance*. Given two theories which are internally consistent, have strong empirical support and encompass variables that the nurse is able to modify, what else should influence the choice of which theory to use? Assuming that both are focused on the same nursing problem, presumably the nurse would act on the one which would bring about the *strongest, most favorable outcome*. Take, for example, psychoanalytic theory and behavioral modification theory, both of which may address the problem of obesity. Although one theory addresses the childhood origins of obesity and the other the environmental factors influencing overeating, both can be used to assist patients to lose weight. However, behavior modification appears to bring about more major and enduring changes in eating habits. In this experiment no comparison is being made of the internal consistency of empirical support of the two theories; the point is to illustrate the efficacy of one theory over another in achieving desired behavioral outcomes.

Nursing as a health profession and as a scientific discipline has come a long way, but it still has much to achieve. As a discipline, it needs to struggle through and beyond the preparadigm stage of scientific development. This will entail challenges and risks, but the process should help create a corps of nurse-scientists able to develop knowledge which reflects sensitivity to problems in clinical practice, and a corps of their clinical counterparts capable of evaluating and using this knowledge.

REFERENCES

Gibbs, J. (1972). *Sociological theory construction.* Hinsdale, IL: Dryden Press.

Hage, J. (1972). *Techniques and problems of theory construction in sociology.* New York: John Wiley & Sons.

Hardy, M. (1978). Perspectives on theory. In M. Hardy & M. Conway (Eds.). *Role theory: Perspectives for health professionals.* New York: Appleton-Century-Crofts.

Kaplan, A. (1964). *The conduct of inquiry.* New York: Chandler Press.

Kuhn, T. (1970). *The structure of scientific revolutions* (2nd ed.). Chicago: University of Chicago Press.

Merton, R. (1957). The bearing of sociological theory on empirical research. In R. Merton (Ed.). *Social theory and social structure.* New York: Free Press.

Riehl, J., & Roy, C. (1974). *Conceptual models for nursing practice.* New York: Appleton-Century-Crofts.

Rogers, M. E. (1970). *An introduction to the theoretical basis of nursing.* Philadelphia: F. A. Davis.

Rudner, R. (1966). *Philosophy of social science.* Englewood Cliffs, NJ: Prentice-Hall.

Reactions

Advances in Nursing Science, 1(3), viii-ix.

To the Editor:

. . . I would like to have Margaret Hardy's explanation, description, or definition of paradigm as a concept before she gives us examples of two classes of paradigms. Incidentally, I found her article most thought provoking and significant. . .

BETTY D. PEARSON, RN, PhD
Associate Dean
Graduate Program in Nursing
School of Nursing
The University of Wisconsin
Milwaukee, Wisconsin
1978

Response

Advances in Nursing Science, 2(3), viii-x.

To the Editor:

This letter is in response to Dr. Betty Pearson's letter... Kuhn's term "paradigm" is central to my article "Perspectives on Nursing Theory" (*Advances in Nursing Science, 1*(1), 37-48). The term paradigm has been used frequently and with a wide variety of meanings by Kuhn (1962, 1970) as he developed his ideas on the growth of scientific knowledge. Although the term paradigm is central to his work, he left it undefined. He does say that the established usage of the term—meaning model or pattern—is not his usage (Kuhn, 1972, p. 23).

Masterman (1970), in an analysis of Kuhn's original work in 1962, identifies paradigm as being used in at least 21 different senses. Masterman clusters these 21 different meanings of paradigm into three groups. One of these, the metaphysical or metaparadigm, is the only type of paradigm that Kuhn's philosophical critics have referred to (Masterman, 1970, p. 65) and it is the type of paradigm central to my ANS 1:1 article. From this article I would like to quote what I consider to be a general definition of a metaphysical or metaparadigm.

The ... metaparadigm ... is a gestalt or total world view within a discipline; it provides a map which guides the scientist through the vast, generally incomprehensible world. It gives focus to scientific endeavor ... The metaparadigm is the broadest consensus within a discipline. It provides the general parameters of the field and gives scientists a broad orientation from which to work. (Hardy, 1978, p. 38)

This definition of paradigm as a gestalt, cognitive orientation or general perspective that has broad consensus within a discipline is based on several descriptive phrases used by Kuhn. Here I will cite phrases referring to the gestalt nature of paradigm. In a recent paper (Hardy, 1979), I focus on the significance of a paradigm having consensus within a discipline. Kuhn (1962), for example, refers to paradigm as a set of beliefs, as a successful metaphysical speculation, as a standard, as a way of seeing, as an organizing principle overriding perception itself, as a map, and as something that determines a large area of reality. Masterman points out that Kuhn's metaparadigm is neither "basic theory" nor a "general metaphysical viewpoint" (Masterman, 1970, p. 61). The metaparadigm is far broader than scientific theory and is prior to it. It is an ideologic, philosophic, and cognitive entity that has gained the consensus of scientists in a discipline.

In response to Dr. Pearson's request, I have gone to considerable length in quoting both Kuhn and Masterman. I have done so because philosophy is not my field of specialization and those with more expertise in this area may make different inferences than I, and secondly, because I think that the meaning of metaparadigm is not easy to grasp, particularly for those of us who are heavily steeped in the tradition of scientific theory, hypothesis testing, and research. Finally, I think it is an important concept for those of us in nursing who are attempting to identify nursing knowledge as opposed to knowledge in the basic and social sciences.

MARGARET E. HARDY, PhD
Boston, Massachusetts
1978

REFERENCES

Hardy, M. E. (1978). Perspectives in nursing theory. *Advances in Nursing Science, 1,* 37–48.

Hardy, M. E. (1979, April). *Paradigms as tools for structuring the professional science of nursing.* Paper presented at the 1979 Rozella M. Schlotfeldt Lectureship, Case Western Reserve University, Cleveland.

Kuhn, T. (1962). *The structure of scientific revolutions.* Chicago: University of Chicago Press.

Kuhn, T. (1970). *The structure of scientific revolutions* (2nd ed.). Chicago: University of Chicago Press.

Masterman, M. (1970). The nature of paradigm. In I. Lakatos & A. Musgrave (Eds.). *Criticism and the growth of knowledge.* London: Cambridge Press.

The Author Comments

Perspectives on Nursing Theory

This article reflects my thinking regarding the knowledge needed by doctoral students to evaluate theories that are germane to nursing. The ideas in this article were first presented at a nursing conference at Case Western Reserve in response to an invitation from Dr. Rosemary Ellis to speak to doctoral students. The notions of metaparadigm and theory development were important metatheoretical ideas for students to understand to effect the status and progress of knowledge in nursing. The ideas in this article, including the often-used diagrammatic model of the structure of a theory, were borrowed from sociology. This diffusion of knowledge from sociology helped launch the explosion of theory development activity that occurred in nursing during the decade this article was written and continues to this day.

— MARGARET E. HARDY

Congruence Between Existing Theories of Family Functioning and Nursing Theories

Ann L. Whall

Family theories have largely been accepted "as is" by nursing practitioners and researchers. The implications regarding the use of these existing theories need to be evaluated both in terms of the syntax of the discipline and the future courses that wholesale adoption may dictate. This discussion examines the relationship between specific family theories and the nursing theories of King, Peplau, and Rogers.[1-3]

Relationships Among Theories

According to Schwab, the knowledge base of a discipline may be divided into substantive and syntactical structures.[4] The substantive knowledge of a discipline is mostly concerned with the proper subject of inquiry,

and the syntactical knowledge is concerned with determining the acceptability of that subject base and the way in which the substantive knowledge is used. Schwab further describes the long-term syntax of a discipline as the way in which the discipline synthesizes and examines the substantive knowledge. Thus, syntactically a discipline examines the subject area for adequacy of concepts, for identification of weaknesses, and for devising reformulations. Existing theories of family functioning have been developed primarily within the disciplines of sociology and psychology. These family theories are mostly midrange in level (more specific than grand theory but not to the level of specificity of microlevel theory, which is situation-prescribing and -producing). This is especially the case in

About the Author

ANN L. WHALL is a native Michiganian and three-time graduate of Wayne State University in Detroit. She is an Advanced Nurse Practitioner in Michigan and has completed postdoctoral studies in geropsychiatry and neuroscience and, most recently, as a Fulbright Distinguished Scholar in the United Kingdom, examining expert nurses' use of implicit memory in dementia care. Throughout her career, Dr. Whall has been "driven by the desire to explicate the depth and exquisite nature of nursing knowledge, which has historically been unrecognized exterior to nursing." As a diploma graduate, she was denied admittance to graduate programs that were exterior to nursing on the belief that nursing was "manual art, not a science." Her works have since been published widely, and she has held several visiting professorships and completed multiple research studies and related publications, often with an identifiable emphasis upon the metatheoretical nature of nursing knowledge. Dr. Whall enjoys classical music, golfing, interacting with her 3 children, and developing international connections within nursing.

sociology; the psychological theories of family function tend, in contrast, to be midrange to micro-level in nature.

Within these disciplines, family theories form a substantive knowledge base that is viewed from the context of each discipline. The discipline of nursing has largely adopted the existing theories of family functioning from sociology and psychology. The use of this theoretical base takes place across clinical areas of nursing.[5-7] In general, these theories have not been viewed from the syntax of nursing theory.

This discussion is premised on the assumption that the discipline of nursing considers family functioning a proper subject of inquiry or a substantive knowledge base for nursing. Nursing conceptual frameworks, or theories, with their broad level of applicability, can be used as the theoretical umbrella or syntax by which existing theories of family functioning may be examined for adequacy as well as weakness, for the purposes of reformulation and revision. The consideration of existing theories from a discipline other than nursing in light of nursing knowledge is supported by nursing theorists.

According to Fawcett, for an existing theoretical structure to be viewed as a nursing theory, that theory must first be evaluated and reformulated in terms of congruence and consistency with the central concepts of nursing theory (person, environment, health, and nursing).[8] This is consistent with Hardy's position that because nursing draws upon biopsychosocial knowledge, it is free to draw upon knowledge developed by these disciplines; but nursing has an obligation to alter theories it draws upon to fit the problems associated with nursing.[9] Ellis also addressed this issue when she discussed theories of, in, and for nursing.[10] Existing theories used in nursing are to be examined in light of current nursing knowledge. Fawcett also makes the point that once reformulation of the major concepts of an existing theory has occurred, along with evaluation of the relational statements, the resultant formulations can be designated as nursing theory.[8]

The major nursing theories are mostly at the conceptual framework level in terms of theory development; nursing theories are not, therefore, generally situation-producing or -prescriptive. According to Fawcett, it is crucial that prescriptive theories borrowed from other fields be carefully scrutinized in terms of the basic concepts of nursing theory. The discussion here attempts to address this issue and move forward the scrutiny of borrowed family theory.

Family Functioning Theory

Theories of family functioning from the discipline of psychology appear to have the most applicability to

nursing practice. Most sociological theories are deductive and midrange; in contrast, some psychological theories of family functioning are inductive and situation-prescribing. Psychological theories of family functioning thus tend to be more useful to nursing practice. Rather than discussing what is, psychological theories tend to prescribe what will be of assistance to a particular family. Because nursing as a discipline is concerned with caring, helping, and nurturing, lack of specificity in many a priori midrange sociological formulations leads to delay or impasse in utilization. Duffey and Muhlenkamp point out that the usefulness of theoretical structures is of prime importance in the evaluation of theories.[11] The psychologically based theories referred to here are those of the family theorists considered somewhat psychoanalytic in approach, such as Framo[12] and Boszormenyi-Nagy;[13] those considered communicationist in approach, such as Haley,[14] Satir,[15] and Jackson;[16] and those using a systems approach, such as Napier and Whitaker,[17] and Minuchin et al.[18] These theorists discuss specific approaches, interventions, and goals in dealing with family functioning.

Nursing Theory

All nursing theories deal somewhat with four central concepts: person, environment, health, and nursing. Because nursing theories are generally at the broad conceptual framework level of theory development, for the purposes of this discussion nursing theory is considered to be the syntax of nursing.[8,9] The nursing theories referred to are those of King, Peplau, and Rogers.[1-3]

The syntax of nursing theory indicates the way to handle the four central concepts; the existing theory or substantive knowledge area can thus be viewed in terms of congruence and consistency with person, environment, health, and nursing. Given that existing theories do not discuss nursing as such, aspects of the nursing process which are addressed, such as goal and mode of intervention, can also be evaluated. It is important to note that the nursing theories vary in the way in which the central concepts are handled.

Most nursing theories define *person* in some holistic fashion. However, the way in which the term *holistic* is interpreted by nursing theorists varies; some believe that aspects of a person may be addressed separately, while others insist upon terms that handle only the whole person. Nursing theorists also consider environment in various field-figure arrangements, either as separate, as a unified entity with person, or as a somewhat unified entity.

The term *health* is also discussed in different ways by the nursing theorists. Some describe the health-illness continuum; others discuss health in more holistic terms, such as optimum well-being. Both linear and holistic approaches to family health are represented in the existing theories of family functioning. Likewise, the concepts of person and environment are primarily handled in either a linear or holistic manner. The congruence between nursing theory and existing theories of family functioning forms the basis of the following discussion.

Holism and Linearity

Maslow states that if one is to perceive holistically, then it is necessary to assess holistically or in some manner that considers the total and not the parts.[19] In a discussion of reductionist tendencies, he says that "good knowers," or those who know not only through cognitive operations but also through the senses, do not split mind from body, but attempt to perceive the whole person.[19] Once the Cartesian position that mind and body may be considered separately is accepted, it follows that the parts may be assessed separately. Maslow explains that the latter approach leads to reductionism, or the belief that a sum of the parts equals the whole.

Linear conceptualizations place person, health, or environment on a plane. The health-illness continuum is a familiar linear conceptualization. If the person is seen as progressing through time and space in such a fashion that past problems may be returned to and addressed, then the whole of the person is not perceived. Obviously, because no one gets younger, all persons progress through time and space. For this linear conceptualization to remain consistent, the person is perceived separately from the environment of time and space. Therefore, the separatism of many linear models does not handle the concepts of person and environment as a whole.

When the conceptualization is such that problems may be returned to, addressed, and corrected, then for a while the time and space environment is ignored. The person is thus viewed as independent from the environmental field, and it is then possible to discuss the person adapting in a time-lag sequence to the environment. Problems of the environment can be addressed as separate from the person and vice versa.

The helper, who can be viewed as separate from the field, may "fix-up" the environment or the client separately, without joining the field. From this linear field-independent perspective, active participation of client with helper becomes questionable. In the world of strict linear formulations, the helper may be separate from the client, the client separate from the environment, and all on a continuum in which progression and retrogression are possible. This approach appears antithetical to Maslow's holistic approach. Because the whole person is generally considered the proper subject matter for nursing,[1-3,20] it is important to consider the implications of the use of linear concepts.

Congruence of Family Functioning and Nursing Theories

Existing theories of family functioning primarily use holistic or linear approaches, view environment as separate or as a whole with person, and address health as a linear continuum or as part of the whole of time and space. Minuchin et al classify theories of family functioning as primarily holistic or linear. Theories of family functioning are divided into three general types: psychoanalytic, communicationist, and systems.[18] The Minuchin et al classification system is used to organize the following discussion.

Psychoanalytic Approach

In the commonly held psychoanalytic view, each of the family architects, the parents, brings into the present family unit needs formulated via the heritage of their early life experiences.[12] The parents, as individuals, are thus the prime unit of consideration. Early events in the lives of the parents are of prime importance; these early events must be addressed for there to be a change in the present family unit.[13] This view considers personhood as deterministically foretold by prior events.

The type and magnitude of past events can determine the type of mate selected, the career chosen, and even the selection of friends. The psychoanalytic view is thus primarily a linear approach in which energy may be stopped (fixated), progress (be worked through), or even go backward (regression). The marriage partners are mostly seen as separate, in terms of influence from the present environmental field. The present family is clearly not the prime focus of intervention because resolution of present difficulties lies in the working through of past problems.

As in the classical psychoanalytic approach, theories of family functioning using this theory base consider the therapeutic relationship to be of prime importance. Because much of the problem is unconscious and therefore unavailable to the client, the client depends upon the helper to discover and work through past problems.

In this view the family is an aggregate of individuals with complementary needs. The question is not one of whole family unit versus individual interventions, but one of preeminence and a working out of symptoms of the most needy individual through the rest of the family members. Theories of family functioning that demonstrate this view begin with a working through of the "tension states" or underlying problems of the marital partners. Once these tensions are resolved, the family unit is expected to function well. Health is thus viewed as a working through of past difficulties so that it is no longer necessary to attempt to repetitively work through the past problems in to the present.

Nursing Theory

Nursing theories congruent with the psychoanalytic view would consider person, environment, and health in some composite fashion—person as a biopsychosocial being with the psychological portion preeminent. Health is seen as a continuum with the possibility of assisting the client back to health through the interpersonal relationship. Because of past experiences, the client is unable to clearly discern problems and thus depends upon the nurse for clarification; the client is therefore less active. The helper assists each client to work through present problems that reflect past deficits. The goal and focus of the intervention is insight developed via the interpersonal relationship.

Although there are some inconsistencies, Peplau's approach to nursing theory is generally congruent with the psychoanalytic approach to family functioning.[2] Peplau defines *person* as an organism that strives to reduce tension generated by needs and defines *nursing* as a significant interpersonal process. The person is viewed as a biopsychosocial being with emphasis upon the psychological aspects. This composite view of person is compatible with a linear view of tension reduction. The client responds to the nursing intervention, primarily the interpersonal relationship, with a reduction in tension. The tension is generated primarily from past needs. A notable incongruence between Peplau's approach and the psychoanalytic approach is that Peplau insists upon participation of the client in such things as mutual goal setting and action. The family is not addressed as a specific unit. This is considered consistent with Peplau's discussion of person as an individual striving to work through individual needs.

Communicationist Approach

Minuchin et al identify a second group of family theorists as communicationists, including Haley,[14] Bateson,[21] and Satir.[15] Due to the theorizing of Harry Stack Sullivan, a shift in thinking took place, with interest focusing upon the pattern of signals by which information is transferred within dyads and triads.[18] The communicationists emphasize present communication patterns in terms of pattern, sequence, and hierarchy, rather than the past nature of people.[13] The person is perceived as actively involved in the present, not the past and the cause-effect influence of early relationships. The communicationists stress the ways in which the person interacts, not only in terms of parts but also the whole. The field within which the person functions becomes highlighted. The helper and client influence and become influenced by one another; the split between action and reaction becomes less with the concept that actions and reactions occur together in the same field. Persons interact with the environment in terms of patterns and cues. The unit of intervention thus changes from helper and individual client to helper uniting with the field, and in particular, the dyadic and triadic relationships in which the client is involved.[15]

The communicationist approach is viewed as an extension of the prior psychoanalytic view, from individual to interactional patterns among people. Double bind communication patterns, scape-goating processes, pseudomutualities and silencing strategies within the dyads or triads of the family are of prime importance. The locus of difficulty lies in transmission processes. Homeostasis considerations prevail as equilibrium concepts imply that equality of relationships is health. The goal becomes clarification of relationships among all people within the dyadic and triadic patterns. The helpers' authority is subject to challenge, for as part of the field, the helper is an active participant in the communication sequences. The communicationist approach, emphasizing mutual action and reaction among people, may imply a time lag, thus suggesting linearity. However, the linearity is much less clear than in the psychoanalytic approach. The field is emphasized and field and person are treated as one.

Nursing Theory

King's theory, which focuses on transactions within the dyad of nurse and client, is most consistent with the approach of the communicationists. King states that person (*man* in her terminology) is a reacting being with awareness of the environment.[1] The response or reaction is a comprehensive response of mind and body; the nurse and client work together toward a mutually acceptable goal. Health implies continuous adaptation to internal and external stresses. The relationship between nurse and client is prime. Although the environment is discussed as one with the individual, families are not specifically addressed. The therapeutic relationship is central and the person and nurse are viewed as part of the same field. Although King sometimes uses linear terms such as reaction and adaptation, the linearity of person is less clear than in psychoanalytic conceptualizations. As with the communicationists, King's model implies field dependence. The interpersonal orientation implies that the client and nurse are of the same field.

Systems Approach

The systems theories of family functioning emerged in the late 1950s and are considered extensions of the communicationist approach. The unit of intervention in systems theory is a dramatic departure from previous theory. Not only is the family unit perceived holistically, but it must be analyzed and approached holistically, not reductively. No longer are subsystem dyads considered primary and sometimes seen alternatively. In the pure systems approach, the family is always seen together. Sometimes three and four generations are included in the approach, and all problems are handled in total family sessions. According to a systems framework, the family is a type of unitary living organism.[18] The family is a living system relating to the systems of community, country, and universe. Just as one organ of the body relates to and is influenced by every other organ, the family system is influenced by internal subsystems as well as the larger community system. The family grows and changes, giving birth to new and different forms, just as an organism grows, changes, and reproduces. The family is a system in that it is a series of interrelated parts. Family rules govern the system and the individual's margin of choice. An important point is that family systems theorists generally imply a closed system perspective. Dysfunction or illness is defined as the closing down of the family system in much the same way as the clos-

ing down of the body's circulatory system is dysfunctional for the whole body. In terms of mode of intervention, the helper works with the system and becomes part of the system. By changing a key element of the system, not always the most negative portion, the total system changes and hopefully dysfunctions are alleviated.

Nursing Theory

In terms of a nursing conceptual framework, Rogers is perhaps closest to the family systems approach.[3] The greatest departure perhaps is that Rogers considers the person from an open rather than a closed systems perspective. The person is always open or in mutual, simultaneous interaction with the environment. As do family systems theorists, Rogers sees boundaries as more perceptual than real, everything is connected to everything else. According to both Rogers and the family systems theorists, pattern and organization characterize the system. Change in one portion of the system affects changes in the whole, and these changes create reverberations in the system in wavelike fashion.

The unit of intervention for both Rogers and family system theorists is the total *family system*. Both consider the fields of nurse and family environments as coextensive and infinite energy fields. There is also congruence between the approaches of Rogers and family systems theory in terms of working within the system as opposed to external manipulation in a psychoanalytic sense. Health in Rogers' terms is a value judgment, because disease conditions are not entities by themselves but manifestations of the total pattern of the family system. The goal of nursing is to promote a symphonic interaction between persons (subsystems of the family), the family system, and the environment. The focus is thus redirection of patterns and organization within the family.[22]

Behaviorist Approach

The behaviorist approach to family is not discussed at length here because it is not well developed. However, compatible positions might be found between the behaviorist approaches to family and nursing theorists such as Roy who discuss adaptation.[19] According to Minuchin et al, the behaviorist views the family as a unit to decondition individual behavior, producing certain signals that organize the patient's behavior. The person is considered as somewhat separate, not one with the field.[18] Thus the unit of intervention is the individual. The behaviorist helper appears separate from the system. The view is one of person interacting with the environment to bring about an adopted state on the health-illness continuum. The linear causality focus of the behaviorist does not appear compatible with the communications or systems theorists who view person as part of total system or field.

Importance of Theory Reformulation

Reformulation of the theories of family functioning so as to achieve consistency with nursing approaches is important. With some of the theories of family functioning, such as the systems approach, reformulation in terms of nursing theory may be readily achieved. The perspective, however, would be changed from a closed to an open systems perspective. In the case of the psychoanalytic approach, reformulation in terms of the nursing theory that requires client independence may not be as readily achieved. If nursing is to follow a holistic approach to person, environment, and health—and the major nursing theories would lead one to believe this is the direction with the most support—then linear conceptualizations in both existing theories and nursing theories need to be evaluated. Newman states the true holistic approach is not to be confused with the summing of many facts, but with factors reflective of the whole.[22] Reformulation of linear aspects may be necessary.

The important point is that the existing theory is to be examined for reformulation in terms of the nursing theory. In the past, the nursing approach was often reformulated for congruence with existing theories from other disciplines.

REFERENCES

1. King I: *Toward a Theory of Nursing: General Concepts of Human Behavior.* New York, John Wiley & Sons, 1971.
2. Peplau H: *Interpersonal Relations in Nursing.* New York, Putnam, 1952.
3. Rogers M: *The Theoretical Basis of Nursing.* Philadelphia, FA Davis, 1970.
4. Schwab J: Structure of the disciplines: Meanings and significances, in Ford G (ed): *The Structure of Knowledge and the Curriculum.* Chicago, Rand McNally & Co, 1964, pp 6–30.
5. Miller J, Janosik E: *Family Focused Care.* New York, McGraw-Hill, 1980.
6. Hymovich D, Barnard M: *Family Health Care.* New York, McGraw-Hill, 1979.
7. Smoyak S: *The Psychiatric Nurse as a Family Therapist.* New York, John Wiley & Sons, 1975.
8. Fawcett J: The what of theory development, in *What, Why and How of Theory Development.* New York, National League for Nursing, 1978.
9. Hardy M: Evaluating nursing theory, in *What, Why and How of Theory Development.* New York, National League for Nursing, 1978.
10. Ellis R: Characteristics of significant theories. *Nurs Res* 17:217–222, May-June 1968.
11. Duffey M, Muhlenkamp A: A framework for theory analysis. *Nurs Outlook* 22:570–574, September 1974.
12. Framo J: Rationale and techniques of intensive family therapy, in Boszormenyi-Nagy I, Framo J (eds): *Intensive Family Therapy: Theoretical and Practical Aspects.* New York, Harper & Row, 1965.
13. Boszormenyi-Nagy I: Intensive family therapy as process, in Boszormenyi-Nagy I, Framo J (eds): *Intensive Family Therapy: Theoretical and Practical Aspects.* New York, Harper & Row, 1965.
14. Haley J: *Problem Solving Therapy.* San Francisco, Jossey-Bass, 1978.
15. Satir V: *Conjoint Family Therapy.* Palo Alto, Calif, Science & Behavior Books, 1967.
16. Jackson D: The question of family homeostasis. *Psychiatr Q Suppl* 31: 79–90, 1957.
17. Napier A, Whitaker C: *The Family Crucible.* New York, Harper & Row, 1978.
18. Minuchin S, Rosman B, Baker L: *Psychosomatic Families.* Cambridge, Mass, Harvard University Press, 1978.
19. Maslow A: *The Psychology of Science.* South Bend, Ind, Gateway, 1966.
20. Roy C: *Introduction to Nursing: An Adaptation Model.* Englewood Cliffs, NJ, Prentice-Hall, 1976.
21. Bateson G: The birth of a matrix or double bind and epistemology, in Berger M (ed): *Beyond the Double Bind.* New York, Brunner/Mazel, 1978.
22. Newman M: *Theory Development in Nursing.* Philadelphia, FA Davis, 1979.

The Author Comments

Congruence Between Existing Theories of Family Functioning and Nursing Theories

As a public health nurse, I was cognizant of the historical value placed upon the family as a unit of care within nursing. Yet, in the nursing literature in the late 1970s, there was little knowledge presented from a nursing perspective. Most was derived "as is" from nonpractice-oriented disciplines that were exterior to nursing. I wrote this article based on my dissertation research after being challenged by my dissertation chairperson, Dr. Joyce Fitzpatrick, to explicate the differences between the nursing perspective and that of others. The members of the Nursing Theory Think Tank also challenged the existence of a nursing perspective upon family. This article was also a response to that challenge.

—ANN L. WHALL

CHAPTER 15

Theory: Of or For Nursing?

Elizabeth M. Barrett

Various authors of nursing literature refer to nursing theory in one of two ways. Some say theory "of" nursing and some say theory "for" nursing. This "of-for" debate has been the subject of many discussions in nursing. "Of" means knowledge that is original to the discipline and describes the unique phenomenon of concern to nursing. "For" means a synthesis of knowledge from other disciplines is applied in nursing practice. "Of" implies an explication of *new* knowledge coming from nursing. "For" implies an application of *previously developed* knowledge.

The crux of the issue is whether or not nursing is viewed primarily as a basic science meaning *to know* what is clearly unique to nursing, or an applied science, meaning *to do* what is required in the practice of nursing. Differences in these positions have their roots in the debate concerning unique versus borrowed knowledge that began appearing in the literature over 30 years ago (Johnson, 1959). However, as nursing's knowledge base has continued to emerge, the issue has become more complex.

Rogers (1970, 1990), Parse (1981), and Newman (1986), nursing theorists in the simultaneity paradigm (Parse, Coyne, & Smith, 1985) represent the theory "of" nursing view very explicitly. These theorists define nursing as a basic science concerned with unitary, irreducible human beings and their environments. While rooted in new scientific world views, nursing science clearly does not derive from other basic or applied sciences. Rather, it is an emergent, a new product (Rogers, 1988).

Two theorists in the totality paradigm, Roy (1988) and Orem (1988), also use theory "of" nurs-

Nursing Science Quarterly, 4(2), 48-49
Copyright © 1991 Chestnut House Publications. Reprinted with permission.

About the Author

ELIZABETH ANN MANHART BARRETT was born in Hume, IL. She holds a PhD in nursing science from New York University, a master of science in nursing, a master of arts, and a bachelor of science in nursing, summa cum laude, from the University of Evansville, Evansville, IN. She has 5 children and 15 grandchildren. Dr. Barrett is Professor Emerita of Nursing, Hunter College, City University of New York. Currently, she maintains a private nursing practice of health patterning in New York City and is also a research consultant. The primary focus of Dr. Barrett's research and other scholarly activities is *Rogers' Science of Unitary Human Beings*. Reflecting Rogers' worldview, she developed a theory of power, an instrument to measure the power construct, and the practice methodology of Health Patterning.

ing terminology although they take a somewhat different position from the simultaneity paradigm theorists. Thus, the "of-for" issue does not clearly separate into simultaneity-totality views. Instead, the notion crosses paradigms. While some totality paradigm theorists are beginning to call nursing a basic science, a close look at their work indicates a primary focus on application of knowledge rather than development of new knowledge. Since the simultaneity and totality paradigms present very different views of the nature of nursing science, using theory "of" nursing when describing totality paradigm perspectives could lead to confusion.

Roy (1988) describes a basic and clinical science "of" nursing. The basic science of nursing that she describes, focuses on human life processes; the clinical science of nursing focuses on diagnosis and treatment of the patterning of the life processes in wellness and illness. The clinical science evolves from the basic science.

Orem (1988) outlines yet a different perspective and does not explicitly state that nursing is a basic science. Rather, her theory "of" nursing means "nursing science is practical science" that "provides knowledge that gives direction for the activities of practitioners" (p. 77). The action of nurses is central to practical nursing science which emerges from a process of gathering knowledge from different sciences "in order to conceptualize and express the unity that is nursing" (p. 79).

Orem (1988) maintains that practical science brings together what nurses need to know with what nurses need to do. This, she believes, will give rise to "a general theory of nursing that is descriptively explanatory of nursing as a form of care" (p. 78).

There are also totality paradigm theorists who explicitly represent the theory "for" nursing view. King (1971, 1981, 1989), like Johnson (1980), has consistently proposed a theory "for" nursing. This perspective arose from the argument that reformulation of borrowed knowledge will lead to "new" concepts and theories of nursing intervention that will produce predictable results in clients (Johnson, 1959). The borrowed knowledge generally reflects the older world views of traditional science. King (1989) proposes that the general systems conceptual framework that she used to derive her theory "for" nursing cuts across disciplines. She contends that it can be used to generate theories "for" nursing as well as for any other discipline in higher education and for any profession that focuses on human beings. "Knowledge is similar but the way each professional group uses knowledge is different" (p. 154).

The simultaneity paradigm theorists explicitly represent the theory "of" nursing view. Some totality paradigm theorists explicitly represent the theory "for" nursing position; others do not stay with the strict meaning in defining theory "of" nursing as presented in this column.

Regardless of differences in epistemology and ontology, what is common to both theory "of" and theory "for" nursing is that the authors firmly embrace nursing as a science that differs in varying degrees from other sciences. However, the distinct nature of this knowledge has significant implications, since from this disciplinary foundation flows not only the practice of nursing but also the contribution of nursing knowledge to the larger community of science.

Uniformity of perspective is neither possible nor desirable. Nor is it within the scope of this column to articulate the positions of all nursing theorists. Rather, the purpose is to issue a clarion call for greater specificity of differences and precise, correct use of terms.

We make our views precise by the language we use to convey meaning. If one believes that nursing is a basic science, then the correct terminology called for is theory "of" nursing. If one believes that nursing is an applied science, then the correct terminology is theory "for" nursing. Knowing what we mean and meaning what we say will further advance clarity in the "of-for" debate. Then, perhaps, we will move into the 21st century with more explicit answers to the question, "What constitutes substantive knowledge in nursing science?"

REFERENCES

Johnson, D. E. (1959). The nature of a science of nursing. *Nursing Outlook, 7,* 292.

Johnson, D. E. (1980). The behavioral system model for nursing. In J. P. Riehl & C. Roy (Eds.), *Conceptual models for nursing practice* (2nd ed.) (pp. 207–216). New York: Appleton-Century-Crofts.

King, I. M. (1971). *Toward a theory for nursing.* New York: Wiley.

King, I. M. (1981). *A theory for nursing: Systems, concepts, process.* New York: Wiley.

King, I. M. (1989). King's general systems framework and theory. In J. P. Riehl-Sisca (Ed.), *Conceptual models for nursing practice* (3rd ed.) (pp. 149–158). Norwalk, CT: Appleton & Lange.

Newman, M. A. (1986). *Health as expanding consciousness.* St. Louis: Mosby.

Orem, D. E. (1988). The form of nursing science. *Nursing Science Quarterly, 1,* 75–79.

Parse, R. R. (1981). *Man-living-health: A theory of nursing.* New York: Wiley.

Parse, R. R., Coyne, A. B. & Smith, M. J. (1985). *Nursing research: Qualitative methods.* Bowie, MD: Brady.

Rogers, M. E. (1970). *An introduction to the theoretical basis of nursing.* Philadelphia: Davis.

Rogers, M. E. (1988). Nursing science and art: A prospective. *Nursing Science Quarterly, 1,* 99–102.

Rogers, M. E. (1990). Nursing: Science of unitary, irreducible, human beings: Update 1990. In E. A. M. Barrett (Ed.), *Visions of Rogers' science-based nursing* (pp. 5–11). New York: National League for Nursing.

Roy, C. (1988). An explication of the philosophical assumptions of the Roy Adaptation model. *Nursing Science Quarterly, 1,* 22–34.

The Author Comments

Theory: Of or For Nursing?

The purpose of this article was to clarify the nature of the debate concerning whether nursing is a basic science concerned with theory *of* nursing or an applied science concerned with theory *for* nursing. The *of-for* debate, then and now, concerns knowledge reflecting nursing theories and frameworks. Whether one supports the *of* or *for* side of the debate, the key is related to fortifying these nursing schools of thought as guides to practice and research. As we move further into the 21st century, the article may prompt scholars to examine the disciplinary effect of abandoning theory *of* or *for* nursing by those who say that nursing theories and frameworks are going, going, and will soon be gone, only to be remembered as relics of a bygone age. Indeed, in some circles, "nursing science" has become a euphemism disguising theory *without* nursing or atheoretical perspectives. Beware; nursing science guided by theory *of* or *for* nursing may be an endangered species!

—ELIZABETH ANN MANHART BARRETT

An Analysis of Changing Trends in Philosophies of Science on Nursing Theory Development and Testing

Mary C. Silva

Daniel Rothbart

The effects of changing trends in philosophies of science on nursing theory development and testing are analyzed. Two philosophies of science—logical empiricism and historicism—are compared for four variables: (a) components of science, (b) conception of science, (c) assessment of scientific progress, and (d) goal of philosophy of science. These factors serve as the basis for assessing trends in the development and testing of nursing theory from 1964 to the present. The analysis shows a beginning philosophic shift within nursing theory from logical empiricism to historicism and addresses implications and recommendations for future nursing theory development and testing.

Both philosophy of science and nursing theory are in a state of transition. At times this transition is characterized by contradictory, divergent, and confusing points of view that lead to probing questions about the nature of science in general and nursing theory and science in particular. What are the goals and components of science? How should science be conceptualized and scientific knowledge assessed? Have nursing theory development and testing kept pace with changing trends in philosophies of science?

The goal of this analysis is to show the influences of changing trends in philosophies of science on nursing theory development and testing and to encourage dialogue among nurses about the future directions of nursing theory.

From Advances in Nursing Science, *January 1984, 6(2), 1-13. Copyright © 1984 by Aspen Systems Corporation. Reprinted with permission from Lippincott Williams & Wilkins.*

About the Authors

MARY CIPRIANO SILVA was born and raised in the small town of Ravenna, OH. She earned a BSN and an MS from Ohio State University and a PhD from the University of Maryland. She also undertook post-doctoral study at Georgetown University in health care ethics. The focus of her scholarship and key contributions to nursing has been in philosophy, metatheory, and health care ethics. She is a Professor and Director, Office of Healthcare Ethics, Center for Health Policy, Research, and Ethics, at George Mason University, Fairfax, VA. When not working, she attends foreign films, the Shakespeare Theatre, and fine and performing arts events.

DANIEL ROTHBART received three degrees in philosophy: a BA in 1972 from Fairleigh Dickinson University, an MA in 1975 from the State University of New York at Binghamton, and a PhD in 1978 from Washington University in St. Louis. Dr. Rothbart has lectured on medical ethics and philosophy of science throughout both the U.S.A. and Europe. He was appointed a visiting research scholar at the University of Cambridge in England a few years ago. He has published articles, chapters, and a book titled *Metaphor and the Growth of Scientific Knowledge*. He has been a member of the faculty at George Mason University since 1979.

Philosophies of Science

Since the 1940s, two major schools of philosophical thought have influenced philosophy of science: logical empiricism (1940s-1960s) and historicism (1960s to the present). The most influential proponents of logical empiricism (the orthodox view) included Braithwaite (1953), Ayer (1959), Nagel (1961), Scheffler (1963), Hempel (1965, 1966), and Rudner (1966). These proponents understood the nature of scientific knowledge as an application of logical principles of reasoning.

Although the logical empiricist view dominated the study of philosophy of science for more than two decades, a wave of criticism began in the early 1960s. Logical empiricism was subjected to intense philosophical scrutiny, revolving around the general contention that the orthodox view became too purified in its idealistically formal approach to science. In providing logical rigor and formalization to the nature of scientific knowledge, logical empiricism removed itself from the actual practice of working scientists; the orthodox view approached logic more closely than it did science according to critics. These critics began to reexamine the actual practices of scientists, the patterns of reasoning, and the sociological influences during a historical era.

The history of science became an essential element of any adequate philosophical analysis, prompting a new philosophy of science known as historicism.

Major historicists include Hanson (1958), Kuhn (1962, 1970), Lakatos (1968), Toulmin (1972), Laudan (1977), and Feyerabend (1978). Although Kuhn is the best known of these historicists, based on the influential work *The Structure of Scientific Revolutions* (Chicago: University of Chicago Press, 1962, 1970), his philosophical proposals have been widely criticized by other historicists, and Kuhn himself (1977) has had second thoughts about certain aspects of this work.

Therefore, to draw the distinctions between logical empiricism and historicism, it is desirable to focus on the work of Laudan rather than Kuhn. The reasons are threefold: (a) Laudan's works represent the forefront of philosophy of science today; (b) his views are largely shared by other historicists; and (c) his works have gone almost unnoticed by nurse theorists and researchers.

To show fundamental differences regarding theory development, testing, and assessment between logical empiricism and Laudan's version of historicism, these two philosophies are compared for four significant variables: (a) the components of science, (b) the conception of science, (c) the assessment of scientific

Table 16-1
A Comparison of Logical Empiricism and Historicism
on Four Parameters of Science

Parameters	Logical Empiricism	Historicism
Components of science	Concepts, theoretical assumptions, empirical generalizations	Concepts, scientific theories, research traditions
Conception of science	Science as product	Science as process
Assessment of scientific progress	Accept theories as probably true Reject theories as probably false	Number of solved problems within a discipline
Goal of philosophy of science	Logical explanation of nature of scientific knowledge	Historical explanation of the nature of scientific knowledge

Note: Although this table highlights the major differences between two philosophies of science, there are some shared views. For example, historicists primarily define science as a human process, but they also examine the products of solved scientific problem

progress, and (d) the goal of philosophy of science. Table 16-1 summarizes the basic differences between logical empiricism and historicism. These comparisons show the shifting trends within philosophy of science. From this table one can also surmise implications for the emergent development of new nursing theory.

Components of Science

The components of science, as defined by logical empiricists, are well documented in both the philosophical literature and the nursing literature. Logical empiricists attempt to understand science in terms of theories and the relationships among the components of a theory. A scientific theory is intended to systematically unify all the diverse phenomena of a particular discipline. The unification is achieved by encompassing descriptions of phenomena within an abstract set of statements known as a deductive system.

A deductive system is composed of three major components that are arranged in descending order of abstractness. First, the system's most abstract statements are its assumptions, which introduce the theory's basic concepts through the use of theoretical terms. Secondly, from these theoretical assumptions, propositions are deduced as part of the second level of abstraction. Together these assumptions and propositions systematically organize the entities and processes that presumably "lie behind" the observable phenomena. To

complete the theory it is necessary to bridge these principles to empirical generalizations. Toward this goal, bridge principles, still within the second level of abstraction, indicate how the theoretical entities and processes relate to empirical phenomena. Without these principles no empirical explanations or prediction would be possible and the system would be immune to empirical testing. Thirdly, these bridge principles in turn produce empirical generalizations within the lowest level of abstraction. In summary, the components of a scientific system, according to logical empiricists, are a set of statements that are systematically unified within a deductive system and that link theoretical concepts to empirically observable properties through the use of bridge principles (Braithwaite, 1953).

In contrast to the logical empiricists who attempt to understand science in terms of theories, historicists like Laudan (1977) attempt to understand science in terms of research traditions, each of which includes many theories. Although theories are seen by logical empiricists to be specific, short-lived, stable in formulation, and testable, historicists believe research traditions to be global, long-lived, and changeable within the boundaries of an acceptable ontological commitment.

By definition, a research tradition is a broadly based foundation of many theories and is an accepted way of viewing the fundamental phenomena within a discipline. It provides a global backdrop from which theories are constructed and evaluated through a set of guidelines for identifying the fundamental objects of a particular research tradition. Laudan does recognize, however, that the domains of science are not always clear; thus, classification of knowledge into a particular research tradition may be ambiguous. Every discipline has several research traditions, as illustrated by the nursing research traditions of holism and particularism. According to Laudan (1977), three specific components make up a research tradition: (a) specific theories, (b) ontological commitments, and (c) methodological commitments. Some of the specific theories within a given research tradition are new and others are modified versions of older theories that "fit" within the tradition. The function of any theory is to solve scientific problems within the discipline, from the perspective of the research tradition's, ontological commitments. If, for example, one ontological commitment of a research tradition is holism, various theories within this research tradition might address the problem of how to view the person as a holistic being without looking at parts.

In addition to specific theories and ontological commitments, the third component, methodological commitments, is also essential for a research tradition. Methodological commitments define the legitimate methods of inquiry and experimental procedures that are inseparably linked to a research tradition's ontology. To follow the logic of the above example, would not the case study method of inquiry better preserve the ontological commitment to holism than the elemental design method of inquiry with its built-in reductionism?

The components of a scientific system, according to historicists like Laudan, are multiple research traditions, each containing theories that produce a set of ontological viewpoints and methods of inquiry that are not only essentially compatible with the research tradition but also capable of solving problems within it.

Conception of Science

Based on this comparison of the components of science for logical empiricism and historicism, it is apparent that the two schools assume very different views about what science means. Logical empiricists do not understand science in terms of the human activities of working scientists (e.g., experimenting and compiling data). Instead, they conceive of science only in terms of the results of these activities. The term *science* refers only to a product; i.e., a set of statements that purportedly constitute the body of scientific knowledge. The product includes scientific terminology and definitions, propositions, hypotheses, theories, and laws. This conception of science as product rests on the philosophical goal of articulating the logical foundations of scientific knowledge (Rudner, 1966). Within this viewpoint, it is important to recognize that logical empiricists are not interested in how scientific hypotheses are conceived but rather in how they can be sufficiently supported by empirical evidence. Their emphasis is one of theory validation, not theory discovery (Rudner, 1966).

In contrast, historicists understand science as a process of human behavior and thought exhibited by practicing scientists. Historicists would be interested in different questions. What reasoning patterns do practicing scientists use to accept or reject a theory? To what extent are scientists influenced by the theory's empirical findings in contrast to the theory's logical elegance in such a decision? How do external factors such as religious convictions influence the scientist's decision-making judgments? To the historicist, every facet of the scientific process is subject to philosophical examination, including the process of explaining how fruitful theories are conceived by practicing scientists. With greater understanding of this process, historicists hope to develop models for future theory construction. Within this scientific viewpoint, valid data for theory construction include:

- the psychological factors of individual scientists
- the social forces on the community of scientists at a particular time
- the overall historical environment, especially the "nonscientific" influences on scientists.

Assessment of Scientific Progress

The assessment of scientific progress within the logical empiricist tradition rests on the ability to justify a scientific theory by examining the requirements for the theory's truth and the conditions of its falsehood. If a scientist can demonstrate the truth of a theory, the scientist has acquired scientific knowledge.

Certain criteria identify theory as false or true. Generally, if a theory's predictions are repeatedly disconfirmed, the logic of testing requires a rejection of the problematic dimensions of the theory, assuming that the observations are correct (Hempel, 1966). But logical empiricists have more difficulty explaining the method of proving that a theory is true. According to the logic of theory testing, no finite number of experiments can conclusively prove that a theory is true. If a theory passes many severe tests, it is only empirically confirmed; that is, the theory's probability of truth has increased. Therefore, to logical empiricists, scientific progress is assessed by the degree of probability that the theory is true, based on the number and severity of empirical tests it passes.

In addition, logical empiricists consider theoretical reduction an important scientific goal. In theoretical reduction, one theory can be absorbed by or reduced to some other inclusive theory. The philosophical advantage of reduction lies not only with the simplicity of fewer theoretical concepts and laws but also with the insight into the ultimate character of reality (Nagel, 1961).

For historicists, the question of whether philosophy of science should try to explain when, if ever, a theory is true or false is the subject of considerable debate. Many agree with Laudan (1977), who argues that philosophy should not search for distinguishing characteristics of true theories, primarily because practicing scientists rarely evaluate theories in terms of truth or falsity. The history of science includes many instances in which a theory was accepted even though it contained scientific anomalies or produced false experimental predictions. Conversely, some theories have been rejected even though they received the most empirical confirmation. Thus, Laudan argues that questions about truth are essentially irrelevant to scientific progress. The relevant element is the theory's problem-solving effectiveness; a theory's progress is defined by the degree to which it solves more scientific problems than its rivals. As stated by Laudan, *"the solved problem*—empirical or conceptual—*is the basic unit of scientific progress"* (Laudan, 1977, p. 66).

Historicists such as Laudan find reductionism counterproductive to the goal of solving scientific problems. Research traditions should not be seen as competitors trying to mutually undermine each other rather as collaborators toward the goal of solving scientific problems. This process of synthesizing research traditions, thus expanding them, is called the "integration of research traditions," according to Laudan (1977). Two ways in which this integration may occur are described:

1. One research tradition can be grafted onto another without any major modifications in the components of either.
2. Two or more research traditions may each sacrifice fundamental elements that have been refuted while combining their remaining elements in a new way.

An important scientific motivation for integrating research traditions is the goal of explaining different dimensions of the same phenomena under study. For example, in nursing, the integration of divergent research traditions from biology, psychology, and sociology can account for the ontological perspective that individuals are bio-psychosocial beings, which is common in nursing. This pattern of conjoining fundamental perspectives from different traditions is common when scientists develop new interdisciplinary fields of study to account for previously unexplained scientific problems. The integration of research traditions and corresponding theories is shown in Figure 16-1.

Laudan's analysis of integration departs significantly from the logical empiricist contention that science progresses through the elimination of theories by reduction. But the process of integration does not involve elimination by reducing one tradition to another, because both traditions retain their identity. Integration aims at extracting the progressive components of each tradition in a way that produces solutions to previously unsolved problems.

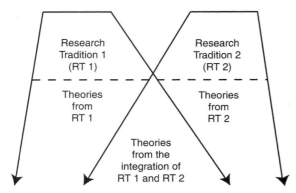

Figure 16-1 *A conceptualization of the integration of research traditions and corresponding theories within historicism.*

Goal of Philosophy of Science

According to logical empiricists, the ultimate goal of philosophy of science is to present a formalized account of the nature of scientific knowledge. This includes an application of logical principles to questions about the nature of science, since logic provides the eternal principles for relationships between scientific statements. By examining these relationships, the foundation of science is intended to systematically reveal the logical requirements for all scientific knowledge.

Historicists share with logical empiricists the belief that the philosopher's task is to construct a general account of the nature of scientific knowledge. But for historicists like Laudan, such a task must conform to the human elements of scientific evolution and growth. To meet this goal, historicists engage in studies of the actual activities, behavior patterns, and reasoning processes of working scientists. The belief is that philosophy of science must show how science, as it is actually practiced, can yield knowledge about the world. Such examination of the actual practice of scientists is used by historicists as evidence against logical empiricism, because the growth of scientific knowledge seems at times to be aided by illogical and nonrational decision making. It is believed that illogical processes can contribute to create growth of knowledge within a discipline.

Nursing Theory Development and Testing

Since 1964, nurse scholars have become more aware of the influences of philosophy—in particular philosophy of science—on the development of nursing theory. A review of significant and representative nursing theory literature within three time periods shows the status of nursing theory in regard to logical empiricist and historicist trends in philosophy of science.

1964 to 1969

An important influence on nursing theory development during the 1960s was support given by the Division of Nursing of the U.S. Department of Health, Education, and Welfare (now the Department of Health and Human Services) to nursing schools to sponsor programs on the nature and development of nursing science. An analysis of metatheoretical papers from the proceedings of two such conferences—the Symposium on Theory Development in Nursing held at Case Western Reserve University in 1968 and the Conference on the Nature of Science in Nursing held at the University of Colorado in 1969—gives insight into how nurse scholars and others during the late 1960s conceptualized the derivation of nursing knowledge.

In 1968, Dickoff and James presented a version of their position paper on a theory of theories, introducing the idea that significant nursing theory must be situation producing. Although they modified the orthodox view about the purpose of theory—that is, they postulated that theory could be capable of both more than and less than prediction—they, nevertheless, explicitly stated their faithfulness to the logical empiricist tradition. They forthrightly spoke of their work as a broader interpretation of the writings of such philosophers as Nagel (1961) and Hempel (1965, 1966). The language they used to describe theory supports logical empiricism. They spoke of concepts, propositions, set; they assessed scientific progress in terms of truth; and they insisted on a product orientation to science (i.e., production of desired situations).

In 1969, Abdellah discussed the nature of nursing science. Although no mention was made per se of the writings of philosophers who supported logical empiricism, Abdellah's views of what constitutes a scientific theory were nevertheless consistent with their writings; that is, terms must be operationally defined and preferably observable and quantifiable. Postulates are validated by testing deductions, which either helps to confirm the theory or leads to modifications of the postulates. Abdellah concludes that the reward of nurse scientists for their efforts is the discovery and affirmation of truth. Thus, as with Dickoff and James (1968), the criterion for the assessment of scientific progress is an increase in scientific truths.

Other writings (Dickoff, James, & Widenbach, 1968a, 1968b) related to nursing theory development and testing during the late 1960s all tended to have a logical empiricist perspective, with the exception of Leininger's (1969) introductory comments to the Conference on the Nature of Science in Nursing, which offered an ethnoscience research methodology to the discovery of scientific knowledge. This approach stresses the viewing of behavior from the subject's perspective rather than the researcher's. This accommodation to subjectivism is more compatible with historicism than with the objectivism of logical empiricism.

1970 to 1975

In the first half of the 1970s, two major trends in nursing theory occurred:

1. Metatheoretical formulations relevant to nursing theory and testing within the logical empiricist tradition were developed to a high degree by such investigators as Jacox (1974) and Hardy (1974).
2. A number of conceptual frameworks for nursing were published; for example, the work of Rogers (1970), King (1971), Orem (1971), and Roy (1974).

According to Jacox (1974), the goal of science is the discovery of truths, and the purpose of scientific theory is description, explanation, and prediction of part of our empirical world. In discussing theory construction, Jacox uses the language of the logical empiricists, including concepts, propositions, axioms, and theorems. Hardy (1974) is even more oriented to the formal logic

underlying logical empiricism, discussing nine possible relationships that can exist between concepts and presenting a diagrammatic and matrix presentation of a situation that shows (a) the concepts, (b) the sign of the relationship between concepts, and (c) the nature of the relationships between concepts.

These two articles represented a culmination of the metatheoretical notions about logical empiricism in nursing theory. The irony, of course, is that at the time these and similar reports were making a profound impact on the derivation of theory in nursing, the logical empiricist view-points espoused in them were being strongly repudiated by a growing number of philosophers of science. In other words, nursing's theoretical link to philosophy of science was, from the historicist perspective, about a decade behind the times.

The irony continues in regard to the second trend—the publication of a number of important conceptual frameworks for nursing. Several conceptual frameworks published in the early 1970s were essentially devoid of any explicit linkage to philosophy of science (King, 1971; Orem, 1971). This is in no way meant to diminish the quality or significance of these seminal works but only to point out that a situation existed in which the most influential nursing literature on theory construction and testing followed rather than preceded the derivation of the conceptual frameworks, apparently because the metatheoretical movement in nursing was, for the most part, a separate movement from the conceptual framework movement.

1976 to Present

Since 1976, the following trends have occurred:

1. a continued and relatively stable commitment to logical empiricism, although a beginning trend toward historicism is apparent;
2. a revision of several conceptual frameworks for nursing and the introduction of some new frameworks; and
3. a questioning of the adequacy of strictly quantitative research methods to test nursing theory deductions.

The relatively stable commitment to logical empiricism is reflected in the current writings of several nurse authors (Chinn & Jacobs, 1983; Fawcett, 1983; Menke, 1983; Walker & Avant, 1983). However, there are some new trends. For example, in 1979 when Newman introduced a new theory of health, the viewpoint was one of logical empiricism. However, in a recent work (1983), a shift in her thinking is evident. Reflecting the thoughts of Kuhn (a historicist), Newman defines science as "a process of knowing, a process of challenging, and a continuing revolution" (Newman, 1983, p. 387). This emphasis on process (not product) and revolution (not logic) is a noticeable shift in viewpoint from logical empiricism to historicism.

In a recent publication, Hardy (1983) also extensively cited Kuhn in discussing nursing theory. The primary emphasis is on metaparadigms; however, Hardy also seems to agree, at least implicitly, with Kuhn's definition of the development of scientific knowledge as both nonrational and noncumulative. This represents a marked shift in viewpoint from the 1974 Hardy article, which, of all the metatheoretical articles, represented the most rigorous and logically structured formulations in support of logical empiricism. These contradictions in the works of Hardy and other metatheorists are indicative of the pull between orthodox and new ideas in philosophy of science and in nursing theory development and testing.

Although several other nurse authors (Carper, 1978; MacPherson, 1983; Meleis, 1983; Menke, 1983; Munhall, 1982) briefly address Kuhn's *The Structure of Scientific Revolutions,* with the exception of Meleis (1983) they do not discuss Kuhn's more recent writings or mention Laudan's work, which represents the forefront of philosophy of science today. However, Laudan's work is briefly mentioned in an article by Watson (1981) and cited in the bibliographies of books by Parse (1981) and Chinn and Jacobs (1983). Although this attention to the work of Laudan is scant, it is encouraging because it begins to bring the development of nursing theory knowledge in line with current trends in philosophy of science.

The second trend occurring between 1976 and the present is the expansion and revision of the works of those nurse authors who in the early 1970s had developed conceptual frameworks for nursing. For example, first editions of books and other publications were rewritten, expanded, or revised by Orem (1980), King (1981), Roy (1981), Roy and Roberts (1981), and Rogers (1980). Several of these nurse theorists, in an attempt to bring their works more in line with what the nurse metatheorists of the mid-1970s were espousing—logical empiricism—revised their works to explicitly identify such elements as concepts and propositions that are inherent in the orthodox viewpoint.

Thus, an interesting situation has been created: While these nurse theorists have been updating trends in philosophy of science as espoused in the nursing literature of the mid-1970s, those who espoused these views have begun to question them and some no longer espouse them. This is not to say that individuals should not alter their viewpoints but to point out again the seeming separateness of the metatheoretical and conceptual framework movement in nursing and the effect of this separateness on perpetuating traditional or singular viewpoints about philosophy of science.

Two other conceptual frameworks were developed in books published in 1976 by Paterson and Zderad and in 1981 by Parse. Neither book has received much attention in the nursing literature, although there is some evidence that this is changing (Chinn & Jacobs, 1983; King 1981). Could it be that both of these books have a strong existential-phenomenological perspective that, until recently, was out of the mainstream of the thinking of orthodox nurse scientists about philosophy of science? The underlying assumptions these three authors hold about the nature of science are much more in keeping with nontraditional views about philosophy of science than with traditional views. In particular, they see science as process; they envision a strong link between the theory's ontological commitment and its methodological commitment; and they place little emphasis on precise, logical formulations.

The third trend is a shift in emphasis from quantitative to qualitative research methods to test nursing theory deduction. In the late 1970s, nurse scholars (Silva, 1977) began to question the limits of quantitative research methods because they too often sacrificed meaningfulness for rigor. Out of this questioning, articles suggesting alternative approaches to logical empiricism began to appear in the nursing literature (Munhall, 1982; Oiler, 1982; Omery, 1983; Swanson & Chenitz, 1982; Tinkle & Beaton, 1983; Watson, 1981). These approaches were sought because of the inadequacy of logical empiricism to deal with certain phenomena in nursing, in particular, those phenomena dealing with humanism and holism. By exploring alternative philosophies of science and research methodologies that are compatible, it seems possible to study these phenomena in a more meaningful and creative way and, in so doing, to help bridge the gaps among philosophies of science, nursing theory, and nursing research. Historicism is one of the alternative philosophies that holds promise in helping to bridge these gaps.

Implications and Recommendations for the Future

Since every scientific theory is tied to some philosophical framework as the basis for understanding and assessing theory, it is important for the theorists within a given discipline to be aware of the discipline's philosophical orientation. Therefore, nursing theorists should continue to explore the philosophical underpinnings of their discipline in order to integrate the latest advances in nursing theory development and testing with a coherent philosophical foundation.

This review of the trends in nursing theory from 1964 to the present shows not only that nursing theory is presently in a state of transition, but also that many of the changes in nursing theory reflect a reorientation of the underlying philosophy of the discipline. This is evident in the beginning metatheoretical shift away from a strongly empirical and logical orientation to theory construction reminiscent of logical empiricism and toward a more holistic and humanist approach more in line with historicism. There are several implications for nursing theory development and testing:

- Laudan dismisses as counterproductive the logical empirical goal of reducing one theory to another. Rather than trying to restrict the range of possible theories, Laudan encourages theory expansion through a process of integrating components from different research traditions, which results in a multidimensional understanding of the phenomena. Based on this historicist orientation, there should not be a single, conceptual framework for nursing. This orientation suggests, rather, the expansion of nursing theory through the integration of progressive components of the various existing nursing conceptual frameworks, which results in multiple frameworks. This process should be a cooperative endeavor and, if adhered to, should encourage a cooperative rather than a competitive attitude among nurse scholars. In the future some of the conceptual frameworks for nursing may be integrated so that the unimportant elements are sacrificed and the important elements are combined in a new way.

- The historicist's conception of science as a human process, rather than a product of some endeavor, suggests that nursing theory should always be understood as a stage in its evolution and growth. Although nursing theory is experiencing shifts in its evolution, the result of the transition will not be some final and static body of knowledge. Like any scientific discipline, nursing theory construction will never culminate in some static set of eternal truths but will represent one episode in its evolving history.

- Historicism strongly encourages a careful study of the actual practices, belief systems, and external factors influencing a community of scientists within a given discipline. This has a direct bearing on the type of data relevant for any theory construction. Thus, data for nursing theory development and testing will include the common practices of nurse clinicians, the social and psychological factors affecting the profession of nursing, the widely held beliefs of the community of nurses, and the reasoning patterns of individual nurse theorists. A result of integrating these data will be a nursing theory that more explicitly addresses the human dimensions of nursing and the practitioners of nursing.

- Scientific progress for Laudan reduces to the number of solved problems within a discipline. Therefore, the assessment of progress in nursing theory development and testing will be less rigid and more practical than suggested by a logical empiricist orientation. That is, there will be less emphasis on truth and error as the criteria for assessing scientific progress and more emphasis on the actual solution to nursing care problems. This shift should help to bridge the gap between those persons who are primarily nurse scholars and those who are primarily nurse clinicians. The clinician, of course, is in an ideal position to both understand and assess whether, and to what degree, a nursing care problem has been solved. Within this framework, the nurse clinician should be highly valued as an integral part of the process of nursing theory development and testing.

Based on the changing trends in philosophies of science and nursing theory, four recommendations are made:

1. Creation of liaisons between departments of nursing and departments of philosophy to help nurse scholars, theoreticians, researchers, and clinicians stay abreast of changes in philosophy of science;
2. Establishment of closer, cooperative working relationships among nurse metatheorists, theoreticians, researchers, and clinicians with a common goal of solving problems of significance in nursing;
3. Exploration of innovative, qualitative methods for testing nursing theory that are in keeping with the historicist tradition; and
4. Continued and explicit emphasis in nursing theory courses on the interrelationships among philosophies of science, nursing theory, and nursing research.

If the above recommendations are implemented, they should help to establish and maintain an open dialogue, which portends a healthy and promising future for the advancement of nursing science.

REFERENCES

Abdellah, F. G. (1969). The nature of nursing science. *Nursing Research, 18,* 390–393.

Ayer, A. J. (1959). Editor's introduction. In A. J. Ayer (Ed.), *Logical positivism* (pp. 3–28). New York: Free Press.

Braithwaite, R. B. (1953). *Scientific explanation: A study of the function of theory, probability and law in science.* London: Cambridge University Press.

Carper, B. A. (1978). Fundamental patterns of knowing in nursing. *Advances in Nursing Science, 1*(1), 13–23.

Chinn, P. L., & Jacobs, M. K. (1983). *Theory and nursing: A systematic approach.* St. Louis: C. V. Mosby.

Conference on the Nature of Science in Nursing (1969). *Nursing Research, 18,* 388–411.

Dickoff, J., & James, P. (1968). A theory of theories: A position paper. *Nursing Research, 17,* 197–203.

Dickoff, J., James, P., & Wiedenbach, E. (1968a). Theory in a practice discipline: Part I. Practice-oriented theory. *Nursing Research, 17,* 415–435.

Dickoff, J., James P., & Widenbach, E. (1968b). Theory in a practice discipline: Part II. Practice-oriented research. *Nursing Research, 17,* 545–554.

Fawcett, J. (1983). Hallmarks of success in nursing theory development. In P. L. Chinn (Ed.), *Advances in nursing theory development* (pp. 3–17). Rockville, MD: Aspen Systems.

Feyerabend, P. (1978). *Against method: Outline of an anarchistic theory of knowledge.* London: Verso.

Fitzpatrick, J. J., & Whall, A. L. (1983). *Conceptual models of nursing: Analysis and application.* Bowie, MD: Brady.

Hanson, N. R. (1958). *Patterns of discovery: An inquiry into the conceptual foundation of science.* London: The Syndics of the Cambridge University Press.

Hardy, M. E. (1974). Theories: Components, development, evaluation. *Nursing Research, 23,* 100–107.

Hardy, M. E. (1983). Metaparadigms and theory development. In N. L. Chaska (Ed.), *The nursing profession: A time to speak* (pp. 427–437). New York: McGraw-Hill.

Hempel, C. G. (1965). *Aspects of scientific explanation and other essays in the philosophy of science.* New York: Free Press.

Hempel, C. G. (1966). *Philosophy of natural science.* Englewood Cliffs, NJ: Prentice Hall.

Jacox, A. (1974). Theory construction in nursing: An overview. *Nursing Research, 23,* 4–13.

King, I. M. (1971). *Toward a theory for nursing: General concepts of human behavior.* New York: John Wiley & Sons.

King, I. M. (1981). *A theory for nursing: Systems concepts, process.* New York: John Wiley & Sons.

Kuhn, T. S. (1962). *The structure of scientific revolutions.* Chicago: The University of Chicago Press.

Kuhn, T. S. (1970). *The structure of scientific revolutions* (2nd ed.). Chicago: The University of Chicago Press.

Kuhn, T. S. (1977). Second thoughts on paradigms. In F. Suppe (Ed.), *The structure of scientific theory* (pp. 459–482). Urbana, IL: University of Illinois Press.

Lakatos, I. (1968). Changes in the problem of inductive logic. In I. Lakatos (Ed.), *The problem of inductive logic* (pp. 315–417). Amsterdam: North-Holland.

Laudan, L. (1977). *Progress and its problems: Toward a theory of scientific growth.* Berkeley, CA: University of California Press.

Leininger, M. M. (1969). Nature of science in nursing. *Nursing Research, 18,* 388–389.

MacPherson, K. I. (1983). Feminist methods: A new paradigm for nursing research. *Advances in Nursing Science, 5*(2), 17–25.

Meleis, A. I. (1983). A model for theory description, analysis, and critique. In N. L. Chaska (Ed.), *The nursing profession: A time to speak* (pp. 438–452). New York: McGraw-Hill.

Menke, E. M. (1983). Critical analysis of theory development in nursing. In N. L. Chaska (Ed.), *The nursing profession: A time to speak* (pp. 416–426). New York: McGraw-Hill.

Munhall, P. L. (1982). Nursing philosophy and nursing research: In apposition or opposition? *Nursing Research, 31,* 176–177, 181.

Nagel, E. (1961). *The structure of science: Problems in the logic of scientific explanation.* New York: Harcourt Brace & World.

Newman, M. A. (1979). *Theory development in nursing.* Philadelphia: F. A. Davis.

Newman, M. A. (1983). The continuing revolution: A history of nursing science. In N. L. Chaska (Ed.), *The nursing profession: A time to speak* (pp. 385–393). New York: McGraw–Hill.

Oiler, C. (1982). The phenomenological approach in nursing research. *Nursing Research, 31,* 178–181.

Omery, A. (1983). Phenomenology: A method for nursing research. *Advances in Nursing Science, 5*(2), 49–63.

Orem, D. E. (1971). *Nursing: Concepts of practice.* New York: McGraw-Hill.

Orem, D. E. (1980). *Nursing: Concepts of practice* (2nd ed.). New York: McGraw-Hill.

Parse, R. R. (1981). *Man-living-health: A theory of nursing.* New York: John Wiley & Sons.

Paterson, J. G., & Zderad, L. T. (1976). *Humanistic nursing.* New York: John Wiley & Sons.

Rogers, M. E. (1970). *An introduction to the theoretical basis of nursing.* Philadelphia: F. A. Davis.

Rogers, M. E. (1980). Nursing: A science of unitary man. In J. P. Riehl & C. Roy (Eds.), *Conceptual models for nursing practice* (2nd ed.) (pp. 329–337). New York: Appleton-Century-Crofts.

Roy, C. (1974). The Roy adaptation model. In J. P. Riehl & C. Roy (Eds.), *Conceptual models for nursing practice* (pp. 135–144). New York: Appleton-Century-Crofts.

Roy, C. (1981). *Introduction to nursing: An adaptation model.* Englewood Cliffs, NJ: Prentice-Hall.

Roy, C., & Roberts, S. L. (1981). *Theory construction in nursing: An adaptation model.* Englewood Cliffs, NJ: Prentice-Hall.

Rudner, R. S. (1966). *Philosophy of social science.* Englewood Cliffs, NJ: Prentice-Hall.

Scheffler, I. (1963). *The anatomy of inquiry: Philosophical studies in the theory of science.* New York: Knopf.

Silva, M. C. Philosophy, science, theory: Interrelationships and implications for nursing research. *Image, 9,* 59–63.

Swanson, J. M., & Chenitz, W. C. (1982). Why qualitative research in nursing? *Nursing Outlook, 30,* 241–245.

Symposium on Theory Development in Nursing (1968). *Nursing Research, 17,* 196–222.

Tinkle, M. B., & Beaton, J. L. (1983). Toward a new view of science: Implications for nursing research. *Advances in Nursing Science, 5*(2), 27–36.

Toulmin, S. (1972). *Human understanding* (Vol. 1). Princeton, NJ: Princeton University Press.

Walker, L. O., & Avant, K. C. (1983). *Strategies for theory construction in nursing.* Norwalk, CT: Appleton-Century-Crofts.

Watson, J. (1981). Nursing's scientific quest. *Nursing Outlook, 29,* 413–416.

Reaction . . .

Nursing Theory Development: Another Look

To the Editor:

    In their article, "An Analysis of Changing Trends in Philosophies of Science on Nursing Theory Development and Testing" (*Advances in Nursing Science 6*(2), January 1984), Silva and Rothbart conducted a historical analysis of the development of nursing theories that contrasted with the changing philosophies of science from 1964 to the present. Although their analysis is interesting, it leaves the reader suspended regarding their opinion on why these trends occurred and whether they should be considered aberrant behavior or developmentally expected. The authors are clearly advocating a historical approach to the basis of nursing theory, but their treatment of external factors responsible for the devotion of nurse researchers to logical empiricism is not convincing.

    One must first examine the rationale on which theory building was based and ask why it was constructed on the altar of positivism. If one looks at the beginning nursing theorists, it becomes apparent that they felt a theory must have some reality base (Abdellah, 1969; Johnson, 1959). They sought ideas that would be clearly explainable in the everyday observations of nursing care. Taking cues from the biomedical model, they attempted to ground theory in observations, trying to find or discover nursing truths.

That is still a sticking point today. Are there priority nursing principles that data collectors such as Benner (1984) may yet find? This is not to endorse total devotion to empirics, but a large anomaly has developed in that we are devoting much time to theory development without adequate data collection. It must be understood that, in a developing discipline, it was easier to justify spending time and money on classic methods rather than on trying to solve as-yet undefined problems.

One note of caution regarding the historical approach is that it requires a careful study of external factors. A reality is that, as doctoral programs—the profession's breeding ground for young researchers—increase in number, most teaching will continue to be done by faculty steeped in quantitative methodology. Faculty teaching in doctoral programs are people who have little background in qualitative versus quantitative research. The result will be continued emphasis on logical positivism in nursing.

Meleis (1985) has a valid criticism with which I agree. What dictates that nursing must follow the tradition of philosophy of sciences? This question deserves consideration. Nursing theory is not necessarily subject to the laws of the hard sciences. Instead, macrotheorists must examine what nursing is and ask: is it a science, an art, or neither? Observers of nursing progress must also assess how that profession embraces or relinquishes its theories. In a community in which its researchers are separated by a wide gap from its practitioners, the observer must choose carefully when deciding what factors influence its frameworks. Are nursing theorists creating new frameworks or just describing frameworks that fit the observable phenomena?

Studying the development of nursing theory is fascinating but can be hazardous to one who relies on traditional referent points of scientific progress. One must be careful to take into account the distinctiveness of the nursing perspective and the unique approach nursing may use to articulate its place among the disciplines.

JOHN G. TWOMEY, JR., RN, MS
Doctoral Student in Nursing
University of Virginia
Charlottesville, Virginia
1984

REFERENCES

Abdellah, F. G. (1969). The nature of nursing science. *Nursing Research, 18,* 390–393.

Benner, P. (1984). *From novice to expert: Excellence and power in clinical nursing.* Reading, MA: Addison-Wesley.

Johnson, D. E. (1959). A philosophy of nursing. *Nursing Outlook, 7,* 198–200.

Meleis, A. (1985). *Theoretical nursing: Development and progress.* Philadelphia: J. B. Lippincott.

The Authors Comment

An Analysis of Changing Trends in Philosophies of Science on Nursing Theory Development and Testing

The ideas for this article arose when Dr. Silva was introduced to logical empiricism as the accepted mode of scientific inquiry, which she found limiting. Because every discipline has more than one point of view that changes with time, Dr. Silva asked Dr. Rothbart what major shifts had occurred in the philosophy of science during the decade before publishing this article. In reviewing writings from nursing, Dr. Rothbart revealed that nursing had a somewhat outdated philosophic emphasis on logical empiricism. He went on to describe historicism and the profound effect it could have on constructing nursing theory and research methods. Although philosophy of science has continued to change, the historicist views of Kuhn, Laudan, and others continue to influence how nursing and other disciplines practice their science.

—MARY CIPRIANO SILVA
—DANIEL ROTHBART

CHAPTER 17

A Non-Theorist's Perspective on Nursing Theory: Issues of the 1990s

Freda G. DeKeyser
Barbara Medoff-Cooper

The basis of all nursing endeavors, including practice and research, lies in theory. While nursing theo-rists are postulating and debating, practicing nurses are continuing with their daily routines and are often unaware that the world of nursing theory is changing. It is important, however, for all nurses to keep abreast of the latest developments in nursing theory. This article discusses some of the key develop-ments within nursing theory based on a review of the nursing literature from 1990 through 1999.

The basis of all nursing endeavors, including practice and research, lies in theory. While nursing theorists are postu-lating and debating, practicing nurses are continuing with their daily routines and are often unaware that the world of nursing theory is changing. It is important for all nurses to keep abreast of the latest developments in nursing theory. As Fawcett (1999) points out, "Many disciplines exist to generate, test and apply theories that will improve the qual-ity of people's lives. Every such theory-development effort is based on a particular frame of reference that provides an intellectual and socio-historical context for theoretical thinking, for research, and ultimately, for practice" (p. 1). Theory development is then seen as a basis for the advance-ment of research as well as practice. Few studies have in-vestigated attitudes of practicing nurses toward nursing the-ory. A study conducted in 1991 (Laschinger) found that 367 Canadian staff nurses considered nursing theory devel-opment and its use important to the advancement of the nursing profession. While this study is rather old, no other study was found which asked staff nurses their attitudes to-ward nursing theory. Laschinger concludes that the cadre of nurses familiar with theory-based nursing practice will

From Scholarly Inquiry for Nursing Practice: An International Journal, *15(4), pp. 329-341. Copyright © 2001, Springer Publishing Company. Used with permission.*

About the Authors

FREDA DEKEYSER was born in New York. She received her BSN from New York University, MA and PhD from the University of Maryland at Baltimore, and a Postdoctoral Fellowship from Johns Hopkins University. Dr. DeKeyser's clinical area is critical care. Her research also focuses on critical care, as well as psychoneuroimmunology. Several years ago, Dr. DeKeyser moved with her family to Jerusalem, Israel, where she was appointed coordinator of nursing research of a new clinical master's program, the first one in Israel. She has actively worked toward advancing the academic level of research among nurses, as well as advancing the awareness of nurses and fellow health care practitioners toward nursing research, especially clinically based research.

BARBARA MEDOFF-COOPER was born in Philadelphia at the Hospital of the University of Pennsylvania. Her education includes a BSN from the College of New Jersey, an MS in pediatric nursing from the University of Maryland, and a PhD in educational psychology/child development research from Temple University. Dr. Medoff-Cooper was a Robert Wood Johnson Clinical Nurse Scholar at the University of Pennsylvania and then joined the faculty as an assistant professor. Currently, she is the Helen M. Shearer Professor of Nutrition and the Director for the Center for Nursing Research in the School of Nursing, University of Pennsylvania. Her program of research has focused on the neurobehavioral development of high-risk infants, which has included both feeding behaviors and infant temperament. Dr. Medoff-Cooper's two key contributions to the discipline are the Early Infancy Temperament Questionnaire and the development of feeding norms for both high-risk and healthy neonates.

only increase due to the increased numbers of nursing programs including nursing theory in their curriculum. This reported increase in exposure to nursing theory is even more appropriate today, more than 10 years later.

The purpose of this article is not to teach or review nursing theory. It is assumed that the reader has some general knowledge of nursing theory and its importance to nursing. Instead this discussion is aimed at exposing the reader to some, not all, of the issues which concerned authors who wrote about nursing theory over the previous decade. This article addresses some of the key developments within nursing theory based on a review of the nursing literature from 1990 through 1999. The authors are not nurse theorists themselves but rather nurses who base their practice and research on contemporary nursing theory. Therefore, it is anticipated that this discussion will be useful and accessible to a wide range of nurses.

A Medline and CINAHL search was performed on articles published between January 1990 and December 1999 which referred to nursing theory. Many issues related to nursing theory were presented in the literature. It is beyond the scope of this article to review all of the literature published during the 1990's dealing with nursing theory. Topics which were more commonly discussed and/or had relevance to practicing nurses were chosen for review and discussion. Some of the issues discussed are controversies that have been debated for several decades; others are new areas of discussion. The controversial areas discussed are: is nursing theory dead?; unique as opposed to borrowed theory in nursing; and the theory-practice gap. Newer issues discussed are the use of philosophy as opposed to theory; types of knowing; and changes in the metaparadigm of nursing.

Continuing Controversies

Is Nursing Theory Dead?

Over the decade of the '90s nursing theory seemed to take an increasingly smaller role in the content of nursing schools' curricula and in the literature. It seemed that nursing theory was "out" and possibly even dead. Theories that are dead are those that lie on a shelf somewhere, in some journal or book, without being used or applied. Several reasons cited in an article by Nolan, Lundh, and Tishman (1998) for the disenchantment with nursing theory are: that theories were considered too abstract and general; grand theories attempted to explain everything while explaining nothing; and there was little empirical evidence to back theories up. Most nurses had exposure to such nursing theory in their undergraduate courses and were expected to uncritically accept theories that did not necessarily agree with traditional nursing values such as holism and attention to cultural needs (Whall, 1993).

According to Fawcett (1999), nursing models and theories are by definition abstract and general and, therefore, cannot meet clinicians' expectations for concrete prescriptions directed toward the solution of problems. Grand nursing theories were developed thoughtfully, using creative intellectual leaps in order to go beyond existing knowledge. They were not based on empirical research (Fawcett, 1999). Consequently, many nurses became disappointed by the grand theories.

Due to these arguments, many abandoned the use of grand theory or conceptual models and a movement began which stressed the intuitive side of nursing, a "know how" rather than a "know that" approach. This movement is reflected in the development of theories such as that of Benner (1984) that led to a more practice-based approach rather than a purely theoretical one (Nolan, Lundh, & Tishelman, 1998). Theory derived from practice is based on the Heidegerrian view that actions are more basic than thinking. This approach reflects the presence of embodied intelligence; people learn at an unconscious level by doing instead of at a conscious level by thinking. This view is in contrast to that of Descartes, who claimed that we know the world through observation and that we consciously place these observations into mental representations by thinking (Ward, 1993). This new approach is philosophically different from that of the traditional nursing theories. Previous nursing theorists observed their nursing world and then designed their theories based on their use of reason. For example, Betty Neuman logically derived her Health Care Systems Model

(1972) from her observations as a nurse and nurse educator. These new approaches, similar to that of Benner, do not focus on conclusions based on reasoning alone but on the experience itself.

Another response to the grand theories or conceptual models was the introduction and incorporation of middle-range theories. Middle-range theories are made up of a limited number of concepts and are written at a relatively concrete and specific level. Unlike grand theories, middle-range theories are generated and tested by means of empirical research (Fawcett, 1999). These types of theories are thought to be more useful in everyday practice (Nolan, Lundh, & Tishelman, 1998), possibly due to their lower level of abstraction and greater substance (Lenz, Pugh, Milligan, Gift & Suppe, 1997). Cody (1997a) categorizes middle-range theories as incipient nursing theories. Others (e.g., Liehr & Smith, 1999) state that middle-range theories are extremely appropriate for the current historical context that calls for the development of a knowledge base supported by art and science as well as by practice and research. An example of a middle-range theory in nursing is the theory of unpleasant symptoms (Lenz, Pugh, Milligan, Gift, & Suppe, 1997).

While it is possible to conclude that nursing as a discipline has moved away from the use of grand theories or conceptual models, there are some who carry on the work of individual grand theorists such as Rogers or Orem. Some claim that middle-range theories can be developed from these grand theories thereby making the grand theories more "user friendly" (Fawcett, 1999). Others see grand theories or conceptual models as the means by which practitioners can develop systematic reasoning and as a tool to develop a sense of collective self for the discipline of nursing (Kozol-McLain & Maeve, 1993). Grand theory has been described as a method to help nurses find the trees, while middle-range and other less abstract theories are used to describe more details such as the reason the leaves grow in a certain pattern (Oberst, 1995). Finally, some are concerned with the rapidity with which nursing has adapted to changes in the economic market place versus the extremely slow adaptation of the field to changes in theory and philosophy (Cody, 1997b).

In summary, while the majority of articles reviewed tended to devalue the use of grand theories at this time, there are still major supporters of such theories. In addition, middle-range theories and other less abstract schools of thought have revitalized the development of nursing theory. In the long run, the issue of whether nursing theory is dead or alive is less important than whether nurses can incorporate theory into their daily lives. This is possible whether the theory is at the grand or middle-range levels. Many nurses, usually as students, learn, think about, and eventually internalize conceptual models and nursing grand theories. These thoughts get filtered and modified through the prism of experience. Nurses in clinical practice may find themselves in a specific situation and reflect that the situation reminds them of a nursing theory or conceptual model. For example, a pediatric nurse might find him- or herself confronting issues related to control with a 2-year-old and with a 15-year-old. The 2-year-old might want to play with a specific toy only when the toy is unavailable. The 2-year-old wants to control the environment and be able to play with the desired toy when she wants to play with it. A 15-year-old might want to smoke cigarettes in his room despite rules against it. He wants to control his actions and be able to do what he wants to do where he wants to do it. While these two behavioral issues look similar, they are actually quite different. Martha Rogers (1970) describes such situations within the concept of helicy. Certain situations may appear to be the same with similar characteristics but because space-time moves forward and there is no going back, these situations are inherently different. Therefore, specific clinical situations can shed light on the most abstract concepts and theories. Middle-range theories are used often as the theoretical basis for many research studies. For example, the middle-range theory of Psychoneuroimmunology has been used by one of the authors in her research (DeKeyser, Wainstock, Rose, Converse, & Dooley, 1998). Psychoneuroimmunology theory describes interactions between psychosocial factors and the neurological and immune systems. This theory has direct bearing on the nature of the author's research. For example, Psychoneuroimmunology theory suggests that stress and anxiety impact on immune function. Several research studies were conducted by the author which attempted to evaluate this interaction. Therefore, we personally find that while grand theories and conceptual models influence our way of thinking about nursing in general, middle-range theories can be more easily applied to our work on a day-to-day basis.

Unique Versus Borrowed Theory

There is an ongoing debate as to whether nurses should use only theories that are developed by nurses or whether it is of value to borrow theories from other disciplines and adapt these theories to nursing. An example of a borrowed theory is the use of Self-Efficacy Theory to describe many nursing-related phenomena. For example, Chever and Hardin (1998) evaluated the effects of traumatic events, social support and self-efficacy on adolescents' self-health assessments. Self-Efficacy Theory, however, though widely used in nursing research, was developed by Bandura (1977), a psychologist.

Those who take the more conservative approach, refusing to accept external theories, cite several reasons for their stand. One argument is that only nursing science can describe the phenomena of nursing (Phillips, 1996). Also, non-critical acceptance of theories from other disciplines has led to the potential for overlooking the cultural needs of clients as well as the acceptance of values which may be contrary to nursing (Whall, 1993). Cody (1996a) adds that theories from varying sources do not necessarily coincide with one another. Northrup (1992) states that nursing theories need to be placed within a larger context that is consistent with the values of knowing nursing. The use of borrowed theory makes the foundation of nursing into a grab bag where nurses have minor knowledge of many theories but have in-depth knowledge of none, thus making nurses into the Jack or Jill of all trades and master of none (Cody, 1996a). Some maintain that the empirical gains won, such as advances in clinical practice, are offset by the conceptual losses brought about by compromise (Northrup, 1992). One author commented how ironic it is that many disciplines have called for interdisciplinary theory and research yet only nursing is willing to leave its roots to accomplish this (Cody, 1997a). Practically speaking, when nurses are constantly borrowing from other disciplines they have less energy to devote to sustaining, growing and developing their own (Cody, 1996a).

While still in its early stages, nursing needed to establish itself as a unique discipline, separate from others such as medicine and to develop its unique knowledge base in order to achieve academic and professional status (Cody, 1996a; Nolan, Lundh, & Tishelman, 1998). Nurses were trained to do (i.e., to practice nursing) and not to know. What nurses needed to know they learned from other disciplines and so became more familiar with these (Cody, 1996a). Northrup (1992) suggests that when nursing began to develop as a discipline it borrowed from others; however, she states that with continuing research nursing will develop to be unique. One example of this development is cited by Cody (1997b) who stated that theory-based guides for practice have been created over the previous decades that are unique to nursing science and distinct from other sciences. These purists, therefore, believe that while initially nursing theorists were forced to borrow from other fields, with time nursing theory will develop without the influence of other disciplines.

On the other hand, other authors claim that nursing cannot develop independently and use only its unique theory due to historical as well as practical reasons. The original nurse scientists received their academic training in fields other than nursing. They learned the tools necessary to build theory and research in those other fields. These tools were those of the home discipline (Cody, 1996a; Monti & Tingen, 1999). Nurse educators have handed down these tools to subsequent generations of nurse scientists. As a result, many nurse scientists have been trained to borrow and incorporate theories from other fields.

Another view is that nursing cannot develop its own theory because nursing deals with the complexity of humans. This wish for a unique theory can be called "physics envy." In physics, a pure basic science, it is possible to develop theories unique to the discipline. Theories dealing with the complexity and variability of humans, however, must draw upon more than one discipline (Levine, 1995).

Finally, others state that theories are relevant to nursing if they relate to nursing and the source of the theory is irrelevant. Oberst (1995) contends that as long as a theory helps nurses solve nursing problems, the theory is applicable and useful and thereby helps the discipline progress. Its origin is of little consequence. Nursing can be viewed as unique if it uses knowledge in a unique manner (Nolan, Lundh, & Tishelman, 1998). Booth, Kenrick and Woods (1997) strongly adhere to the conception of knowledge as a "web of belief" as described by Quine. According to this view, knowledge consists of various elements interconnected like a spider's web. The web is anchored where reality converges with beliefs through experiences. Experience is seen as the testing ground for knowledge. Therefore, the knowledge and experiences of other disciplines which are associated with nursing could be accommodated within the 'web' of nursing knowledge without compromising the core of nursing.

We agree with the position of Sims as cited by Timpson (1996) that knowledge gained from borrowed theories is changed once used within the context of the nursing discipline. The borrowed knowledge can eventually emerge as nursing theory because it is used in a way unique to nursing. Both of the present authors have used borrowed theories as the basis for their research (for example, Medoff-Cooper, McGrath, & Bilker, 2000). In both our cases theories from other disciplines, biology and psychology, have added to the richness of the theoretical underpinnings of our programs of research and allowed for a more operational/direct use of theory. As researchers and practitioners, we agree with the position that knowledge cannot be owned by one discipline or another. What makes a discipline unique is not only what problems it addresses but how it addresses, as well as solves, those problems with the knowledge it has.

Theory Practice Gap

During the 1990s and for many years before that, there was a heightened awareness in the nursing literature of the gap between nursing theory and practice. Differences between the language used to describe practice as opposed to the language of theory have been one major cause noted for this gap (Levine, 1995; Tolley, 1995). Another reason cited is that the people who develop theories have for the most part not been practitioners. Clinical nurses have not historically developed nursing theory and that trend continues to this day (Tolley, 1995). In a call for increased attention to nursing science in advanced practice graduate curricula, Huch (1995) states that students need more than one theory course to be able to apply theory to practice. Levine (1995) states that many practicing nurses were trained by those who believed that there was a chasm between practice and theory. Therefore curricula were developed such that theory and clinical practice were taught in courses independent of one another.

Engebretson (1997) adds that an understanding of the theory-practice gap can be informed by the dichotomy between medicine and nursing. Nursing theory has traditionally been developed within nursing academia, while nursing practice has dwelled within the medical model. These conflicting world views have contributed to the gap.

Some authors caution the developers of nursing diagnoses. They predict a similar progression to the one that occurred in the development of nursing theory. Many theorists designed their own language or words to describe nursing when developing their nursing theories, thereby making theory inaccessible to many. While there is a need to establish the uniqueness of nursing, at the same time these theorists may be isolating nursing by creating a language that is idiosyncratic (Nolan, Lundh, & Tishelman, 1998). In addition, practicing nurses utilize diagnoses, interventions and outcome classification systems. They deal with the specific details or "the parts." The concept of holism, however, is very prevalent among nurse theorists. Therefore, according to this view many clinical practices are incongruent with theoretical holism (Engebretson, 1997).

Some disagree with the usefulness of practice theory in general (Koziol-McLain & Maeve, 1993). They state that a theory that defines or delineates practice is by its very nature a prescriptive theory. These types of theories are problematic because the clinical environ-

ment is constantly changing. By accepting a theory, one has, in essence, accepted a stable structure that does not exist in a realistic setting.

A recent development associated with the theory-practice gap is the inclusion of action research in nursing. Action research is thought to be a means of narrowing the theory-practice gap by researching clinical problems and introducing improvements based on the research into practice (Clark, 2000). It involves four major characteristics; collaboration between researchers and practitioners, a solution of practical problems, change in practice and the development of theory. It contains three major phases, the first being a fact-finding phase where a goal or action intention is defined. This phase also includes observations to discover the true theoretical nature of the situation. The second, or action, phase, involves an action or intervention where data are collected to help achieve the designated goal. Each action taken is part of a larger plan to bring about a specific change. Activities can be either practical or theoretical. The third phase is that of evaluation. Action research simultaneously attempts to implement a practical change while generating an action theory (Greenwood, 1994). An action theory is then developed that is prescriptive and situation specific. Therefore, action research is both practical and theoretical. It attempts to solve clinical problems and then develops theories based on an evaluation of the problem and the attempts at solving it.

Theory by its very nature is abstract. Practice by its very nature is not. Therefore, an inherent gap must exist between theory and practice. Perhaps, then, the problem is not that there is a gap between theory and practice but our expectations of what theory can do for us as practitioners. Perhaps we as practitioners should see theory as a guide and not as a prescription. Theory cannot tell us what to do in a specific situation but it can be used in clinical practice as a general guide to help us channel our thinking. In turn, clinicians should learn to abstract the lessons they have learned from their practice. Here is the opportunity for clinicians to translate lessons learned from practice into theory and thereby contribute to the discipline of nursing as well as to nursing theory development.

New Issues

The phrase, "There is nothing new under the sun," can certainly be applied to the discussions of nurse theorists. While controversy around the issues related above has been prominent in the nursing literature for a while, there are several issues which while not new, have gained increased attention during the 1990s.

Nursing Philosophy Versus Theory

An interesting shift in thought is the movement from discussions about theories of nursing to more recent discussions about the philosophy of nursing. Brunk (1995) describes theory development in nursing as progressing through several stages. The first involved defining the domain of nursing. The second and third phases were the mechanical aspects and conceptual development of nursing phenomena. More recently, philosophical discussions about the nature of nursing have been published. Edwards (1997) states that philosophy of nursing contains three components:

1. Conceptual clarification and assessment of arguments;
2. Consideration of traditional philosophical problems which have relevance to nursing theory and practice; and,
3. A focus on the framework of propositions which constitute nursing discourse and on the concepts from which those propositions are comprised.

Northrup (1992) has suggested that the nursing literature has blurred the distinction between philosophy and theory. Philosophy is concerned with inquiries into the nature of reality, what nursing should be (Northrup, 1992). Philosophical issues are related to a perspective on life. Such perspectives sometimes resemble those of the grand theories such as those of Rogers (1970). Theory, on the other hand, clarifies a domain of a discipline while describing, explaining, predicting or controlling. It has been recommended that future knowledge development in nursing concentrate on philosophies of nursing as opposed to theories of nursing (Koziol-McLean & Maeve, 1993).

Uys and Smit (1994) caution nurses against confusing two different concepts related to philosophy and nursing. They discriminate between "a philosophy of nursing" and "philosophy of nursing." "A philosophy of nursing" refers to a set of beliefs, principles and values which can direct practice while "philosophy of nursing" is a theoretical analysis. The "philosophy of nursing" endeavor is used to define the object of study within the discipline and limit it, analyze basic questions and concepts, and criticize its ideology. "A philosophy of nursing" can, and perhaps should, be held and elucidated by every individual nurse as something personal. "Philosophy of nursing" is not personal but rather is an "objective" evaluation of the discipline of nursing as a source of knowledge.

This more recent trend in theoretical writing has great promise for nurse theoreticians, practitioners and researchers. It is not our view that further development of nursing theories should be stopped. We have a sense, however, that a common philosophy, as opposed to a theory of nursing, might be more accepted and reach a more common consensus among nurses. It seems that nurses can agree, more or less, as to what nursing should contain. Perhaps a further delineation of not only the philosophy of nursing but also of a philosophy of nursing would be of use.

Types of Knowing

Another recent development is the movement from purely abstract theories to those with greater direct clinical relevance. A re-emphasis on a classic article by Carper (1978) has emerged (for example, as described in Cody, 1996b; Koziol-McLain, & Maev, 1993; Nolan, Lundh, & Tishelman, 1998; Rose & Parker, 1994; Tolley, 1995). In her article, Carper describes four ways of knowing related to clinical knowledge. The four ways include: empirics, esthetics, personal knowledge, and moral knowledge. Empirics deal with the science, while esthetics focuses on the art of nursing. Esthetics can only be expressed. It cannot be published or written down and only the client receiving nursing care can observe this form of knowledge. Personal knowledge involves knowledge of the self. This is tacit knowledge that is difficult to teach but is basic to nursing practice. This type of knowledge is the basis of interactions with clients and makes these interactions more reciprocal in nature. Personal knowledge cannot be described. It can only be actualized. Moral knowledge is concerned with the ethics of nursing. The legitimization of all types of knowledge and the attempt to set them on an equal level with empirical knowledge was the theoretical basis for movements such as practice-based theories and action theories.

Cody (1996b) claims that the major impact of Carper's work was to stress that knowledge in nursing can be gained from sources other than those that are empirical or scientific. Cody also suggests that a major aspect of Carper's work is that these sources of knowledge are interrelated and dynamic.

Nolan, Lundh, and Tishelman (1998) cite the increasing popularity of Carper's theory as evidence of the widening gap between theory and practice. They state that nurses have used the theory to advance the importance of the "art" of nursing, or nursing practice, over the "science" of nursing or nursing theory.

As practitioners and researchers, we have experienced these types of knowing and agree with their importance to nursing. We hope, however, that these categories will lead to the advancement of nursing knowledge and not become a weapon to be used by one side in a theoretical debate.

Changes in the Meta-Paradigm of Nursing

The meta-paradigm of nursing has also shifted over the past decade. While each theorist can be associated with a specific interpretation of the four main concepts of the field—person, health, environment and nursing—new aspects related to these concepts have emerged. A summary of these changes is provided by Thorne and colleagues, (1998). These authors point out that for much of nursing's history the patient's body was the primary focus. In the 1970s the holistic movement impacted nursing such that a more holistic view of the person was more accepted. Other more recent theorists, however, de-emphasized the physical body and felt that the entire energy field or lived experience was more important.

Another concept shift is related to the increased emphasis on health promotion and illness prevention. This perspective includes illness as a personal experience.

While health is still considered within nursing theories to be the intended outcome of nursing actions, other nursing outcomes have emerged, such as quality of life. The authors of this review also point to the surroundings between different conceptualizations of health. Some view health as an aspect or dimension of a person which is a normative state or process. Others view health as a reflection of the whole person and not just one aspect. Health has also been viewed from a social critical theory standpoint. According to this approach, nurses must take into account the unique criteria by which people evaluate their own lives and circumstances. What might be considered healthy for one person might be sick for another. What might be considered as a health care decision born of free will for one might be considered forced or denied by another.

While most nursing theories have stated that the environment is important, in fact many deal only with the person and not the society. In keeping with more modern views, it was suggested that the nursing environment should be defined as a multi-layered construct. Two conceptualizations of the environment were also summarized. The environment can be seen as contiguous and inseparable from the person. The other view is that the environment is the surroundings or circumstances of the individual to which the person must adapt. In the first case the person and the environment are essentially one, while in the second, they are connected yet separate.

Finally, the view of the role of the nurse has come into question. The movement to formalize nursing diagnoses, as well as the traditional role of the nurse, has defined the nurse as an expert who helps clients achieve optimal health care. This view is in contrast to the consumer movement that has empowered clients to become experts themselves using media such as the internet. There also exists a conflict between the social mandate of the nurse which is "to do" as opposed to the role of the nurse as viewed by others, to simply "be there." This last conflict relates to whether nurses should be active caregivers or be more passive and allow clients to take the active role in their health care.

It has been suggested (Thorne et al., 1998) that caring be added to "the big four" concepts of nursing. The concept of caring is an attempt to define nursing's unique place in the health care world. This attempt also helps to decrease the theory-practice gap by making theory more meaningful to those practitioners who do their caring in a very technological environment. While the concept of caring is important to nursing, disagreements have arisen as to its place within nursing. Is caring nurse-centered? Patient-centered? Or both? Others stated that the caring debate was distracting nurses from finding the real boundaries of nursing. Caring is the domain of many roles and is not unique to nursing. Therefore why should nursing take on this concept as its own? The last argument against emphasizing the concept of caring in nursing is a political one. In a society that does not value caring, and in fact devalues it because of its association with gender, it is not wise for nurses to position themselves as the primary providers of caring. The role of caring within the framework of nursing remains rather controversial.

Summary

Many of the issues discussed over the past decade related to nursing theory are a continuation of those addressed previously while several have begun to cover new ground. It is safe to say that nursing theory is not dead. It remains an essential component of research and practice. As the discipline has matured, the focus of theory development has changed to more realistically reflect the practice and research environment. There is a place within the discipline of nursing for borrowed theory that can be adapted to our profession. There is no doubt, however, that theory unique to nursing provides the perspective necessary for nursing inquiry and practice. Theory is becoming more integrated into practice in many environments but there is much work to be done to narrow the theory-practice gap.

New ways of exploring old issues within the discipline have been advanced, such as action research and the various ways of knowing. More recent approaches to the meta-paradigm of nursing have moved from the more abstract to realistically reflect issues such as health promotion and disease prevention as well as the political reality. In conclusion, can theorists and non-theorists talk to one another? We believe that they can and that doing so will advance the art and science of nursing.

REFERENCES

Bandura, A. (1977). Self-efficacy: Toward a unifying theory of behavioral change. *Psychological Review, 84,* 1911–1215.

Benner, P. (1984). *From novice to expert: Excellence and power in clinical nursing practice.* Menlo Park, CA: Addison-Wessley.

Booth, K., Kenrick, M., & Woods, S. (1997). Nursing knowledge, theory and method revisited. *Journal of Advanced Nursing, 26,* 804–811.

Brunk, Q. (1995). Setting the stage for the 21st century. *Clinical Nurse Specialist, 9,* 317.

Carper, B. (1978). Fundamental patterns of knowing in nursing. *Advances in Nursing Science, 1,* 13–23.

Cheever, K., & Hardin, S. (1998). Effects of traumatic events, social support, and self-efficacy on adolescents' self-health assessments. *Western Journal of Nursing Research, 21,* 673–684.

Clark, J. E. (2000). Action research. In D. Cormak (Ed.), *The research process in nursing* (4th ed., pp. 183–198). Oxford, UK: Blackwell Science Ltd.

Cody, W. K. (1996a). Drowning in eclecticism. *Nursing Science Quarterly, 9,* 86–87.

Cody, W. K. (1996b). Occult reductionism in the discourse of theory development. *Nursing Science Quarterly, 9,* 140–142.

Cody, W. K. (1997a). Of tombstones, milestones, and gemstones: A retrospective and prospective on nursing theory. *Nursing Science Quarterly, 10,* 3–5.

Cody, W. K. (1997b). The many faces of change: discomfort with the new. *Nursing Science Quarterly, 10,* 65–66.

DeKeyser, F. G., Wainstock, J. M., Rose, L., Converse, P. J., & Dooley, W. (1998). Distress, symptom distress and immune function in women with suspected breast cancer. *Oncology Nursing Forum, 25,* 1415–1426.

Edwards, S. D. (1997). What is philosophy of nursing? *Journal of Advanced Nursing, 25,* 1089–1093.

Engebretson, J. (1997). A multiparadigm approach to nursing. *Advances in Nursing Science, 20,* 21–33.

Fawcett, J. (1999). *The relationship of theory and research.* Philadelphia: F. A. Davis Company.

Greenwood, J. (1994). Action research: A few details, a caution and something new. *Journal of Advanced Nursing, 20,* 13–18.

Huch, M. H. (1995). Nursing science as a basis for advanced practice. *Nursing Science Quarterly, 8,* 6–7.

Koziol-McLain, J., & Maeve, M. K. (1993). Nursing theory in perspective. *Nursing Outlook, 41,* 79–81.

Laschinger, H. S. (1991). Nurses' attitudes about nursing models in practice. *Journal of Nursing Administration, 21,* 12, 15, 18.

Lenz, E. R., Pugh, L. C., Milligan, R. A., Gift, A., & Suppe, F. (1997). The middle-range theory of unpleasant symptoms: An update. *Advances in Nursing Science, 19,* 14–19.

Levine, M. E. (1995). The rhetoric of nursing theory. *Image, 27,* 11–14.

Liehr, P., & Smith, M. J. (1999). Middle-range theory: Spinning research and practice to create knowledge for the new millenium. *Advances in Nursing Science, 21,* 81–91.

Medoff-Cooper, B., McGrath, J., & Bilker, W. (2000). Nutritive sucking and neurobehavioral development in infants from 34 weeks PCA to term. *Maternal Child Nursing, 25,* 64–70.

Monti, E. J., & Tingen, M. S. (1999). Multiple paradigms of nursing science. *Advances in Nursing Science, 21,* 64–80.

Neuman, B. (1972). The Betty Neuman model: A total person approach to viewing patient problems. *Nursing Research, 21,* 264–269.

Nolan, M., Lundh, U., & Tishelman, C. (1998). Nursing's knowledge base: Does it have to be unique? *British Journal of Nursing, 7,* 271–276.

Northrup, D. T. (1992). Disciplinary perspective: Unified or diverse? *Nursing Science Quarterly, 5,* 154–155.

Oberst, M. T. (1995). To what end theory? *Nursing in Research and Health, 18,* 83–84.

Phillips, J. R. (1996). What constitutes nursing science? *Nursing Science Quarterly, 9,* 48–49.

Rogers, M. E. (1970). *An introduction to the theoretical basis of nursing.* Philadelphia: F. A. Davis Company.

Rose, P., & Parker, D. (1994). Nursing: An integration of art and science within the experience of the practitioner. *Journal of Advanced Nursing, 20,* 1004–1010.

Thorne, S., Canam, C., Dahinten, S., Hall, W., Henderson, A., & Kirkham, S. R. (1998). Nursing's metaparadigm concepts: disimpacting the debates. *Journal of Advanced Nursing, 27,* 1257–1268.

Timpson, J. (1996). Nursing theory: Everything the artist spits is art? *Journal of Advanced Nursing, 23,* 1030–1036.

Tolley, K. A. (1995). Theory from practice for practice: Is this a reality? *Journal of Advanced Nursing, 21,* 184–190.

Uys, L. H., & Smit, L. H. (1994). Writing a philosophy of nursing? *Journal of Advanced Nursing, 20,* 239–244.

Ward, R. (1993). The search for meanings in nursing: Could facet theory be a way forward? *Journal of Advanced Nursing, 18,* 549–557.

Whall, A. L. (1993). Let's get rid of all nursing theory. *Nursing Science Quarterly, 6,* 164–165.

The Authors Comment

A Non-theorist's Perspective on Nursing Theory: Issues of the 1990s

As the person responsible for continuing education at a school of nursing, I searched for a seminar topic that was general enough to be of interest to all faculty members. Most nurses who received a master's degree have taken at least one course in nursing theory. However, few, if any, return to the subject once they have graduated, nor do they attempt to see how theory relates to their practice. I began to search the literature and found little that summarized what was new in nursing theory or how these advances were related to practice. I asked Dr. Medoff-Cooper to help me prepare and present this seminar. On one of her visits to the Hadassah-Hebrew University School of Nursing as a visiting professor, we jointly presented the material as a seminar to the faculty. The presentation and the ensuring conversation with the faculty made us believe that perhaps the content was part of a bigger discussion. From this came the impetus for the article.

—FREDA DEKEYSER
—BARBARA MEDOFF-COOPER

CHAPTER .18

Nursing Reformation: Historical Reflections and Philosophic Foundations

Pamela G. Reed

Nursing is in the throes of reform. We are speaking more openly about graduate education as the level of entry for practice, more boldly about the art and spiritual dimensions of nursing care, more matter-of-factly about the necessity of science-based practice, and more creatively about nursing's philosophy and unique methods of building knowledge. Reform means to amend or improve by change of form or removal of faults or abuses (Webster's New Collegiate Dictionary, 1993). But will the changes be radical enough to make a positive difference for those within the discipline, those contemplating a career choice, and those who work and are served within healthcare systems?

When we contemplate the roots of professional nursing in reference to contemporary nursing, it is evident that we have not yet mined the full implications of nursing initiated by Nightingale (1859/1969) in the 19th century and carried forward by other visionaries during the 20th century. Nursing has evolved into a disintegrated profession, due largely to factions of variously educated nurses. The purpose of this dialogue is to propose ideas for clarifying philosophic foundations for reforming nursing in the 21st century.

Key words: nursing, philosophy, pragmatism, reformation

Nursing Science Quarterly, Vol. 13 No. 2, April 2000, 129–136
Copyright © 2000 Sage Publications, Inc. Reprinted with permission.

About the Author

PAMELA G. REED was born in Detroit, MI, in June 1952 and grew up in an environment enriched by the sociopolitical and musical events of Motown. She is a three-time graduate of Wayne State University in Detroit, receiving a BSN in 1974, an MSN in 1976 (with a double major in child-adolescent psychiatric mental health nursing and teaching), and her PhD, with a major in nursing (focus on lifespan development and aging, nursing theory) in 1982. She worked as a psychiatric-mental health clinical nurse specialist and was an Instructor in Nursing at Oakland University, Rochester, MI, from 1976 to 1979. From 1983 to the present, she has been on the faculty at the University of Arizona College of Nursing in Tucson, including 7 years serving as Associate Dean for Academic Affairs. With her doctoral work, she pioneered nursing research into spirituality and its role in well-being. Dr. Reed has developed a theory of self-transcendence and two widely used research instruments, the *Spiritual Perspective Scale* and the *Self-Transcendence Scale*. Her publications reflect her three main passions and contributions to nursing: the conceptual and empirical bases of the significance of spirituality in health experiences, a lifespan developmental perspective of well-being in aging and end of life, and the philosophic dimensions of the development of the discipline. Dr. Reed also enjoys classical music, hiking in the Grand Canyon, swimming, and raising her two daughters, Regina and Rebecca, with her husband, Gary.

Historical Reflections

There is a need to revive the roots of professional nursing's existence. These roots are found in Nightingale's (1895/1969) emancipatory spirit for nursing and for her patients to not only be well, but to use well every power they have; her spiritual commitment concerning the role of nursing; her clarity of a philosophy for nursing that was both scientific and caring; her revolutionary ideas about formally educating nurses, distinct from other healthcare providers; her pragmatism in addressing the health needs of society; and her vision for nursing as a profession. Despite nurse leaders' revolutionary ideas about health reform, university-based education, theory development, and research during the past 100 years, nursing's roots have not developed the discipline as fully as desired.

Service needs of hospitals and physicians have exploited the nursing vision, twisted its roots and choked potential growth that could have been realized in great part through higher education. There is still a proliferation of technical "nursing" training fostered by political interests and profit-driven employers who quell nursing shortages, and the viability of professional nursing, with employment of nonprofessional "nurses." State boards of nursing, with one exception, maintain an outdated, unenlightened, and dispiriting system of nurse licensure. Furthermore, what occupies too much of state boards' time is implementing disciplinary action against nurses whose most common error, amid all that they do, is the implementation of physicians' (medication) orders. The relentless, dependent activity of passing medications, as well as transcribing, filling, and requesting other orders, sustains the need for undereducated "nurses" and erodes the creativity and autonomy that could be nursing.

Professional nurses, by definition, are morally obligated to work within their field and to have a knowledge base adequate for ordering their own actions, especially for direct patient care, whether ambulating patients, talking with a grieving family, or distributing medications. And physicians must take the responsibility for fulfilling their own orders. Nurses who identify with the oppressor by integrating if not embracing medical practice across nursing roles, whether advanced, basic, or technical, rob from the potential to advance nursing care. So do nurses, as CEOs and directors, academic administrators, and teachers, who have the leadership but lack the vision and expertise to implement nursing models of care in their systems, and who lack the courage to speak the language of nursing in their daily work.

The tangled roots of nursing are due also in part to the entry-into-practice debacle from the 1960s and the so-called diversity in educational offerings. Well-meaning and not-so-well-meaning officials are trying to reframe the diverse and disintegrated condition of nursing preparation today with euphemisms that speak of promoting a continuum of practice and therefore a continuum of education, as though something less than a baccalaureate degree provides a foundation for professional nursing education. This continuum may better serve the hospitals than the science.

Increasingly, articles from a range of professional nursing journals such as *Journal of Professional Nursing, Nursing Outlook, Image, Western Journal of Nursing Research, Advances in Nursing Science,* and *Nursing Science Quarterly* speak to the invisibility and low profile of nursing, and to the oppression of nurses. Authors ask readers where all the future nurses have gone, or if nursing even has a future. Others ponder whether nursing will become extinct or, more alarmingly, whether it will exist tomorrow.

The force of nursing has waxed and waned since Nightingale's era, in part, because an enormous number of people who call themselves nurses lack knowledge and education to understand the processes of nursing. Their ontology of practice derives from (mostly medical) authority and habit, as well as intuition and experience. But such an ontology is uninformed and unenriched by the science of nursing and by other patterns of knowing that are acquired only through the process of higher education and continued learning. Without this knowledge, what appear to be nursing actions may instead be nursing imitations.

Imitations focus more on what, when, and how to do something, and less on the why, the underlying scientific and moral base. Perhaps, during the first half of the 20th century, there was no urgency to ask why. Wars and medical advances created many employment opportunities for nurses, although these wars weren't used to advance the profession as did Nightingale (1859/1969) in the Crimea. It is regrettable, as Schlotfeldt (1987) reflected, that nursing's early leaders were so preoccupied with preparing sufficient numbers of nurses to meet societal needs. From 1900 to 1926, schools of nursing increased from 432 to 2,155, whereas medical schools decreased from 160 to 79 in response to the Flexner Report. The scientific exploration of Nightingale's Laws of Nursing or Laws of Health was abandoned and the promise of improved nursing practice unfulfilled.

The second half of the 20th century brought more socio-political changes and accelerated scientific advancement. The teachings of Peplau (1992), Rogers, (1990), Roy (1997), Newman (1995), Watson (1997), Parse (1995) and others awakened nursing to its scholarly heritage and exposed the dogma of a nursing practice that had been separated from its roots, and lacked its own knowledge base. The relevance of a university-based education for professional nursing, envisioned by historical legends Adelaid Nutting, Lavinia Dock, Richard Beard (Dolan, 1968), and others became more widely recognized. However, this recognition seems fragile in the face of yet another nurses' shortage at the end of this century and the continued proliferation of diploma and associate degree graduates in nursing.

Nursing, regarded most basically as a healing process within human systems, has always existed and will always exist, if only underground at times. Nightingale (1859/1969) formalized nursing in the 19th century by initiating efforts to educate people about the nature and facilitation of this process for the betterment of society. The discipline was born out of nothing less than a learned context, a belief in human potential for healing, and a commitment to serving the welfare of human beings. It is unconscionable that the ontology and epistemology of some if not much of nursing practice is manifested in a dominance of technical knowledge and medical orders. There is a need for nursing reform whereby nursing comes clean of the values and beliefs that have misinformed practice and instead identifies with a new philosophy that re-integrates its diversity for the emancipation of the discipline.

An Integrative Philosophy

Despite the increasing dissatisfaction over the current systems of education, licensure, and healthcare, nurses have not been idle in furthering philosophic development of nursing. What must not be overlooked or underutilized in this time of reform is the direction for change provided by a philosophic basis. In the interest of maintaining this momentum, I propose five theses for dialogue in explicating a philosophic basis for a nursing reformation.

The theses address ontologic and epistemologic areas and derive from the current movement toward an integrative philosophy of nursing. This philosophic perspective more purposely links the art and science of nursing, and closes fissures between practice and science that can be exploited by others and diminish the strength of the profession. It is a philosophy that recognizes nursing as a basic discipline (as distinguished from a basic science or art), with a unique focus, and is collaborative with but not dependent upon the orders or knowledge of other professions to provide the substance and purpose of practice and research.

Thesis 1: Nursing Is a Basic Human Healing Process

Previously, I have described nursing as a process inherent to human systems, characterized by ongoing changes in complexity and integration that generate well-being (Reed, 1997). I proposed this substantive definition of nursing, distinguished from the important meaning of nursing as a disciplinary body of knowledge, to provide a shared focus across nursing theory, research, and practice. This definition was developed in answer to the need for what Peplau (as cited in M. J. Smith, 1988) called a simplified rubric that distinguishes a discipline's phenomena from others. The definition, then, puts forth "nursing processes" as the central concern of nursing.

Nursing processes are manifested in a diversity of health experiences among human systems, on all imaginable levels of the person-environment mutual process (individual, patient-nurse, family, community, etc.)

Nursing processes may (or may not) cross boundaries of traditional domains of study, such as the physiologic, psychologic, social, and cultural. As with photosynthesis, pathogenesis, or geologic processes for example, nursing processes can be studied to learn about the patterns and natural laws of, in this case, human well-being. Nursing processes may be elucidated in our theorists' work on pattern recognition, human becoming, adaptation, and knowing participation in change, as well as in other processes discovered to reflect homeodynamic principles of life that generate well-being.

Nursing as process provides a fundamental focus for inquiry and integrates the science and the practice of nursing. This is in contrast to defining nursing primarily as a practice commonly found in the nursing literature (for example, see ANA's, 1995, Social Policy Statement; see also Bishop & Scudder, 1999). Nursing as a "practice" emphasizes the performance and repetition of actions, external to the patient and conducted by someone other than the patient. With the focus on nursing as practice, research logically would delve into the nurse's practice of caring rather than into the patient's potential for healing. Whereas Bishop and Scudder (1999) believe that the "study of nursing should focus on nursing as practiced" (p. 24), I propose that the study should focus on nursing as process, inherent in all human systems.

It is reductionistic and disintegrative to describe nursing primarily as a practice, an art, or a science. The dichotomy between practice and science that is engendered by these descriptors makes the discipline vulnerable to the exploitations that have occurred during the 20th century. It may be more productive to conceptualize nursing first as a healing process, the knowledge of which is developed through the synergy between the science and the art.

Thesis 2: Holism Does Not Define Nursing's Unique Perspective and Contributions

The term *holism* is not adequate for describing what nurses do or what nursing is. Holism is a default term employed too often in place of clearer and more precise language to describe the perspective and unique contribution of nursing. The complexity of meanings and implications regarding holism has made application of the term difficult for both philosophic and practical purposes, despite its intuitive appeal to nursing (Kolcaba, 1997; Owen & Holmes, 1993). Moreover, research into the diffusion of the holistic paradigm in nursing from 1960 to 1990 indicated that the term had various applications in the practice community. Holism referred to a variety of factors including therapeutic modalities, beliefs, and roles of clients and nurses. Moreover, there was no indication of its application in the research community (Johnson, 1990).

As a term, holism is used widely across many disciplines, reflecting various perspectives ranging from mechanistic to unitary (Kolcaba, 1997) and reflecting disparities between written discourse and clinical practice (Owen & Holmes, 1993). The nature of the term is such that qualifying words are often needed to explain holism. For some, holism conjures up vague and sometimes unattainable expectations and stifles attempts to conjecture about nursing phenomena.

It is not inaccurate to describe nursing as a holistic discipline. However, if holism is applicable to only a certain part of the nursing community, as the qualifier in the term holistic nursing implies, then holism is not useful in conveying an integrative perspective for nursing. Alternatively, if the essence of nursing is holism, then use of the term holistic nursing is redundant; the term *nursing* should stand alone. It is more productive to spend our efforts identifying terms that clarify the substance of nursing rather than the substance of holism. These terms will better serve our research and practice endeavors to unite nurses in a deeper understanding of what their discipline is all about.

Thesis 3: Embodiment Is a Core Concept in Understanding Health Experiences

The linguistic focus of postmodernism has emphasized the role of language and discourse in building knowledge. The social, cultural, and political dimensions have garnered recognition of their roles in scientific inquiry. Terms like spiritual, self-transcendence, perception,

and consciousness, which tend to emphasize mind over body, have gained increased attention. Nevertheless, embodiment remains a critical context for nursing inquiry into health experiences (Wilde, 1999).

Dewey (1929) addressed the dichotomy in knowledge development found between discursive and nondiscursive experiences, mind and body. He, along with other pragmatists, argued for the importance of nondiscursive experience and he, in fact, posited that nondiscursive experience is foundational to all thinking. Shusterman (1997) extended Dewey's views in a more integrative manner by arguing the need for philosophy to value the somatic as well as the linguistic and rational experience. This was justified, he said, given philosophy's pragmatic goal of not only grounding knowledge but producing a better experience. He proposed, radically, that somatics should be integrated into the discursive practices of philosophy, and in the practices of other disciplines interested in promoting transformation and betterment of life. Similarly, Schneider (1998) called for a revival of romanticism in science and advocated for a more balanced approach to post-modern inquiry that included exploration of peoples' felt impressions, bodily sensations, and existential awareness.

The integration of somatic experience into nursing inquiry helps bridge the gap between the worlds of the patient, the practitioner, and the researcher. The body is an important manifestation of the human being, around which much in nursing revolves. As Gadow (1980) explained, the self is inseparable from the body, and nursing philosophy cannot address human health experiences in abstraction from the existential ground, the body. The quest for nursing knowledge, then, occurs not only through the discursive modes of philosophic inquiry and the research process, but also by attending to the embodiment of health processes and practices.

Thesis 4: Scientific Knowledge Is Transformed Into Nursing Knowledge Through Contexts of Nursing Practice

This fourth thesis moves us beyond traditional and disintegrative pathways of developing and distributing knowledge, that is, moving from the top down, from theorist and researcher to practitioner. Putnam (1988), a contemporary philosopher who espouses a pragmatic approach to philosophy, explained that the traditional pathway to epistemologic justification, from the theoretical to the more observable concepts, was only one approach to knowledge development. He proposed that theory development proceed in all directions, in any direction that may be handy. Philosopher Nancy Cartwright (1988) elaborated on this idea in explaining that it is not enough to know a given law of nature and deduce other occurrences from that law, as one would using Hempel's (1966) covering law. That is to say that nature is not so well-regulated and independent of context that events can be determined from a given law. Science, she explained, cannot shut down once a law is put forward. Rather, explanations entail ongoing consideration of data from an integration of various ways of knowing, of which we have identified many in nursing: empiric, personal, ethical, aesthetic, unknowing, and intuition, to mention some. Similarly, philosopher Susan Haack (1996) argued against the received (realist) view of truth and the perceived (relativist) view of truth as being the only options for selecting an approach to developing knowledge in a discipline. Instead, she proposed a new term that represented a synthesis of the two dichotomous views, foundationalism and coherence, which she called "foundherentism." Foundherentism was a better justified and more practical approach to building knowledge, in which both experience and beliefs provided an epistemologic basis.

In realizing the meaning of Carper's (1978) nursing epistemology and other postmodern perspectives, nursing began reforming its traditional top-down approach to building knowledge. More nurses are using approaches that privilege the experiences and beliefs of multiple individuals, including researcher, practitioner, and patient.

Professional nurses are people who, in their practice, ethically and skillfully engage patients and themselves in application and testing of knowledge. This engagement transforms scientific knowledge into nursing knowledge (Reed, 1996). The mutual process between nurses and patients or, more broadly, between persons and their environments provides contexts for both the discovery and confirmation of knowledge.

Thesis 5: Nursing Is a Spiritual Discipline

Spiritual is defined as existing in an intentional community with others where otherness is an unreduced intrusion into the experience of each person (S. G. Smith, 1988). While intentions are shared across the community, the individuals are neither diminished nor supplanted by the community. In applying this interpretation of spirituality in nursing, it can be said that the nurse participates with the patient, sharing intentions about health through the intimacy and skill of touch and talk. Intentions are spiritual, focused on health as experienced wholeness.

A spiritual discipline is distinguished from the psychosocial sciences in that it is not merely descriptive of behaviors but rather poses a normative and pragmatic call to action, which is freely chosen. A spiritual person is said to be "called" or "launched outward to others to inhabit a world that transcends one's own world" (S. G. Smith, 1988, p. 62). The spiritual is directed toward "enabling, supporting, growing, loving, respecting, and appreciating" (Lane, 1988, p. 335). A spiritual person, like a poet, discovers new things and ideas from "beyond the horizon of the self" (S. G. Smith, 1988, p. 71) for the benefit and transformation of others.

Regarding a profession as spiritual enhances the meaning of a profession. It is more than compassion; it requires a sense of self-transcendence, connectedness to others, a desire to promote life, and a sense of freedom in choosing these things (Lane, 1988). This perspective nourishes the aesthetic as well as other ways of knowing required within a discipline.

The spiritual, then, is a philosophic basis for praxis, uniting values and knowledge with actions in accord with patients' needs for healthcare. In so doing, the spiritual is integrative and promotes unity within a discipline.

Toward Scholarship and Praxis in Nursing

Paradoxically, postmodernism has provided us with an awareness of our freedom to turn toward philosophic foundations to create a possibility for unity within a complex discipline characterized by much diversity. We have come to understand that there is no dichotomy between the theoretical and observable. Kant (1781/1964), Popper (1965), and contemporary philosophers of science have argued convincingly that there is no observation in the absence of theory and values. In nursing, this epistemologic view translates into the realization that some of the distinctions drawn between practitioner and researcher may be reformed in an integrative way to enhance development of nursing knowledge and patient care. This was not so 30 years ago, when Ellis' (1969) idea of practitioner as theorist was dismissed by modernist nurses who regarded science as an endeavor separate from art, values, and practices of nursing.

Contemporary pragmatic approaches to knowledge development diminish the dichotomy between the theoretical and the observable, theory and practice, beliefs and experience. The theses presented here have posited a nursing ontology based upon a relational, embodied, and processual view of health. This view necessitates an epistemology that involves both the scientist's and the practitioner's expertise within what Lerner (1995) called the natural laboratory of the world. Scientific knowledge, which is generated outside of this natural laboratory, is transformed into nursing knowledge by its integration within contexts of nursing practice.

A nursing reformation that derives from an integrated philosophy of nursing is not likely to end in revolt and further divisions. But successful reform will require a type of symbolic home where a diversity of theories and ideas can flourish within a spiritual community of shared values and beliefs. Trainor (1998) distinguished this home from the unshakable foundation of modernism. He described it instead as a home that offers a foundational faith in the connectedness of our ideas to the world and to each other. Nursing reformation will require the participation of theorists, scientists, and practitioners in a shared vision of nursing and of the education needed for nurses to participate in integrated methods of knowledge development. Within this perspective, a reformation may remove faults that divide

nurses and may restore the scholarship and praxis to nursing that Nightingale envisioned.

REFERENCES

American Nurses' Association. (1995). *Nursing: A social policy statement* (Rev. ed.). Washington, DC: Author.

Bishop, A. H., & Scudder, J. R. (1999). A philosophical interpretation of nursing. *Scholarly Inquiry for Nursing Practice, 13,* 17–27.

Carper, B. (1978). Fundamental patterns of knowing in nursing. *Advances in Nursing Science, 1,* 13–23.

Cartwright, N. (1988). The truth doesn't explain much. In E. D. Klemke, R. Hollinger, & A. D. Kline (Eds.), *Philosophy of science* (Rev. ed., pp. 129–136). New York: Prometheus.

Dewey, J. (1929). *Experience and nature* (Rev. ed.). Carbondale: Southern Illinois University Press.

Dolan, J. A. (1968). *History of nursing* (12th ed.). Philadelphia: W. B. Saunders.

Ellis, R. (1969). The practitioner as theorist. *American Journal of Nursing, 69,* 1434–1438.

Gadow, S. (1980). Body and self: A dialectic. In S. Specker & S. Gadow (Eds.), *Existential advocacy: Philosophical foundations of nursing* (pp. 86–100). New York: Springer.

Haack, S. (1996). Evidence and inquiry: Towards reconstruction in epistemology. In M. Warnock (Ed.), *Women philosophers* (pp. 273–299), London: J. M. Dent.

Hempel, C. G. (1966). *Philosophy of natural sciences.* Englewood Cliffs, NJ: Prentice-Hall.

Johnson, M. B. (1990). The holistic paradigm in nursing: The diffusion of an innovation. *Research in Nursing & Health, 13,* 129–139.

Kant I. (1964). *Critique of pure reason* (N. Kemp Smith, Trans). New York: Macmillan. (Original work published in 1781)

Kolcaba, R. (1997). The primary holisms in nursing. *Journal of Advanced Nursing, 25,* 290–296.

Lane, J. A. (1988). The care of the human spirit. *Journal of Professional Nursing, 36,* 332–337.

Lerner, R. M. (1995). The integrations of levels and human development: A developmental contextual view of the synthesis of science and outreach in the enhancement of human lives. In K. E. Hood, G. Greenberg, & E. Tobah (Eds.), *Behavioral development* (pp. 421–455). New York: Garland.

Newman, M. (1995). *Health as expanding consciousness* (2nd ed.). New York: NLN.

Nightingale, F. (1859/1969). *Notes on nursing: What it is and what it is not.* New York: Dover.

Owen, M. J., & Holmes, C. A. (1993). "Holism" in the discourse of nursing. *Journal of Advanced Nursing, 18,* 1688–1695.

Parse, R. R. (1995). *Illuminations: The human becoming theory in practice and research.* New York: NLN.

Peplau, H. (1992). Interpersonal relations: A theoretical framework for application in nursing practice. *Nursing Science Quarterly, 5,* 13–18.

Popper, K. R. (1965). *Conjectures and refutations: The growth of scientific knowledge.* New York: Harper.

Putnam, H. (1988). What theories are not. In E. D. Klemke, R. Holllinger, & A. D. Kline (Eds.), *Philosophy of science* (Rev. ed., pp. 178–183). New York: Prometheus.

Reed, P. G. (1996). Transforming knowledge into nursing knowledge: A revisionist analysis of Peplau. *Image: The Journal of Nursing Scholarship 28,* 29–33.

Reed, P. G. (1997). Nursing: The ontology of the discipline. *Nursing Science Quarterly, 10,* 76–79.

Rogers, M. (1990). Nursing: Science of unitary, irreducible human beings: Update 1990. In E. Barrett (Ed.), *Visions of Rogers' science-based nursing* (pp. 5–12). New York: NLN.

Roy, C. (1997). Future of the Roy model: Challenge to redefine adaptation. *Nursing Science Quarterly, 10,* 49–52.

Schlotfeldt, R. M. (1987). Defining nursing: A historic controversy. *Nursing Research, 36,* 64–65.

Schneider, K. J. (1998). Toward a science of the heart. *American Psychologist, 53,* 277–289.

Shusterman, R. (1997). *Practicing philosophy: Pragmatism and the philosophical life.* New York: Routledge.

Smith, M. J. (1988). Perspectives in nursing science. *Nursing Science Quarterly, 1,* 80–85.

Smith, S. G. (1988). *The concept of the spiritual: An essay in first philosophy.* Philadelphia: Temple University Press.

Trainor, B. (1998). The origin and end of modernity. *Journal of Applied Philosophy, 15,* 133–144.

Watson, J. (1997). The theory of human caring: Retrospective and prospective. *Nursing Science Quarterly 10,* 49–52.

Webster's new collegiate dictionary. (1993). Springfield, MA: Merriam-Webster.

Wilde, M. H. (1999). Why embodiment now? *Advances in Nursing Science, 22,* 25–38.

The Author Comments

Nursing Reformation: Historical Reflections and Philosophic Foundations

The impetus for this article came from a contributing editor of *Nursing Science Quarterly,* Dr. Marilyn Rawnsley, who provided me the wonderful opportunity to write about what I believed was significant as nursing moved into the 21st century. As an educator, an administrator, and a nurse, I was frustrated with the state of nursing practice education, which in its diverse forms was incongruous with visions of the kind of education professional nursing requires, nursing shortages notwithstanding. I grounded my ideas in historical visions of nursing, still unrealized, in terms of a truly independently functioning profession. I wanted to expose some key philosophic issues (presented as my "theses") in reforming nursing from within the discipline to put forth a philosophic basis for professional nursing.

—PAMELA G. REED

Philosophic Foundations of Science and Theory

This section presents current thinking about the philosophic foundations of nursing theory. The articles transport the reader one step deeper into the foundations of nursing science and theory development through clear and comprehensive presentations of the topics of worldviews and prevailing paradigms; epistemology; ontology; and ethics. For each topic, the seminal article and the origins of thinking are presented, followed by articles that extend or challenge the status quo. Beyond Carper, there are new epistemologies. Beyond the nursing metaparadigm, nurses have authored distinctive metaparadigmatic statements about nursing. Beyond ethics, there is a movement toward viewing the ethical as being equally as, if not more important than, the empirical in nursing theorizing. This unit closes with a special subsection on philosophies and knowledge development. Postmodern influences of deconstructing and integrating paradigms and philosophies are generating unprecedented conversations about nursing theory.

From a Plethora of Paradigms to Parsimony in Worldviews

Jacqueline Fawcett

Nursing knowledge development is guided by philosophic claims about the nature of human beings and the human-environment relationship. Those philosophic claims are variously referred to as paradigms or worldviews. Four sets of worldviews have been cited as fundamental to the development of nursing knowledge. One set is the mechanism-organicism dichotomy. The characteristics of those two philosophic approaches to the study of the human-environment relationship were described by Reese and Overton (1970), among others, and are outlined in Table 19-1. Hall (1981) proposed another set of worldviews that reflect philosophic claims about the nature of change in human beings and the human-environment relationship. The characteristics of those views, which are labeled change and persistence, are shown in Table 19-2.

Parse (1987) discussed the features of yet another set of philosophic claims, which she called the totality and simultaneity paradigms. The characteristics of those two paradigms are listed in Table 19-3. Recently, Newman (1992) identified what she claims are the three prevailing paradigms for nursing knowledge development. The characteristics of her three paradigms, the particulate-deterministic, the interactive-integrative, and the unitary-transformative, are summarized in Table 19-4. Newman (1992) explained that "the first of the paired words [in the names of the three paradigms] describes the view of the entity being studied and the second describes the notion of how change occurs" (p. 10).

About the Author

JACQUELINE FAWCETT received her Bachelor of Science degree from Boston University in 1964, her master's degree in parent-child nursing from New York University in 1970, and her PhD in nursing from New York University in 1976. Dr. Fawcett is currently Professor, College of Nursing and Health Sciences, University of Massachusetts-Boston. She is Professor Emerita at the University of Pennsylvania. Starting with her dissertation, Dr. Fawcett conducted a program of research dealing with wives' and husbands' pregnancy-related experiences that was derived from Martha Rogers' conceptual system. Subsequently, she undertook a program of research dealing with responses to cesarean birth derived from the Roy Adaptation Model of Nursing. A third program of research, also derived from the Roy Adaptation Model, focuses on function during normal life transitions and serious illness. Dr. Fawcett is perhaps best known for her metatheoretical work, including many journal articles and several books. Since 1996, Dr. Fawcett has lived in the midcoast region of Maine with her husband, John; two Maine Coon cats, Matinicus and Acadia; and a now-tame feral cat, Lydia Dasher. She and her husband own Fawcett's Art, Antiques, and Toy Museum. She swims laps and walks on a treadmill at a fitness center for exercise and relaxation and sails on a windjammer off the Maine coast during the summer.

Table 19-1
Characteristics of the Organismic and Mechanistic Worldviews

Organicism	Mechanism
Metaphor is the living organism.	Metaphor is the machine.
Human beings are active.	Human beings are reactive.
Behavior is probabilistic.	Behavior is a predictable linear chain.
Holism and expansionism are assumed—focus on wholes.	Elementarism and reductionism are assumed—focus on parts.
Development is qualitative and quantitative.	Development is quantitative.

Table 19-2
Characteristics of the Change and Persistence Worldviews

Change	Persistence
Metaphor is growth.	Metaphor is stability.
Change is inherent and natural.	Stability is natural and normal.
Change is continuous.	Change occurs only for survival.
Intra-individual variance.	Intra-individual invariance.
Progress is valued.	Solidarity is valued.
Realization of potential is emphasized.	Conservation and retrenchment are emphasized.

Table 19-3
Characteristics of the Simultaneity and Totality Paradigms

Simultaneity	Totality
Human beings are synergistic; more than and different from the sum of their parts.	Human beings are bio-psycho-social-spiritual organisms.
Human beings are in mutual rhythmical interchange with the environment.	Human beings interact in a linear way with the environment.
Health is a process of becoming; it is living a set of value priorities.	Health is physical, mental, social and spiritual well-being. Human beings strive toward an optimal level of health through manipulation of the environment.

Table 19-4
Characteristics of the Particulate-Deterministic, Interactive-Integrative, and Unitary-Transformative Paradigms

Particulate-Deterministic	Interactive-Integrative	Unitary-Transformative
Phenomena are isolatable, reducible entities with definable, measurable properties.	Reality is multidimensional and contextual.	Human beings are unitary and evolving as self-organizing fields.
Entities have orderly and predictable connections.	Entities are context-dependent and relative.	Human fields are identified by pattern and by interaction with the larger whole.
Change occurs as a consequence of antecedent conditions that can be predicted and controlled.	Change is a function of multiple antecedent factors and probabilistic relationships.	Change is unidirectional and unpredictable.
Relationships are linear and causal.	Relationships move from linear to reciprocal.	Systems move through stages of organization and disorganization to more complex organization.
Only objective, observable phenomena are studied.	Both objective and subjective phenomena are studied, with emphasis on objectivity, control, and predictability.	Emphasis is on personal knowledge and pattern recognition.

Toward Parsimony in Worldviews

An analysis of the characteristics of the four sets of worldviews revealed some similarities and yielded a single parsimonious set of three worldviews: reaction, reciprocal interaction, and simultaneous action. More specifically, the analysis revealed that the particulate-deterministic paradigm is similar to mechanism, persistence, and totality. The combination of characteristics from those perspectives yielded the reaction worldview (Box 19-1).

Furthermore, the analysis indicated that the interactive-integrative paradigm is similar to organicism and

---

BOX **19-1**

The Reaction Worldview

- Humans are bio-psycho-social-spiritual beings.
- Human beings react to external environmental stimuli in a linear, causal manner.
- Change occurs only for survival, as a consequence of predictable and controllable antecedent conditions.
- Only objective phenomena that can be isolated, defined, observed, and measured are studied.

BOX **19-2**

The Reciprocal Interaction Worldview

- Human beings are holistic.
- Parts are viewed only in the context of the whole.
- Human beings are active.
- Interactions between human beings and their environments are reciprocal.
- Reality is multidimensional, context-dependent, and relative.
- Change is a function of multiple antecedent factors.
- Change is probabilistic and may be continuous or may be only for survival.
- Both objective and subjective phenomena are studied through quantitative and qualitative methods of inquiry.
- Emphasis is placed on empirical observations, methodological controls, and inferential data analytic techniques.

BOX **19-3**

The Simultaneous Action Worldview

- Unitary human beings are identified by pattern.
- Human beings are in mutual rhythmical interchange with their environments.
- Human beings change continuously, evolving as self-organized fields.
- Change is unidirectional and unpredictable as human beings move through stages of organization and disorganization to more complex organization.
- Phenomena of interest are personal becoming and pattern recognition.

reflects elements of the totality view. In addition, that paradigm can incorporate elements of both change and persistence. Taken together, those perspectives yielded the reciprocal interaction worldview (Box 19-2).

Finally, the analysis suggested that the unitary-transformative paradigm is similar to organicism but even more similar to simultaneity. Furthermore, the elements of change are most evident in that paradigm. Combining the characteristics of those perspectives resulted in the simultaneous action worldview (Box 19-3).

Conclusion

The triad of worldviews presented in this column represents an attempt to draw together the characteristics of four different existing sets of paradigms or world-

views, representing nine perspectives, in a logical manner. Nursing's early scientific development began with the reaction worldview and evolved through the reciprocal interaction worldview to the simultaneous action worldview. Most contemporary scientific nursing knowledge resides in the reciprocal interaction and simultaneous action paradigms. The schema presented here is a relatively parsimonious structure that reflects the different philosophic claims under-girding nursing's scientific knowledge development. This attempt at drawing existing sets of paradigms together is open to debate, and readers are invited to a dialogue on the issue.

REFERENCES

Hall, B. A. (1981). The change paradigm in nursing: Growth versus persistence. *Advances in Nursing Science, 3*(4), 1–6.

Newman, M. A. (1992). Prevailing paradigms in nursing. *Nursing Outlook, 40*, 10–13, 32.

Parse, R. R. (1987). *Nursing science: Major paradigms, theories, and critiques.* Philadelphia: Saunders.

Reese, H. W., & Overton, W. F. (1970). Models of development and theories of development. In L. R. Goulet & P. B. Baltes (Eds.), *Life span developmental psychology. Research and theory* (pp. 115–145). New York: Academic Press.

The Author Comments

From a Plethora of Paradigms to Parsimony in Worldviews

This article was written in response to what I regarded as a growing diversity of perspectives about worldviews under girding nursing conceptual models and theories. The author's preceding schemata of worldviews failed to acknowledge the existing schemata and, instead, presented their views as if they arose in isolation from what came before. Inasmuch as I believe that knowledge is cumulative and that new ideas come from an understanding of existing ideas, I attempted to integrate the various existing worldviews into a parsimonious schema of three worldviews. I have found my schema particularly useful to my understanding of the philosophic underpinnings of nursing conceptual models and theories. I have incorporated this schema into my frameworks for analysis and evaluation of conceptual models of nursing and analysis and evaluation of nursing theories (see my book, *Analysis and Evaluation of Contemporary Nursing Knowledge: Nursing Models and Theories*, Philadelphia: F. A. Davis; 2000). I believe that a better understanding of worldviews is a crucial component of theory development in the 21st century.

—JACQUELINE FAWCETT

CHAPTER 20

Prevailing Paradigms in Nursing

Margaret A. Newman

The variability and ambiguity of things called paradigms, both within and outside nursing, have left me at times feeling very confused. In nursing we often refer to the medical paradigm as opposed to the nursing paradigm, or curing versus caring, or health as the absence of disease versus health as an evolving pattern of the whole.[1] Parse[2] has categorized nursing theories in what she has labeled the totality paradigm versus the simultaneity paradigm. Others speak to a quantitative paradigm versus a qualitative paradigm. These perspectives reflect to some degree various philosophies of science. What is the basis for the naming of a paradigm: the discipline it represents, the subject matter it addresses, the thought processes it reflects, dimensions of time-space, the nature of the data collected, or what? One of the international doctoral students at Minnesota asked me why nursing is so caught up

in consideration of paradigms. In answer to her question, my thoughts were that it has something to do with the history of the development of nursing science (e.g., our alignment and subsequent disalignment with medicine). When you take a look at the various ways in which we refer to the paradigms, not to mention for the moment the term *metaparadigm*, it is no wonder that graduate students have difficulty sorting it out.

Nursing is not alone in having to deal with the paradigm issue. Guba's recent book, *The Paradigm Dialog*,[3] is based on a 1989 conference devoted to this debate in education and related fields. Guba introduced the discussion with an ontologic, epistemologic, and methodologic analysis of four paradigms he identified as relevant: positivism, postpositivism, critical theory, and constructivism. A resume of the basic belief systems associated with these

Adapted from a paper presented at the 1991 National Forum on Doctoral Education,
Amelia Island, Fla., June 1991. Nursing Outlook, 40*(1), 10-13, 32. Copyright © 1992 Elsevier Science. Reprinted with permission.*

About the Author

MARGARET A. NEWMAN was born in Memphis, TN, on October 10, 1933. She received her first degree (BSHE, 1954) in home economics at Baylor University. She entered nursing at the University of Tennessee, Memphis, in 1959 and received a BSN in 1962. Her graduate study included an emphasis on medical-surgical nursing at the University of California, San Francisco (MS, 1964) and a further emphasis on rehabilitation nursing and nursing science at New York University (PhD, 1971). Except for a short tenure as director of nursing for the clinical research center at the University of Tennessee, the emphasis of her work has been in education (at New York University, Penn State University, and the University of Minnesota). The focus of her scholarship has been on theory development in nursing. The books *Health as Expanding Consciousness* (1986, 1994) and *A Developing Discipline* (1995) represent her major contribution to nursing theory. She is an avid fan of live theater and music, with subscriptions to two local theater groups' offerings and the St. Paul Chamber Orchestra.

paradigms (Table 20-1) provides a background for sorting out the paradigm issues in nursing.

Extant Views in Nursing Research

A wide range of beliefs about what constitutes reality and how to go about finding it is reflected in the research taking place in nursing. Sime, Corcoran-Perry, and I have developed our own version of the scientific paradigms we see at work in nursing research.[4] We pursued this task for the purpose of delineating how the seemingly disparate work of various members of our faculty can indeed relate to a common focus. We tried not to introduce three new labels, but we did not see

Table 20–1
Basic Belief Systems of Positivism, Postpositivism, Critical Theory, and Constructivism

	Ontology	Epistemology	Methodology
Positivism	Realist: Reality exists "out there" Driven by natural laws	Objectivist: Inquirer adopts distant and non-interactive posture	Experimental Empiric Controlled Testing of hypotheses
Postpositivism	Critical realist: Same as positivism except cannot be known because of lack of ability to know	Modified objectivist: Objectivity an ideal that can be only approximated Guarded by critical community	Modified experimental Emphasis on critical "multiplism" (elaborated triangulation)
Critical theory	Critical realist: Reality influenced by societal structures	Subjectivist: Values mediate inquiry Goal is to free participants from effect of ideology	Dialogic, transformative Intended to eliminate false consciousness and facilitate transformation
Constructivism	Relativist: Reality is mental construction, socially and experimentally based Many interpretations possible Multiple realities	Subjectivist: Inquirer and respondent are fused into single entity Findings are creation of process between the two	Hermeneutic, dialectic Aims to identify the variety of constructions that exist and bring them to as much consensus as possible

Excerpted from Guba EG. The alternative paradigm dialog. In: Guba EG, ed. The paradigm dialog. Newbury Park, Calif: Sage, 1990:17–27.

our categorizations fitting neatly into those already described. Eventually, rather than referring to them as I, II, and III, we succumbed to assigning descriptive labels to depict the key dimensions in each: I—particulate-deterministic, II—interactive-integrative, and III—unitary-transformative. The idea here is that the first of the paired words describes the view of the entity being studied and the second describes the notion of how change occurs.

From the particulate-deterministic paradigm, which holds closely to the positivist view, phenomena are

viewed as isolatable, reducible entities having definable properties that can be measured. These entities have orderly and predictable connectedness to each other. Change is assumed to be a consequence of antecedent conditions—conditions that, if sufficiently identified and understood, could be used to predict and control change in the phenomena. Relationships within and among entities are viewed as linear and causal.[4]

From a particulate-deterministic view, only the most objective, observable manifestations of health, such as physiologic parameters, would be considered suitable subject matter for research. A phenomenon such as caring, considered by some as the essence of nursing, either would have to be removed from its context and given an operational definition or would be considered by some as outside the realm of science.

The interactive-integrative paradigm (similar to postpositivism) maintains allegiance to the need for control and predictability in research but views reality as multidimensional and contextual. It acknowledges the importance of experience and includes both subjective and objective phenomena but holds to the objectivity, control, and predictability of the positivist view. It moves away from linearity and acknowledges that in some instances understanding without predictability is enough. Change is viewed as "a function of multiple antecedent factors and probabilistic relationships."[4] Knowledge is context dependent and relative. From this perspective, nursing phenomena are viewed

as both objective and subjective in reciprocal interaction.

The unitary-transformative paradigm presents a significant shift in the view of reality. The human being is viewed as unitary and evolving as a self-organizing field, embedded in a larger self-organizing field.

It is identified by pattern and by interaction with the larger whole . . . .Change is unidirectional and unpredictable as systems move through stages of organization and disorganization to more complex organization. Knowledge is personal, involves pattern recognition, and is a function of both viewer and the phenomenon viewed . . . .Inner reality depicts the reality of the whole.[4]

Nursing would be studied as a unitary process of mutuality and creative unfolding.

Historically we seem to have moved from addressing primarily the health of the body as affected by environmental factors to interplay of body-mind-environment factors in health, and, more recently, to health as an experience of the unitary human field phenomenon embedded in a larger unitary field. These three perspectives, biophysical science, biopsychosocial science, and human science relate to different paradigms. The biophysical sciences are single-paradigm sciences with broad consensus among their members; biopsychosocial sciences involve multiple competing paradigms encompassing both objective and subjective phenomena and relating to different views on the nature of human beings and society.[5] Human science embraces a view of the human being as a unitary phenomenon and represents a major paradigm shift from the previous two (Table 20-2).

Table 20–2
Shift in Emphasis of Nursing Science

Health Focus	Science Category	Paradigm
Body ← environment	Biophysical	Single
Body-mind-environment	Biopsychosocial	Multiple
Unitary field	Human	Emergent

Focus of the Discipline

There is another consideration in nursing science. Nursing science is a professional discipline and as such has a commitment to alleviate the problems of society. The nature of the reality we are dealing with must incorporate knowledge of the process of making things better for society—a knowledge of praxis: "thoughtful reflection and action that occurs in synchrony, in the direction of transforming the world."[6]

What is our commitment then? Some would say "the promotion of health." At least two objections to that focus are that (1) it is phrased in the language of intervention and objectivity and therefore excludes the unitary-transformative paradigm; and (2) it is not an exclusive domain of nursing. Others would say "caring." Similar objections might apply: (1) from a positivist view, caring may not be amenable to scientific study; and (2) it is of a universal nature that is not limited to one discipline.

Sime, Corcoran-Perry, and I found that as we progressed in our exploration of prevailing paradigms, our intent became to identify the unifying focus of nursing as a professional discipline. After much discussion among ourselves and other colleagues and review of the literature, particularly over the past decade, we came to the conclusion that the focus of nursing as a professional discipline can be characterized as "caring in the human health experience."[4] This focus synthesizes the phenomena of nursing at the metaparadigm level and makes explicit the nature of the social mandate of nursing. *Caring* designates the nature of the nursing practice participation. *Human health* experience brings together the focus on *human* health and modifies it to mean the human health *experience*. The experiential dimension characterizes the phenomenon as something beyond the traditional objective-subjective perspective. The whole phrase taken together signifies the social mandate to which nursing has responded throughout our history and circumscribes the boundaries of the discipline.

Each major concept of this focus, taken alone, manifests itself in different ways. Morse and her associates[7] have done a comprehensive review of the variety of ways in which caring has been defined and studied. Their work illustrates the different paradigmatic positions prevalent in nursing today. The same is true for research related to the concept of health. Most of this research emanates from the dominant objective-subjective paradigms.[8] At the same time, research that connects caring and the health experience in a mutual, transformative process is emerging as a powerful force within the explication of our discipline.

Are We A Multiple-Paradigm Discipline?

This question leads to the question of whether the aforementioned focus can be addressed within the objectivist, interventionist tradition. Benner's answer would seem to be "no." Benner[9] points out that within a social scientific context, caring is "decontextualized" and "operationalized" and becomes just one more therapeutic technique. I take that to mean that this way of viewing caring does not capture the essence of caring.

When we[4] began work on "The Focus of the Discipline" paper, we thought of ourselves as each being representative of one of the three paradigms, but the more we discussed the underlying assumptions of each and came to accept the disciplinary focus of caring in the human health experience, the more each of us became convinced of the necessity of the unitary, transformative paradigm for development of the knowledge of our discipline. We ourselves were transformed in the process. We concluded that knowledge emanating from the first two paradigms is relevant but not sufficient for the full elaboration of nursing science.

Others tend to agree. Pender[10] describes the shift in nursing to human science, which views persons as unified wholes and focuses on the *experience* of health. She calls for a unitary perspective but still uses the language of objectivity in calling for valid and reliable measures. Parse[2] says that a discipline encompasses more than one paradigm to guide inquiry, yet clearly takes her stand in what she calls a simultaneity paradigm, one that embraces mutuality and transformation as the nature of human processes.

We seem to be hedging. Are we afraid to give up the certainty in knowing that the positivist view offers? In discussing the movement to new paradigms, Skrtic[5] points out that the "divorce of science from its contemporary raw empiricist base, and its realliance with judgment, discernment, understanding, and interpretation as necessary elements of the scientific process" means giving up the false certainty of logical positivism and facing the anxiety of less certain forms of knowing.

My original intent was to try to fairly, accurately present each of the prevailing paradigms and to say "Let's agree to disagree and go on about our business." Identifying the paradigms is the easy part. The hard part is acknowledging the pervasive nature of a paradigm, the fact that the values inherent in a paradigm are deeply embedded in the adherents and become normative, indicating what is important and what should be done about it. Paradigms have been compared with cultures in that they represent shared knowledge of what is and what ought to be and *adherents cannot imagine any other way to behave.*[11] This begins to explain some of the uneasiness we experience when an adherent of a paradigm other than our own speaks to the importance of that way of thinking and behaving.

Some argue for accommodation among paradigms; others assert that they have nothing in common. Skrtic[5] takes the position that "the point is not to accommodate or reconcile the multiple paradigms . . . ; it is to recognize them as unique, historically situated forms of insight; to understand them and their implications; to learn to speak to them and through them . . . ." Moccia[12] has described the deeper meaning of what is involved in attempts to accommodate different paradigms: the contradiction of trying to control and not to control, the expectation of being able to predict and at the same time acknowledging the process as innovative.

For almost a decade now, thanks to Munhall,[13] we have been aware of the discrepancies between our values as a profession and our practices as scientists. Now it is important to recognize the inconsistencies within our science, inconsistencies we are passing on to students. Lincoln[14] has experienced the same conflicting values:

I have often told questioners that research training programs should be two-tracked, with training in conventional and emergent-paradigm inquiry models, followed by training in quantitative and qualitative methods both, completed with computer applications for both quantitative and qualitative data.

But with what I have intuitively come to understand about the pervasiveness of the paradigm we use to conduct inquiry, I now think that training in multiple paradigms (at least in more than a historical sense) is training for schizophrenia. If we want to change new researchers' paradigms, we must do more than legitimate those paradigms in the inquiry outlets, such as journals. We have to train people in them, intensively. We probably ought not to be dividing their attention with other than historical accounts of conventional science. We probably ought to recognize the profound commitments people make to worldviews and create centers where such training can go on . . . .[14]

A movement has begun within nursing education to create centers with a particular focus—perhaps to emphasize one paradigm as dominant. The question is: Are we willing to allow, even encourage, that to occur? Or do we want to give all of the paradigms equal time and emphasis in all the programs? Or perhaps a third alternative might be to promote pockets of parallel emphases from different paradigmatic perspectives within a single program.

Some think that positivism is dead—others see it as alive and well and still dominating the scientific community. In graduate curricula, for instance, is it not true that most "basic" research courses emphasize the tenets of controlled, objective science? Does that not say that this is the way it is and anything else is alternative or deviant? And how many of our courses on theory development begin with the isolation of concepts, development of propositional sets, and derivation of causal relationships? If a faculty seeks to convey a different perspective, they would need to examine their basic ontologic and epistemologic beliefs and develop courses that are consistent with those beliefs.

A Paradigm Shift

Evidence of a paradigm shift exists in nursing. Johnson's bibliometric analysis of nursing literature since 1966 depicts a shift from a scientific medical model to a model based on holism.[15] Sarter's analysis of four contemporary nursing theories reveals commonly shared themes, emphasizing holism, process, and self-transcendence.[16] She suggests that it represents an emerging paradigm. The shift perhaps has not been as revolutionary as Kuhn would have predicted. A recent headline in the *Brain/Mind Bulletin* is apropos: has various advantages and disadvantages, depending on individual program needs.

"Can you remember where you were when the paradigm shifted?"[17] Assuming that the shift has occurred, it is incumbent on us to reevaluate the values and structures that shape our discipline.

The Challenge

The challenge before us is twofold: the need to identify and agree on the central question in nursing, the focus of discipline, and the need to clarify the scientific values and methods that will address that question.

REFERENCES

1. Newman MA. Health as expanding consciousness. St. Louis, Mo.: CV Mosby, 1996.
2. Parse RR. Nursing science: major paradigms, theories, and critiques. Philadelphia, Pa.: Saunders, 1987.
3. Guba EG, ed. The paradigm dialog. Newbury Park, Calif.: Sage, 1990.
4. Newman MA, Sime AM, Corcoran-Perry SA. The focus of the discipline of nursing. ANS 1991;14(1):1-6.
5. Skrtic TM. Social accommodation: toward a dialogical discourse in educational inquiry. In: Guba EG, ed. The paradigm dialog. Newbury Park, Calif.: Sage, 1990:125-35.
6. Wheeler CE, Chinn PL. Peace & power: a handbook of feminist process. 2nd ed. New York: National League for Nursing, 1989:1.
7. Morse JM, Solberg SM, Neander WL, Bottorff JL, Johnson JL. Concepts of caring and caring as a concept. ANS 1990; 13(1):1-14.
8. Newman MA. Health conceptualizations. Ann Rev Nurs Res 1991;9:221-43.
9. Benner P. Nursing as a caring profession. Paper presented at meeting of the American Academy of Nursing, October 16-18, Kansas City, Mo., 1988.
10. Pender NJ. Expressing health through lifestyle patterns. Nurs Sci Q 1990;3(3):115-22.
11. Firestone WA. Accommodation: toward a paradigm-praxis dialectic. In: Guba EG, ed. The paradigm dialog. Newbury Park, Calif.: Sage, 1990:105-24.
12. Moccia P. A critique of compromise: beyond the methods debate. ANS 1988;10(4):1-9.
13. Munhall P. Nursing philosophy and nursing research: in apposition or opposition? Nurs Res 1982;31(3):176-7;181.
14. Lincoln YS. The making of a constructivist: a remembrance of transformations past. In: Guba EG, ed. The paradigm dialog. Newbury Park, Calif.: Sage, 1990:67-87.
15. Johnson MB. The holistic paradigm in nursing: the diffusion of an innovation. Res Nurs Health 1990;13:129-39.
16. Starter B. Philosophic sources of nursing theory. Nurs Sci Q 1988;1(2):52-9.
17. Can you remember where you were when the paradigm shifted? Brain/Mind Bulletin 1991;16(7).

The Author Comments

Prevailing Paradigms in Nursing

This article is a follow-up to the treatise on the "focus of the discipline" and provides a general paradigmatic background for viewing the nursing paradigms. More importantly, it presents the methodologic and curricular dilemmas posed for students and educators when the unitary-transformative paradigm is acknowledged as essential to the development of nursing knowledge. I no longer see "human" as adequate for describing the science of nursing, because the unitary focus is on a continuous human-environmental field and the praxis nature of the knowledge encompasses the action component of the nurse-patient process.

—Margaret A. Newman

CHAPTER 21

Toward a New View of Science: Implications for Nursing Research

Mindy B. Tinkle
Janet I. Beaton

It was her first dissertation committee meeting. The topic of discussion was her proposed research methodology. Two of the committee members (well-known for their "hard" research) began to dialogue about the "softness" of the approach in the proposal before them—the lack of control, the lack of quantitative measurement, and the lack of manipulation of variables. Before long, the committee was in accord about the relatively low scientific merit of this type of research methodology as opposed to an experimental approach. The student found herself agreeing to shift her methodology to one involving experimental manipulation.

The above scenario typifies the view held by many members of the scientific community that hard research is more rigorous, more objective, and hence more worthy of being done than so-called soft research. It highlights the value placed on the experimental method at the expense of devaluing other approaches involving naturalistic observation and qualitative patterning of phenomena. Bakan has cogently described this valuing of method as the "disease of methodolatry, worship of method." He states that "when there is worship of these methods themselves rather than that to which they are directed, then indeed does science become idolatrous" (Bakan, 1966, p. 8).

This value orientation is only a part of a much broader conception of what is proper or real science. It is a view that is influencing the development of nurs-

From Advances in Nursing Science, *January 1983, 5(2), 27–36. Copyright © 1983. Aspen Systems Corporation. Reproduced with permission of Lippincott Williams & Wilkins.*

About the Authors

MINDY TINKLE was born in Abilene, TX, and received her BS from Texas Woman's University, MSN from the University of Texas Health Science Center at San Antonio, and PhD in nursing from the University of Texas at Austin. She is also a Women's Health Certified Nurse Practitioner (WHCNP). She is currently the Intramural Program Director for Research and Training at the National Institute of Nursing Research (NINR) at the National Institutes of Health. In her current role, she coordinates the NINR's Summer Genetics Institute, a 2-month intensive research training program in molecular and clinical genetics. The focus of her scholarship is on women's health promotion and genetics.

JANET ISABEL BEATON was born in Winnipeg, Manitoba, Canada, and received her basic nursing education degree from the University of Manitoba in 1969. Her graduate preparation was completed at the University of Washington (MA, 1972) and at the University of Texas (PhD, 1986). In both of her graduate programs, her area of specialization was maternal-infant research, and she fully expected that research work in this area would be her career path. However, in 1992, after 7 years as associate dean of the graduate program, she became Dean of the Faculty of Nursing at the University of Manitoba. Consequently, she believes that her biggest contributions to the profession have been in nursing administration. During her term as Dean, nursing education in the province was consolidated at the University of Manitoba. Satellite programs were developed in rural and northern areas, which substantially increased access to nursing education and enhanced career opportunities for young people in these traditionally underserved areas.

ing's body of knowledge. As nursing's sophistication in research and theory building grows, it is imperative that the dominant concept of what is proper science with its concomitant values not to be borrowed and adopted without introspection about the adequacy of this approach to meet nursing's most substantive problems.

Two Views of Science

Paradigm I

Sampson (1980) has eloquently described the long-standing controversy between two camps in regard to the definition of science. He has labeled these two positions paradigm I and paradigm II, a distinction that will be used throughout this article. Paradigm I, often termed hard science, (Baumrind, 1980), the positivist-empiricist approach, (Baumrind, 1980) or natural-law thought, (Wolf, 1971), is the dominant conception of science. This paradigm adopts the view

that there is a body of facts and principles to be discovered and understood that are independent of any historical or social context. This search for truth seeks principles that are abstract, general, and universal. The critical assumption of this position is the belief in the existence of an independent, autonomous ordering of facts that are historical and acontextual.

Several authors have expounded on the constellation of characteristics that distinguish paradigm I science (Baumrind, 1980; Parlee, 1979; Sampson, 1980; Sheriff, 1979). The experimental methodology is typically employed with the purpose of inferring unambiguously the existence and direction of causal relations. The assumption of linearity is also synonymous with this view. Research is generally conducted in artificial contexts, and the influence of sociohistorical factors is considered a source of error. Context-free generalizations are then formulated to apply to all individuals with little regard to situation.

Paradigm II

In contrast, paradigm II views science as necessarily historical. Facts and principles are inextricably embedded in a particular historical and cultural setting. All forms of knowledge are historically generated and rooted. According to this paradigm, truth is dynamic and is to be found only in the interactions between persons and concrete sociohistorical settings (Sampson, 1980).

Guided by this view, research is often conducted in naturalistic settings, using observational methods. Investigations are often unguided by any hypotheses and uncontaminated by structured experimental designs imposed prior to data collection (Bronfenbrenner, 1977). The influence of sociohistorical factors is not considered a source of error, but rather an integral part of the phenomenon being studied.

Basis for Dominant Approach

Beyond a mere description of these two conceptions of science lies a subtle paradox. The dominant paradigm I view of science, while loudly proclaiming its objective and universal nature, is itself an evolutionary product of a particular sociohistorical context. Sampson, in a synthesis from the works of several writers, has proposed that contemporary paradigm I science has grown and developed as a result of the nourishment it has received from a "male-dominant, Protestant-ethic oriented, middle-class, liberal, and capitalistic society" (Sampson, 1980, p. 1332). The philosophy of rugged individualism and the Protestant work ethic have significantly influenced scientific thought by dictating a science that is divorced from the influences of social context and by advocating an instrumental, utilitarian approach to scientific inquiry.

Similarly, the point that paradigm I science is a male model of scientific pursuit has been made by several authors (Baumrind, 1980; Bernard, 1973; Parlee, 1979; Sampson, 1980; Sheriff, 1979). Carlson (1971) has used Bakan's (1966) original terminology of agency and communion to describe paradigm I and II science. Agentic or more masculine science (paradigm I) can be described as individualistic, achievement-mastery oriented, and detached from feelings or impulses. Communal or more feminine science (paradigm II) can be characterized as attached, organic, reflective, and relational.

Bernard (1973) makes the crucial point that the dominant male ideal of science has been catapulted to the position of standard science. It has become the touchstone against which scientific endeavors are measured. The sociohistorical, relational conception of science has meanwhile been relegated to an inferior and secondary, if not suspect, position. By maintaining this power balance, paradigm I science is able to reaffirm its value orientation and maintain the status quo. By ignoring the sociocultural context in which facts and scientific truths are embedded, paradigm I science perpetuates its own values and traditions. New information is fitted into pre-existing schemas. On the other hand, paradigm II science places environmental and cultural influences within the purview of proper science, thereby fostering social criticism, innovation, and change.

With growing numbers of nurses pursuing graduate education, the belief that paradigm I science is the best way of perceiving and doing proper science may become solidly entrenched. Values about the research process, including the appropriate framing of research questions and methodologies, are generally formed in graduate school. Many nurses gain their knowledge about research from other fields in which the dominant paradigm I view is exclusively held. Nurses may also be schooled in the research process by other nurses who were themselves taught the positivist-empiricist approach. The entrenchment of the belief that there is only one acceptable method for the acquisition of scientific truth can have profound implications for the development of nursing's body of knowledge and for its relationship as a practice discipline to the rest of society.

Implications for Nursing

Uncritical, unilateral acceptance of the paradigm I view of science has important implications for nursing research and practice. These implications extend from the type of variables deemed important concerns for nursing research to the impact that research findings ultimately have on health care delivery and social policy.

The paradigm I conception of science asserts that scientific truths, by virtue of their abstract, universalistic nature, are value free; that is, they exist independently of the particular sociohistorical context in which they are discovered. As has already been discussed, there is a relationship between models for the acquisition of scientific knowledge and the value orientation of a society. Not only do scientific paradigms reflect the dominant values of society, but they also serve to reinforce and reaffirm those values. It follows that scientific research will never and can never be entirely value free.

Relevance of Values

For those who embrace the paradigm I conception of scientific truth as ahistorical and acontextual, questions of the values and biases underlying research endeavors have no meaning. Indeed, they are largely irrelevant. Implicit value assumptions are not made explicit. They are either taken for granted as a priori truths or are ignored altogether. The danger in denying the influence that values can exert on scientific truth lies in the fact that it can produce a distorted view of social reality.

In psychology, for example, the pervasive yet subtle manner in which implicit methodological biases have worked against the accumulation of accurate knowledge about women has only recently been recognized (Frieze, Parsons, Johson, et al., 1978). Frieze et al. have stated that "one of the latent functions of most research on women and sex differences has always been to support the researcher's political position on the status of women in society" (Frieze, Parsons, Johson, et al., 1978, p. 15). Conclusions thus reached could hardly be said to represent acontextual universal truths. Yet, frequently they have been presented and accepted as such by the scientific community and have all too frequently hindered rather than furthered an understanding of women and the social issues affecting them.

Recognition Research Biases

As a social phenomenon, nursing is no less value laden than psychology, patients are no less vulnerable to distorted representation than are women, and the dangers of actually preventing or ignoring needed changes in the contextual variables affecting patient care are no less real. To accurately evaluate the results of research studies, nursing must make explicit the values on which its research methodologies are based. Otherwise, nursing will be blind to its own biases.

If, for example, patients are found not to participate in decision making regarding their care, the question could be raised as to whether this is a reflection of the natural order of things—i.e., that patients are by definition passive—or whether it is a function of other social, cultural, or economic factors that are amenable to change. When patient passivity is coupled with an underlying belief that decision making in health care is a professional prerogative for which patients should not really assume responsibility, such a finding can be used to reaffirm and justify the status quo. Patients are passive because that is their choice. Therefore, there is no reason to involve them in decision making or to question further the cause of their passivity beyond an investigation of intrapsychic variables.

This is not to say that an understanding of intrapsychic variable is not important nor that it is impossible to control for the influence of contextual variables to arrive at a valid conclusion that patients do indeed wish to remain passive with regard to decision making. Rather, situation-person interactions are less likely to be considered important within a scientific frame of reference that is focused exclusively on a paradigm I conception of proper science. Similarly, the influence of implicit professional biases is less likely to be acknowledged as a factor of the interpretation of research results. In this regard, paradigm I science has the potential to be less objective than that of paradigm II.

Frame of Reference

The acontextual nature of the paradigm I conception of science negates the involvement of the consumer in determining which questions are important areas for nursing research. Research interests will necessarily reflect the investigator's rather than the consumer's interests, values, and frame of reference. Considerations of social relevancy are unimportant to a science that emphasizes the pursuit of scientific truth as ahistorical and asocial.

No science is in reality value free. The only values that can be reflected by paradigm I research are those of the investigator. Consequently, not only is it likely that such research will suffer from a profound professional bias regarding what are the really important issues, it will also be severely limited in the scope of the issues that can be researched. When question generation is dependent solely on the values and experience of the investigator, a narrow science emerges (Wallston, 1981). It is also a science that tends to tacitly accept the status quo because those are the values on which it is based. Such an orientation is apt to favor retention of traditional modes of research and practice rather than experimentation with new ideas and methodologies.

Professional Relationships

At its most basic level, nursing is a relational profession. It exists by virtue of its commitment to provide care to others. If the concerns and perceptions of the recipients of nursing services are considered unimportant factors in nursing research, then nurses may indeed be providing nursing care that is more meaningful to themselves than to patients. Similarly, if research studies regarding patient behavior fail to ascertain the patients' perception of the rationale for their own actions, interpretation of research results will reflect only a one-sided bias in favor of what the nurse thinks the patient thinks.

Studies that fail to acknowledge the research subject's perception of the environment are said to lack ecological validity (Bronfenbrenner, 1977). According to Bronfenbrenner, the ecological validity of a study "refers to the extent to which the environment experienced by subjects in a scientific investigation has the properties it is supposed or assumed to have by the investigator" (Bronfenbrenner, 1977, p. 516). Research dominated by a paradigm I conception of science would have difficulty meeting Bronfenbrenner's criteria for ecological validity because it would not be concerned with the research subjects' definition of their situation. Nursing studies that fail to consider the patient's perspective could therefore be considered ecologically invalid.

Studies of the Real World

The goal of paradigm I science is to minimize the influence of contextual variables so that the results of a study may be generalized to all individuals without regard to age, sex, or situation (Baumrind, 1980). This goal is usually sought by means of experimental control and manipulation of situational variables. Unfortunately, this often results in research that is so tightly controlled that it bears little resemblance to what actually transpires in the real world (Baumrind, 1980; Bronfenbrenner, 1977). Rather than increasing the generalizability of research findings, the interpretation of the results of such studies must be limited to the artificial contexts in which they occur. In this regard, the methods employed by paradigm I science are self-defeating.

If a goal of nursing research is to provide findings that will have an impact on the delivery of health care services, then the exclusive use of methodologies typical of paradigm I science is obviously inappropriate. Similarly, research findings resulting from methodologies that ignore the importance of person-situation interactions are of limited utility in the formulation of social policy. The necessary data on which to base policy recommendations will not exist. If nursing is concerned about the strength of its voice in decision making regarding improvements in health care services, then it would do well to evaluate carefully the limitations placed on this ability by a paradigm I conception of the constituents of proper science.

Nursing's View of Science

Following the delineation of the implications an overvaluation of paradigm I science has for nursing, it is germane to examine the views of science most commonly held by nursing theorists and researchers. After a review of some of the classic metatheoretical pieces and papers on nursing research, a striking conflict emerges. This conflict involves a wide discrepancy between the conceptualization of nursing and the definition of science. Almost without exception the nurse authors, in talking about the goals and purposes of nursing, the content of nursing theory, and the criteria by which to evaluate nursing theory, emphasize the importance of sociohistorical contexts or person-environment interactions. There is strong evidence of a deep commitment to nursing conceptualized in a relational sense.

However, as the authors turn from conceptualization of nursing and nursing theory to definitions of science and the research process, the overvaluation of paradigm I science is blatant. Indeed, this view of science is presented as synonymous with true science, as little or no debate about an alternative view is evident. To illustrate this conflict, an overview of the major ideas posited in the nursing literature concerning theory, science, and the research process will be briefly sketched.

Human as Holistic Being

The overarching conceptualization of nursing that can be abstracted from many of nursing's theorists is centered around the view of human as a holistic being (Ellis, 1968; Fawcett, 1978; Johnson, 1974; Neuman, 1974; Rogers, 1970). Nursing involves treating those factors affecting the patient's health that emerge from each one's unique biopsychosocial context. There is concern for the whole person. Ellis (1968) suggests that nursing must examine and treat the variables that affect a patient's health in combination or in interaction with each other versus separately or in isolation. This combination of variables is often represented as greater than the sum of each part, a systems model approach (Ellis, 1968; Rogers, 1970).

The impact of the environment on patients and their health status is a recurrent theme in the nursing literature. Fawcett (1978) postulates that as skill in theory development matures, nursing theories will emerge

that fully appreciate the continuous person-environment interaction and its relationship to health. The patient's environment is not restricted to one setting; it includes several levels of analysis—the individual level, the family level, and the community level. King (1964) extends the patient's environment within the domain of nursing beyond the community level to include those more distant social institutions that impinge on individual functioning.

Sociocultural Context

The import of the patient's sociocultural context is evident in the evaluative criteria for nursing theories. Johnson (1974) suggests that the criteria of "social congruence," "social significance," and "social utility" be used to assess the significance of a theory for nursing. These criteria address specifically the embeddedness of the individual as well as the nursing profession itself in a unique and specific social context. Hardy (1974) alludes to this dynamic and changing social context in discussing the tentative nature of theories. She posits that theory cannot be assessed without an examination of the cultural and societal values that are inextricably linked with theory development.

A synthesis of these perspectives on the goals of nursing and the context and evaluative criteria for nursing theory portrays a profession committed to the values embraced by the paradigm II view of science. These values include an appreciation of both the sociohistorical context in which an individual exists and the organismic or relational nature of the practice of nursing. However, these values are not congruent with the definitions of science and the descriptions of the research process most prevalent in the nursing literature. The paradigm I conceptualization is the model for proper science.

Empirical Reality

Jacox (1974) and Johnson (1974) describe the main purpose of science as the discovery of truths about the world. There is a knowable empirical reality to be discovered. Scientific knowledge is expressed in general, abstract, and universal laws. These universal statements are devoid of any sociohistorical context. Silva (1977) further asserts that the scientist is primarily concerned with establishing cause and effect relationships.

The experimental method is also held in the highest regard. Several authors describe a progression for research designs based on the amount of knowledge available in a discipline (Fawcett, 1978; Hardy, 1974). According to this progression, descriptive or qualitative research should be undertaken when there is little information available or when a science is young. Correlational research can then follow when the essential characteristics of a phenomenon under study are known. Finally, and most important, the experimental method can be utilized when these two lower levels have been explored. The experimental method is portrayed as the most appropriate design in testing theory (Brown, 1964).

Superiority of Paradigm I

There is some evidence within the nursing literature that this exclusive approach to science might be somewhat dissonant with dominant nursing values. However, following the explication of an alternative method of pursuing science, the superior or more rigorous nature of the experimental approach is usually reaffirmed. For example, Quint (1967) proposes that grounded theory or the field approach of Glaser and Strauss (1967) have much to offer in the development of nursing knowledge but views the outcome of these types of research only as the grounds for more rigorous or refined scientific endeavors. Walker identifies the strength of this grounded theory approach as an opportunity for the researcher "to really see what's going on out there" (Walker, 1980, p. 5). However, she warns that the findings from an investigation of this sort should only be used in the context of discovery and not in the context of verification. As Sampson (1980) points out, this distinction grants final authority and superiority to paradigm I science.

Clearly what is needed is a more balanced and convergent perspective on what constitutes proper science. It is not that paradigm I values should be dismissed as useless and false, but rather that these values should no longer be dominant in nursing education and nursing research endeavors.

Toward a Convergent Definition of Science

The preceding discussion should not be interpreted as a total condemnation of paradigm I science. Nor should it be interpreted as the wholehearted endorsement of paradigm II. It is the position of the authors that neither paradigmatic stance by itself is sufficient. Indeed what is proposed is a blending of both methodologies to produce a science that retains a critical concern for the objectivity traditionally associated with paradigm I while ensuring that the research it produces has some validity in the real world and that the influence of contextual variables on research findings is acknowledged and made explicit. Such a synthesis requires the granting of equal status to each paradigmatic view, not the negation of one in favor of the other (Sampson, 1980).

If as a profession nursing does indeed possess its own body of knowledge, it would seem reasonable to expect that it may well have to develop its own unique research strategies to develop that body of knowledge. Nursing's research methodologies should reflect its theoretical propositions about the nature of its science. Borrowing methodologies from other disciplines with a different conceptual base may not only retard the development of nursing theory but will almost certainly dilute its uniqueness as well.

Nursing would do well to learn from other disciplines to avoid the pitfalls of "physics envy" and the concomitant devaluing of "soft" research to validate itself as a scientific discipline. In psychology, for example Wallston (1981) has pointed out how an overvaluing of agentic approaches has retarded the understanding and integration of major concepts related to the study of women. She calls for the synthesis of agentic and communal science as a means of gaining additional information.

"Whole" Person in Context

Nursing theories and models for practice expound on the importance of considering the "whole" person in the sociocultural-biological context. Yet how often do nursing research questions, designs, and methodologies reflect this perspective? Too often nursing has taken a stance based on the prior belief that one methodological approach is by definition necessarily superior to another. All too often that belief had reflected nurses' desire to prove themselves as real scientists rather than a concern for the ability of one scientific paradigm over another commits the researcher to the view that there is only one right way to do research. Such a position is only slightly removed from a procedure manual approach to nursing research.

Dialectical Synthesis of Approaches

When paradigms I and II are granted equal status, the door is opened to a critical dialogue from which a dialectical synthesis of the two approaches can emerge. Sampson (1980) has argued that this new synthesis will not consist of the use of paradigm II methods in the context of discovery and the use of paradigm I methodologies in matters of verification. Rather, a convergence of paradigm I and paradigm II conceptions of science will involve the "higher organization of the opposites in both paradigms" (Sampson, 1980, p. 1312). Perhaps the true opportunity for nursing to develop a body of knowledge that is uniquely its own lies in this type of synthesis.

The development of a more convergent definition of science has the potential to enhance the impact that nursing research has on health care delivery and social policy. A new emphasis on contextual variables would force a closer examination not only of those theories that nursing currently utilizes to explain what happens in practice settings, but of the practices and their settings as well. A more functional integration of theory and practice can be achieved, and change and innovation in nursing practice can be facilitated. Similarly, when there is an increased awareness of the importance of contextual variables, policy implications are more likely to be considered and recommendations made.

The real value of a convergent definition of science for nursing, however, lies in the opportunity it provides to draw from a variety of sources to develop new methods and approaches specifically tailored to investigate questions of concern to nursing while remaining flexible and creative enough to avoid the "disease of methodolatry."

REFERENCES

Bakan, D. (1966). *The duality of human existence: An essay on psychology and religion.* Chicago: Rand McNally.

Baumrind, D. (1980). New directions in socialization research. *American Psychologist, 35,* 639–652.

Bernard, J. (1973). My four revolutions: An autobiographical history of the ASA. *American Journal of Sociology, 78,* 773–791.

Bronfenbrenner, U. (1977). Toward an experimental ecology of human development. *American Psychologist, 32,* 513–531.

Brown, M. (1964). Research in the development of nursing theory. *Nursing Research, 13,* 109–112.

Carlson, R. (1971). Sex differences in ego functioning: Exploratory studies of agency and communion. *Journal of Consulting and Clinical Psychology, 37,* 267–277.

Ellis, R. (1968). Characteristics of significant theories. *Nursing Research, 69,* 1434–1438.

Fawcett, J. (1978). The relationship between theory and research: A double helix. *Advances in Nursing Science, 1,* 49–62.

Frieze, I. H., Parsons, P. B., et al. (1978). *Women and sex roles.* New York: Norton.

Glaser, B. G., & Strauss, A. L. (1967). *Discovery of grounded theory: Strategies for qualitative research.* Chicago: Aldine.

Hardy, M. E. (1974). Theories: Components, development, evaluation. *Nursing Research, 23,* 100–107.

Jacox, A. (1974). Theory construction in nursing: An overview. *Nursing Research, 23,* 4–13.

Johnson, D. E. (1974). Development of theory: A requisite for nursing as a primary health profession. *Nursing Research, 23,* 372–377.

King, I. M. (1964). Nursing theory—problems and prospect. *Nursing Science, 2,* 394–403.

Neuman, B. (1974). The Betty Neuman health care systems model: A total person approach to patient problems. In J. Riehl & C. Roy (Eds.), *Conceptual models for nursing practice.* New York: Appleton-Century-Crofts.

Parlee, M. B. (1979). Psychology and women. *Signs, 5,* 121–133.

Quint, J. C. (1967). The case for theories generated from empirical data. *Nursing Research, 16,* 109–114.

Rogers, M. E. (1970). *An introduction to the theoretical basis of nursing.* Philadelphia: F. A. Davis.

Sampson, E. E. (1980). Scientific paradigms and social values: Wanted—A scientific revolution. *Journal of Personality and Social Psychology, 35,* 639–652.

Sheriff, C. W. (1979). Bias in psychology. In J. A. Sherman & E. T. Beck (Eds.), *The prism of sex: Essays in the sociology of knowledge.* Madison, WI: University of Wisconsin Press.

Silva, M. C. (1977). Philosophy, science, theory: Interrelationships and implications for nursing research. *Image, 9,* 59–63.

Walker, L. O. (1980, June). Inductive approaches to theory development in nursing. Unpublished manuscript.

Wallston, B. S. (1981). What are the questions in psychology of women? A feminist approach to research. *Psychology of Women Quarterly, 5*(4), 597–615.

Wolf, K. H. (1971). Introduction. In K. Mannheim, *From Karl Mannheim.* New York: Oxford University Press.

The Authors Comment

Toward a New View of Science: Implications for Nursing Research

Janet and I were spurred to write this article when we were both enrolled in the doctoral program at the University of Texas at Austin School of Nursing and taking a marvelous graduate course on the psychology of women. We wrote our article at a time when nursing was beginning to examine the overvaluation of quantitative methods. At this point in our science, we are past this seminal issue and, instead, are more concerned with an integrative approach, with more emphasis on how best to use these methods to answer our questions. Nurse investigators have linked with scientists in other disciplines who are doing excellent qualitative work and are also often included on research teams to provide that qualitative perspective.

—Mindy Tinkle
—Janet Isabel Beaton

CHAPTER 22

A Multiparadigm Approach
to Nursing

Joan Engebretson

Nursing theory development has made good progress in differentiating the domain of nursing from medicine; many of these theories are categorized as holistic theories. Nursing classification systems are also being developed to organize extant nursing practice. The dissonance between the two has been one of the most difficult contemporary issues for the leadership of nursing. A framework is proposed that would account for these disparate approaches. This proposed framework for the domain of healing is in keeping with the metaparadigm of health and uses a multiple paradigm approach. Nursing interventions are discussed in relation to the framework. It invites a dialogue in keeping with the scholarship of holism. Practice and scholarship implications are discussed.

Key words: *classification systems, culture, holism, paradigm, theory*

Nursing theory has, since the 1960s, sought to define the profession of nursing and to differentiate its scope of practice from that of biomedicine.[1] This search has led to some discrepancies between theory development that differentiates nursing action from biomedical nursing practice, the latter of which uses many nursing actions derived from biomedicine. Differentiating autonomous nursing practice was a necessary step, because historically many nursing functions were derived from biomedicine, since nurses have practiced in biomedically dominated settings.

One primary differentiating feature was holism, which was contrasted with biomedical reductionism. The movement to declare nursing holistic is now well

Reprinted from Advances in Nursing Science *1997;20(1):21-33*
Copyright © 1997 Aspen Publishers, Inc. Reprinted with permission of Lippincott Williams & Wilkins.

About the Author

JOAN C. ENGEBRETSON was born in Wisconsin, on November 12, 1943, and grew up in Minnesota. She received a BSN from St. Olaf College, an MS from Texas Woman's University, and a DrPH from the University of Texas Health Science Center at Houston School of Public Heath. She worked as a public health nurse both in Oakland, CA, and Boston, MA, and has been a faculty member at University of St. Thomas, Houston, TX, and University of Texas Health Science Center at Houston, School of Nursing and School of Public Health. Her clinical focus has been maternal-child and women's health. Her academic focus includes health promotion, culture, theory, and qualitative methodologies in research. Her research has included the development of a pacifier for low-birth-weight infants, women's anticipations of hormonal therapy for perimenopause, ethnographic studies of healing, clinical trials of Reiki Touch therapy, patient's beliefs and experiences related to chronic diseases, and the incorporation of complementary therapies and approaches to healing. Her primary focus is related to a better understanding of various perspectives and strategies of healing that nurses can incorporate into patient care to promote health throughout the health-illness continuum. Throughout her life, she has developed interests in travel, cooking, reading, and photography.

accepted; however, a holistic framework must be inclusive of, not only differentiated from, biomedicine. In alignment with holism, the appropriate construct for the nursing profession is healing. Health is a derivative of healing, or making whole, and part of the metaparadigm of nursing.

Another element of professional evolution is the development of diagnostic, intervention, and outcomes classifications systems. These are often grounded in nursing practice and thus reflect both nursing activities as well as predominant sociocultural ideologies. There is often a disjuncture between the differentiating and defining theories and the more pragmatic classifications systems.[2] In an effort to reconcile grand conceptual models and practice, this article presents a conceptual framework for discussion as a step toward the consolidation of a holistic approach to nursing. The intent is to support both unique autonomous actions and to incorporate medically derived actions. Using the construct of healing, a multiparadigm model is presented to incorporate both the medical model and other cultural healing models on which nurses may ground their actions. This integration is at the level of paradigm, which allows the incorporation of and expansion beyond the biomed-

ical model and avoids the pitfalls of the derivative-differentiation polarity.

Nursing has over the past 30 years made great strides in the development of nursing theories and conceptual models. These activities have been necessary to define the professional domain to its members and to society at large. Theory guides the practice and the activities that are unique to the profession, informs research efforts, and provides direction for future development.[3]

Contemporary Controversies

Despite the progress made, the use of nursing theories in practice has been a matter of controversy. One area of controversy is the dichotomy between medicine and nursing, with many theories focusing on unique nursing functions and in some cases redefining actions associated with medical models. This position has often still held the medical model as the orthodox standard against which nursing defined itself by negation or differentiation, thereby maintaining dependence on the medical model.

Closely related to the nursing-medicine dichotomy is the rupture between academia and practice. Academia and much of theory development focused on the autonomous nature of nursing, differentiating it from medicine. Extant nursing practice often eschewed the nursing theories learned in school, and practicing nurses functioned in a more pragmatic manner reflective of the medical model.[4] Many times the praxis of nursing is covertly, if not overtly, aligned with the medical model. This alliance with the medical model is understandable considering the hegemony of the medical bio-scientific model in U.S. culture. Barnum[4] noted that normative theory evolves from practice rather than academic theory development and that inconsistencies develop when practice (theory) is not intellectually analyzed and scrutinized according to logical coherence.

A third, related problem area is the disjuncture between nursing theories and the diagnosis, intervention, and outcome classification systems. The two strongest competitors in the theory business are holistic theories and nursing process,[1,4] which often represent opposing philosophies regarding content, methodology, and interpretation. Holistic theories are global, espouse a transcendental view of humans, and are committed to not viewing subject matter as an accumulation of parts.[4]

Nursing process approaches are much more concrete and practice based and have focused on nursing action and classification systems.[5] The International Council of Nurses,[6] the Omaha Project,[7] the Iowa Project,[8] and separate projects by Grobe[9] and Saba[10] have recently developed nursing classification systems.

Recent debates in nursing have also reflected controversies over the usefulness of a unified theory vs multiple theories. Reed[11] proposed an approach that links science, philosophy, and practice in the development of nursing knowledge. She advocated a metanarrative that involves a dialogue of practice and philosophy. This metanarrative provides an excellent format for the development of nursing theory that is holistic in nature and can integrate multiple paradigms from the patient's perspective and from the nurse. It is in this spirit of inviting a dialogue and providing a format for a dialectic discussion between paradigms that the author presents the multiparadigm model.

Holism and Nursing

Grand theory, or the concept level of theory development, has evolved into a metaparadigm with four propositional statements related to the concepts person-health, person-environment, health-nursing, and person-environment-health.[12] The global level defines the frameworks within which the more restricted structures develop.

Consistent with the concept heal—health, the related ideologies for nursing theory development would come from healing, rather than be restricted to medicine. Healing and health stem from the root word *hale*, or to make whole.[13] This etymology grounds the concept heal—health in holism. Barnum[4] identified holistic theories as the fastest growing trend in nursing. Holistic concepts in nursing have been evident since the time of Florence Nightingale and evolved in nursing theories through the influence of Teilhard de Chardin, Jan Smuts, and Ludwig von Bertalanffy.[14] Anthropology, another discipline based on holism, provides another source of information on healing that can inform nurses in the development of holistic theory. Traditionally, in many cultures, healers, shamans, and medicine people reflected the broader concept of healing rather than the science-based concept of cure.

Holistic health has recently become very popular among both lay and professional groups. Characteristics of holistic health have been described in many studies.[15-19] Two common mistakes occur in the analysis of holism from a modernist perspective based in a scientific or reductionistic paradigm. Alster's[15] analysis of holistic health is an example of such an attempt; it reaches the syllogistic conclusion that holistic health cannot be studied scientifically because it is not scientific.

The opposite pitfall is to romanticize traditional or primitive healing systems and unfavorably compare science and biomedicine. This antiscience position is often seen in lay literature that attributes all social ills to scientific–rational thinking while extolling a holistic framework as the alternative. A consistent holistic framework incorporates science but does not hold that paradigm as sufficient for explaining the human experience or for bringing about health or healing. The model proposed in this article recognizes the holistic nature of nursing and expands the domain from disease treatment to the broader concept of health by incorporating several paradigms and their adjunctive ideological perspectives on humans, health, and therapeutic actions.

Historical Context of Western Medicine

Healing systems reflect and influence the cultural values of the parent culture. Contemporary biomedicine has been informed by and influential in the development of modernism. Modernity had its philosophical origins in the 17th century with the emphasis on rationality by the protagonists Galileo and Descartes.[20] Kuhn[21] described the shift of vision that enabled people to see and think about phenomena in a different manner and that he labeled a "paradigm shift." Modernity is characterized by the development of science and technology, the valorization of reason and humanity's dominion over nature. The scientific paradigm of modernity has dominated medicine and health care.

The establishment of the scientific model as the foundation for biomedicine paralleled the development of modernity. The scientific paradigm is characterized by philosophical dualism between the material and nonmaterial, and the corresponding designation of matter as the subject of science and the nonmaterial or metaphysical as the domain of religion. Descartes is often credited with conceptualizing the mind–body dualism and the corresponding value of the mind–soul as the superior demarcation of the human.

Throughout the following centuries, especially in England, increasing cultural value was placed on the scientific, material, rational, and technical.[22,23] Metaphysical and nonmaterial issues associated with religion were progressively devalued, especially among intellectuals.[24] Medicine, which historically had been based in a metaphysical model and supported by religion, became the domain of science and was severed from its metaphysical and religious roots. This split allowed medicine to make unprecedented technological advances through the application of scientific reason. But a contemporary surge of public interest in alternative healing modalities suggests that the biomedical scientific approach by itself is insufficient for healing.

Development of the Multiparadigm Model

The multiparadigm model was developed from the author's ethnographic work with healers and nurses. Field work, including participant observation, long interviews, free listing, and pile sorts, was used in a study exploring and comparing the conceptual frameworks of health and healing between nurses and healers.[25] A matrix of healing modalities that incorporated biomedicine and examples of alternative models emerging in the United States in the late 1980s and early 1990s was developed to focus the study on healers using healing touch[26] and used to orient nurse practitioners to alternative healing modalities that their clients might be using.[27]

This matrix was then developed into the Heterodox Explanatory Paradigms Model for health practice that incorporated multiple healing modalities.[28] The philosophical coherence of the model and the related positioning of modalities was presented as a framework for developing integrated health care models. Because nurses and healers have similar conceptual frameworks of healing,[25] this model could be adapted for nursing as a possible framework toward a more holistic model.

Philosophical Design

The multiparadigm model (Fig. 22-1) developed from the author's previous work[25-28] represents a multiparadigm approach to healing. Philosophical dualism between the material and nonmaterial is represented on both axes. Four paradigms of healing are incorporated and philosophically arranged from the most material to the most nonmaterial along the horizontal axis, which represents a philosophical continuum from logical pos-

Material ↑

Nonmaterial ↓

Modalities	Mechanical	Purification	Balance	Supranormal
Physical manipulation	Biomedical surgery	Colonics Cupping	Magnetic healing Polarity	Drumming Dancing
Applied and ingested substances	Pharmacology	Chelation	Humoral medicine	Flower remedies Hallucinogenic plants
Energy	Laser Radiation	Bioenergetics	Tai chi Chi gong Acupuncture Acupressure	Healing touch Laying on of hands
Psychological	Mind–body	Self-help (confessional type)	Mindfulness	Imagery
Spiritual	Attendance at organized religious functions	Forgiveness Penance	Meditation Chakra Balancing	Primal religious Experience Prayer

Figure 22-1 *Explanatory paradigms.*

itivism to metaphysics. Consistent with the positivist–metaphysical continuum, the mechanical paradigm is on the extreme left, reflecting the logical positivism of its philosophical scientific foundation. The paradigms are progressively more nonmaterial, ending in the most metaphysical paradigm, supranormal, at the extreme right. The vertical axis represents the Cartesian body–mind dualism in healing activities. Activities that are most material or physical are at the top. Moving down, activities become progressively less material and more psychological or spiritual.

Horizontal Axis

The four paradigms are mechanical, purification, balance, and supranormal. The mechanical paradigm is best represented by examples from biomedicine, which is primarily a mechanistic, materialistic paradigm exemplified by the focus on discovering explanatory mechanisms to understand a healing activity. The positivist philosophy bases knowing on objective, material data perceived by the senses.[29] It is characterized by determinism, mechanism, and reductionism. Disease is assumed to be reducible to disordered body functions and a disease-specific etiology.[30] Treatment and intervention are disease specific.

The purification paradigm has examples cross-culturally and throughout Western history. This paradigm is characterized by healing actions that cleanse or purify. The name of the prestigious English medical journal *Lancet* is a remnant of the bloodletting and purges that dominated Western medicine before technical advances in surgery and antibiotics in the 20th century. Health and healing activities related to cleanliness or purification either physically or symbolically have been documented in many ritual practices.[31] The hygienic health reform movement of the late 19th century[32,33] incorporated many practices that were understood as cleansing and keeping the body pure.

The balance paradigm is best represented by Eastern or humeral systems. In Eastern systems health–healing is viewed as the proper balance of yin and yang and unimpeded flow of Chi (or Ki or Qi).[34] Humeral medicine, or the balance of vital forces or humors, is evident in Hippocratic, Galenic, and Ayurvedic medicine.[35] Nineteenth-century vitalism also incorporated this approach. Health is attained or maintained by creating a balance in daily living through types of foods, activities, temperature, and so forth. Personality types, environment, and circumstances are considered in determining the corrective balance. One example is the hot and cold classification in Mexican folk medicine. The balance paradigm is on the right half of the model and therefore cannot be fully understood through a materialist mechanistic paradigm.

The supranormal paradigm incorporates all magicoreligious and psychic phenomena used to promote health or create healing. Spiritual, symbolic, and other nonmaterial understandings of healing are in this column. The supranormal paradigm is philosophically the most metaphysical, going beyond physics, sense experience, or any discipline and involving ultimates.[36] This paradigm incorporates psychic, spiritual, and other types of healing such as prayer, distant healing, and other spontaneous healing that cannot be explained by mechanistic models or one of the other paradigms.

Vertical Axis

The vertical axis describes types of healing activities that progress along the continuum from body to mind–soul, from material to nonmaterial. The first row contains physical manipulations, and examples are given for each paradigm. Physical manipulation may be performed either by the patient or on the patient by a healer.

In row 2 applied and ingested substances are listed according to each paradigm. Such substances include all foods, herbs, and pharmaceuticals that are ingested, inhaled, or topically applied.

Using energy, the third activity, is a concept that is poorly understood in biomedicine but important in other paradigms. Many healing activities are understood and conducted as an active manipulation of energy. The concept of energy, or the transfer from matter to energy to matter, has been proposed by some scientists (eg, Bohm, Capra[37]) as the basis for quantum physics and as a possible link in understanding the material and nonmaterial worlds. This could be a promising area in linking the material, physical body with nonmaterial thought, spirit, and so on. The concept of energy has been proposed by some nurses as the basis for understanding the benefits of touch therapies.[38-40]

Psychological activities deal with functions of cognition and of the mind. Mind to body medicine has been a rapidly growing area of research. With the discovery of neurotransmitters and hormonal–neural pathways, mechanisms have been discovered by which thoughts and feelings can manifest in physiological changes.[41] Theory has been developed and researched regarding the association of personality characteristics with illness, in particular hostility and heart disease.[42] Psychoneuroimmunology is another promising field where theory is developing. Associations have been demonstrated between various personality characteristics and mortality and morbidity.[43,44]

Spiritual activities are at the polar opposite of the continuum from physical manipulation. Spiritual actions are distinct from cognitive activities. Spirituality, being the most distant from the physical or material, is the least understood from a modernist perspective. Some studies have found that attendance at religious activities is related to improved health or healing.[45] Attendance at religious activities represents a mechanistic conceptualization of spiritual activity, whereas a primal spiritual experience as described by Cox[46] would be a more metaphysical approach.

The model has, at present, four paradigms, but others could be added along the continuum. Restriction to a two-dimensional format is often interpreted as containing mutually exclusive cells. A more appropriate geographic conceptualization would be as general areas on a double-axis continuum, with no specific boundary between areas. Modalities in the model are examples only, and many other modalities could fit in each location. The modalities describe healing activities only. An individual practitioner–healer could, and often does, use many modalities.

The positioning of modalities according to philosophical continuums also reflects the degree of passivity or activity of the healer. Starting from the upper left corner, where the modalities are most material, the healer is most active and the recipient most passive. Moving diagonally down and across, the person who is healing is progressively more active and the role of the healer increasingly that of facilitator, consistent with healing philosophy, which posits that real healing is done by the "healee."

One area that is a vital part of the nursing metaparadigm and other healing systems is the environment, especially social relationships. Although not specifically addressed in the model, an additional line at the bottom could be added to address social activities.

Application to Nursing

The multiparadigm model is holistic and avoids the medicine-nursing and practice-academia dichotomies by placing the Western biomedical model in context with other paradigms of healing. It speaks to the domain of healing, which is the stated domain of nursing. This model can provide a framework for nursing diagnoses and interventions that easily integrates biomedical model functions with complementary functions that either are autonomous nursing activities or might constitute appropriate referrals. The model also incorporates paradigms that can be useful in understanding cross-cultural healing practices and systems.

Implications for Practice

Operating from a multiparadigm model allows nurses to adapt whatever paradigm or modality fits the situation. This flexibility is helpful in working with patients who practice health- and healing-related activities from other paradigms. A multiparadigm approach that incorporates models of health–healing can help providers better understand beliefs and practices of patients that may be poorly comprehended in the biomedical model.

Most health practices originate in the popular sector,[47] which includes family and social networks. This sector has beliefs about health maintenance and hierarchies of resort that direct types of health–healing activities, healer consultants, and adherence to treatments. The orientation of the popular sector often incorporates other paradigms than the scientific–mechanistic approach of biomedicine. By understanding the explanatory paradigm of health practices, the practitioner is bet-

ter able to communicate and collaborate with the client and family in the management of health–healing.

Many interventions listed in the various nursing classification systems may be positioned in this model. Examples from one of these systems, the Nursing Interventions Classification (NIC),[8] have been identified in Fig. 22-2, along with other modalities that could be referral sources for the client. Examples are easily placed in the mechanistic and purification paradigms but more difficult to place in the balance and supranormal paradigms. Thus, the model can display areas where nursing has developed actions and where referrals are more appropriate. It is important to note that a holistic paradigm is impossible to implement in its entirety by any one person or discipline; therefore, nurses should be able to understand how other providers fit into an overall plan of care.

By understanding these modalities through the appropriate paradigm, practitioners may select whatever modality is appropriate for the client, either by interventions or referral to other providers. For example, existing NIC actions in the mechanical paradigm for physical manipulation could incorporate positioning, exercise therapy including range of motion, and ambulation. Applied and ingested substances include medication administration of all types. Although energy is poorly understood in the mechanical model, it is present on the NIC as laser precautions. Energy, if better understood, could have potential for much broader use.

Psychological interventions in the mechanical (medical) model include cognitive restructuring and reality therapies. Spiritual interventions may include assisting a patient with religious practices such as attending chapel or praying. This is not specifically listed in NIC but is covered under activity therapy.

Examples of nursing actions in the purification paradigm using physical manipulation include bathing and other hygiene activities. Wound and bladder irrigations are good examples of applied and ingested substances. Many medications have cleaning or purification action, such as emetics, expectorants, and purgatives. Psychological and emotional catharsis are examples of psycho-

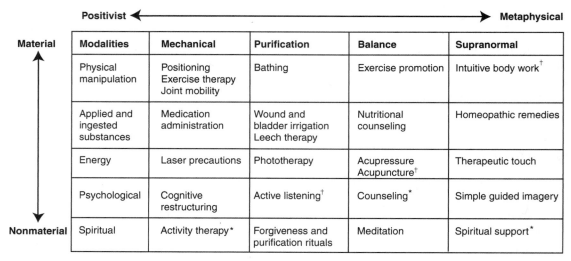

Figure 22-2 *Nursing activities and interventions.*

logical purification. These are not specifically listed, although could be covered under the NIC active listening.

Spiritual purification includes a number of rituals that serve to purify and cleanse the individual, such as confession, seeking of forgiveness, ritual bathing, and use of incense. These would need to be developed or referred because there is no NIC entry related to this.

Nursing interventions are being expanded into the balance and supranormal paradigms through the work of nurses who have expanded their individual practice and those who are using many of the more recent nursing theories, such as Rogers,[48] Watson,[49] Parse,[50] or Newman,[51] to direct their practice. Exercise promotion is listed in NIC and could be expanded and developed with a better understanding of the balance paradigm. Nutritional counseling is based on providing a balance of nutrients and could also be expanded to incorporate use of some herbs for the promotion of health. Approaching these from the perspective of balance rather than mechanical cure allows for an expansion into health and attention to individual life systems. Acupuncture or acupressure are not on the NIC but could be a source of referral. While currently not part of the balance paradigm, counseling, simple relaxation therapy, or self-modification assistance have the potential for development into that paradigm. Meditation also has potential for development.

Nursing interventions in the supranormal paradigm cluster in the nonmaterial areas. Intuitive body work, if not done by a nurse, could constitute a referral. Likewise, activities using homeopathic remedies or flower essences are included as they are understood to work through the spiritual level.

Therapeutic touch is well developed in nursing and is understood as a supranormal use of energy. Guided imagery is a supranormal psychological technique that is listed in the NIC. Spiritual support, including prayer, could be further developed to fully express this paradigm.

Implications for Research and Scholarship

By constructing a paradigm map with health–healing activities, nurses can determine appropriate paradigms to guide their understanding and research of particular modalities. Locating it on the model can serve as a guide for better understanding a particular modality; it also provides a direction for further scholarship and research. An exploration of both axes can enhance understanding. For example, nursing actions in the mechanical paradigm are often best understood by a better comprehension of the medical—scientific model, and research using the positivist philosophy is often appropriate. Many of the NIC classifications can be understood from this paradigm.

Working with a modality such as guided imagery could be enhanced by exploring both the supranormal paradigm and the psychological literature. Healing touch, a modality with a rich history in nursing, is located at the nexus of energy and the supranormal, the two axes least understood by biomedical science. Nurses who have conducted research using this modality or the existential psychological theories can attest to the frustration in conducting research without documented material and measurable mechanisms of action that are compatible with the mechanical paradigm. Research in these areas can be enhanced by learning more about the approaches of anthropology, theology, some psychology, and other humanity disciplines consistent with the supranormal paradigm. Investigation of energy through quantum physics (energy) and Eastern healing are also proximal areas that can illuminate the understanding of touch therapies.

The model can serve as an agenda for research and scholarship. In some modalities, links have been or can be developed that enable more mechanistic studies. In others, their position invites more qualitative or naturalistic methodologies of inquiry. Nursing theories may develop links that connect modalities for practice. For example, some of the developmental theories may have links across paradigms on the psychological axis. Although methods may be successfully combined, caution must be taken in attempting to link paradigms. Many paradigms are based on contradictory beliefs that are impossible to adhere to simultaneously.[52]

The multiparadigm model provides a holistic approach to bridging the gulf between holistic theories and biomedical nursing praxis. The dialectic method is appropriate scholarship for holistic frameworks.[4,53] In this approach, the whole is seen as governing relationships and providing coherence to the parts. The dialectic process would describe a nursing issue from one position—for example, the mechanical paradigm—and then counter that description with an oppositional position, the supranormal. After debate and dialogue, a third position emerges. This position can, in similar fashion, be refined by the same process. Placing the polar opposites in one model invites a dialectic methodology, appropriate for holistic nursing scholarship. The challenge remains for nurses to continue to develop theory that links modalities and explanatory paradigms. These links are being developed along nursing themes of health, environment, and individual potentials for healing. The model could help to provide a geographic map to locate these dialogues.

REFERENCES

1. Chinn PL, Kramer MK. *Theory and Nursing: A Systematic Approach.* St. Louis, Mo: Mosby; 1995.
2. Fitzpatrick JJ, Whall AL. *Conceptual Models of Nursing Analysis and Application.* 3rd ed. Stamford, Conn: Appleton & Lange; 1996.
3. Newman MN. *A Developing Discipline: Selected Works of Margaret Newman.* New York, NY: National League for Nursing Press; 1995.
4. Barnum BJS. *Nursing Theory: Analysis, Application, Evaluation.* Philadelphia, Pa: Lippincott; 1994.
5. Snyder M. Defining nursing interventions. *Image J Nurs Schol.* 1996;28(2):137–141.
6. International Council of Nurses. *Nurses' Next Advance: An International Classification for Nursing Practice.* Geneva, Switzerland: ICN; 1993.
7. Martin KS, Scheet NJ. *The Omaha System: Applications for Community Health Nursing.* Philadelphia. Pa: W. B. Saunders; 1992.
8. McCloskey JC, Bulechek GM. *Nursing Interventions Classification (NIC).* St. Louis, Mo: Mosby; 1996.
9. Grobe SJ. The nursing lexicon and taxonomy: implications for representing nursing care data in automated patient records. *Holistic Nurs Pract.* 1996;11(1):48–63.
10. Saba VK. The classification of home health nursing. *Caring.* 1992;11(3):50–57.
11. Reed, PG. A treatise on nursing knowledge development for the 21st century: beyond postmodernism. *ANS.* 1995;17(3): 70–84.
12. Fawcett J. *Analysis and evaluation of nursing theories.* Philadelphia, Pa: F. A. Davis; 1993.

13. *Webster's Ninth New Collegiate Dictionary.* Springfield, Mass: Merriam-Webster; 1990.

14. Owen MJ, Holmes CA. Holism in the discourse of nursing. *J Adv Nurs.* 1993;18;1688–1695.

15. Alster, KB. *The Holistic Health Movement.* Tuscaloosa, Ala: University of Alabama Press; 1989.

16. English-Lueck JA. *Health in the New Age: A Study in California Holistic Practices.* Albuquerque, NM: University of New Mexico Press; 1990.

17. Gordon, JS. The paradigm of holistic medicine. In: Hastings AC, Fadiman J, Gordon JS, eds. *Health for the Whole Person.* Toronto, Ontario: Bantam Books; 1980.

18. Lowenberg JS. *Caring and Responsibility.* Philadelphia, Pa: University of Pennsylvania Press; 1989.

19. Mattson PH. *Holistic Health in Perspective.* Palo Alto, Calif: Mayfield; 1982.

20. Toulmin S. *Cosmopolis: The Hidden Agenda of Modernity.* Chicago, Ill: University of Chicago Press; 1990.

21. Kuhn T. *The Structure of Scientific Revolutions.* Chicago, Ill: The University of Chicago Press; 1972.

22. Tarnas R. *The Passion of the Western World: Understanding the Ideas That Have Shaped our World View.* New York, NY: Ballantine Books; 1991.

23. Lavine TZ. *From Socrates to Sartre: The Philosophic Quest.* New York, NY: Bantam; 1984.

24. Johnson P. *Intellectuals.* New York, NY: Harper Perennial; 1988.

25. Engebretson J. Comparison of nurses and alternative healers. *Image J Nurs Schol.* 1996;28(2):95–100.

26. Engebretson J. *Cultural Models of Healing and Health: An Ethnography of Professional Nurses and Healers.* Houston, Tex: University of Texas-Houston, School of Public Health; 1992. Dissertation.

27. Engebretson J, Wardell D. A contemporary view of alternative healing modalities. *Nurse Practitioner.* 1993;18(9):51–55.

28. Engebretson J. Models of heterodox healing. *Alternat Ther Health Med.* In press.

29. Andrews MM, Boyle JS. *Transcultural Concepts in Nursing Care.* 2nd ed. Philadelphia, Pa: Lippincott; 1995.

30. Freund PES, McGuire MB. *Health, Illness and the Social Body: A Critical Sociology.* Englewood Cliffs. NJ: Prentice-Hall; 1991.

31. Douglas M. *Purity and Danger: An Analysis of the Concepts of Pollution and Taboo.* London, England: Ark Paperbacks; 1989.

32. Brown PS. Nineteenth-century American health reformers and the early nature cure movement in Britain. *Med History.* 1988;32:174–194.

33. Whorton JC. *Crusaders for Fitness: The History of American Health Reformers.* Princeton, NJ: Princeton University Press; 1982.

34. Kaptchuk TJ. *The Web that Has No Weaver: Understanding Chinese Medicine.* New York, NY: Congdon and Weed; 1993.

35. Helman CG. *Culture, Health and Illness: An Introduction for Health Professionals.* 3rd ed. Wolburn, Mass: Butterworth-Heinemann; 1994.

36. Reese WL. *Dictionary of Philosophy and Religion: Eastern and Western Thought.* Atlantic Highland, NJ: Humanities Press; 1991.

37. Horgan J. *The End of Science, Facing the Limits of Knowledge in the Twilight of the Scientific Age.* Reading, Mass. Addison Wesley; 1996.

38. Dossey BM, Keegan L, Guzzetta CE, Kolkmeier LG, *Holistic Nursing: A Handbook for Practice.* Gaithersburg, Md: Aspen Publishers; 1995.

39. Slater VE. Toward an understanding of energetic healing, part 1: energetic structures. *J Holistic Nurs.* 1995;13: 209–224.

40. Slater VE. Toward an understanding of energetic healing, part 2: energetic process. *J Holistic Nurs.* 1995;13:225–238.

41. Rossi E. *The Psychobiology of Mind-Body Healing.* New York, NY: W. W. Norton; 1993.

42. Orth-Gomer K, Schneiderman N. *Behavioral Medicine Approaches to Cardiovascular Disease Prevention.* Hillsdale, NJ: Erlbaum; 1996.

43. Dreher H. *The Immune Power Personality.* New York: Dutton; 1995.

44. Schneiderman N, McCabe P, Baum A. *Perspectives in Behavioral Medicine: Stress and Disease Processes.* Hillsdale, NJ: Erlbaum; 1992.

45. Larson DB. Religion and spirituality—the forgotten factor in public health: what does the research share? Presented at the 12th annual meeting of the American Public Health Association, November 18, 1996; New York, NY.

46. Cox H. *Fire from Heaven.* Reading, Mass: Addison-Wesley; 1995.

47. Kleinman A. *Patients and Healers in the Context of Culture.* Berkeley, Calif: University of California Press; 1980.

48. Rogers ME. *An Introduction to the Theoretical Basis of Nursing.* Philadelphia, PA: F. A. Davis; 1970.

49. Watson J. *Nursing: Human Science and Human Care: A Theory of Nursing.* New York, NY: National League for Nursing.

50. Parse RR. *Man-Living-Health: A Theory of Nursing.* New York, NY: Wiley; 1981.

51. Newman MA. *Health as Expanding Consciousness.* 2nd ed. New York, NY: National League for Nursing; 1984.

52. Nagle LM, Mitchell GJ. *Theoretic Diversity: Evolving Paradigmatic Issues in Research and Practice.* Gaithersburg, Md: Aspen Publishers; 1991.

53. McKeon ZK. *On Knowing the Natural Sciences.* Chicago, Ill: University of Chicago Press; 1994.

The Author Comments

A Multiparadigm Approach to Nursing

As a public health nurse, I listened to what people believed about health, disease, and healing, and I became interested in cultural orientations to health. An understanding of these orientations, values, and beliefs that underlie health behaviors is central in working with clients in promoting their health. Conducting fieldwork with lay healers, who incorporated strategies and philosophies from cross-cultural and historical approaches to healing, and exploring related literature from anthropology provided a perspective for the multiparadigm model of healing. This perspective allowed for the development of an integrative healing model that includes the biomedical paradigm as opposed to other approaches that compare all healing methods from the biomedical perspective. Incorporating multiple approaches to healing and understanding the differences at the paradigm level will not only be relevant to providing the best health care to a global society but also provide an inclusive model for nursing that incorporates biomedical approaches rather than distinguishing nursing as oppositional to medicine.

—JOAN C. ENGEBRETSON

CHAPTER 23

Toward a Complementary Perspective on Worldviews

Susan K. Leddy

This column has dual purposes. The first purpose is to argue that fragmentation of knowledge in nursing science can be related to the dominant way of thinking of worldviews as competitive dualities. Then, inspired by a rereading of Bohm (1980), the second purpose is to advance a complementary perspective on worldviews to foster an alternative way of thinking with potential for encouraging creative thinking and knowledge synthesis.

Key words: dialectics, nursing science, worldviews

Competitive Dualities and Worldviews

Philosophic beliefs about the nature of the existence of human beings and their environments, the human-environment relationship, what accounts for change and stability, and what constitutes knowledge are basic to the development of nursing knowledge and practice. These beliefs represent diverse worldviews that provide "different ways of being aware of the universe" (Phillips, 1995, p. 149). These beliefs also provide the philosophic base for the conceptual models, or paradigms, that represent various frames of reference that can guide the scientific and practical activities needed to develop knowledge (Fawcett, 1995).

Bohm (1980) also stresses the influence of one's worldview on ways of thinking and the development of knowledge. For example, he says that

Reprinted from Nursing Science Quarterly, Vol. 13 No. 3, July 2000, 225-233.

About the Author

SUSAN LEDDY was fortunate to have the best nursing education possible, earning a BS from Skidmore College (1960, nursing), an MS from Boston University (1965, teaching M/S nursing), and a PhD from New York University (1973, nursing science). She later did postdoctoral work at Harvard University (1985, educational administration) and the University of Pennsylvania (1994 to 1996, psychosocial oncology). She has been a National League for Nursing consultant and a department, school, and college chair and dean. Dr. Leddy has taught nursing at all educational levels, most recently, teaching nursing science and research in the doctoral program at Widener University. Her scholarship has been grounded in a unitary worldview and a belief in theory as a foundation for the development of knowledge. Currently, her primary interests are exploring energy theory and health. Her hobbies include exotic travel, weaving, quilting, knitting, watercolor painting, and enjoying her 13-month-old granddaughter Katie.

when we look at the world through our theoretical insights, the factual knowledge that we obtain will evidently be shaped and formed by our theories . . . . Given perception and action, our theoretical insights provide the main source of organization of our factual knowledge. Indeed, our overall experience is shaped in this way. (p. 5)

Bohm emphasizes that worldviews and ways of thinking, as well as the nature of knowledge that is generated, are intricately interrelated. In fact, he goes even further to suggest that one's perspective shapes the experience of reality.

An important issue in ontology is whether reality exists or is constructed. The influence of science, so highly valued in our culture, can be attributed to the desire for a rational system of truths from which accurate information about the world can be deduced with certainty and precision. Science values rationality, logical thinking, and numerical measurement. Subjective feelings have little value. It is believed that effects can be attributed to a specific cause. Therefore, given that all "facts" have a specific cause, the cause can be discovered through objective and verifiable observation. Science is based on the belief that it is possible to discover true and accurate knowledge of reality.

In contrast, for Bohm (1980), the nature of reality is essentially a way of looking at the world, or world-

view, because for him an underlying and unseen pattern is the primary order of reality. Bohm (1980) suggests that "a theory is primarily a form of *insight*, i.e. a way of looking at the world, and not a form of *knowledge* of how the world is" (p. 4). In a similar vein, he proposes that the degree of clarity of these insights or theories are domain specific; that is, what is clear within the context of some domains may be less than clear when extended beyond those parameters. Bohm further contends that "our theories are to be regarded primarily as ways of looking at the world as a whole (i.e. worldviews) rather than as 'absolutely true knowledge of how things are'" (p. 5). These conceptions of reality as related to perspective provide an interesting alternative to the dominant scientific paradigm and challenge the assumed superiority of competitive dualistic thinking as a primary mode of thinking.

There are two basic philosophic positions for beliefs about reality. Monistic beliefs, such as in Vedanta philosophy, consider ultimate reality as an individual oneness of being. All phenomena are considered to be illusionary manifestations of one unitary consciousness. If everything is flow and mutual transformation, then everything has multiple aspects. Because there is no time, space, or causation, division is only an illusion. Different aspects of the same thing are considered in terms of relation, not reality. Each requires the other to manifest its total nature. However, according to Ajaya

(1983), accepting the monistic assumption of the universe as an illusion does not rule out the possibility of employing a dualistic approach to comprehending "the structure, form and dynamics of this illusion" (p. 38). Ajaya maintains that within the monistic worldview, a dualistic approach can be "useful for describing a limited range of phenomena" (p. 115). However, he states that "the more encompassing perspective recognizes both the uses and the limitations of the more restricted perspective, while the more limited point of view is adamantly intolerant of a viewpoint that is beyond its range of understanding" (p. 116).

Contrasting with the monistic view of reality is a dualistic perspective. In one dualistic perspective such as represented in the predominant Western way of thinking, the opposition of contraries, logic, and critical thinking based on competitive dualities is emphasized. In this reductive approach to thinking, the focus is on distinctions between independent concepts. Through a cognitive interaction comprising contrast and comparison, distinct boundaries between concepts are delineated. According to this logic, contraries are seen as mutually exclusive or diametrically opposed to one another. The thinking is *either/or;* thus, contradictions are not allowed, and both cannot be true. For example, health considered as being "good" and disease considered as being "bad" are frequently viewed as mutually incompatible. Therefore, from an either/or standpoint, a person with a disease diagnosis cannot be healthy.

Competitive dualistic thinking has predominated within nursing as the discipline has embraced science. Inevitably, this ingrained way of thinking has permeated extant discussions of worldviews in nursing science. For example, Newman and colleagues have differentiated a three-part schema of particulate/deterministic-interactive/integrative-unitary/transformative worldviews (Newman, 1992; Newman, Sime, & Corcoran-Perry, 1991). Parse classified worldviews into a two-part schema known as totality and simultaneity paradigms (Parse, 1987; Parse, Coyne, & Smith, 1985). Fawcett (1993) described a different three-part schema of reaction-reciprocal interaction-simultaneous action worldview perspectives. Because these worldviews are independent in the sense

that they are not interchangeable, each worldview can be interpreted as competitive relative to the other or others within a given schema. For example, Fawcett (1993) clearly indicates that each worldview in her schema is distinct from the others.

All dualistic forms of thinking "interpret experience as an interaction between two fundamental principles" (Ayaja, 1983, p. 11). However, contrasting with the previous view of contraries as mutually exclusive, independent concepts is the perspective that "pairs of opposites are creations of the mind . . . .Different aspects of the same thing, they are terms of relation, not of reality" (Ajaya, 1983, p. 56). And Sabelli (1989) indicates that "opposites are not extremes in a continuum but separate dimensions in a multidimensional space" (p. 316). As relative phases, they have no fixed values but are different points of view of the same larger reality. Given that neither one could exist without the presence of the other, and given that both come from the same source, truth is always partial (Sabelli, 1989).

Sabelli (1989) describes multiple patterns or modes of dualistic thinking as alternatives to the competitive perspective. For example, in a conflictual mode of thought such as Marxist social philosophy or Darwinist theory, alternatives are not absolute but different, and through dialectic contradiction or struggle, there may be mutual annihilation of both. In a hierarchical mode of thought, the emphasis in the interaction of apparent polarities is on falsification of one position through dominance/submission over the other. Therefore, "truth" overcomes falsity. In contrast, within a harmonic mode of thought, apparent opposites are viewed as complementarities, a *both/and* dialogue in which each contains the other as opposing but interrelated aspects of a whole. The emphasis in a harmonic perspective is on dialogue rather than on conflict.

There are a number of approaches to complementary dualities in the literature. The predominant Eastern way of thinking emphasizes concepts as a synthesis of opposites, or a transformation into one another, in which each thing or phenomenon is both itself and its contrary. For example, health is viewed as a value-free concept that incorporates wellness, illness, well-being, and disease into a larger whole. In the Eastern view, dualities are balanced in mutually supportive, cyclical interplay.

Relational Perspectives of the Whole

From a different point of view known as systems theory, components are perceived in relation to one another. The emphasis in this worldview is on the way components function as a whole. Capra (1996) explains the underlying principle of this way of thinking as a shift from perceiving living systems in terms of distinct parts to perceiving them as integrated wholes whose "essential, or 'systemic,' properties are properties of the whole, which none of the parts have" (p. 36). These systemic properties are said to "arise from the 'organizing relations' of the parts—that is, from a configuration of ordered relationships that is characteristic of that particular class of organisms, or systems" (p. 36). A further characteristic of systems thinking is explained as "the *ability to shift one's attention back and forth* [italics added] between systems levels. Throughout the living world we find systems nesting within other systems" (p. 37).

A most significant perspective that lends support to the thesis of this column lies in the insights of Gestalt psychology, in which objects are perceived in a mutually supportive and reversible relationship between figure and ground. Capra (1996), in discussing this Gestalt perspective using the language of systems, concludes that

> what we call a part is merely a pattern in an inseparable web of relationships. Therefore the shift from the parts to the whole can also be seen as a shift from objects to relationships. In a sense, this is a figure/ground shift. (p. 37)

In other words, Capra disputes a mechanistic approach that considers the relationships of objects as limited to their interactions and therefore of secondary importance in describing reality. Instead, he proposes that relationships are primary: "In the systems view we realize that the objects themselves are networks of rela-

tionships, embedded in larger networks . . . .The boundaries of the discernible patterns ('objects') are secondary" (p. 37).

Bohm's (1980) discussion of different ways of thinking, in relation to the subject being thought about, helps to clarify the connection. Allowing for a critical distinction between thinking about concrete issues that have a technical, functional, or practical purpose in comparison to pondering philosophical matters concerned with understanding a self-world reality, Bohm recognizes the validity of different modes of thought. For example, although he concedes that a thinking process that separates or divides is an appropriate as well as useful way of thinking about certain activities that have a limited scope (such as technical or practical issues), he disputes any claims that such ways of thinking can be meaningfully extended to include ideas about persons and their relations with the universe. He proposes that such a worldview eventually leads past perceiving divisions as a convenient way of processing discrete data and becomes an experience of self-world reality. Such a way of consistently perceiving separately existent fragments in oneself and one's world shifts the perspective. Bohm (1980) warns that "being guided by a fragmentary self-world view, man then acts in such a way as to try to break himself and the world up, so that all seems to correspond to his way of thinking" (p. 2).

A competitive mode of thinking can be a strength in the effective explication and clarification of distinctions, such as in worldviews. In teaching doctoral students, I have found that a useful strategy to clarify content and foster critical thinking is a consideration of the specific distinctions between worldviews. Students then can identify which perspective seems closest to their own usually unexamined views of reality. Inevitably, however, students comment that they are steeped, through nursing education and experience, in the dominant ways of thinking, that is, in the totality or the reciprocal-interaction modes. Although the simultaneity and unitary/transformative worldviews appear to have intrinsic appeal, given that students have to choose between the perspectives, they invariably choose to accept what is comfortable because it is familiar.

Thus, one unintended consequence of competitive thinking can be the perpetuation of the status quo worldview in nursing science. Information can become fragmented, compartmentalized into separate bodies of knowledge, "schools of thought" by worldview or conceptual model. Competitive thinking can contribute to divisiveness and possible right/wrong or better/worse thinking. For example, some individuals may regard the totality worldview as an outmoded way of thinking and the simultaneity worldview as a better way of thinking rather than examining them as alternative perspectives. Competitive thinking leads to questions such as, Which view of reality is the "right" one? Because reality can only be glimpsed and never really "known," this appears to be an arbitrary and futile exercise. Thinking in opposites can be considered an oversimplification that prevents perceiving the world in its complexity, promotes conflict, and prevents the discovery of creative alternatives (Sabelli, 1989). In contrast, a complementary approach to thinking appears to offer the potential for fostering creative thinking, insight, and the synthesis of a body of nursing knowledge.

Complementary Thinking

Bohm (1980) theorized that the nature of reality is a coherent whole "which is never static or complete, but which is in an unending process of movement and unfoldment" (p. ix). Bohm labeled this whole the *implicate order,* an enfolded "unbroken wholeness of the totality of existence as an undivided flowing movement without borders" (p. 172). However, Bohm also explained that "we can, for convenience, always picture the *explicate order . . .* as the order present to the senses" (p. 186). Thus, the explicate order comprises various patterns of manifestations that are perceived by human beings as recurrent, stable, and separable.

Bohm (1980) said, "The notion that all these fragments are separately existent is evidently an illusion . . . . In essence, the process of division is *a way of thinking about things* [italics added] that is convenient and useful" (pp. 1-2). Again, stressing the significance of the domain perspective, he states that "all our different ways of thinking are to be considered as different ways of looking at the one reality, each with one domain in which it is clear and adequate" (p. 8).

One possible implication of these ideas is to understand extant worldviews as different ways of perceiving reality, rather than as views of differing realities. Each provides partial insight into the whole, because "content and process are not two separately existent things, but, rather, they are two aspects of views of one whole movement" (Bohm, 1980, p. 18). Interpreting that complementary worldview within a nursing science perspective offers a new way of seeing the connections. For example, in a complementary worldview, the totality, particulate/deterministic, and reaction perspectives can be viewed as reflecting content of the perceived explicate order. The simultaneity, unitary/transformative, and simultaneous action perspectives hint of an unending process of movement and unfolding of the implicate order.

As a result, although the observer's perspective may shift between content and process, both are recognized as aspects of reality. For example, both bio-psycho-social-spiritual aspects and unitary pattern manifestations characterize the human being. Cyclical interaction and mutual process can be said to characterize the human-environment interface. Health incorporates functioning, adapting, and becoming, as well as the constructing of meaning. And in the short-term, change may be predictable, while evolution proceeds unpredictably toward increasing complexity.

One way to conceptualize this approach is a ground/figure example from Gestalt psychology. Most people have seen pictures of what appears at first to be undifferentiated dots that can, with concentration, be viewed as a vase or as a profile of a young woman, depending on the focus of the viewer. The whole picture contains both possible figures. By shifting the perspective of the ground, either the vase or the face in profile can be the figure. Such is also the case with content and process. Both are essential for the total "picture," but which becomes the figure depends on the focus of the viewer.

Methods to Promote Complementary Thinking

Dialectical thinking is one method that can be used to develop a complementary perspective on worldviews. In particular, dialectical methods of reasoning can be used "to address apparent contradictions and their synchronization" (Reigel, 1976, p. 689). Rafael (1996) states that "from a Hegelian perspective, dialectic is a logical progression of thought that exposes and examines contradictions and reconciles them through a process of thesis, antithesis, and synthesis" (p. 4). Rawnsley (1993) indicates that Hegel's "underlying assumption of harmony in diversity is postulated as a relationship of essential opposites, a structure or pattern in which what appears antagonistic is merged into a qualitatively different possibility through synthesis into a higher abstraction" (p. 3). The intent of this method of thinking is to synthesize contraries into a more inclusive concept.

Ajaya (1983) uses a different approach to dialectical thinking to describe "progressively more comprehensive frames of reference" (p. 115), in which "the more encompassing perspective recognizes both the uses and the limitations of the more restricted perspective" (p. 116). Given that the perception of dualities as opposites is a creation of the mind, Ajaya proposes that a "more comprehensive understanding that transcends the polarity" (p. 163) be sought. He proposes that a neutral point, not a midpoint, be identified, "encompassing awareness of the extremes, the continuum, and the unifying center from which the polarity emerges" (p. 163). For example, complementary thinking occupies a neutral point that encompasses both separate and unified views.

Paradoxical thinking is another method that can be used to explicate a complementary worldview. Ajaya (1983) portrayed dualistic thought as an intermediate phase between reductive and monistic thought in regard to polarities. In contrast to Hegel and Ajaya, who have different perspectives on dialectics as a method of transforming opposites by synthesizing them into a larger whole, Parse (1992) conceptualizes paradox as

"two sides of the same rhythm that coexist all at once . . . .Paradox refers to apparent opposites. These rhythmical patterns are not opposites. Both sides of the rhythm are present simultaneously" (p. 38). As meaning is structured in the process of becoming, the contradiction of opposites is experienced, further differentiated, and preserved as a rhythmical shifting of views (Mitchell, 1993). Morse, Bottorff, and Hutchinson (1995) also point out that meaning is developed through the examination of a word with its opposite: "For instance, in has no meaning without out, nor up without down. Similarly, comfort has no meaning without discomfort, nor comfortable without uncomfortable" (p. 18).

Parse's approach to paradox can be contrasted with dialectical thinking. In dialectical methods of thinking, differentiating or contradicting characteristics are resolved by being subsumed or synthesized into one more inclusive concept. For example, a 24-hour "day" subsumes daytime, nighttime, twilight, daybreak, and so forth. In contrast, paradoxical thinking preserves the differentiating characteristics in a mutually supportive, cyclical interplay. As paradoxical thinking fosters nuance and a rhythmical shifting of focus between alternatives to clarify continuities and distinctions, sensitivity to paradox should facilitate creative thinking, whereas dialectical thinking promotes synthesis.

Implications for Nursing

I frequently ask students to consider the implications of their proposals, in what has become a trademark, "So what!" Thus, it could be asked, what difference does it make if a complementary rather than a competitive perspective toward worldviews is adopted? What are the advantages for nursing of methods of thinking based on complementary perspectives?

Kim (1996b) has reviewed four different modes with which nursing scientists engage in producing knowledge for nursing practice. A coherence mode refers to a commitment to "a specific philosophical, epistemological, and paradigmatic orientation" (p. 112). A scientist working with a coherence mode is therefore guided by this orientation in knowledge development. Furthermore, Kim maintains that within the coherence mode the focus is on building a paradigm. In contrast, she describes a scientist operating in an integrative mode as seeking to incorporate new knowledge to expand the current foundation for the purpose of increasing the explanatory power of the framework. In addition, Kim describes a scientist working in the pragmatic/eclectic mode as geared toward therapeutic and pragmatic goals that are rational and pragmatic. In this mode, the focus is on solving significant clinical problems. Finally, in the reflective mode identified by Kim, the scientist evaluates viable knowledge in terms of its validity in the practice situation. The focus in this mode "is on knowledge development as a situationally generative process" (p. 112).

It should be made clear that my personal scientific commitment is to the development of knowledge from the perspective of the coherence mode. I believe that an inclusive, overarching, ontological framework is essential as the philosophical basis for synthesis of knowledge from apparently disparate theories and conceptual models into a coherent science. It therefore follows that I would think it desirable, if possible, to accommodate competitive worldviews in such an inclusive, overarching, ontological framework.

Kim (1996a) suggests that pluralism as an approach to nursing knowledge development and the application of theory into practice "points to a possibility, not of coherence and patterning, but of chaos, fragmentation, and arbitrariness" (p. 63). Although competing ontological perspectives are only one probable basis for the current state of the science, Kim states concern that absence of a unifying structure for such pluralism can impede knowledge development and create confusion. She maintains that "nursing must seek or develop a unifying framework that can pull together its effort in knowledge development in order to prevent nursing's demise to an epistemic chaos" (1996c, p. 15).

In addition to providing a comprehensive framework for knowledge synthesis, a complementary perspective on worldviews has the advantage of facilitating the exploration of contextual background and multiple facets of concept, content, and process. The emphasis shifts from competition to inclusion. Instead of bits of incomplete and unconnected information, a much more meaningful gestalt of knowledge can be generated. Therefore, through a complementary perspective, the worldview can provide both a blueprint for developing knowledge and a perspective for synthesizing knowledge into a meaningful whole.

In nursing, critical thinking leading to clinical decision-making is the primary—some might say exclusive—way of thinking taught in educational programs. This is the premise, even though support is lacking for the impact of nursing education on critical thinking. Little evidence links critical thinking to clinical judgment, and support for a strong relationship between critical thinking and success in nursing education is lacking (Kintgen-Andrews, 1991).

Bohm (1980, p. 5) stresses the influence of one's worldview on ways of thinking and the development of knowledge. Given the emphasis on atheoretical rationality and logical thinking throughout their education, is it any wonder that many nurses have fragmented knowledge and therefore practice with rule-based cognitive rigidity? I submit that an overarching ontological framework for theories would make possible education that is more likely to develop a coherent organization of knowledge for nursing practice. Critical thinking is only one facet of integrative thinking (P. Fasnacht, personal communication, August 1999), which is a thinking method that fosters creative tension leading to linkages between concepts, envisioning, and the creation of patterns. Such thinking methods, essential to the development of cognitive flexibility and creativity so necessary for truly professional nursing practice, should be fostered in nursing curricula at all levels.

Summary

In this column, it has been argued that fragmentation of knowledge in nursing science can be related to the dominant way of thinking of worldviews as competitive dualities. To move toward resolving that conflict, the thesis has been set forth to claim that a complementary perspective on worldviews as an ontological framework can promote knowledge synthesis and alternative thinking methods in nursing science. Implications of the potential for a complementary perspective for encouraging integrative and creative thinking for professional nursing practice has been presented.

REFERENCES

Ajaya, S. (1983). *Psychotherapy East and West: A unifying paradigm.* Honesdale, PA: Himalayan Institute.

Bohm, D. (1980). *Wholeness and the implicate order.* London: Routledge & Kegan Paul.

Capra, F. (1996). *The web of life.* New York: Anchor Books.

Fawcett, J. (1993). From a plethora of paradigms to parsimony in worldviews. *Nursing Science Quarterly, 6,* 56–58.

Fawcett, J. (1995). *Analysis and evaluation of conceptual models in nursing* (3rd ed.). Philadelphia: Davis.

Kim, H. S. (1996a). Reflections on building a cumulative knowledge base for nursing: From fragmentation to congruence. In *Proceedings of the Nursing Knowledge Impact Conference* (pp. 63–67). Boston: Boston College.

Kim, H. S. (1996b). Summary of future directions. In *Proceedings of the Nursing Knowledge Impact Conference* (pp. 111–117). Boston: Boston College.

Kim, H. S. (1996c). Viable options for applying theory to practice. In *Proceedings of the Nursing Knowledge Impact Conference* (pp. 15–21). Boston: Boston College.

Kintgen-Andrews, J. (1991). Critical thinking and nursing education: Perplexities and insights. *Journal of Nursing Education, 30,* 152–157.

Mitchell, G. J. (1993). Living paradox in Parse's theory. *Nursing Science Quarterly, 6,* 44–51.

Morse, J. M., Bottorff, J. L., & Hutchinson, S. (1995). The paradox of comfort. *Nursing Research, 44,* 14–19.

Newman, M. A. (1992). Prevailing paradigms in nursing. *Nursing Outlook, 40,* 10–13, 32.

Newman, M. A., Sime, A. M., & Corcoran-Perry, S. A. (1991). The focus of the discipline of nursing. *Advances in Nursing Science, 14,* 1–6.

Parse, R. R. (1987). *Nursing science: Major paradigms, theories, and critiques.* Philadelphia: Saunders.

Parse, R. R. (1992). Human becoming: Parse's theory of nursing. *Nursing Science Quarterly, 5,* 35–42.

Parse, R. R., Coyne, A. B., & Smith, M. J. (1985). *Nursing research: Qualitative methods.* Bowie, MD: Brady.

Phillips, J. R. (1995). Can researchers transcend bad science? *Nursing Science Quarterly, 8,* 148–149.

Rafael, A. R. F. (1996). Power and caring: A dialectic in nursing. *Advances in Nursing Science, 19*(1), 3–17.

Rawnsley, M. M. (1993). Dialectics and the diverse discourse in nursing science. *Nursing Science Quarterly, 6,* 2–4.

Riegel, K. F. (1976). The dialectics of human development. *American Psychologist, 31,* 689–698.

Sabelli, H. C. (1989). *Union of opposites: A comprehensive theory of natural and human processes.* Lawrenceville, VA: Brunswick.

The Author Comments

Toward a Complementary Perspective on Worldviews

This article evolved out of a sense of frustration with the current status quo in nursing science. Students, even at the doctoral level, are unwilling, or unable, to engage in imaginative risk taking, thinking "out of the box." Much current research is atheoretical, with an emphasis on concrete "right or wrong" outcomes. My point in the article is that by reframing thinking perspectives, engaging in dialectical and paradoxical thinking, and renewing emphasis on clear conceptual and theoretical foundations, there is potential to stimulate creative thinking, knowledge synthesis, coherent scholarship, and the development of a real scientific rationale for practice.

—Susan Leddy

Fundamental Patterns of Knowing in Nursing

Barbara A. Carper

It is the general conception of any field of inquiry that ultimately determines the kind of knowledge the field aims to develop as well as the manner in which that knowledge is to be organized, tested and applied. The body of knowledge that serves as the rationale for nursing practice has patterns, forms and structure that serve as horizons of expectations and exemplify characteristic ways of thinking about phenomena. Understanding these patterns is essential for the teaching and learning of nursing. Such an understanding does not extend the range of knowledge, but rather involves critical attention to the question of what it means to know and what kinds of knowledge are held to be of most value in the discipline of nursing.

Identifying Patterns of Knowing

Four fundamental patterns of knowing have been identified from an analysis of the conceptual and syntactical structure of nursing knowledge (Carper, 1975). The four patterns are distinguished according to logical type of meaning and designated as: (a) empirics, the science of nursing; (b) aesthetics, the art of nursing; (c) the component of a personal knowledge in nursing; and (d) ethics, the component of moral knowledge in nursing.

Empirics: The Science of Nursing

The term *nursing science* was rarely used in the literature until the late 1950s. However, since that time there

From Advances in Nursing Science. *October 1978, 1 (1), 13-23. Copyright © 1978 Aspen Systems Corporation,*
Reprinted with permission from Lippincott Williams & Wilkins.

About the Author

BARBARA A. CARPER is Professor Emerita and former Associate Dean for Academic Affairs at the College of Nursing, University of North Carolina—Charlotte. Dr. Carper received her baccalaureate degree from Texas Woman's University and her MEd and EdD from Columbia University Teacher's College. She also earned a Clinical Certification in Anesthesia from the University of Michigan in 1962. She spent 1981 through 1982 at Harvard University as a Visiting Scholar in Medical Ethics. Her areas of expertise include ethics and nursing theory development. One of her legacies to nursing is her widely cited, critiqued, and admired publication *Fundamental Patterns of Knowing*. Retirement now allows Dr. Carper to enjoy traveling with her husband, as well as to be active in the community and on the local Hospice Ethics Committee.

has been an increasing emphasis—one might even say a sense of urgency—regarding the development of a body of empirical knowledge specific to nursing. There seems to be general agreement that there is a critical need for knowledge about the empirical world, knowledge that is systematically organized into general laws and theories for the purpose of describing, explaining and predicting phenomena of special concern to the discipline of nursing. Most theory development and research efforts are primarily engaged in seeking and generating explanations which are systematic and controllable by factual evidence and which can be used in the organization and classification of knowledge.

The pattern of knowing which is generally designated as "nursing science" does not presently exhibit the same degree of highly integrated abstract and systematic explanations characteristic of the more mature sciences, although nursing literature reflects this as an ideal form. Clearly there are a number of coexisting, and in a few instances competing, conceptual structures—none of which has achieved the status of what Kuhn (1962) calls a scientific paradigm. That is, no single conceptual structure is as yet generally accepted as an example of actual scientific practice "which include[s] law, theory, application, and instrumentation together . . . [and] . . . provide[s] models from which spring particular coherent traditions of scientific research" (Kuhn, 1962, p. 10). It could be argued that some of these conceptual structures seem to have

greater potential than others for providing explanations that systematically account for observed phenomena and may ultimately permit more accurate prediction and control of them. However, this is a matter to be determined by research designed to test the validity of such explanatory concepts in the context of relevant empirical reality.

New Perspectives

What seems to be a paramount importance, at least at this stage in the development of nursing science, is that these preparadigm conceptual structures and theoretical models present new perspectives for considering the familiar phenomena of health and illness in relation to the human life process; as such they can and should be legitimately counted as discoveries in the discipline. The representation of health as more than the absence of disease is a crucial change; it permits health to be thought of as a dynamic state or process which changes over a given period of time and varies according to circumstances rather than a static either/or entity. The conceptual change in turn makes it possible to raise questions that previously would have been literally unintelligible.

The discovery that one can usefully conceptualize health as something that normally ranges along a continuum has led to attempts to observe, describe and classify variations in health, or levels of wellness, as expressions of a human being's relationship to the internal and external environments. Related research has sought to identify behavioral responses, both physiological and psychological, that may serve as cues by which one can infer the range of normal variations of health. It has also attempted to identify and categorize significant etiological factors which serve to promote or inhibit changes in health status.

Current Stages

The science of nursing at present exhibits aspects of both the "natural history stage of inquiry" and the "stage of deductively formulated theory." The task of the natural history stage is primarily the description and classification of phenomena which are, generally speaking, ascertainable by direct observation and inspection (Northrop, 1959). But current nursing literature clearly reflects a shift from this descriptive and classification form to increasingly theoretical analysis which is directed toward seeking, or inventing, explanations to account for observed and classified empirical facts. This shift is reflected in the change from a largely observational vocabulary to a new, more theoretical vocabulary whose terms have a distinct meaning and definition only in the context of the corresponding explanatory theory.

Explanations in the several open-system conceptual models tend to take the form commonly labeled functional or teleological (Nagel, 1961). For example, the system models explain a person's level of wellness at any particular point in time as a function of current and accumulated effects of interactions with his or her internal and external environments. The concept of adaptation is central to this type of explanation. Adaptation is seen as crucial in the process of responding to environmental demands (usually classified as stressors), and enables an individual to maintain or reestablish the steady state which is designated as the goal of the system. The development models often exhibit a more genetic type of explanation in that certain events, the developmental tasks, are believed to be causally relevant or necessary conditions for the normal development of an individual. Thus, the first fundamental pattern of knowing in nursing is empirical, factual, descriptive and ultimately aimed at developing abstract and theoretical explanations. It is exemplary, discursively formulated and publicly verifiable.

Aesthetics: The Art of Nursing

Few, if indeed any, familiar with the professional literature would deny that primary emphasis is placed on the development of the science of nursing. One is almost led to believe that the only valid and reliable knowledge is that which is empirical, factual, objectively descriptive and generalizable. There seems to be a self-conscious reluctance to extend the term knowledge to include those aspects of knowing in nursing that are not the result of empirical investigation. There is, nonetheless, what might be described as a tacit admission that nursing is, at least in part, an art. Not much effort is made to elaborate or to make explicit this aesthetic pattern of knowing in nursing—other than to vaguely associate the "art" with the general category of manual and/or technical skills involved in nursing practice.

Perhaps this reluctance to acknowledge the aesthetic component as a fundamental pattern of knowing in nursing originates in the vigorous efforts made in the not-so-distant past to exorcise the image of the apprentice-type educational system. Within the apprentice system, the art of nursing was closely associated with an imitative learning style and the acquisition of knowledge by accumulation of unrationalized experiences. Another likely source of reluctance is that the definition of the term art has been excessively and inappropriately restricted.

Weitz (1960) suggests that art is too complex and variable to be reduced to a single definition. To conceive the task of aesthetic theory as definition, he says, is logically doomed to failure in that what is called art has not common properties—only recognizable similarities. This fluid and open approach to the understanding and application of the concept of art and aesthetic meaning makes possible a wider consideration of conditions, situations and experiences in nursing that may properly be called aesthetic, including the creative process of discovery in the empirical pattern of knowing.

Aesthetics Versus Scientific Meaning

Despite this open texture of the concept of art, aesthetic meanings can be distinguished from those in science in several important aspects. The recognition "that art is expressive rather than merely formal or descriptive," according to Rader, "is about as well established as any fact in the whole field of aesthetics" (Rader, 1960, p. xvi). An aesthetic experience involves the creation and/or appreciation of a singular, particular, subjective expression of imagined possibilities or equivalent realities which "resists projection into the discursive form of language" (Langer, 1957). Knowledge gained by empirical description is discursively formulated and publicly verifiable. The knowledge gained by subjective acquaintance, the direct feeling of experience, defines discursive formulation. Although an aesthetic expression requires abstraction, it remains specific and unique rather than exemplary and leads us to acknowledge that "knowledge—genuine knowledge, understanding—is considerably wider than our discourse" (Langer, 1957, p. 23).

For Wiedenbach (1964), the art of nursing is made visible through the action taken to provide whatever the patient requires to restore or extend his ability to cope with the demands of his situation. But the action taken, to have an aesthetic quality, requires the active transformation of the immediate object—the patient's behavior—into a direct, nonmediated perception of what is significant in it—that is, what need is actually being expressed by the behavior. This perception of the need expressed is not only responsible for the action taken by the nurse but reflected in it.

The aesthetic process described by Wiedenbach resembles what Dewey (1958) refers to as the difference between recognition and perception. According to Dewey, recognition serves the purpose of identification and is satisfied when a name tag or label is attached according to some stereotype or previously formed scheme of classification. Perception, however, goes beyond recognition in that it includes an active gathering together of details and scattered particulars into an experienced whole for the purpose of seeing what is there. It is perception rather than mere recognition that re-

sults in a unity of ends and means which gives the action taken an aesthetic quality.

Orem speaks of the art of nursing as being "expressed by the individual nurse through her creativity and style in designing and providing nursing that is effective and satisfying" (Orem, 1971, p. 155). The art of nursing is creative in that it requires development of the ability to "envision valid modes of helping in relation to 'results' which are appropriate" (Orem, 1971, p. 69). This again invokes Dewey's (1958) sense of a perceived unity between an action taken and its result—a perception of the means and the end as an organic whole. The experience of helping must be perceived and designed as an integral component of its desired result rather than conceived separately as an independent action imposed on an independent subject. Perhaps this is what is meant by the concept of nursing the whole patient or total patient care. If so, what are the qualities that enable the creation of a design for nursing care that eliminate or would minimize the fragmentation of means and ends?

Aesthetic Pattern of Knowing

Empathy—that is, the capacity for participating in or vicariously experiencing another's feelings—is an important mode in the aesthetic pattern of knowing. One gains knowledge of another person's singular, particular, felt experience through empathic acquaintance (Lee, 1960; Lippo, 1960). Empathy is controlled or moderated by psychic distance or detachment in order to apprehend and abstract what we are attending to, and in this sense is objective. The more skilled the nurse becomes in perceiving and empathizing with the lives of others, the more knowledge or understanding will be gained of alternate modes of perceiving reality. The nurse will thereby have available a larger repertoire of choices in designing and providing nursing care that is effective and satisfying. At the same time, increased awareness of the variety of subjective experiences will heighten the complexity and difficulty of the decision making involved.

The design of nursing care must be accompanied by what Langer refers to as sense of form, the sense of "structure, articulation, a whole resulting from the relation of mutually dependent factors, or more precisely, the way the whole is put together" (Langer, 1957, p. 16). The design, if it is to be aesthetic, must be controlled by the perception of the balance, rhythm, proportion and unity of what is done in relation to the dynamic integration and articulation of the whole. "The doing may be energetic, and the undergoing may be acute and intense," Dewey (1958) says, but "unless they are related to each other to form a whole," what is done becomes merely a matter of mechanical routine or of caprice.

The aesthetic pattern of knowing in nursing involves the perception of abstracted particulars as distinguished from the recognition of abstracted universals. It is the knowing of a unique particular rather than an exemplary class.

The Component of Personal Knowledge

Personal knowledge as a fundamental pattern of knowing in nursing is the most problematic, the most difficult to master and to teach. At the same time, it is perhaps the pattern most essential to understanding the meaning of health in terms of individual well-being. Nursing considered as an interpersonal process involves interactions, relationships and transactions between the nurse and the patient-client. Mitchell points out that "there is growing evidence that the quality of interpersonal contacts has an influence on a person's becoming ill, coping with illness and becoming well" (Mitchell, 1973, p. 49-50). Certainly the phrase "therapeutic use of self" which has become increasingly prominent in the literature implies that the way in which nurses view their own selves and the client is of primary concern in any therapeutic relationship.

Personal knowledge is concerned with the knowing, encountering and actualizing of the concrete, individual self. One does not know *about* the self; one strives simply to *know* the self. This knowing is a standing in relation to another human being and confronting that human being as a person. This "I-Thou" encounter is unmediated by conceptual categories or particulars abstracted from complex organic wholes (Buber, 1970). The relation is one of reciprocity, a state of being that cannot be described or even experienced—it can only be actualized. Such personal knowing extends not only to other selves but also to relations with one's own self.

It requires what Buber (1970) refers to as the sacrifice of form—i.e., categories or classifications—for a knowing of infinite possibilities, as well as the risk of total commitment.

> Even as a melody is not composed of tones, nor a verse of words, nor a statue of lines—one must pull and tear to turn a unity into a multiplicity—so it is with the human being to whom I say You . . . .I have to do this again and again; but immediately he is no longer You. (Buber, 1970, p. 59)

Maslow (1956) refers to this sacrifice of form as embodying a more efficient perception of reality in that reality is not generalized nor predetermined by a complex of concepts, expectations, beliefs and stereotypes. This results in a greater willingness to accept ambiguity, vagueness and discrepancy of oneself and others. The risk of commitment involved in personal knowledge is what Polyani calls the "passionate participation in the act of knowing" (Polyani, 1964, p. 17).

The nurse in the therapeutic use of self rejects approaching the patient-client as an object and strives instead to actualize an authentic personal relationship between two persons. The individual is considered as an integrated, open system incorporating movement toward growth and fulfillment of human potential. An authentic personal relation requires the acceptance of others in their freedom to create themselves and the recognition that each person is not a fixed entity, but constantly engaged in the process of becoming. How then should the nurse reconcile this with the social and/or professional responsibility to control and manipulate the environmental variables and even the behavior of the person who is a patient in order to maintain or restore a steady state? If a human being is assumed to be free to choose and chooses behavior outside of accepted norms, how will this affect the action taken in the therapeutic use of self by the nurse? What choices must the nurse make in order to know another self in an authentic relation apart from the category of patient, even when categorizing for the purpose of treatment is essential to the process of nursing?

Assumptions regarding human nature, McKay observes, "range from the existentialist to the cybernetic, from the idea of an information processing machine to one of a many splendored being" (McKay, 1969, p. 399). Many of these assumptions incorporate in one form or another the notion that there is, for all individuals, a characteristic state which they, by virtue of membership in the species, must strive to assume or achieve. Empirical descriptions and classifications reflect the assumption that being human allows for prediction of basic biological, psychological and social behaviors that will be encountered in any given individual.

Certainly empirical knowledge is essential to the purposes of nursing. But nursing also requires that we be alert to the fact that models of human nature and their abstract and generalized categories refer to and describe behaviors and traits that groups have in common. However, none of these categories can ever encompass or express the uniqueness of the individual encountered as a person, as a "self." These and many other similar considerations are involved in the realm of personal knowledge, which can be broadly characterized as subjective, concrete and existential. It is concerned with the kind of knowing that promotes wholeness and integrity in the personal encounter, the achievement of engagement rather than detachment; and it denies the manipulative, impersonal orientation.

Ethics: The Moral Component

Teachers and individual practitioners are becoming increasingly sensitive to the difficult personal choices that must be made within the complex context of modern health care. These choices raise fundamental questions about morally right and wrong action in connection with the care and treatment of illness and the promotion of health. Moral dilemmas arise in situations of ambiguity and uncertainty, when the consequences of one's actions are difficult to predict and traditional principles and ethical codes offer no help or seem to result in contradiction. The moral code which guides the ethical conduct of nurses is based on the primary principle of obligation embodied in the concepts of service to people and respect for human life. The discipline of nursing is held to be a valu-

able and essential social service responsible for conserving life, alleviating suffering and promoting health. But appeal to the ethical "rule book" fails to provide answers in terms of difficult individual moral choices which must be made in the teaching and practice of nursing.

The fundamental pattern of knowing identified here as the ethical component of nursing is focused on matters of obligation or what ought to be done. Knowledge of morality goes beyond simply knowing the norms or ethical codes of the discipline. It includes all voluntary actions that are deliberate and subject to the judgment of right and wrong—including judgments of moral value in relation to motives, intentions and traits of character. Nursing is deliberate action, or a series of actions, planned and implemented to accomplish defined goals. But goals and actions involve choices made, in part, on the basis of normative judgments, both particular and general. On occasion, the principles and norms by which such choices are made may be in conflict.

According to Berthold, "goals are, of course, value judgments not amenable to scientific inquiry and validation" (Berthold, 1968, p. 196). Dickoff, James and Wiedenbach also call attention to the need to be aware that the specification of goals serves as "a norm or standard by which to evaluate activity . . . [and] . . . entails taking them as values—that is, signifies conceiving these goal contents as situations worthy to be brought about" (James & Weidenbach, 1968, p. 422).

For example, a common goal of nursing care in relation to the maintenance or restoration of health is to assist patients to achieve a state in which they are independent. Much of the current practice reflects an attitude of value attached to the goal of independence, and indicates nursing actions to assist patients in assuming full responsibility for themselves at the earliest possible moment or to enable them to retain responsibility to the last possible moment. However, valuing independence and attempting to maintain it may be at the expense of the patient's learning how to live with physical or social dependence when necessary; e.g., in instances when prognosis indicates that independence cannot be regained.

Differences in normative judgments may have more to do with disagreements as to what constitutes a "healthy" state of being than lack of empirical evidence or ambiguity in the application of the term. Slote suggests that the persistence of disputes, or lack of uniformity in the application of cluster terms, such as health, is due to "the difficulty of decisively resolving certain sorts of value questions about what is and is not important." This leads him to conclude "that value judgment is far more involved in the making of what are commonly thought to be factual statements than has been imagined" (Slote, 1966, p. 220).

The ethical pattern of knowing in nursing requires an understanding of different philosophical positions regarding what is good, what ought to be desired, what is right; of different ethical frameworks devised for dealing with the complexities of moral judgments; and of various orientations to the notion of obligation. Moral choices to be made must then be considered in terms of specific action to be taken in specific, concrete situations. The examination of the standards, codes and values by which we decide what is morally right should result in a greater awareness of what is involved in making moral choices and being responsible for the choices made. The knowledge of ethical codes will not provide answers to the moral questions involved in nursing, nor will it eliminate the necessity for having to make moral choices. But it can be hoped that:

> The more sensitive teachers and practitioners are to the demands of the process of justification, the more explicit they are about the norms that govern their actions, the more personally engaged they are in assessing surrounding circumstances and potential consequences, the more "ethical" they will be; and we cannot ask much more (Greene, 1973, p. 221).

Using Patterns of Knowing

A philosophical discussion of patterns of knowing may appear to some as a somewhat idle, if not arbitrary and artificial, undertaking having little or no connection with the practical concerns and difficulties encountered in the day-to-day doing and teaching of nursing. But it represents a personal conviction that there is a need to examine the kinds of knowing that provide the discipline with its particular perspectives and significance. Understanding four fundamental patterns of knowing makes possible an increased awareness of the complexity and diversity of nursing knowledge.

Each pattern may be conceived as necessary for achieving mastery in the discipline, but none of them alone should be considered sufficient. Neither are they mutually exclusive. The teaching and learning of one pattern do not require the rejection or neglect of any of the others. Caring for another requires the achievements of nursing science, that is, the knowledge of empirical facts systematically organized into theoretical explanations regarding the phenomena of health and illness. But creative imagination also plays its part in the syntax of discovery in science, as well as in developing the ability to imagine the consequences of alternate moral choices.

Personal knowledge is essential for ethical choices in that moral action presupposes personal maturity and freedom. If the goals of nursing are to be more than conformance to unexamined norms, if the "ought" is not to be determined simply on the basis of what is possible, then the obligation to care for another human being involves becoming a certain kind of person—and not merely doing certain kinds of things. If the design of nursing care is to be more than habitual or mechanical, the capacity to perceive and interpret the subjective experiences of others and to imaginatively project the effects of nursing actions on their lives becomes a necessary skill.

Nursing thus depends on the specific knowledge of human behavior in health and in illness, the aesthetic perception of significant human experiences, a personal understanding of the unique individuality of the self and the capacity to make choices within concrete situations involving particular moral judgments. Each of these separate but interrelated and interdependent fundamental patterns of knowing should be taught and understood according to its distinctive logic, the restricted circumstances in which it is valid, the kinds of data it subsumes and the methods by which each particular kind of truth is distinguished and warranted.

The major significances to the discipline of nursing in distinguishing patterns of knowing are summarized as: (a) the conclusions of the discipline conceived as subject matter cannot be taught or learned without reference to the structure of the discipline—the representative concepts and methods of inquiry that determine the kind of knowledge gained and limit its meaning, scope and validity; (b) each of the fundamental patterns of knowing represents a necessary but not complete approach to the problems and questions in the discipline; and (c) all knowledge is subject to change and revision. Every solution of an existing problem raises new and unsolved questions. These new and as yet unsolved problems require, at times, new methods of inquiry and different conceptual structures; they change the shape and patterns of knowing. With each change in the shape of knowledge, teaching and learning require looking for different points of contact and connection among ideas and things. This clarifies the effect of each new thing known on other things known and the discovery of new patterns by which each connection modifies the whole.

REFERENCES

Berthold, J. S. (1968). Symposium on theory development in nursing: Prologue. *Nursing Research, 17,* 196–197.

Buber, M. (1970). *I and thou.* (W. Kaufman, Trans.). New York: Scribner.

Carper, B. A. (1975). Fundamental patterns of knowing in nursing. (Doctoral dissertation, Columbia University Teachers College). *Dissertation Abstract International, 36,* 4941B. (University Microfilms No. 76-7772).

Dewey, J. (1958). *Art as experience.* New York: Capricorn.

Dickoff, J., James, P., & Wiedenbach, E. (1968). Theory in a practice discipline: Part I, Practice-oriented theory. *Nursing Research, 17,* 415–435.

Greene, M. (1973). *Teacher as stronger.* Belmont, CA: Wadsworth.

Kuhn, T. (1962). *The structure of scientific revolutions.* Chicago: University of Chicago Press.

Langer, S. K. (1957). *Problems of art.* New York: Scribner.

Lee, V. (1960). Empathy. In M. Rader (Ed.), *A modern book of esthetics* (3rd ed.). New York: Holt, Rinehart and Winston.

Lippo, T. (1960). Empathy, inner imitation and sense-feeling. In M. Rader (Ed.), *A modern book of esthetics* (3rd ed.). New York: Holt, Rinehart and Winston.

Maslow, A. H. (1956). Self-actualizing people: A study of psychological health. In C. E. Moustakas (Ed.), *The self.* New York: Harper and Row.

McKay, R. (1969). Theories, models and systems for nursing. *Nursing Research, 18,* 393–399.

Mitchell, P. H. (1973). *Concepts basic to nursing.* New York: McGraw-Hill.

Nagel, E. (1961). *The structure of science.* New York: Harcourt, Brace and World.

Northrop, F. S. C. (1959). *The logic of the sciences and the humanities.* New York: World.

Orem, D. E. (1971). *Nursing: Concepts of practice.* New York: McGraw-Hill.

Polanyi, M. (1964). *Personal knowledge.* New York: Harper and Row.

Rader, M. (1960). Introduction: The meaning of art. In M. Rader (Ed.), *A modern book of esthetics* (3rd ed.). New York: Holt, Rinehart and Winston.

Slote, M. A. (1966). The theory of important criteria. *Journal of Philosophy, 63,* 211–224.

Weitz, M. (1960). The role of theory in aesthetics. In M. Rader (Ed.), *A modern book of esthetics* (3rd ed.). New York: Holt, Rinehart and Winston.

Wiedenbach, E. (1964). *Clinical nursing:* A helping art. New York: Springer.

The Author Comments

Fundamental Patterns of Knowing in Nursing

The genesis for this article, which was part of my doctoral dissertation, was my perplexity and confusion as an inexperienced teacher regarding what should be included in the nursing curriculum. Both student and teacher became disoriented in a maze of seemingly disparate disarticulated facts. My search for some meaningful guide to a sense of the whole to counteract this fragmentation led me to design a study to qualitatively analyze the types of knowledge that exemplified nursing. The resulting dissertation and article allowed nurses the freedom to begin asking questions about nursing and move beyond the assumptions about the essence of nursing and stimulate new thinking about the discipline. I never anticipated how popular the article would become!

—BARBARA A. CARPER

CHAPTER 25

Nursing Epistemology:
Traditions, Insights, Questions

Phyllis R. Schultz

Afaf I. Meleis

Epistemology is the study of what human beings know, how they come to know what they think they know and what the criteria are for evaluating knowledge claims. Nursing epistemology is the study of knowledge shared among the members of the discipline, the patterns of knowing and knowledge that develops from them, and the criteria for accepting knowledge claims. Three types of knowledge specific to nursing as a discipline are described here: clinical knowledge, conceptual knowledge and empirical knowledge. Different criteria for evaluating each type are suggested.

Nursing epistemology is the study of the origins of nursing knowledge, its structure and methods, the patterns of knowing of its members, and the criteria for validating its knowledge claims. Just as women are aware increasingly that their perceptions, observations and reasoning about the world contribute understandings that are unique, so too nurses, as members of a discipline and profession made up mostly of women, are changing in consciousness as knowledge for and from the practice of nursing continues to grow. This paper explores the epistemology of nursing; it grows out of the belief that, as nurses, our ways of knowing have not yet been fully articulated but that they will emerge if we allow ourselves to see the world through the eyes of practicing nurses and their clients.

The term "epistemology" comes from philosophy, where it is defined as the study of knowledge, or theory of knowledge (Flew, 1984). As a practice discipline and profession, nursing is often described as both an "art" and a "science." Articulating its epistemology is therefore a complex task: The study of nursing knowledge must range from the seemingly intuitive "knowing" of the experienced and expert nurses to the systematically verified knowledge of empirical researchers.

From IMAGE: Journal of Nursing Scholarship 20*(4), 217–221. Copyright © 1988.*
Sigma Theta Tau International Pub.

About the Authors

PHYLLIS SCHULTZ was born on March 9, 1938. She holds BSN, MN, MA, and PhD degrees from colleges and universities in North Dakota, Georgia, and Colorado and completed postdoctoral studies at the University of California, San Francisco. Her 40-year nursing career included 19 years in various clinical positions, including intensive care, primary care, and community health, coupled with 21 years in higher education at the University of Colorado Health Sciences Center and the University of Washington. Her scholarship focused on examining the theoretical, empirical, and clinical foundations of community nursing and administration as unique practice fields within the nursing domain. She considers her 1987 article "When the client is more than one" key to advancing nursing knowledge in these fields, and she is coauthor of several review chapters and articles since then that have contributed to the literature in the discipline. Currently, she is learning how to be a long-distance grandmother as well as exploring ways of "being" after a lifetime of "doing."

AFAF I. MELEIS, a nurse and medical sociologist, is currently the Margaret Bond Simon Dean of Nursing at the University of Pennsylvania School of Nursing. She completed her undergraduate nursing education at the University of Alexandria, Egypt (1961), and came to the United States as a Rockefeller Fellow (1962) to pursue her graduate education. She earned an MS in nursing (1964), an MA in sociology (1966), and a PhD in medical and social psychology (1968) from the University of California, Los Angeles. Her scholarship focuses on theory and knowledge development, including her theory on living with transitions, immigrant and international health, and women's role integration and health. She is the author of more than 150 articles and 40 chapters and numerous monographs, proceedings, and books, including the widely used book, *Theoretical Nursing: Development and Progress.* Currently, Dr. Meleis serves as President of the International Council on Women's Health Issues. She has received several national and international awards and honorary doctorates, including the 1990 Medal of Excellence for professional and scholarly achievements, presented by Egyptian President Hosni Mubarak, and an Honorary Professorship from the Department of Health Sciences, the Hong Kong Polytechnic University.

The epistemology of any field of inquiry depends on the nature of the phenomena studied and on the propensities of the inquirers who are developing knowledge in the field. Nursing epistemology, then, is the study of how nurses come to know what they think they know, what exactly nurses do know, how nursing knowledge is structured and on what basis knowledge claims are made.

What is Knowing/ What is Known?

For any person, knowing begins with the processes of observation, perception and experience in encountering the world and being in the world. These processes give rise to describing and interpreting phenomena, including anticipating, with some degree of accuracy, what is likely to happen at some future time. It is helpful to think of "knowing" as a process and the knowledge that comes from that process as the product (Benoliel, 1987; Chinn & Jacobs, 1987).

According to Benoliel, "Knowing can be viewed as an individual's perceptual awareness of the complexities of a particular situation and draws on inner knowledge resources that have been garnered through experience in living" (p. 151). It rarely can be expressed through discourse but is experienced through the acts of persons (Benner, 1983; Chinn & Jacobs, 1987). By contrast, knowledge as product is often expressed in some form of communication such as informal conversations, formal oral presentations, written articles and texts or art forms such as paintings, poetry, novels or music.

In a practice discipline, knowing is also working on solutions to problems that are important for the welfare of clients. It includes the ability to identify the questions at the forefront of inquiry in the field, the issues involved in answering these questions, the ways to go about answering the answerable questions and the ways to handle the unanswerable questions. Knowing is also having the wisdom to recognize which questions have top priority, which are secondary and which are trivial; it is recognizing which questions can be answered in the near future and which have to be deferred.

In epistemology, Chisholm (1982) formulated the questions about knowing:

1. "What do we know? What is the extent of our knowledge?"
2. "How are we to decide whether we know? What are the criteria of knowledge?" (p. 50) Chisholm identified three epistemological positions as possible answers to these questions: skepticism, methodism and particularism. Skeptics say that these are unanswerable questions because we cannot answer either set without presupposing an answer to the other. This position is untenable for a practice discipline because we have to take care of real people with real health problems.

By "methodism," Chisholm (1982) meant that to have knowledge is to have a preferred method of inquiry and procedures for recognizing reliable or credible knowledge (i.e., one begins by answering the second set of questions (set 2). Chisholm explicitly identified empiricism as a "type of 'methodism'" (p. 67). Recent debates in nursing about qualitative and quantitative data collection with their corresponding metaphysical and epistemological foundations reflect a type of methodism in nursing (Schultz, 1987). This methodism has led some nurse inquirers to subscribe to science in general and to empiricist science in particular as the preferable epistemological position in nursing.

The allegiance to empiricism can explain some of the sense of separation that has arisen among nurse inquirers who hold different epistemological positions and use different methods of inquiry. Some rely on reflection and reasoning; others elect structured observation and hypothesis testing; still others prefer phenomenological dialogue and reflective interpretation. Academicians tend to insist on knowledge that is formal, orderly, validated and communicable. Practitioners trust knowledge that results in appropriate actions with clients in specific situations. To espouse the methodist's epistemological position is to fail to recognize the legitimacy of these multiple ways of knowing; it is to resist accepting the complexity and holistic character of nursing (Benoliel, 1987; Chinn & Jacobs, 1987; Visintainer, 1986).

By "particularism," Chisholm (1982) meant "We can know and know that we know some particular thing at a particular point in time" (p. 74). This position starts from the premise that there are some things we know, whether or not we agree on the methods and procedures for knowing (Chisholm, 1982; Schultz, 1987). Philosophers begin with rather ordinary, everyday cases of knowledge such as "I know how to drive a car" and "I know that seven plus five equals twelve." Similarly, "I know that the sentence, Some mushrooms are poisonous, is true" (Lehrer, 1974). These three statements can be classified as (a) recounting a practical skill, (b) communicating a conceptual insight and (c) articulating an empirical hypothesis.

As nurses, we begin with particular cases of knowledge from (a) our practice, (b) our theories, or (c) our research. Statements about what we "know" are reflected implicitly or explicitly in the writings of our clinicians, theorists and researchers, for example:

1. The experiences of persons in health and illness are revealed in characteristic patterns. These patterns tend to be repetitive, orderly, predictable, and unified; they reflect organization.
2. Some individuals have health and illness experiences that do not fit the general pattern. Thus another case of what we "know" in nursing is that it is

predictable that individuals may be unpredictable in their health and illness experiences.

3. Human health and illness can be perceived and understood through uncovering the meanings that individuals, groups and societies derive from their experiences.

4. The health and illness of persons are interactive with environments.

5. Nursing acts influence the responses of persons in health and illness; nursing and the experiences of persons with health and illness are interactive.

Statements such as these about what we "know" in nursing are what we want to begin with in formulating the criteria of knowledge in our discipline. But before we explore such criteria, we will discuss patterns of knowing revealed in the nursing literature, and those from a study of women (Belenky et al., 1986), which may contribute to our understanding of the types of knowledge in present-day nursing.

Patterns of Knowing in Nursing

The complexity of nursing's epistemology was clearly demonstrated by Carper's (1978) delineation of four fundamental patterns of knowing in nursing: empirics, ethics, esthetics and personal knowledge. Each of these four patterns has recently been specified epistemologically by Chinn and Jacobs (1987). Here we will elaborate only on personal knowledge, because of our belief in the importance of the practitioner as the knower in nursing's development of knowledge.

Personal knowledge was described by Carper (1978) as self-knowledge, or awareness of the self. This description seems to leave out the knowledge from practice that Benner (1983) termed "practical knowledge," following the reasoning of Polanyi (1964) in his *Personal Knowledge*. For Polanyi, "personal" referred to a characteristic of the knower; "knowledge," to a mental process:

I regard knowing as an active comprehension of the things known, an action that requires skill . . .

Comprehension is neither an arbitrary act nor a passive experience, but a responsible act claiming universal validity. (p. xiii)

Thus to know the self is part of comprehending "the things known." Knowing what one knows is also part of comprehending.

Polanyi (1964) distinguished between knowledge as theory and knowledge as practical skill. He termed knowledge that may not be articulated through language as "tacit knowing"; knowledge that is communicable through discourse he termed "explicit knowing." Another way to phrase this distinction is "knowing how" and "knowing that," which Benner (1983) found useful in explaining what expert nurses know. Expert nurses may enter a caring encounter with awareness of the self as therapeutic agent (Carper, 1978) and with a foundation of formal concepts, theories, facts and skills learned in their education (the knowing that). According to Benner (1983), as the encounter, or event, unfolds, they refine, elaborate or disconfirm this "foreknowledge"; the encounter then deserves to be termed "experience" and contributes to the knowing how. These three aspects of personal knowledge—knowing the self, knowing that and knowing how—are the sum of what one knows. All three are brought to the caring situation and are used to identify and solve the problems of the discipline.

Unfortunately, we know very little about personal knowing, especially about knowing the self and knowing how, in part because they can only be articulated retrospectively (Chinn & Jacobs, 1987). The knowing how from practice may, however, be brought to consciousness and made communicable through innovative methods of inquiry such as interpretive, grounded theory or phenomenological research (Benner, 1983; 1985; Pyles & Stern, 1983; Ray, 1987). For example, using a grounded theory approach, Pyles and Stern described the "nursing gestalt," by which expert critical care nurses identify impending cardiogenic shock and prevent untimely death. They learned that novice nurses must work with expert critical care nurses (the Gray Gorilla concept) to acquire their know how for practice. Their findings corroborated those of Benner's (1983) study of the knowledge embedded in clinical practice.

Also, in a study of critical care nursing using phenomenology as method, Ray (1987) discovered that the essence of nursing in critical care involves technological and ethical caring; it is an experiential dialectic between technical competence (doing no harm) and compassion (in response to suffering), which are mediated through ethical choice (preserving autonomy and ensuring justice).

Efforts to bring to consciousness the self-knowledge and knowing how of nursing practice may be aided by examination of women's ways of knowing identified by Belenky et al. (1986). The patterns they discovered were not supposed to be hierarchical, although unfortunately their descriptions appear to be so. In applying their framework to nurses, we will assume that different patterns of knowing exist simultaneously. The five patterns of women's knowing that Belenky et al. identified are silence, received knowledge, subjective knowledge, procedural knowledge and constructed knowledge. Each of the five patterns is explained in the following:

Silence. Persons "experience themselves as mindless and voiceless and subject to the whims of external authority" (p. 16). Belenky et al. add that silent women know at the "gut level" but have not cultivated their capacity for abstract thought; nor do they attempt to articulate why they do what they do. They accept the voices of authority for direction in their work and life because of others' power, not necessarily expertise. Others are "right"; the silent one is "wrong" and "dumb."

According to Colliere (1986) silent nurses may not know how to conceptualize their daily experiences; they follow the voices of others because of fear of others' power. They do not have the language to generalize from what they know so that their knowledge can be communicated. They have learned to be silent. Their work, their patterns of knowing and their knowledge are invisible.

Received knowledge. Persons "perceive themselves as capable of receiving, even reproducing, knowledge from all-knowing external authorities but not capable of creating knowledge on their own" (p. 15). Individuals who use this way of knowing rely on others for the words to communicate what they know. For this type of knower, knowledge is observable; there is no ambiguity in it, and it depends on the expertise of others.

Many nurses have contented themselves with using the words of others to express and guide their knowing. American nurses have used medical knowledge, psychological and sociological knowledge, philosophical knowledge and administrative knowledge to communicate what they know. Following the same pattern, nurses in other countries have used nursing theories developed in the United States to communicate the nature of their practice.

Subjective knowledge. Knowledge is "conceived of as personal, private, and subjectively known and intuited" (p. 15). The subjective pattern of women's knowing reminds us of the debates in nursing today about the usefulness and reliability of experiential knowing (i.e., knowledge from practice). Knowers such as this in nursing offer us their subjective wisdom from their own inner voices, which may enhance our understanding of complex situations, but their knowledge is transient, and not cumulative. Such knowers may find it difficult to articulate the processes that they have gone through in knowing because knowing for them is intuitive, experienced, not thought out and something felt rather than cognitively appraised or constructed.

Procedural knowledge. These knowers depend on careful observation, structured procedures and systematic analyses. In short, they are rationalists. They use objectivity as a measure of what can be known as well as repeated observations under controlled situations for corroboration. They distance themselves from experience in order to know. Though they use subjective awareness to provide insights, they adhere to the idea that objectivity yields the knowledge that is most reliable.

Nurse researchers and academicians are the strongest adherents of this way of knowing. Following strict procedures for inquiry is considered the way to secure reliable knowledge for teaching the principles and practices of nursing and for further inquiry. As we emphasize increasingly research-based practice, clinicians are joining the ranks of the rational, procedural knowers in nursing.

Constructed knowledge. A pattern of knowing in which persons "view all knowledge as contextual, experience themselves as creators of knowledge, and value both subjective and objective strategies of knowing" (p. 15). These knowers integrate the different ways of knowing and the different voices (including the silent voice). To them, "all knowledge is constructed, and the knower is an intimate part of the known" (p. 37).

Nurses who subscribe to this view of knowing see theories as approximations of reality that are ongoing and always in process; their frames of reference are constructed and reconstructed (Visintainer, 1986), and posing questions is as important as attempting to answer questions. These nurses believe that knowing is achieved as much through openness and curiosity and through examination of the assumptions and context within which questions are posed as through adherence to procedures or systematic observation and replication.

For nurses who subscribe to this view of knowing, the development of knowledge is a never-ending process. There are glimmers of certain knowledge if one understands the whole of a situation including formal knowledge of the phenomenon. Experts (i.e., experienced knowers) develop a connected knowing through conversing with each other and through identifying patterns, consistencies and order in the evidence provided by the various ways of knowing (Benoliel, 1987; Schultz, 1987). Their knowledge is corroborated by knowledge from other disciplines.

Types of Nursing Knowledge and Criteria of Credibility

From our reflections on the traditional patterns of knowing in nursing and on women's ways of knowing, we have identified three types of knowledge specific to nursing as a discipline: clinical knowledge, conceptual knowledge and empirical knowledge. Discussed below are their relationships to the different patterns of knowing and possible criteria of credibility for each type.

Clinical Knowledge

Clinical knowledge results from engaging in the gestalt of caring, from bringing to bear multiple ways of knowing in order to solve the problems of patient care. Florence Nightingale knew the needs of the soldiers who fought in the Crimean War because she worked with them day and night; she was able to see the results of limited resources and exposure to the unhygienic environment. She realized that not only were diseases afflicting the soldiers, but the care they failed to receive affected their recovery.

Clinical knowledge is manifested primarily in the acts of practicing nurses; it is individual and personal. Historically, it has often been voiceless except in descriptions of the art of nursing, which have come to be viewed as less important and credible since nursing has been developing formal empirical foundations for practice. Clinicians experience patients' situations and "do" (i.e., they act based on these experiences).

Historically, clinical knowledge has been the product of a combination of personal knowing and empirics. It has usually involved intuition and subjective knowing, although these have tended to be ignored, denigrated or denied (Rew & Barrow, 1987). In the past, the empirical base was often "received empirics" from medicine or the social and behavioral sciences. Increasingly, however, empirical studies by nurses inform clinical practice. Further, intuition and subjective knowing are regaining their legitimacy as necessary components of humane care (Watson, 1985). The aesthetic and ethical patterns of knowing are also contributing to the development of clinical knowledge in response to the changing needs of persons interacting with technological and organizational environments.

Traditionally, clinical knowledge has been communicated retrospectively, through the publication of articles on specific client problems. These accounts, in national journals of nursing and increasingly in international journals, report individual case descriptions or summaries of multiple cases that provide answers for questions and problems in practice. These published accounts often reflect received knowledge and procedural knowledge and are characterized by prescriptions for practice.

The credibility of clinical knowledge has been based on the usefulness of its communicated wisdom—"It works." This criterion meets the requirement of purposefulness of a practice discipline (Chinn & Jacobs, 1987). Do we need other modes of corroboration? Can the art of nursing yield as reliable and reproducible knowledge as does the "science" of nursing? Should it? Perhaps models of practice, the discovery of patterns within and across clients and testimonials of subjective knowledge might be appropriate criteria for the credibility of clinical knowledge. These are unanswered questions.

Conceptual Knowledge

Conceptual knowledge is abstracted and generalized beyond personal experiences; it explicates the patterns revealed in multiple client experiences in multiple situations and articulates them as models or theories. Concepts are defined, and statements about the relationships among them are formulated. These propositions are supported by empirical and/or anecdotal evidence or defended by inferences and logical reasoning. This type of knowledge is manifested in the works of nurse theorists who seek answers to questions such as, Who is our client? What is it that nurses do that influences persons' health (Meleis, 1985)? These theorists develop comprehensive formulations of the nursing world. They use knowledge from other disciplines but through reflection and imagination evolve perspectives on that knowledge that are unique to nursing. They are influenced by procedures followed in the development of other fields but adhere to procedures supportive of the values and purpose of nursing.

Conceptual knowledge is the product of reflection on nursing phenomena. It emanates from curiosity and evolves from innovation and imagination in inquiry, along with persistence and commitment to the accumulation of facts and reliable generalizations. This type of nursing knowledge requires logical reasoning and comes primarily from individuals who take the position

that knowledge is constructed within a context, and its development is a never-ending process.

Empirical knowing has influenced the development of conceptual knowledge in nursing through a dynamic interplay between systematic observation (empirics) and theorizing (reflecting, describing, synthesizing) (Weekes, 1986). The results of an inquirer's own research and that of others are used to support the propositional structure of frameworks or theories. But imagination and risk taking are important in their origination.

Will aesthetic knowing lead to formal conceptualizations of nursing that reflect its art? Will conceptual frameworks and models emerge from ethics as a pattern of knowing to describe this dimension of nursing? The answers to these questions depend on the degree to which nurse inquirers can view multiple ways of knowing as equally valuable in contributing to the mission of nursing.

The credibility of conceptual knowledge rests, in part, on the extent to which nurses find useful models and theories in communicating what they know. Whether or not a particular conceptual formulation holds up to critical appraisal depends also on its coherence and logical integrity—two criteria for evaluating theories (Meleis, 1985; Chinn & Jacobs, 1987).

Conceptual knowledge is often communicated in the form of propositional sentences. Thus it is the propositions and their relationships to each other that are evaluated for credibility. Chisholm's six levels of epistemic preferability illustrate the criteria for evaluating propositional credibility. Schultz (1987) explicated these levels with a proposition exemplifying a nursing knowledge claim:

> Nursing acts influence persons' energy exchange for healing and health. For the person who believes this claim the statement is (1) self presenting to him or her at a particular point in time; (2) the claim has some presumption in its favor because it is not contradicted by other beliefs; (3) the claim is judged to be acceptable because it is not disconfirmed by the set of propositions having some presumption in their favor; (4) the claim is epistemi-

cally in the clear because it is not disconfirmed by the set of acceptable propositions and therefore (5) the claim is beyond reasonable doubt. Having met these conditions, the claim is judged to be (6) evident or certain (p. 141).

These are stringent criteria. Since nurses attend to individual experiences as well as to general patterns of experience, we may need to formulate different criteria of credibility for the conceptualization of nursing phenomena.

Empirical Knowledge

Empirical knowledge results from research. By research, we do not mean simply the empiricist approach per se but also historical, phenomenological, interpretive and critical theory approaches (Chinn, 1986). Empirical knowledge is manifest in published reports and is often used to justify actions and procedures in practice. It forms the basis for new studies and thereby contributes to the cumulative body of knowledge of a discipline. It often stimulates theoretical conceptualizations.

Researchers rely, in part, on received and procedural knowledge to inform their inquiries, but the hypotheses they test may originate in subjective knowledge; that is, their experiences with and reflections on nursing phenomena may give rise to hunches that lead to innovative methods or approaches to inquiry. If the empirical inquirer is also a practitioner, self-knowledge and practical knowledge may be brought to bear on the methods of inquiry. It is less clear how the aesthetic or ethical patterns of knowing contribute to the development of empirical knowledge except that usually (a) researchers adhere to ethical precepts in the conduct of their studies and (b) nurse inquirers are turning to the arts and humanities for approaches to systematic inquiry.

Advocates of different types of research approaches and methods have carved out criteria to validate their findings that are congruent with the particular designs and epistemological orientations that they follow (Gortner, 1984; Sandelowski, 1986). For all, however, the credibility of empirical knowledge rests on the degree to which the researcher has followed procedures accepted by the community of researchers and on the log-

ical derivation of conclusions from the evidence without bias or prejudice (Schultz, 1987; Gortner & Schultz, 1987). Of particular importance is whether or not the researcher is cognizant of previous research findings, knowledgeable about the procedures by which they were discovered, and dedicated to basing new research efforts on previous knowledge (Benoliel, 1987).

In addition to the procedural criteria accompanying various research designs and methods, the credibility of empirical knowledge is assessed by the systematic review and critique of research published in annual reviews (Werley & Fitzpatrick, 1983-1986; Fitzpatrick & Taunton, 1987), by consensus conferences focused on corroborating what is known about specific phenomena (e.g., pain) (National Institute of Health, 1987), and by invitational conferences to clarify the state-of-the-art on a topic and suggest new directions to be taken (Duffy & Pender, 1987). The epistemic preferability criteria enumerated above for conceptual knowledge claims may also be useful for assessing the credibility of empirical knowledge claims.

Ultimately credibility criteria must be consistent with nurses' various ways of knowing and types of knowledge. Can criteria be developed to accommodate the epistemological plurality of nursing, its complexity and holism? Is there one set of criteria or are there several? These are unanswered questions, but let us consider the possibility that the criteria for accepting knowledge vary for each type of knowledge.

Conclusion

Throughout this paper, we have deliberately avoided using the concept of "truth." Unfortunately inquirers from differing and contradictory perspectives have a propensity to put forth the view that their way of knowing yields *the* truth rather than *a* truth. Perhaps it is inappropriate to use the language of truth in nursing or in any practice discipline that deals with complex human experiences. Perhaps comprehending the context and patterns of human experiences, adjusted for individual differences, is more appropriate for claiming universal validity (Polanyi, 1964; Visintainer, 1986). Perhaps it is not sufficient to speak of facts alone, rather we should speak of experiences, intuition *and* facts. Perhaps it is not enough to rely on research as the medium for knowledge development; conceptualization and expert knowledge from clinical practice may be equally powerful and credible.

If we agree that there are different ways of knowing, different unknowns to be known, different propensities of knowers for knowing and different aspects to be known about the same phenomenon, then perhaps we can develop appropriate criteria for knowing from what we do know and, then, for knowing what we want to know.

REFERENCES

Belenky, M. F., Clinchy, B. M., Goldberger, N. R., & Tarule, J. M. (1986). *Women's ways of knowing.* New York: Basic Books.

Benner, P. (1983). Uncovering the knowledge embedded in clinical practice. *IMAGE: The Journal of Nursing Scholarship, 15*(2), 36–41.

Benner, P. (1985). Quality of life: A phenomenological perspective on explanation, prediction, and understanding in nursing science. *Advances in Nursing Science, 8*(1), 1–14.

Benoliel, J. Q. (1987). Response to "Toward holistic inquiry in nursing: A proposal for synthesis of patterns and methods." *Scholarly Inquiry for Nursing Practice: An International Journal, 1*(2), 147–152.

Carper, B. A. (1978). Fundamental patterns of knowing in nursing. *Advances in Nursing Science, 1*(1), 13–23.

Chinn, P. L. (1986). *Nursing Research Methodology.* Rockville, MD: Aspen Publications.

Chinn, P. L., & Jacobs, M. K. (1987). *Theory and nursing: A systematic approach* (2d ed.). St. Louis: The C. V. Mosby Company.

Chisholm, R. M. (1982). *The foundations of knowing.* Minneapolis: University of Minnesota Press.

Colliere, M. F. (1986). Invisible care and invisible women as health care-providers. *International Journal of Nursing Studies, 23*(2), 95–112.

Duffy, M. E., & Pender, N. J. (1987). *Conceptual issues in health promotion research.* Indianapolis: Sigma Theta Tau Publications.

Fitzpatrick, J. J., & Taunton, R. L. (1987). Annual Review of Nursing Research (Vol. 5). New York: Springer Publishers.

Flew, A. (1984). *A dictionary of philosophy* (2d Ed.). New York: St. Martin's Press.

Gortner, S. R. (1984). Knowledge in a practice discipline: Philosophy and pragmatics. In C. Williams (Ed.), *Nursing research and policy formation: The case of prospective payment* (pp. 5–16). Kansas City, MO: American Academy of Nursing.

Gortner, S. R., & Schultz, P. R. (1987). Approaches to nursing science methods, *IMAGE: Journal of Nursing Scholarship, 20*(1), 22–24.

Lehrer, K. (1974). *Knowledge.* London: Oxford University Press.

Meleis, A. I. (1985). *Theoretical nursing.* Philadelphia: J. B. Lippincott Co.

National Institute of Health Consensus Development Conference (1987). The integrated approach to the management of pain. *Journal of Pain and Symptom Management, 2* (1), 35–44.

Polanyi, M. (1964). *Personal knowledge: Towards a post-critical philosophy.* New York: Harper Torchbooks.

Pyles, S. H., & Stern, P. N. (1983). Discovery of nursing gestalt in critical care nursing: The importance of the gray gorilla syndrome. *IMAGE: The Journal of Nursing Scholarship, 15*(3), 51–57.

Ray, M. A. (1987). Technological caring: A new model in critical care. *Dimensions of Critical Care Nursing, 6*(3), 166–173.

Rew, L., & Barrow, E. M. (1987). Intuition: A neglected hallmark of nursing knowledge. *Advances in Nursing Science, 10*(1), 49–62.

Sandelowski, M. (1986). The problem of rigor in qualitative research. *Advances in Nursing Science, 8*(3), 27–37.

Schultz, P. R. (1987). Toward holistic inquiry in nursing: A proposal for synthesis of patterns and methods. *Scholarly Inquiry for Nursing Practice: An International Journal, 1*(2), 135–146.

Visintainer, M. A. (1986). The nature of knowledge and theory in nursing. *IMAGE: Journal of Nursing Scholarship, 18*(2), 32–38.

Watson, J. (1985). *Nursing: Human science and human care.* Norwalk, CT: Appleton-Century-Crofts.

Weekes, D. P. (1986). Theory-free observation: Fact or fantasy. In P. L. Chinn, (Ed.). *Nursing Research Methodology.* Rockville, MD: Aspen Publications, 11–22.

Werley, H. H., & Fitzpatrick, J. J. (1983–1986). *Annual Review of Nursing Research* (Vols. 1–4).

The Authors Comment

Nursing Epistemology: Traditions, Insights, Questions

We wrote this article to explore nurses' various ways of knowing and how the knowledge that flows from these ways can provide solutions to the urgent problems germane to client welfare as well as be credible in the larger context of science in practice disciplines. In Schultz's view, it is "an especially good example of careful in-depth reasoning about our discipline." We were challenged to identify what credibility might mean for types of nursing knowledge. Critical to our concerns was a need to legitimize what clinical nurses "know" and to place that type of knowing and knowledge in its rightful place within the discipline. Many of the questions we posed about credibility criteria for different types of nursing knowledge remain unanswered. They await pursuit by nurse scholars in the 21st century.

—Phyllis Schultz
—Afaf I. Meleis

CHAPTER 26

'Unknowing': Toward Another Pattern of Knowing in Nursing

Patricia L. Munhall

As I sit on this hard bench I suddenly yearn for one last long look, and not only of the phenomenon of little Joe and little Michael, but of the others too: Ellen, four, and Annie, seven months, sharing a peach . . . . As I watch them now as adults the fact that I will never see their toddler selves again is tormenting.

—JANE SMILEY,[1] *Ordinary Love and Good Will,* 1989

When you are thirty, the child is two. At forty, you realize that the child in the house, the child you live with, is still, when you close your eyes, or the moment he has walked from the room, two years old. When you are sixty and the child is gone, the child will also be two, but then you will be more certain. Wet sheets, wet kisses. A flood of tears. As you remember him the child is always two.

—ANN BEATTIE,[2] *Picturing Will,* 1989

The foregoing literary excerpts illustrate the power of individual perceptions and the different structures of subjectivity that call for a fifth pattern of knowing in nursing to be acknowledged, that of "unknowing." Many nurses have endorsed in our nursing literature, and in some curricula, a structural, categorical approach to knowledge, reflected in Carper's *Fundamental Patterns of Knowing in Nursing.*[3] These four patterns of knowing are part of Fawcetts' proposed "metaparadigm" for nursing.[4]

This article focuses on the state of mind of unknowing as a condition of openness. "Knowing," in contrast, leads to a form of confidence that has inherent in it a state of closure. The "art" of unknowing is discussed as a de-centering process from one's own organizing principles of the world.[5] Unknowing is not simple, but it is essential to the understanding of sub-

Reprinted from Nursing Outlook *1993;41:125-8. Copyright © 1993 by Mosby-Year Book, Inc. Reprinted with permission of Elsevier Science.*

About the Author

Born in New York City, PATRICIA L. MUNHALL received her master's degree from New York University and her doctorate from Columbia University. She went on for psychoanalytic training and has become a nationally certified psychoanalyst. The majority of her professional life has been in academia as Professor of Nursing. Tricia has been intrigued with the philosophy that underpins qualitative methods of research and continues to pursue the study of phenomenology, having written a text on the approach for health care sciences. She has written more than 50 articles, and her book on qualitative research is in its fourth edition. In addition, she has written 10 phenomenologic collections of women's, men's, and family experience. Tricia is an international speaker and consultant. The circle is completing now, with a private practice in phenomenologic psychoanalysis. In 1996, she founded and is now President of the International Institute of Human Understanding. For more information on this organization, please go to http://www.iih.org.

jectivity and perspectivity. These concepts are discussed, and a suggestion is offered that for understanding to emerge the perceptual field that evolves when two or more personal universes come together must be clearly focused upon by the involved individuals. It also is proposed that in this perceptual field of two or more subjective perspectives, called the "intersubjective space," all sources of human understanding, empathy—and also conflict—can and will evolve.

The Art of Unknowing

Unknowing, paradoxically, is another pattern of knowing. Knowing that one does not know something, that one does not understand someone who stands before them and that perhaps this process does not fit into some preexisting paradigm or theory is critical to the evolution and development of knowledge.

To engage in an authentic encounter, one must stand in one's own socially constructed world and unearth the other's world by admitting, "I don't know you. I do not know your subjective world."

When a nurse stands with another human being, forming impressions, making a diagnosis, formulating a perception, and knowing what is best, that nurse may indeed practice an efficient type of nursing based on the empirical, ethical, personal, and esthetic patterns of knowing.

Still, knowing of this kind leads to a form of confidence that has inherent in it a state of closure. To be authentically present to a patient is to situate knowingly in one's own life and interact with full unknowingness about the other's life. In this way unknowing equals openness (Figure 26-1).

This is by no means easy. Unknowing as an art is not presently acknowledged and calls for a great amount of introspection. However unknowing remains essential to the understanding of intersubjectivity and perspectivity. In other words, it is essential that we understand our self and our patient to be two distinctive beings, one of whom we do not know.

Placing aside a cogent argument that might speak to just how well nurses know themselves, there can be little doubt that they do not know the patient. Each patient has a unique perspective of their situated context and a unique perspective of who they are as person in the world. This is their perspectivity, their worldview, their reality. When nurses and patients meet, two perspectives of a situation need to be recognized. Thus the process of intersubjectivity begins to create the perceptual field (Figure 26-2).

Intersubjectivity

Intersubjectivity is not a difficult concept to understand, though many writings about it seem intent at making the

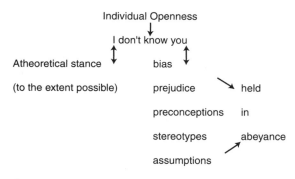

Figure 26-1 *The art of unknowing.*

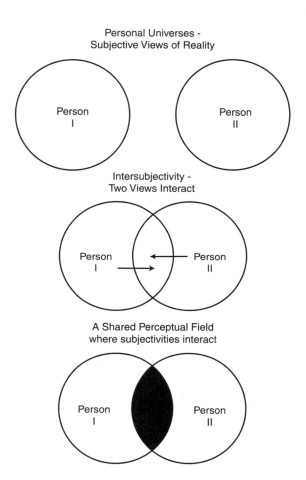

Figure 26-2 *Personal universes, intersubjectivity, and a shared perceptual field.*

concept complex. What is challenging is practicing it in a wide-awake manner.

Intersubjectivity is the verbal and nonverbal interplay between the organized subjective world of one person and the organized subjective world of another.[5-9] It is one person's subjectivity intersecting with another's subjectivity. In each person's subjective world is organization of feeling, thoughts, ideas, principles, theories, illusions, distortions, and whatever else helps or hinders a person. Individuals do not know about another's subjective world unless they are told about it, and even then one cannot be sure. Figures 2 and 3 illustrate visually the concept of intersubjectivity.

In Figure 26-3 the illustration depicts where many nurse theorists say nursing takes place. Sometimes this is called the "in-between,"[6] but visually it depicts a connection that for the purpose of this article is called a "shared perceptual field." When this shared perceptual field is pulled out by the nurse, it becomes a whole, as shown in Figure 26-4.

It is in this field that caring, understanding, empathy, conflict, and misunderstandings take place. This, then, is no small matter. For caring to be realized, this perceptual field that emerges, this intelligible whole or intersubjective space, must be clearly focused on, mutually analyzed, and mutually interpreted. The mutuality here reflects the nurse and patient communicating, reflecting, and validating the meaning of the patient's experience. The unknowing stance of the nurse is primarily motivated by the intent

to come to know the patient's world. The patient "knows" the nurse as one who is engaging in the process of coming to know so that the nurse can better understand, empathize, and care in an authentically individualized manner.

A De-Centering Process

This art of unknowing when two subjective worlds intersect is discussed as a de-centering process, one that de-centers us from our own organizing principles of the world.[5] This unknowing art enables empathy of the sit-

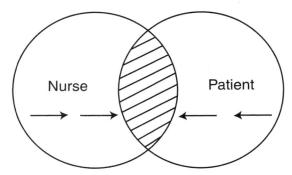

Figure 26-3   *The nurse-patient shared perceptual field.*

uated context where nurses understand the actual essence of meaning the patients' experiences hold for them.

Figure 26-5 might be what Sartre[10] thought of as utmost importance in understanding and evaluating his conception of the human situation. This is called "being for others." Sartre feared in this the loss of self, but what is portrayed here as de-centering is a temporary suspending of self as the nurse allows the patient's subjective structure of reality to become known. The nurse is metaphorically eclipsed by a patient in order to

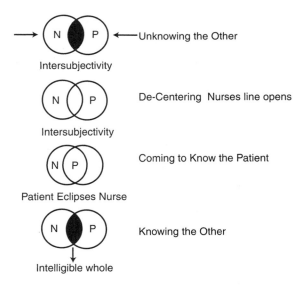

Figure 26-4   *Perceptual field.*

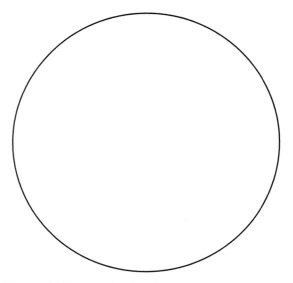

Figure 26-5   *Knowing the other.*

"know" the patient. Nurses encourage patients to reveal their perspectives without interruption or the introduction of alternative interpretations. Nurses allow patients to be seen and heard.

These ideas of unknowing and decentering are very practical realities to nursing practice and research. Without extensive examination and introspection of and about the substance of the intersubjective space, two dangers might occur that are counterproductive to understanding and to patients' health, growth, and becoming. Nurses must understand that their perceptions of the world and of health may or may not assist the patient. Stemming from the nurses' subjectivity, if not eclipsed temporarily by the patients', are two dangers of knowing. They are intersubjective conjunction and intersubjective disjunction.[5]

Intersubjective Conjunction

In the instance of intersubjective conjunction nurses are alerted to this circumstance by feelings of comfort with the patient. Nurses need to understand that this comfort is originating from their own perceptions of knowing. We have yet to explore the meaning of this comfort for the patient. Although this initial compatability may feel good, it could cause problems unless an attitude of questioning and unknowing precedes the continuation of the perceived shared subjective stance.

In intersubjective conjunction it seems the two subjective interpretations of the world match. The patient is an analogue model of the nurse, or vice versa. Thoughts such as "We think alike" "We feel alike" "We see things the same way" "We agree on what's to be done" and "We have good rapport" should alert the nurse to this situation.

What is occurring is that both persons share closely similar perceptions of the experience. However, before going further, it is suggested here that the nurse proceed with an air of mystery and an attitude open to alternative interpretations.

Difficulties Inherent in Intersubjective Conjunctions

Closure is the main difficulty inherent in intersubjective conjunctions. While two persons (in this instance a patient and a nurse) may share common attitudes, the reasons and the histories may be very different. So shared assumptions of reality, or conjunction, may:

- Close further exploration
- Achieve the status of objective reality (when it may not be so)
- Represent a shared defensive solution
- Represent a shared illusion or delusion
- Close off testing other alternatives
- Eliminate exploring origin of perception

An example of this could be a nurse and a patient sharing negative feelings about various things—people, places, or an experience. Their agreement becomes an agreed on truthful objective reality. In actuality, these shared perceptions could be a way that both these individuals project inner difficulties onto the outside world. The danger, of course, is that the inner difficulties go left unexplored and the conjunction becomes collusion. It is critical in this intersubjective space to go beyond or underneath the agreed on perceptions of the experience.

The Art of Unknowing in Intersubjective Conjunction

Unknowing can be the impetus to finding out. Where there is agreement about the world, nurses should de-center, hold their beliefs in abeyance, and allow others to tell their stories. Nurses allow others to enlarge their construction of their social reality. Before, nurses said, "I know how you're feeling," which is doubtful. The knowing part comes from allowing the other to be known from individual perceptions, not those of the nurse. So agreement in the intersubjective space does not mean mutual knowing. Unknowing is essential to "knowing," just as in intersubjective disjunction.

Intersubjective Disjunction

In the instance of intersubjective disjunction there is disparity and disagreement with the subjective perceptions of the two socially constructed realities of individuals. It is in this disjunction that misunderstanding and conflict may be counterproductive and non-therapeutic for patients. In disjunction, nurses believe that their interpretation of a situation is the better one and that the patient's interpretation would be improved if it were altered. Rather than assuming an unknowing posture regarding the patient's perception, the nurse attempts to change the subjective meaning for the patient. In contrast, then, to conjunction, in which there is agreement about the world (which may be obstructional as well), in disjunction there is disagreement, and this too may be extremely counterproductive to understanding and empathy.

Difficulties Inherent in Intersubjective Disjunction

The danger in disjunction or disagreement is mainly one of the projection of a nurse's perception on a patient. Once again, there is closure to the meaning and desires of an individual person—the patient. Disagreed upon assumptions of reality, or disjunction, may:

- Close further exploration
- Become self-fulfilling
- Alter the patient's perception of reality

- Give the patient the impression that he is wrong
- Interfere with patient's defense mechanisms

An example of this could be "knowing what is best" for the patient. A case that comes to mind is a nurse who discouraged a patient from marrying a man who was obviously a poor choice for this patient. The patient did not marry; instead she had a series of psychotic episodes. Would they have happened anyway? We do not know. But de-centering here to find out what was going on with this patient from her perspective was essential. Instead of diagnosing and prescribing, the nurse needed to unknow, listen, and understand the meaning of this patient's perceptions.

The Art of Unknowing in Intersubjective Disjunction

Where there is disjunction, there is the potential for misunderstanding the meaning an experience has for a patient. If the nurse "knows" what is best and attempts to communicate this to the patient, the patient may feel misunderstood, conflicted, and may become resistant to the "knower." After all, the patient is a "knower" as well.

Again, nurses must hold their own beliefs and assumptions aside. For instance, if a nurse believes the situation to be hopeless and a patient is hopeful despite all evidence, to be empathic and to help the patient feel understood, the nurse too should attempt a hopeful attitude. Many nurses can speak to a patient they had every cause to believe to be hopeless as far as improving or becoming more differentially integrated only to find that their "knowing" was based on usual cases in similar circumstances. The danger here is obvious, in that the self-fulfilling prophecy may be operating and the patient may begin to perceive his circumstance as the nurse does.

The Fifth Pattern of Knowing: Unknowing

"Knowledge screens the sound the third ear hears, so we hear only what we know."[11]

Our listening characteristics are often those of diagnosing and prescribing. The diagnosing and prescrib-

ing comes from our knowledge and our subjective perceptions. This may lead to premature closure to other possibilities, interpretations, and perceptions. The fact that this occurs is a result of someone else's knowing. Someone else teaching us to know, to put together, to make sense.

"The compulsion to make sense is a resistance to unknowing."[11] The pattern of unknowing can lead to a much deeper knowledge of another being, of different meanings, and interpretations of all our various perceptions of experience. The intent of bracketing in qualitative research is one in which the researcher assumes the posture of the naive listener.

Huxley[12] states:

Sit down before fact like a little child, and be prepared to give up every preconceived notion, following humbly wherever and to whatever abyss nature leads, or you shall learn nothing.

Summary

Knowing is wonderful, but it is just a guiding means. Unknowing is a condition of openness. This unknowing in the intersubjective space of two people or people of two cultures allows others to be. This art of unknowing may enable a nurse to understand, with empathy, the actual essence of the meaning an experience has for a patient. This pattern of unknowing focused herein on the intersubjective whole between patient and nurse is applicable as well to learning in a more formal sense. To be open to learning one needs to posture oneself in a position of unknowing to hear a colleague, a teacher, a student. To provide and find openness is to be able to say, "I never thought about it that way," and at once experience the wonderment of coming upon an "unknown."

REFERENCES
1. Smiley J. Ordinary love and good will. New York: Random House, 1989;120.
2. Beattie A. Picturing Will. New York: Random House, 1989;53.

3. Carper B. Fundamentals patterns of knowing. *Adv Nurs Sci 1978*;vol:13–23.
4. Fawcett J. The metaparadigm of nursing: present status and future refinements. *Image 19;16(3)*:84–7.
5. Atwood D, Stolorow R. Structures of subjectivity. New Jersey: Lawrence Erlbaum Associates, 1984;47–53.
6. Paterson JD, Zderad ZJ. Humanistic nursing. New York: National League for Nursing, 1990.
7. Watson J. Nursing: human science and human care. Norwalk, Connecticut: Appleton-Century-Crofts, 1985.
8. Moccia P. Theory development and nursing practice: a synopsis of a study of the theory-practice diabetic. In: Moccia P,

ed. New approaches to theory development. New York: National League for Nursing, 1986.
9. Benner P, Wrubel J. The primacy of caring stress and coping in health and illness. Menlo Park, California: Addison-Wesley, 1989.
10. Sartre JP. Being and nothingness. New York: Washington Square Press, 1966.
11. Kurtz S. The art of unknowing. New Jersey: Aronson, Inc., 1989;6–7.
12. Huxley JH. Space, time and medicine. Boulder, Colorado: Shambhala, 1982;225.

The Author Comments

'Unknowing': Toward Another Pattern of Knowing in Nursing

I believe I "found" myself in the study of phenomenology and psychoanalysis and in the process of combining these two philosophies in teaching, research, and writing in nursing. I was inspired to write this article by the existence of theories used as generalizations, cultural studies that stereotyped individuals, and statistical inferences and protocols used without human and environmental contextual analysis. This, I believe, has relevance to the use of nursing theory in the 21st century. The article's main theme is that despite our knowledge, we do not know much about our encounters with "other" human beings, unless the "other" shares from his or her subjective world. I have not reread this article lately, but I believe it may have the quote, "Knowledge screens the third ear." I try to live and practice according to the infinite possibilities of human interpretations, so different from my own, and try not have my listening screened by "knowing."

—Patricia Munhall

Patterns of Knowing: Review, Critique, and Update

Jill White

Carper's patterns of knowing in nursing have been consistently cited in the nursing literature since they appeared in 1978. The degree to which they represent nursing knowledge in the mid-1990s is explored, and a major modification is suggested—the addition of a fifth pattern, sociopolitical knowing. The article also suggests modifications to the model for nursing knowledge put forward by Jacobs-Kramer and Chinn to enable this model to be used more effectively as a framework for exploring processes of inquiry into nursing knowledge and practice.

Key words: *empirics, esthetics, ethics, patterns of knowing, personal knowing, sociopolitical*

In 1978 Barbara Carper[1] published "Fundamental Patterns of Knowing in Nursing" in the first edition of *Advances in Nursing Science*. Based on her doctoral work, the article described her typology of patterns of knowing in nursing. These patterns she named empirics, esthetics, ethics, and personal knowing.

Carper's patterns of knowing have been much cited and commented on, albeit somewhat uncritically, in the writing of nurses over the ensuing years. As with much of nursing's written heritage, there is little connection between the number of citations and the extent of critical development that has taken place. An important exception to this, however, was the work of Jacobs-Kramer and Chinn[2] a decade after Carper's article first appeared. Jacobs-Kramer and Chinn extended Carper's framework by producing a model that elucidated their understanding

Advances in Nursing Science *1995:17(4):73–86. Copyright © 1995 Aspen Publishers, Inc.*
An earlier version of this paper was presented at "Shaping Nursing Theory and Practice," Second National Conference of La Trobe University, Department of Nursing, Melbourne, Victoria, Australia, October 1993. Reprinted with permission of Lippincott Williams & Wilkins.

About the Author

JILL WHITE was born in Wagga Wagga, a country town in southeast Australia. She grew up viewing health care, particularly the hospital, as central to the well-being of the community. However, it was also clear that in the 1950s, the power over illness rested firmly with the doctors and, to a lesser extent, with the nurses, with the virtual exclusion of anyone personally significant to the patient. This, even as a junior Red Cross member, made no sense to her. Making sense of how nurses work together with people in health and illness has become her passion. This led her into nursing, nursing education, and the politics of nursing and health care. Her life has been significantly enriched by her husband Richard and two terrific stroppy wonderful teenaged children.

of the creation and development, the expression and transmission, and the assessment of each of Carper's patterns of knowing. Their intention was for such an elucidation to facilitate the integration of these patterns of knowing in nursing into clinical practice.

The lack of recent dialogue about the patterns themselves or about the model may reflect the decreased interest in the use of models generally in nursing, part of a move from reductionist thinking. The continued citation of both Carper and Jacobs-Kramer and Chinn, however, suggests their work is still being used in teaching.

The "patterns" of Carper[1] and "model" of Jacobs-Kramer and Chinn[2] do provide convenient conceptual organizers for introducing students to different ways of knowing in nursing. The patterns and model can be used to facilitate exploration of nursing practice and to enhance understanding of the rich history of modern nursing writing. They enable the contributions of nurses from the past to be analyzed in terms of the dominant social, political, and philosophical contexts of their time and enable nurses to trace with understanding the cumulative and disparate knowledge development that contributes to the discipline of nursing.

Given that the patterns and the model are still being used in education, it is appropriate that they be reviewed and critiqued within the context of nursing knowledge development in the mid-1990s. This article offers such a review, critique, and update.

In her seminal article "Fundamental Patterns of Knowing in Nursing," Carper[1] identified the following patterns:

- empirics, or the science of nursing;
- ethics, or the moral component;
- the component of personal knowledge; and
- esthetics, or the art of nursing.

In this article the author explores each of these patterns in turn, looking first at what Carper had to say, then at the extension of this pattern within the Jacobs-Kramer and Chinn model, and finally at questions that arise with reference to the current literature and each particular pattern. Table 27-1 summarizes the essential elements of Jacobs-Kramer and Chinn's model of nursing knowledge.

Empirics: The Science of Nursing

Carper described empirics as

> knowledge that is systematically organized into general laws and theories for the purpose of describing, explaining and predicting phenomena of special concern to the discipline of nursing.... The first fundamental pattern of knowing in nursing is empirical, factual, descriptive, and ultimately aimed at developing abstract theoretical explanations. It is exemplary, discursively formulated, and publicly verifiable.[1(pp14-15)]

The key element here is that the "ultimate aim" of this knowing is "theory" development. Inherent in theory development is the ontological position that nature has a single or dominant reality commonly experienced and about which one can draw generalizable abstract expla-

Table 27-1
Summary of Essential Elements: Model of Nursing Knowledge

Dimension	Empirics	Ethics	Personal	Esthetics
Creative	Describing Explaining Predicting	Valuing Clarifying Advocating	Encountering Focusing Realizing	Engaging Interpreting Envisioning
Expressive	Facts	Codes	Self: authentic and disclosed	Art-act
	Theories Models	Standards Normative-ethical theories		
	Descriptions to impart under- standing	Descriptions of ethical decision making		
Assessment: critical question	What does this represent? How is this representative?	Is this right? Is this just?	Do I know what I do? Do I do what I know?	What does this mean?
Process-context	Replication	Dialogue	Response and reflection	Criticism
Credibility index	Validity	Justness	Congruity	Consensual meaning

Source: Jacobs-Kramer M. Chinn P. Perspectives on knowing: a model of nursing knowledge. *Schol Inq Nurs Pract.* 1988;2(2):129–139.

nations. This clearly encompasses the traditional view of scientific knowledge with its stance of objectivity and context-free replicability. This view was the dominant one in the nursing research and writing at the time of Carper's doctoral work. However, it is debatable at this time whether this pattern encompasses all research-based knowing, which Jacobs-Kramer and Chinn expressed as "facts, theories, models and descriptions that impart understanding."[2(p132)]

The realist ontological position, whose assumptions allow generalization, may also be seen as including grounded theory and ethnographic research, which generate generalizable abstractions. However, the relativist position of the interpretive paradigm as represented by phenomenology, for example, also seeks to provide "descriptions that impart understanding" but would not be consistent with Carper's definition of having an ultimate aim of developing abstract theoretical explanations that could be "systematically organized into general laws and theories."[1(p14)]

It is therefore suggested that the definition of the empirical pattern of knowing needs to be modified to accommodate the relativist ontological positions of knowledge development using methodologies such as phenomenology. If not modified, nursing needs to acknowledge the limitations of this definition in encompassing empirical knowing that seeks not to generalize, but rather through interpretation or description to put before the reader context-embedded stories whose purpose is to enrich understanding.

The inclusion of the word "understanding" by Jacobs-Kramer and Chinn[2] within the aim of the empirical pattern of knowing may be confusing; "understanding" is more commonly associated with the aim of research within the interpretive paradigm. The ontological position of the interpretive paradigm embraces the notion of multiple realities that cannot be generalized and puts this paradigm outside Carper's definition of this pattern of knowing. As discussed later, interpretive and critical research is encompassed more appropriately elsewhere.

Jacobs-Kramer and Chinn's model suggests that the pattern of empirics is expressed through "facts, theories, models and descriptions."[2](p132) This expressive dimension may be extended to include the common mode of expression and transmission via books for academic theoretical instruction and professional journals for stimulation of professional debate.

Jacobs-Kramer and Chinn's[2] assessment dimension asks the critical questions, "What does this represent?" and "How is it representative?" The process of assessment is by replication, and the index of credibility they suggest is validity—that the knowledge can be demonstrated to be what it is thought to be. The assessment dimension is dealt with in their article in a brief paragraph that makes it somewhat difficult to fully grasp the intent of the critical questions; a critical question, one would assume, inquires about the relationships between the variables under study and the generalizability of the relationships.

In the case of grounded theory, a critical question would be the relationship to the core concepts of the other concepts and the nature of these relationships. The process of judging the trustworthiness of the results would require both sufficient detail to enable replication and application and the seeking out and offering up to professional debate of the findings. As Kuhn said, "There is no standard higher than assent of the relevant community."[3](p94) The remaining process for ascertaining credibility is the "fit" of the new knowledge with the extant knowledge in the area at the time.

It is within this assessment dimension that the case for empirics, not including work using the interpretive or critical paradigm, gains credence. Here, clearly, the standards of credibility are not related to validity, replication, or relationships between variables or categories. If the empirical pattern were to be expanded to accommodate knowledge created through interpretive or critical work, an entirely new assessment would be required with different critical questions, processes, and credibility indices.[4] Possible modifications to the pattern of empirics within the model of nursing knowledge are proposed in Table 27-2.

Table 27-2
Empirics: Essential Elements

Dimension	Original Model[2]	Modifications
Creative	Describing Explaining Predicting	Describing Explaining Predicting
Expressive	Facts Theories Models	Facts Theories and models described in books and professional journals

	Descriptions to impart
	     understanding
		Descriptions that indicate
		     relationships

Assessment: critical question	What does this represent? How is it representative?	What relationships were found? Under what conditions do these relationships hold?
Process-context	Replication	Replication and application Professional debate Fit with extant knowledge
Credibility index	Validity Reliability	Validity Reliability

Ethics: The Moral Component

"The fundamental pattern of knowing identified here as the ethical component of nursing is focused on matters of obligation or what ought to be done."[1(p20)] In exploring this pattern Carper acknowledged the important place of knowledge of norms and ethical codes: "The examination of the standards, codes, and values by which we decide what is morally right should result in a greater awareness of what is involved in making moral choices and being responsible for the choices made."[1(p21)]

However, Carper goes on to caution that the complexity of the ethical issues in modern health care practice means that "moral choices to be made must be considered in terms of specific actions to be taken in specific concrete situations."[1(p21)] In extending this caution, Carper represents one of the earliest nursing writers to speak of the situational and relational importance of moral decision making, which has become fundamental to the ethic of care now so prevalent in the nursing literature.

There has been a plethora of publications in the area of moral knowing. Principal among these are the works of Benner,[5,6] Benner and Wrubel,[7] Bishop and Scudder,[8,9] Cooper,[10,11] and Watson.[12,13] Not directly within nursing but highly relevant are the works of Gilligan,[14,15] Noddings,[16] Pellegrino,[17,18] and Zaner.[19,20]

Much of this work has its origins in Gilligan's[14] critique of Kohlberg's[21] hierarchy of moral decision making. Gilligan challenged Kohlberg's contention that believing in "the primacy and universality of individual rights" was the highest form of moral development and that this represented a morally superior position to Kohlberg's penultimate stage, which embodies a "very strong sense of being responsible to the world."[14(p444)] Gilligan suggested that the focus on individual justice is a predominantly male orientation, whereas women more commonly adopt the contextual, relational, care orientation that focuses on social and moral good.

Moss[22] provided an excellent exploration of the impact of Gilligan's work over the past 15 years, particularly in relation to nursing. Together with Moss, Bishop and Scudder,[9] Benner,[6] and Watson[12,13] suggested that the moral ideal of doing what is good (that is, adopting a caring orientation), rather than that which is just, will most fruitfully be revealed through the exploration of practice rather than simply through reference to "rule-books." This, they suggested, will happen through processes of reflection, discussion, and storytelling of life and nursing practice.[6,9] Bishop and Scudder made a particularly salient point for nurses within this discussion by questioning the notion that moral decision making is about "solving" dilemmas at all: "One way in which the moral sense differs from traditional nursing ethics is that it directs us to moral dilemmas which cannot be solved but must be lived with and, when possible, ameliorated."[9(p124)]

Zaner, with reference to physicians but equally applicable to nursing, suggested "Moral life is essentially communal at its root, and it is mutuality (in all its complex forms), not autonomy, that is foundational. Nowhere is this more plainly evident than in the contexts of clinical situations dealing with ill persons."[20(p292)] Zaner went on to say that "autonomy and rights" inhibit moral decision making within health care, which requires, foundationally, cooperation and collaboration.

Cooperation is also emphasized in the work of Gadow[23] on existential advocacy. She reinforced the importance of collaboratively making "the effort to help persons become clear about what they want to do, by helping them discern their values in the situation and on the basis of that self examination, to reach decisions which express their reaffirmed, perhaps recreated, complex of values."[23(p44)] Gadow put this effort forward as a moral ideal, not duty, norm, or prescription. It is a moral enterprise through situated engagement.

Jacobs-Kramer and Chinn[2] focused on justice in their assessment dimension of this pattern. An expansion of the assessment dimension is required to accommodate an ethic of care as well as an ethic of justice. Thus, potential modifications to the ethical pattern of knowing are listed in Table 27-3.

The discussion about ethics shows how intimately linked the patterns of moral and personal knowing are.

Table 27-3
Ethics: Essential Elements

Dimension	Original Model[2]	Modifications
Creative	Valuing Clarifying Advocating	Valuing the moral idea of caring Critically appraising values Existential advocacy[23] Sensitizing to other value positions Fostering articulation of everyday notions of good[6]
Expressive	Codes, standards Normative theories Descriptions of decision making	Codes, standards Normative theories Observation Storytelling to explore embedded notions of good
Assessment: critical question	Is it right? Is it just?	Is it good? Is it just? Is it right? Does it embody caring?
Process-context	Dialogue	Dialogue Critical reflection Collaborative values elaboration
Credibility index	Justness	Justness Goodness Caring Congruence with personal values of patient

Moral knowing requires fundamentally an authentic interpersonal involvement for its development.

Personal Knowing

The pattern of personal knowing is concerned with "the knowing, encountering and actualizing of the concrete individual self. One does not know *about* self; one strives simply to *know* the self. This knowing is a standing in relation to another human being and confronting that human being as a person."[1(p18)] The pattern of personal knowing develops when the nurse approaches the patient not as an object or category of illness, but strives instead "to actualize an authentic personal relationship between two persons."[1(p19)] This pattern requires the nurse to allow the person who is the patient-client to "matter." It involves engagement as opposed to detachment.

Mayeroff, whom Carper[1] cited as a source for her notion of personal knowing, saw a special feature of caring for a person as being "able to understand [the person] and his world as if I were inside it."[24(p42)] For Mayeroff relationship is about reciprocity, about helping the other "grow" and through this, growing oneself. However, Mayeroff's words harbor subtle paternalism: "I want it to grow in its own right . . . and I feel the other's growth as bound up with my own sense of well-being."[24(p8)] Such a position mitigates against genuine reciprocity.

Mayeroff's reciprocity was elaborated on and refined in the works of Watson[12] in describing her concept of "transcendental moment," by Taylor[25] in her exposition of the "ordinariness" of nursing, in Morse's[26] work on nurse-patient relationships, and in Moch[27] in her exploration of "personal knowing," and probably most well known within nursing is Benner's[5] seminal work *From Novice to Expert*. Benner's notion of involvement and engagement was further developed collaboratively with Tanner[28] on intuition and with Wrubel[7] on the primacy of caring.

The idea of "being-with," of presence, of letting the person matter and being open to help that person make meaning out of his or her experience, is an essential feature of nursing practice. Without this knowing of self that allows an openness to the knowing of another person, nursing is only technical assistance, not involved care. In Carper's words, "It is concerned with the kind of knowing that promotes wholeness and integrity in the personal encounter, the achievement of engagement rather than detachment, and it denies the manipulative, impersonal orientation."[1(p20)]

In the model of nursing knowledge described by Jacobs-Kramer and Chinn,[2] the pattern of personal knowing is seen as being created by "experiencing the self—encountering and focusing on self while realizing the realities and potentialities."[2(p135)] It also involves "experiencing, encountering and focusing."[2(p135)] These are not easy concepts to grasp. Carper herself said of this pattern that it "is the most problematic, the most difficult to master and to teach. At the same time, it is perhaps the pattern most essential to understanding the meaning of health in terms of individual well-being."[1(p18)]

The creation of personal knowing may be enhanced through the use of art, poetry, literature, and storytelling in an endeavor to more truly "understand [the person] and his world as if I were inside it."[24(p42)] An example of this is poetry about childbirth that helps the midwife "see" inside the patient's world; poems such as Sharon Doubiago's "South American Mi Hija" (in Chester[29]) show the intensity that can allow the soul to grow, whereas stories such as Anais Nin's "Birth" (in Chester[29]) illuminate the potential for the soul to shrivel if a woman is not supported by the right kind of caring. Poems such as "Sunshine Across Living Centre" in Krysl and Watson[30] help nurses "see" the humanity of nurse and patient in interaction. The expressive dimension is the self as authentic (privately known) and disclosed (revealed to others): "Personal knowledge is expressed as ourselves, through the self."[2(p135)]

The assessment of this pattern comes through the "focus on the self as privately known and expressed to others. Assessment of self is a process carried out by the self through a rich inner life."[2(p135)] The critical questions involve exploration for congruence between knowing what we do and doing what we know, between the authentic and disclosed self. The process through which this assessment is made is the reflection and response of others to us, which we reflect on in turn. Agan put it succinctly by suggesting that "credibility of this type of knowing is determined through *individual reflection that is informed by the responses of others* [italics added]."[31(p70)] The credibility index is therefore congruence with the authentic and disclosed self.

Although the volume of literature in this area has provided much clarification and extension of the notion of personal knowing, the "essential elements" identified by Jacobs-Kramer and Chinn[2] are still pertinent. An elaboration could include, within the creative dimension, some examples of the means by which "encountering, focusing and realizing" might be facilitated (eg, poetry, art, literature, and storytelling) and within the process-context dimension, reflection informed by the response of others (see Table 27-4).

Esthetics: The Art of Nursing

Carper suggested that the delay in explicating the esthetic pattern of knowing is associated with nursing's attempt to see itself as scientific and to "exorcise the image of the apprentice-type education system."[1(p16)] This delay has certainly been overcome, and there has been intense interest in this pattern recently. The pattern had its beginnings in the works of many early nursing writers. Wiedenbach[32] suggested that esthetic practice is making "visible through action" the nurse's perception of what the patient needs. Orem[33] spoke of the "creativity and style in design" of the provision of care. Orem also mentioned as necessary in artful practice the ability to "envision" models of helping with regard to the appropriate outcomes. Benner[5] was foremost in the development of the notion of perceiving the whole of a situation, without reference to rational processes, in her work on expert nursing practice. The concept of "intuitive" knowing developed by Benner and Tanner,[28] Rew,[34] and Agan[31] (and mentioned earlier as part of

Table 27-4
Empirics: Personal Knowing

Dimension	Original Model[2]	Modifications
Creative	Encountering Focusing Realizing	Encountering, focusing, and realizing through practice and through art, literature, poetry, and storytelling
Expressive	Self: authentic and disclosed	Self: authentic and disclosed
Assessment: critical question	Do I know what I do? Do I do what I know?	Do I know what I do? Do I do what I know?
Process-context	Response and reflection	Reflection informed by the response of others and our reflection on our response to the life-world of other
Credibility index	Congruity	Congruity

personal knowing) is an important component of perceiving and envisioning.

The design of the art-act combines all patterns of knowing in its esthetic form—it is all of and more than the other patterns: "The design, if it is to be esthetic, must be controlled by the perception of balance, rhythm, proportion and unity of what is done in relation to the dynamic integration and articulation of the whole."[1(p18)]

Carper named "empathy" as an important mode in the esthetic pattern of knowing; however, there is currently debate in the nursing literature over the appropriateness of this concept for nursing. Morse, Bottorff, Anderson, O'Brien, and Solberg suggested that "empathy was uncritically adopted from psychology and is actually a poor fit for the clinical reality of nursing practice."[35(p273)] They recommended exploration of other communication strategies that have been devalued, such as sympathy, pity, consolation, compassion, and commiseration. To these Taylor[25] might add affiliation, fun, and friendship.

Whatever the definitional outcome, the basic requirement of effective and authentic interpersonal engagement remains. This is highlighted in the recent Australian work of Taylor[25] and in the innovative work of

Lumby[36] in her development of a critical feminist methodology for exploring nursing.

According to Jacobs-Kramer and Chinn,

Esthetic knowledge finds expression in the art-act of nursing. Like personal knowledge, the expression of esthetic knowledge is not in language. We can unfold our art and retrospectively recollect and write about its features, and we can record it using electronic media, but the knowledge form itself is not what we write or record. The knowledge form *is* the art-act [italics added].[2(p137)]

They then proceeded to raise an important issue, albeit indirectly, that experience is an important component of esthetic knowing:

As practice contexts are encountered, processes within the creative dimension of esthetics are initiated. Through the process of engagement, interpreting, and envisioning, "past" knowledge is enfolded into esthetics, and clients are uniquely cared for. As caring processes continue, new knowledge merges.[2(pp137-138)]

In putting forward experience as a necessary condition to esthetic practice, it may be necessary to include this context-specific experience as part of the creative and generative dimension, suggested by Jacobs-Kramer and Chinn as including "engaging, interpreting and envisioning." The addition of experience, particularly context-specific experience, suggests that these acts are cumulative, aligning with Benner's[5] position that expertise is context specific and not a transferable skill.

In exploring the assessment dimension within Carper's model of knowledge, Jacobs-Kramer and Chinn followed her inclusion of notions of esthetic appreciation from other art forms. They suggested that the critical question is, "What does this mean?"

> Criticism requires empathy and an intent to fully appreciate what the actors meant to convey. As the art-act is criticized, credibility is discerned by reaching for consensus—a full and rich understanding of the art-act that brings together the perspectives of a community of co-askers who construct and confer meanings.[2(p137)]

Table 27-5 presents the essential elements for the esthetic pattern.

The major point of Jacobs-Kramer and Chinn's model development appears to be the unfolding of a story that suggests that each pattern may be seen by "examination of the art-act that integrates all knowledge patterns as expressed in practice . . . [as it] provides a comprehensive, context-sensitive means for enfolding multiple knowledge patterns."[2(p138)] This, they suggested, leads nursing away from "a quest for structural truth and towards a search for dynamic meaning."[2(p138)]

The model and its exposition of essential elements provide critical questions that may structure our process of inquiry, processes by which the inquiry might take place, and credibility indices to which claims of rigor may be addressed. If it is to be useful in the process of our practice-based inquiry, the model must adequately account for all patterns of knowing and their appropriate processes of inquiry.

Sociopolitical Knowing: Context of Nursing

The patterns and inquiry processes in Jacobs-Kramer and Chinn's[2] model appear adequate to the description of the nurse-patient relationship and the persons of the nurse and the patient. What appears to be missing is the context—the sociopolitical environment of the persons and their interaction. This represents a fifth pattern of knowing essential to an understanding of all the others.

The other patterns address the "who," the "how," and the "what" of nursing practice. The pattern of sociopolitical knowing addresses the "wherein." It lifts the gaze of the nurse from the introspective nurse-patient

Table 27-5
Esthetics: Essential Elements

Dimension	Original Model[2]	Modifications
Creative	Engaging Interpreting Envisioning	Cumulative experience by engaging, interpreting and envisioning and including the "artful enfoldment" of all other patterns
Expressive	Art-act	Art-act
Assessment: critical question	What does this mean?	What does this mean?
Process-context	Criticism	Exhibition and criticism Recognition as authentic to other nurses
Credibility index	Consensual meaning	Consensual meaning

relationship and situates it within the broader context in which nursing and health care take place. It causes the nurse to question the taken-for-granted assumptions about practice, the profession, and health policies.

Sociopolitical knowing may be conceptualized as including understandings on two levels: (1) the sociopolitical context of the persons (nurse and patient), and (2) the sociopolitical context of nursing as a practice profession, including both society's understanding of nursing and nursing's understanding of society and its politics.

The sociopolitical context of the persons of the nurse-patient relationship fundamentally concerns cultural identity, for it is in culture that "self" is intrinsically located. This cultural location influences each person's understanding of health and disease causation, language, identity, and connection to the land. Such understanding goes well beyond Carper's[1] or Mayeroff's[24] notion of personal knowing. It is related to deeply embedded historical issues of connection to and dislocation from land and heritage.

Chopoorian suggested that "nursing ideas lack an archaeology of the social, political, and economic worlds that influence both client states and nursing roles."[37(p41)] She claimed that unequal class structure, power relationships, and political and economic power produce sexism, racism, ageism, and classism, which in turn affect health and result in illness. Chopoorian continued, "Nursing practitioners continually confront the human responses to the underlying social dynamics of poverty, unemployment, undernutrition, isolation and alienation precipitated through the structures of society."[37(pp40-41)]

Violence, drug dependence, and diabetes are examples of responses to what are inherently political rather than simply personal problems, and nurses' efforts to deal with them require nurses to articulate what they see resulting from societies' structures. Stevens suggested that nurses must provide a "critique of domination within fundamental social, political and economic structures and the analysis of how domination affects the health of persons and communities."[38(p58)] This effect includes the position and visibility of nursing

in policy planning and decision making about health issues.

To have a voice in these decisions, nurses must both be articulate about what they know and do and be recognized by others as having something to contribute to debate. Nurses must have an understanding of the gatekeeping mechanisms within the political arena and their function. It is a paradox that when people are involved with nurses and nursing as patients or as concerned friends, the contribution of nurses is prized. Why then is it so quickly forgotten when these same people are influencing health care decisions? Diers and Fagin[39] suggested that the reason is visible in the metaphors the public associates with nursing, which include nurturance, dependence, and intimacy. These images are often reminders of personal pain and vulnerability, the natural reaction to which is suppression. To resurface an understanding of nursing is to resurface the context and all that is associated with it. Nurses must find a way of helping people remember, when they are well and politically able, what they knew of nursing when in crisis. Nurses must find the intersections between the health-related interests of the public and nursing and must become involved and active participants in these interests.

A sociopolitical understanding in which to frame all other patterns of knowing is an essential part of

Table 27–6
Sociopolitical Knowing: Essential Elements

Dimension	Characteristics
Creative	Exposing and exploring alternate constructions of reality
Expressive	Transformation Critique
Assessment: critical question	Whose voice is heard? Whose voice is silenced?
Process-context	Critique and hearing all voices
Credibility index	Shared governance, enlightenment Movement toward equity

nursing's future in an increasingly economically driven world. Nurses must explore and expose alternative constructions of health and health care, find means of enabling all concerned to have a voice in this care provision, and develop processes of shared governance for the future. Table 27-6 illustrates how the sociopolitical dimension might be added to the model of knowing.

As Chinn said of nursing in the next century, "it is time to construct critical analyses of our present that are informed by the ethical and political ideals that we seek. It is time to begin to envision what our future nursing might be like and to create knowledge and skills that we need to begin to make it happen."[40(p56)] Understanding the context of nursing practice is fundamental to this endeavor. Appreciation and exploration of all the patterns of knowing in nursing and their interactions can contribute to the future articulation and development of nursing practice and nurses' place in determining the future of nursing practice and of health care.

REFERENCES

1. Carper B. Fundamental patterns of knowing in nursing. *ANS.* 1978;1(1):13–23. Reprinted with permission from Aspen Publishers, Inc. (c) Copyright 1978.
2. Jacobs-Kramer M, Chinn P. Perspectives on knowing: a model of nursing knowledge. *Schol Inq Nurs Pract.* 1988;2(2):129–139. Used by permission of Springer Publishing Company, Inc., New York 10012.
3. Kuhn T. *The Structure of Scientific Revolutions.* Chicago, Ill: University of Chicago Press; 1970.
4. Sandelowski M. Rigor or rigor mortis: the problem of rigor in qualitative research revisited. *ANS.* 1993;16(2):1–8.
5. Benner P. *From Novice to Expert: Excellence and Power in Clinical Nursing Practice.* Menlo Park, Calif: Addison-Wesley; 1984.
6. Benner P. The role of experience, narrative, and community in skilled ethical comportment. *ANS.* 1991;14(2):1–21.
7. Benner P, Wrubel J. *The Primacy of Caring: Stress and Coping in Health and Illness.* Menlo Park, Calif: Addison-Wesley; 1989.
8. Bishop A, Scudder J, eds. *Caring, Curing, Coping.* University, Ala: University of Alabama Press; 1985.
9. Bishop A, Scudder J. *The Practical, Moral and Personal Sense of Nursing.* Albany, NY: State University of New York Press; 1990.
10. Cooper M. Reconceptualizing nursing ethics. *Schol Inq Nurs Pract.* 1990;4(3):209–218.
11. Cooper M. Principle-oriented ethics and the ethic of care: creative tension. *ANS.* 1991;14(2):22–31.
12. Watson J. *Nursing: Human Science and Human Care.* Norwalk, Conn: Appleton-Century-Crofts; 1985.
13. Watson J. The moral failure of the patriarchy. *Nurs Outlook.* 1990;28(2):62–66.
14. Gilligan C. In a different voice: women's conception of self and morality. *Harvard Educ Rev.* 1979;47:481–517.
15. Gilligan C. *In a Different Voice.* Cambridge, Mass: Harvard University Press; 1982.
16. Noddings N. *Caring—A Feminine Approach to Ethics and Moral Education.* Berkeley, Calif: University of California Press; 1984.
17. Pellegrino E. Being ill and being healed. In: Kestenbaum V, ed. *The Humanity of the Ill.* Knoxville, Tenn: University of Tennessee Press; 1982.
18. Pellegrino E. The caring ethic. In: Bishop A, Scudder J, eds. *Caring, Curing, Coping.* University, Ala: University of Alabama Press; 1985.
19. Zaner R. How the hell did I get here? In: Bishop A, Scudder J, eds. *Caring, Curing, Coping.* University, Ala: University of Alabama Press; 1985.
20. Zaner R. *Ethics and the Clinical Encounter.* Englewood Cliffs, NJ: Prentice Hall; 1988.
21. Kohlberg L. *The Philosophy of Moral Development.* San Francisco, Calif: Harper & Row; 1981.
22. Moss C. Has Gilligan's "Different Voice" made a difference? In: *Nursing Research: Scholarship for Practice.* Geelong, Victoria, Australia: Deakin Institute of Nursing Research, Deakin University; 1992.
23. Gadow S. Existential advocacy: philosophical foundation of nursing. In: Spicker S, Gadow S, eds. *Nursing: Images and Ideals: Opening Dialogue with the Humanities.* New York, NY: Springer; 1980.
24. Mayeroff M. *On Caring.* New York, NY: Harper & Row; 1971.
25. Taylor B. Enhancement of the nursing encounter through a shared humanity. In: *Nursing Research: Scholarship for Practice.* Geelong, Victoria, Australia: Deakin Institute of Nursing Research, Deakin University; 1992.
26. Morse J. Negotiating commitment and involvement in the nurse-patient relationship. *J Adv Nurs.* 1991;16:455–468.
27. Moch S. Personal knowing: Evolving research and practice. *Schol Inq Nurs Pract.* 1990;4(2):155–165.
28. Benner P, Tanner C. Clinical judgment: how expert nurses use intuition. *Am J Nurs.* 1987;87:23–31.
29. Chester L, ed. *Cradle and All.* Boston, Mass: Faber & Faber; 1989.
30. Krysl M, Watson J. Existential moments of caring: facets of nursing and social support. *ANS.* 1988;10(2):12–17.
31. Agan RD. Intuitive knowing as a dimension of nursing. *ANS.* 1987;10(1):64–70.
32. Wiedenbach E. *Clinical Nursing: A Helping Out.* New York, NY: Springer-Verlag; 1985.
33. Orem D. *Nursing: Concepts of Practice.* New York, NY: McGraw-Hill; 1971.

34. Rew L. Intuition and decision-making. *IMAGE J Nurs Schol.* 1988;20(3):150–154.
35. Morse J, Bottorff J, Anderson G, O'Brien B, Solberg S. Beyond empathy: expanding expressions of caring. *Adv Nurs.* 1992;17:809–821.
36. Lumby J. *A Woman's Experience of Illness: The Emergence of a Feminist Method for Nursing.* Geelong, Victoria, Australia: Deakin University; 1993.
37. Chopoorian T. Reconceptualizing the environment. In: Moc-

cia P, ed. *New Approaches in Theory Development.* New York, NY: National League for Nursing; 1986.
38. Stevens P. A critical social reconstruction of environment in nursing: implications for methodology. *ANS.* 1989;11(4): 56–68.
39. Diers D, Fagin C. Nursing as a metaphor. *N Engl J Med.* 1981;309(2):116–117.
40. Chinn P. Looking into the crystal ball: positioning ourselves for the year 2000. *Nurs Outlook.* 1991;39(6):251–256.

The Author Comments

Patterns of Knowing: Review, Critique, and Update

Having been a teacher of nursing theory at a graduate level for some time, I used Carper's work as a conceptual framework for structuring an understanding of research and theory in nursing. However, I became progressively uncomfortable with what I perceived as an absence of "place" for understanding indigenous health practices and other sociopolitical health-related issues. Nursing's apparent invisibility and lack of power within health care was also missing. After class one day over coffee, I "doodled" on a napkin, and those doodles became the bones of this article. Although written some time ago, I believe sociopolitical issues in health care are now of even greater relevance in a world dominated by uncritical globalization, juxtaposed with significant indigenous health issues, disparity of access to health care and education, and religious and cultural intolerance.

—Jill White

From Carper's Patterns of Knowing to Ways of Being: An Ontological Philosophical Shift in Nursing

Mary C. Silva
Jeanne M. Sorrell
Christine D. Sorrell*

Carper's 1978 article in the premiere issue of Advances in Nursing Science *encouraged nurses to consider four fundamental patterns of knowing. Through illustrations from literature and the performing arts, the authors address Carper's patterns of knowing in the context of an emerging philosophical shift. First, they critique the major strengths and limitations of the article. Next, they explore an emerging philosophical shift in nursing from Carper's epistemological focus to ontological reflections on ways of being. Finally, they discuss the significance of the emerging philosophical shift and the ways of being for the science-art of nursing.*

Key words: *Carper, philosophy, epistemology, ontology, ways of knowing and being*

I know noble accents
And lucid, inescapable rhythms;
But I know, too,
That the blackbird is involved
In what I know . . .
When the blackbird flew out of sight,
It marked the edge
Of one of many circles.[1(p21)]

In the autumn of 1978 a new nursing journal devoted to intellectual diversity and creativity made its debut onto the nursing landscape. In volume 1, issue 1 of the journal, an article appeared that changed the way nurses know their world. The journal was *Advances in Nursing Science;* the article was Barbara Carper's "Fundamental patterns of knowing in nursing."[2] Despite the impact of Carper's article from then to now, it rarely has

*Now Christine Sorrell Dinkins

Advances in Nursing Science 1995;18(1):1–13

About the Authors

MARY CIPRIANO SILVA was born and raised in the small town of Ravenna, OH. She earned a BSN and an MS from Ohio State University and a PhD from the University of Maryland. She also undertook post-doctoral study at Georgetown University in health care ethics. The focus of her scholarship and key contributions to nursing has been in philosophy, metatheory, and health care ethics. She is a Professor and Director, Office of Healthcare Ethics, Center for Health Policy, Research, and Ethics, at George Mason University, Fairfax, VA. When not working, she attends foreign films, the Shakespeare Theatre, and fine and performing arts events.

JEANNE MERKLE SORRELL was born in Marshall, MI. She earned a BSN from the University of Michigan, an MSN from the University of Wisconsin, and a PhD from George Mason University. Her scholarly interests focus on philosophic inquiry, writing across the curriculum, qualitative research, and ethical considerations for patients with chronic illness. She has authored and edited numerous manuscripts for publication, including a children's book, *The Magic Stethoscope*, which integrates a fantasy theme to engage children in ways to learn about nursing. Dr. Sorrell is currently Professor and Associate Dean, Academic Programs and Research, College of Nursing and Health Science at George Mason University.

CHRISTINE SORRELL DINKINS was born in Madison, WI. She attended high school at the North Carolina School of the Arts, where she studied music composition, and she continues to compose music today. She earned a BA with honors in philosophy at Wake Forest University, and she holds a PhD in Philosophy from Johns Hopkins University. Dr. Dinkins' primary interests are the philosophic methods of Plato and Heidegger. In her scholarship within health sciences, she is exploring the possibilities of these two methods in hermeneutic research. Dr. Dinkins is Assistant Professor of Philosophy at Wofford College.

been critiqued or examined in light of philosophical shifts in nursing. Therefore, this article

- critiques the major strengths and limitations of the Carper article;
- explores an emerging philosophical shift in nursing from Carper's epistemological focus on patterns of knowing to ontological reflections on ways of being; and
- discusses the significance of the emerging philosophical shift and ways of being for the science-art of nursing.

Critique of the Carper Article

Strengths

In 1978, when Carper's[2] article appeared in *Advances in Nursing Science,* the vast majority of nursing knowledge generated was empiric. Nurses knew well how to objectify and reduce knowledge, how to control for extraneous variables, and how to cast off outliers. What they did not know well were the philosophical underpinnings of their science. Nor did nurses know well that they could come to know in different ways. Carper's article encouraged nurses to view nursing knowledge from three fundamental patterns of knowing beyond empirics: esthetics, personal knowledge, and ethics. Thus, the broadening of the knowing patterns liberated many nurses, allowing them to value and reclaim their lost or dormant creativity. Herein lies one of Carper's greatest contributions.

Another contribution is Carper's insight into how the fundamental patterns of knowing advance nursing knowledge. She understood that philosophical discussions about nursing are not mere intellectual niceties, but are important to how the discipline of nursing should be structured. According to Carper, "there is a need to examine the kinds of knowing that provide the discipline with its particular perspectives and significance. Understanding four fundamental patterns of knowing makes possible an increased awareness of the complexity and diversity of nursing knowledge."[2(p21)] Therefore, for Carper, each pattern of knowing in nursing is necessary for mastery of the discipline, yet each pattern cannot stand alone. The hallowed research principle of mutually exclusive categories fails Carper's vision of the connectedness of the patterns: "The teaching and learning of one pattern do not require the rejection or neglect of any of the others."[2(p22)] Yet each pattern must be understood, attended to, and used wisely so there is a congruence between the pattern and its epistemological goals. Carper stated that she does not view the four patterns of knowing as static, but rather ever emerging. Possibilities exist. Thus, Carper has helped nurses understand that how they come to know is complex, diverse, ever emerging, and ultimately central to how nurses structure the discipline of nursing.

Limitations

Despite the many strengths of the Carper[2] article, there are some limitations. First, there is an incongruency between the wording of the title and the wording of the patterns of knowing. The title "Fundamental patterns of knowing in nursing" suggests a process—how one comes to know—yet the patterns are depicted as four end products: empirics, esthetics, personal knowledge, and ethics. Although the article has an epistemological foundation, the following epistemological question has not been adequately addressed: How does one come to know the knowledge that is empiric, esthetic, personal, or ethical?

A second limitation of Carper's article is that although she clearly stated that the patterns of knowing interact with one another, she presented each pattern as a discrete entity. By so doing, she created a false and clearly unintended illusion that the patterns are mutually exclusive. This unintended illusion is unfortunate because the majority of citations to the Carper article since its publication identify the patterns of knowing as discrete entities.[3-8] Furthermore, Carper also made the point that the patterns of

knowing are not exhaustive; hence, her label "fundamental" patterns of knowing seems appropriate. However, most authors' citations to Carper's work treat the patterns of knowing as if these were exhaustive. So, somehow in Carper's writing of her article and in its interpretation by the majority of authors citing her work, the intended richness of her work has been lost.

Because of this loss of richness, due primarily we believe to Carper's discrete and finite presentation of the patterns of knowing, two-dimensional visions tend to emerge rather than multidimensional ones. As a result of this third limitation, we coined two terms: "the in-between" and "the beyond." By *the in-between* we mean what exists or reveals itself through nonlinear, meditative thinking that moves in all directions and depths. By *the beyond* we mean those aspects of reality, meaning, and being that persons only come to know with difficulty or that they cannot articulate or ever know. Because they are difficult to know, inexplicable, or unknowable (concepts we will return to later), they are puzzling or mysterious. Although Carper's article was clearly intended to have an epistemological focus, aspects of ontology surface (eg, "a state of being"[2(p18)]). By making explicit the implicit ontological threads, Carper could have identified the ontological in-betweens and beyonds in her article without sacrificing her epistemological focus.

Nursing's Emerging Philosophical Shift from Epistemology to Ontology

Since the surge of interest in modern nursing theory in the 1960s and in modern nursing metatheory in the late 1970s and early 1980s, the dominant philosophical thrust has been epistemological. Questions related to kinds, structure, scope, trustworthiness, and justification of knowledge[9,10] were those epistemological questions most often raised by nurse scholars. These nurse scholars' philosophical contributions to the theoretical bases of nursing and nursing practice should not be underestimated. They helped nurses to seek and find an (not "its") identity. These separate identities converged into a variety of patterns that moved nursing largely away from medical and other theoretical perspectives to nursing perspectives, with all their richness and diversity.[11,12]

However, profound changes in society, such as a shift from the knowledge age to the information age, with the emphasis on cyberspace and virtual reality,[13] are altering nurses' perceptions of possible realities. As the world has become increasingly complex, nurses have begun to raise ontological questions regarding the nature and meaning of their own and their clients' realities and beings.[14,15] This questioning differs from the epistemological questioning of the structure and trustworthiness of knowledge. Yet, as reflected by scarcity in the nursing literature, nurses rarely have conceptualized this shift as a philosophical expansion from epistemology to ontology.[16]

This seeming lack of insight has resulted in some philosophical dissonance within nursing theory and research. To place this dissonance within the framework of Carper's[2] article, we reemphasize this: Carper identified the four patterns of knowing as fundamental to the discipline of nursing; however, the patterns have been used to address all types of knowing (epistemological focus) and being (ontological focus) in nursing. Thus, ontological questions have gotten mixed in with epistemological ones. In and of itself, this is not the issue. The issue is that often nurses do not recognize this dissonance and, even when appropriate, do not move beyond epistemological questions to ontological questions that address issues of reality, meaning, and being. Table 28-1 reflects examples of both epistemological and ontological questions based on patterns of knowing identified by Carper; it also expands the questioning to include the concepts of the inexplicable and the unknowable.

In sum, the epistemological focus that characterized the four patterns of knowing described by Carper has begun shifting to an ontological focus. To encourage the reader to see the in-between and the beyond that too often lie concealed in scientific writing, we have used literary and performing arts examples to illustrate the relationship of each of the patterns of knowing to evolving ontological reflections for nursing.

Reflections on Empiric Knowing and Empiric Meaning

An epistemological question related to empirics is, How do I come to know the knowable? (See Table 28-1.) Although Carper[2] focused more on the end products of knowing than on the process of how one comes to know, she did indicate the important role that creative imagination plays in the "syntax of discovery in science."[2(p22)] An illustration of how people come to inform their empiric knowledge with what lies beyond and, consequently, how they find meaning in what they know is presented in Plato's *Republic*.[17] Plato offered the cave allegory as an illustration of stages of knowing that represent different ways of perceiving and relating to one's world. This allegory illustrates the interrelationships between epistemological and ontological awareness. The lower stages serve not only as illustrations of steps on the way to knowledge of the beyond, but also as important components in an ontological understanding of the empiric world as a whole and one's relation to it.

In the allegory the prisoners in the cave see only shadows of real objects, cast on the wall by firelight. Because this is all they can see, they assume that the shadows are real and that the fire is the ultimate source of light. When one prisoner is released, he ascends to the world outside. At first, the brightness of the sun overwhelms him, so he must look down at the ground, where he sees reflections of objects on the surface of the lake and takes those reflections to be real. Eventually, he is able to raise his head, and he finds out at last what is truly real: He sees the objects themselves, and eventually he sees the sun. He then comes to understand that it is the sun that is the ultimate source of light, that which both illuminates all other things and nurtures and allows them to be.

Plato conceptualized a beyond that encompasses the true nature of objects. The realm of meaning of this beyond cannot be understood through an everyday way of relating to things: Understanding comes only through extraordinary effort. In the cave allegory the shadows in the cave and the reflections in the pool represent the facets of the beyond that appear to one in everyday objects. To understand the true nature of things and their relations to each other, to see the sun and know that it nurtures all things, is to see past misleading and limited perceptions of mere objects and to gain access to the world of the in-between and the beyond. Nurses, too, have opportunities to glimpse reflections of the in-between and the beyond in everyday situations, but the meanings inherent in these reflections may be obscured by the "everydayness" that screens our perceptions.

Thus the epistemological question evolves into an ontological question: How do I find meaning in what I know? Plato believed that people cannot understand the world around them without understanding what it is that they know and, more importantly, without understanding how the things they know are interrelated. He would therefore deem it essential, if persons are to distinguish different aspects of knowing, that they understand how these aspects relate to each other. By so doing, they can see the realities in their world and understand their interactions with that world through this interrelatedness between multiple ways of knowing and multiple realms of knowable things.

In Plato's story, when the released prisoner descends back into the cave, his eyes are no longer accustomed to the dark, and he finds he can no longer see things the way his fellow prisoners do. Plato emphasized the importance of not losing sight of early approaches to the knowable so that people can recognize how they are perceiving at any given time. As Carper noted, "there is a critical need for knowledge about the empirical world."[2(p14)] One must not dismiss traditional ways of empiric knowing in nursing, but rather recognize that hidden in the in-between and the beyond of the traditional view of empiric knowledge (science) are other ways of knowing and finding meaning.

Reflections on Esthetic Knowing and Esthetic Being

Carper,[2] in describing esthetics as it relates to the art of nursing, emphasized the importance of form, balance,

rhythm, proportion, and unity as they relate to a whole. Although she did not explicitly state an epistemological question related to esthetic knowing, her characterization of this pattern of knowing in nursing implied, How do I come to know the artistry? (See Table 1.) Thus she contrasted esthetics (art) and empirics (science). Philosophy, however, leads us to view esthetics in an ontological sense, that is, as an important facet of being. Kant[18] characterized esthetics in terms of perceived sensibilities, returning to an earlier definition that emphasized the role of the senses in esthetics. For Kant, it is through delicate, soul-sensitive feelings that we experience the beautiful and the sublime. Santayana,[19] in the title of his book *The Sense of Beauty*, illustrated, too, that the transformative power of art, in all its realities, is through our senses. Within this conception of esthetics, the following ontological question can be stated: What does my perceptual sensibility to art reveal to me?

Carper may have been alluding to the importance of perceptual sensibilities in her focus on the relation of empathy to esthetics when she stated that one gains knowledge of an individual's singular, particular, felt experience through empathic acquaintance. She stated that the nurse who gains expertise in empathizing with others becomes more expert in understanding alternate modes of perceiving reality, thus implying that multiple realities are revealed to us through our perceptual sensibilities.

This ontological question related to esthetics, with its implication that we come to know and to find meaning through our sensibility to art and beauty, suggests the need to look for the in-between and the beyond aspects of esthetic knowing. As the prisoner in Plato's allegory came to know what lay beyond the empiric world and through that knowledge to make meaning through his senses, so can the perceptual sensibilities of esthetic knowing help us find new meanings in everyday experiences and objects. For example, esthetic knowing is illustrated in Heidegger's essay "The origin of the work of art,"[20] in which he describes Van Gogh's painting of an old, worn-out pair of shoes: "But what is there to see here? Everyone knows what shoes consist of."[20(p158)] Heidegger then tells us what there is to see:

As long as we only imagine a pair of shoes in general, or simply look at the empty, unused shoes as they merely stand there in the picture, we shall never discover what the equipmental being of the equipment in truth is . . . .There is nothing surrounding this pair of peasant shoes in or to which they might belong—only an undefined space . . . . And yet. From the dark opening of the worn insides of the shoes the toilsome tread of the worker stares forth . . . .In the shoes vibrates the silent call of the earth.[20(p159)]

Heidegger helps us see that scientific analysis would not lead us to grasp the realization of Van Gogh's work. To create is to bring to light, and creating an authentic work of art will give to being a dwelling not found anywhere else.[20] Only through the in-between and the beyond that the artist has captured in the canvas does the pair of shoes achieve a total, autonomous being. Far beyond any pair of "real" shoes that we encounter, Van Gogh's painting communicates to us the beauty that constitutes the "truth of being" of these simple objects.

When science is seen as separate and perhaps more useful than art, there is increased emphasis on the need for a useful purpose of a being. Carper noted the "sense of urgency"[2(p14)] to develop a body of empiric knowledge specific to nursing, and it is perhaps due to this sense of urgency on the part of nurse scholars, as well as a prejudice against the subjective, that esthetic knowing received little attention in nursing for many years.[21] We propose that esthetics is a significant facet of the ontology of nursing. As with the shoes in Van Gogh's painting, the worn insides of the nurse's shoes—shoes that have carried nurses to exciting new directions through the years—reveal an undefined space in which "the toilsome tread of the worker stares forth."[20(p159)] Nurses' perceptual sensibilities, awakened through such esthetic forms as paintings and sculpture,[22] photography,[23] and writing,[24] help them access the in-betweens and the beyonds that shape the ontology of nursing. Thus, esthetic knowing refers not only to illuminating the art of nursing, as described by Carper, but to how the art of nursing and the openness to perceptual sensibilities can give meaning to the reality of knowing and being.

Reflections on Personal Knowing and Personal Being

Carper[2] stated that personal knowledge as a fundamental pattern of knowing in nursing is the pattern most essential to understanding the meaning of health in terms of individual well-being. In her description of this pattern of knowing, Carper appeared to move closer to ontological concerns than she did in her description of the other three patterns. Whereas the epistemological question implied by this pattern of knowing might be, How do I come to know who I am? Carper emphasized that the focus is not to know "*about* the self," but to "*know* the self."[2(p18)] Thus, her characterization of this pattern of knowing moves close to the ontological question stated simply as, Who am I? (See Table 28-1.)

Yet, for this pattern, too, Carper's characterization of personal knowing remains separate from the other patterns, so that the in-betweens and the beyonds are lost. Perhaps this reflects on why she sees it as the most problematic and the most difficult to master. Can one really know oneself without the in-betweens and the beyonds that come from the overlaps of personal knowing with other patterns of knowing? In fact, Polanyi's description of the "passionate participation in the act of knowing"[25(p19)] that Carper attributed to personal knowing appears to be inextricably related to both esthetic and personal ways of being.

Personal ways of being are reflected in Merleau-Ponty's description of the experiential knowing that evolves out of the individual's perception of the world: "All knowledge takes its place within the horizons opened up by perception."[26(p207)] Each perception is a reflection of a particular hold on reality that is continually remade by time and always in process. The phenomenologist Husserl noted that to make meaning from these continually changing reflections, we need to return to "the things themselves."[27(p17)] Husserl even provided training in "phenomenological seeing"; his conception of phenomenology meant that the foundations

Table 28-1
Epistemological and Ontological Questions Related to
Patterns of Knowing and Ways of Being

Concept	Epistemology	Ontology
Carper's concepts		
Empirical	How do I come to know the knowable?	How do I find meaning in what I know?
Esthetic	How do I come to know the artistry?	What does my perceptual sensibility to art reveal to me?
Personal knowledge	How do I come to know who I am?	Who am I?
Ethical	How do I come to know what I morally ought to do?	Who ought I to be morally?
New concepts		
Inexplicable	How do I come to know the inexplicable?	What meaning does the inexplicable have for me?
Unknowable	How do I come to know the unknowable?	What meaning does the unknowable have for me?

of human experience can be glimpsed by "seeing beyond" everyday experiences to arrive at new understandings of experience.[27(p17)] Thus, phenomenologic seeing can help us to envision the in-betweens and the beyonds that constitute ontological meaning.

This ontological focus is illustrated by the character Jean Valjean in the musical production of Victor Hugo's *Les Misérables*.[28] Through the creative blending of words and music by Alain Boubil and Claude-Michel Schonberg, we sense the agony of the questioning that comes to Valjean in trying to know himself:

If I speak, I am condemned
If I stay silent, I am damned!
Who am I?
Can I condemn this man to slavery?
Pretend I do not see his agony?
This innocent who bears my face
Who goes to judgment in my place.
Who am I?
Can I conceal myself for evermore?
Pretend I'm not the man I was before?
And must my name until I die
Be no more than an alibi?
Must I lie?
How can I ever face my fellow men?

How can I ever face myself again? . . .
Who am I? Who am I?
I am Jean Valjean! . . .
Who am I?
24601![28(p171)]

The drama of *Les Misérables* revolves around Jean Valjean's struggle to know himself, to somehow blend his identity as the prisoner 24601, jailed for stealing a loaf of bread, with his identity as a courageous and virtuous citizen and defender of the victims of society. As we watch and listen to a production of *Les Misérables*, we are transported in between and far beyond the words and notes on a page to arrive at a realization of being of this character that can only be understood through the blending of all of Carper's patterns of knowing.

Nurses have begun returning to "the things themselves." Benner and other researchers[29-31] have implemented important research focused around ontological concerns for nursing. These researchers have helped nursing regain an appreciation for the narrative as a way of understanding ways of being that constitute meaning for nurses. As client, nurse, student, and others tell their personal, unique stories of the "everydayness" of that person's existence, we see the many facets of personal meaning and multiple realities embodied in their narratives, and we glimpse the multiple realities that can come from personal knowing.

Reflections on Ethical Knowing and Ethical Being

Because of the epistemological basis of Carper's[2] article, she correctly addressed the question in Table 28-1, How do I come to know what I morally ought to do? This coming to know ethically was well expressed by Carper: "The fundamental pattern of knowing identified here as the ethical component of nursing is focused on matters of obligation or what ought to be done."[2(p20)] Although this tenet remained her primary focus, she also noted that ethics goes beyond obligation to encompass the judging of moral values related to motives, intentions, and character traits. Thus, Carper presented a complex picture of ethical knowing, reflecting the multidimensional components of ethics. Within that multidimensionality resides a component of ethics—virtue theory as manifested by character traits—that has ontological import. In nursing, the concept of virtue was noted by Liaschenko,[32] and virtue traits such as empathy and compassion were noted by Olsen[33] and by Gaul,[34] respectively.

When in ethics scholars refer to character traits, they address the ontological question, Who ought I to be morally? What one morally ought to be (ontological focus) is substantially different from the knowledge needed to determine the moral validity of what one ought to do (epistemological focus). Aristotle,[35] in *The Nicomachean Ethics,* discussed virtue and virtuous acts. He stated that virtues "must be the expression of a firm and stable character."[35(p187)] Thus, virtues are dispositions to moral "being."

Aristotle also dealt with the concept of motive; that is, a person must be properly motivated for an action to be virtuous:

> Hence we are correct in asserting that a man becomes just by doing just acts and temperate by doing temperate acts, and that without doing them he has no prospect of ever becoming good. But

most men, instead of following this advice, take refuge in theories, and suppose that by philosophizing they will be improved—like a sick man who listens attentively to his physician but disobeys his orders. Bare philosophizing will no more produce health in the soul than a course in medical theory will produce health in the body.[35(pp187-188)]

Thus, Aristotle drew a clear distinction between "knowing that" (an epistemological focus that characterizes the Carper article) and "being that" (an ontological focus related to a disposition to be moral). In short, Aristotle argued that all moral knowing and knowledge is for naught if a person does not behave virtuously.

What then? Often pangs of a lapsed conscience follow. Conscience requires self-reflection and judgment on the morality of one's acts: "It is an internal sanction calling attention to the actual or potential loss of a sense of integrity and wholeness in the self."[36(p476)] It leads one to the in-between and the beyond where people must come to know with difficulty why they violated their conscience, if and how they can articulate this to others, and what the ultimate price or punishment will be. Although Carper did not address conscience in her article, she stressed the importance of nurses making moral choices and alluded to the moral distress that may follow if they are in conflict about their choices.

Note the conflict and anguish of Lady Macbeth as she recalls the night she and her husband plotted to kill King Duncan:

Doctor: What is it she does now? Look at how she rubs her hands.

Gentlewoman: It is an accustomed action with her, to seem thus washing her hands. I have known her continue in this a quarter of an hour.

Lady Macbeth: Yet here's a spot.

Doctor: Hark, she speaks! I will set down what comes from her, to satisfy my remembrance the more strongly

Lady Macbeth: Out, damned spot! out, I say! One; two. Why then 'tis time to do't. Hell is murky. Fie, my lord, fie! a soldier, and afeard? What need we fear who knows it, when none can call our pow'r to accompt? Yet who would have thought the old man to have had so much blood in him?[37(p78)]

Lady Macbeth, in her struggle to determine "Who ought I to be morally?" incriminates herself. All the epistemological "knowing that" about King Duncan and his death fail the ontological facets of moral "being." The psychologic demons cannot be exorcised. Integrity and wholeness are lost; madness ensues.

Reflections on the Inexplicable and the Unknowable

As Table 28-1 shows, Carper[2] did not choose to emphasize the inexplicable and the unknowable, although in her article she embraced an openness to new conceptual structures. We note the two concepts here because nurses frequently deal with them in their work with clients and because these concepts relate strongly to the in-between and the beyond. From an epistemological viewpoint, the question nurses might ask is, How do I come to know the inexplicable and the unknowable? The question takes on a different slant when raised from an ontological perspective: What meaning do the inexplicable and unknowable have for me? Both questions are useful in trying to understand and give meaning to the two concepts.

An example from the world of dance helps elucidate the inexplicable and the unknowable. The particular dance is Martha Graham's *Lamentation*—one of the most powerful and haunting dances ever performed. Its subject was the bearing of unbearable grief. Gardner tried to make explicable the inexplicable grief through his interpretation of this dance:

A solitary, grieving woman was encased in a tube of stretch jersey, with only hands, feet, and face visible. Seated on a low platform throughout, the mummylike figure rocked with anguish from side to side, plunging her hand deep into the dark fabric. Barely perceptible, the body writhed as if attempting to break out of its habit. As the body moved, the tube formed diagonals across the center of the body. The movements, created through the changing forms of the costume, were prayerful and beseeching, not so much a re-creation of grief as its embodiment.[38(pp272-273)]

The power of this inexplicable grief is captured in a poignant story that Martha Graham shared with Agnes de Mille.[39] A mother saw her child hit and killed by a car. For months she could not grieve; she was beyond tears. However, after seeing Martha Graham's performance of *Lamentation,* she relinquished her restraint and wept bitterly. Searing grief such as this occurs both in nursing and in life. It is a lived experience profoundly felt by its bearer but often inexplicable and, to those who have never experienced it, unknowable.

One can experience a facet of the knowable that is inexplicable as this mother did. Such an experience goes beyond our ability to directly understand it or describe it, yet it is so vivid and powerful that one cannot help but know it. The knowable does not hide between our normal areas of awareness as the unknowable does, but presents itself clearly to the one who experiences it. Its indescribability may even lie partially in the fact that such an experience encompasses all levels of awareness. Even though the one who experiences it lacks words to describe it, the all-encompassing nature of the experience allows it to be knowable. For the one who experiences it, the knowable yet inexplicable may have a meaning that is far more significant than the meaning of any explainable experience, not only because of its effect on awareness, but also because of its uniqueness. The fact that it cannot be effectively shared with others through words causes the experience to be inherently different from all other experiences. The inexplicable experience then becomes one's own.

Heidegger, in *On the Way to Language,* cited Stefan George's poem of which the last line is, "Where word breaks off no thing may be."[40(p140)] Heidegger maintained that whatever people cannot explain to others, whatever they cannot name or find words to describe, cannot give rise to thought. Whenever people try to grab on to a perception or idea that they see only as a reflection in a pool, lurking in the shadows away from the mind's well-lit pathways, that perception slips into the in-between or the beyond, and people may not be able to hold on to it long enough to come to know it and make it explicable. To Heidegger, the word itself gives—it gives being.[40]

Nurses must also not ignore the facet of the unknowable that lies completely outside of unconscious thoughts and perceptions. A distant star, for instance, whose light can never be seen, represents the truly unknowable. Even though it cannot in any way be known, its mystery affects us. The realization that there are things in our world that we can never know colors our understanding of our world and our place within it. The meaning of the knowable for us is inescapably bound up with the significance of the unknowable in our lives. In sum, the knowable and the unknowable both can be inexplicable, but the unknowable is always inexplicable. By understanding the concepts of the inexplicable and the unknowable, nurses help clients and themselves envision and find meaning in the in-between and the beyond of their beings.

Significance of the Emerging Philosophical Shift

The philosophical shift from epistemological reflection, as highlighted by the patterns of knowing described by Carper,[2] to ontological reflections on reality, meaning, and being has occurred gradually. Nevertheless, this shift is important because, like an earth tremor, it creates movement, resulting in a foundational shift in the base of a discipline. This movement may alter the discipline for better or for worse, but once the tremor has occurred, the discipline is never the same. Therefore, it seems crucial for nurses to reflect on the significance of the disciplinary tremors and the directions that they want their discipline and profession to take. These are four possibilities:

1. The gap between nursing science and art has begun to close, generating a creative synthesis of the two. We refer to this phenomenon as the "science-art" of nursing. This science-art is bridging the gap between nursing epistemology and ontology. Hence, nurses have before them the potential best of two philosophical worlds. From the 1950s through the 1970s, when epistemology and the scientific method reigned, the science of nursing took root, but its ontology, including its artistry, lay dormant. Since about the 1980s, nurses have seriously begun to explore ontological and artistic concepts. These concepts have most often been reflected in phenomenologic and hermeneutic research and in the poetry, art, and stories created by nurses. Today many nurses are combining the science with the art of nursing, thus creating an integrated foundational base for the discipline.

2. Although, at first glance, discussions of epistemology and ontology appear to be remote from nursing practice, on closer inspection, one sees that they are integral to it and to each other. Both epistemological knowledge and ontological perceptions of reality have helped change how nurses practice nursing, where they practice nursing, when they practice nursing, and why they practice nursing. The difference lies in the type of questions that epistemology and ontology raise. Whereas epistemology leads to questions about knowing, ontology leads to questions about being. How the nurse uses expert knowledge to administer complex chemotherapy treatments is as important as how the nurse uses artistry of being to help a young mother find meaning in her impending death. Often the two converge.

3. Furthermore, how nurses, especially nurse educators, view the emerging philosophical shift and synthesis of epistemology and ontology affects the values transmitted and, consequently, the professional, scientific, and ethical behaviors of students. In the transition from the knowledge age to the information age, nurses must understand that reality has changed. Virtual worlds and environments raise profound ontological questions about what is reality, what is meaning, and what is being. Twentieth-century ontological thinking is outmoded as nurses enter the 21st century.

4. In preparation for the future, both nurses and nursing students must understand how to learn rather than how to hoard knowledge, how to critique rather than how to accept, how to expand rather than how to contract. We emphasize these points because we were struck by the largely unquestioning acceptance of and, frankly, misinterpretation of the four fundamental patterns of knowing described by Carper.[2] Too often the quick fix was sought; that is, nurses only labeled the four patterns without taking into consideration the interrelations of the patterns. Because of this mindset, patterns of knowing in nursing have largely stood still for almost two decades. This situation represents lost creativity and lost opportunity.

By critiquing the Carper article and exploring it and other works through ontological reflections on ways of being and through the in-between and the beyond, we join forces with other nurses who have a sincere desire to hear and respond to disciplinary tremors and, as a result, make a contribution to the foundational bases of nursing. Thus, with these nurses our philosophical journey continues. We challenge you to explore the path of the blackbird and to see all the in-betweens and beyonds that await.

REFERENCES

1. Stevens W. Thirteen ways of looking at a blackbird. In: Stevens H, ed. *The Palm at the End of the Mind.* New York, NY: Vintage Books; 1990. From *Collected Poems* by Stevens. Copyright 1923 and renewed 1951 by Wallace Stevens. Reprinted with permission of Alfred A Knopf Inc.
2. Carper BA. Fundamental patterns of knowing in nursing. *ANS.* 1978;1(1):13–23.
3. Boykin A, Schoenhofer S. Caring in nursing: analysis of extant theory. *Nurs Sci Q.* 1990;3(4):149–155.
4. Boykin A, Schoenhofer SO. Story as link between nursing practice, ontology, epistemology. *IMAGE J Nurs Schol.* 1991;23(4):245–248.
5. Bournaki MC, Germain CP. Esthetic knowledge in family-centered nursing care of hospitalized children. *ANS.* 1993;16(2):81–89.
6. Cooper MC, The intersection of technology and care in the ICU. *ANS.* 1993;15(3):23–32.
7. Jenny J, Logan J. Knowing the patient: one aspect of clinical knowledge. *Image J Nurs Schol.* 1992;24(4):254–258.
8. Moch SD. Personal knowing: evolving research and practice. *Schol Inq Nurs Pract.* 1990;4(2):155–165.
9. Earle WJ. *Introduction to Philosophy.* New York, NY: McGraw-Hill; 1992.
10. Koestenbaum P. *Philosophy: A General Introduction.* New York, NY: Van Nostrand Reinhold; 1968.
11. Newman MA. *Health as Expanding Consciousness.* 2nd ed. New York, NY: National League for Nursing Press; 1994.
12. Orem D. *Nursing: Concepts of Practice.* 5th ed. St. Louis, Mo: Mosby; 1995.
13. Heim M. *The Metaphysics of Virtual Reality.* New York, NY: Oxford University Press; 1993.
14. Tanner CA, Benner P, Chesla C, Gordon DR. The phenomenology of knowing the patient. *Image J Nurs Schol.* 1993;25(4):273–280.
15. Porter EJ. Older widows' experience of living alone at home. *Image J Nurs Schol.* 1994;26(1):19–24.
16. Kikuchi JF. Nursing questions that science cannot answer. In: Kikuchi JF, Simmons H, eds. *Philosophic Inquiry in Nursing.* Newbury Park, Calif: Sage; 1992.
17. Plato; Grube GMA, trans. *Republic.* Indianapolis, Ind: Hackett; 1992.
18. Kant I; Meredith JC, trans. *The Critique of Judgement.* London, England: Oxford University Press; 1964.
19. Santayana G. *The Sense of Beauty.* New York, NY: Dover; 1955.
20. Heidegger M. The origin of the work of art. In: Krell DF, ed. *Martin Heidegger: Basic Writings.* San Francisco, Calif: HarperCollins; 1993.
21. Highley B, Ferentz T. Esthetic inquiry. In: Sarter B, ed. *Paths to Knowledge: Innovative Research Methods for Nursing.* New York, NY: National League for Nursing; 1988.
22. Beckerman A. A personal journal of caring through esthetic knowing. *ANS.* 1994;17(1):71–79.
23. Hagedorn M. Hermeneutic photography: an innovative esthetic technique for generating data in nursing research. *ANS.* 1994;17(1):44–50.
24. Sorrell JM. Remembrance of things past through writing: esthetic patterns of knowing in nursing. *ANS.* 1994;17(1):60–70.
25. Polanyi M. Quoted by: Carper BA. Fundamental patterns of knowing in nursing. *ANS.* 1978;1(1):13–23.
26. Merleau-Ponty M. *Phenomenology of Perception.* London, England: Routledge & Kegan Paul; 1962.
27. Husserl E. Quoted by: Levesque-Lopman L. *Claiming Reality: Phenomenology and Women's Experience.* Totowa, NJ: Rowman & Littlefield; 1988.
28. Behr E. *The Complete Book of Les Misérables.* New York, NY: Arcade; 1989. Reprinted with permission from *The Complete Book of Les Misérables* by Edward Behr. Copyright (c) 1989 by Edward Behr. By permission of Little, Brown and Co.
29. Benner P, ed. *Interpretive Phenomenology: Embodiment, Caring, and Ethics in Health and Illness.* Thousand Oaks, Calif: Sage; 1994.

30. Diekelmann NL. Behavioral pedagogy: a Heideggerian hermeneutical analysis of the lived experiences of students and teachers in baccalaureate nursing education. *J Nurs Educ.* 1993;32:245–250.

31. Kondora LL. A Heideggerian hermeneutical analysis of survivors of incest. *Image J Nurs Schol.* 1993;25(1):11–16.

32. Liaschenko J. Feminist ethics and cultural ethos: revisiting a nursing debate. *ANS.* 1993;15(4):71–81.

33. Olsen DP. Empathy as an ethical and philosophical basis for nursing. *ANS.* 1991;14(1):62–75.

34. Gaul AL. Casuistry, care, compassion, and ethics data analysis. *ANS.* 1995;17(3):47–57.

35. Aristotle; Wheelwright P, trans. *The Nicomachean Ethics.* New York, NY: Odyssey Press; 1951.

36. Beauchamp TL, Childress JF. *Principles of Biomedical Ethics.* 4th ed. New York, NY: Oxford University Press; 1994.

37. Shakespeare W. *The Tragedy of Macbeth.* New York, NY: Simon & Schuster; 1959. The Folger Library General Reader's Shakespeare. Reprinted with permission. Copyright © 1959 by Pocket Books, a division of Simon & Schuster, Inc. Copyright renewed © 1987 by Simon & Schuster, Inc. Reprinted by permission of Simon & Schuster, Inc.

38. Gardner H. *Creating Minds: An Anatomy of Creativity Seen Through the Lives of Freud, Einstein, Picasso, Stravinsky, Eliot, Graham, and Gandhi.* New York, NY: Basic Books; 1993.

39. de Mille A. *Martha: The Life and Work of Martha Graham.* New York, NY: Random House; 1991.

40. George S. Quoted by: Heidegger M. *On the Way to Language.* San Francisco, Calif: Harper & Row; 1982.

The Authors Comment

From Carper's Patterns of Knowing to Ways of Being: An Ontological Philosophical Shift in Nursing

Our inspiration for this article came from the overall unquestioning and misinterpretation of Carper's article, as well as from an emerging shift in nursing philosophy from epistemology to ontology. We encouraged readers not only to consider this shift but also to ponder four concepts: the in-between, the beyond, the inexplicable, and the unknowable. By reflecting on the emerging shift and four concepts, nurses should be better prepared to cope with the virtual reality and cybernetics of the 21st century.

—MARY CIPRIANO SILVA
—JEANNE MERKLE SORRELL
—CHRISTINE SORRELL DINKINS

CHAPTER 29

Unitary Appreciative Inquiry

W. Richard Cowling III

Unitary appreciative inquiry is described as an orientation, process, and approach for illuminating the wholeness, uniqueness, and essence that are the pattern of human life. It was designed to bring the concepts, assumptions, and perspectives of the science of unitary human beings into reality as a mode of inquiry. Unitary appreciative inquiry provides a way of giving fullest attention to important facets of human life that often are not fully accounted for in current methods that have a heavier emphasis on diagnostic representations. The participatory, synoptic, and transformative qualities of the unitary appreciative process are explicated. The critical dimensions of nursing knowledge development expressed in dialectics of the general and the particular, action and theory, stories and numbers, sense and soul, aesthetics and empirics, and interpretation and emancipation are considered in the context of the unitary appreciative stance. Issues of legitimacy of knowledge and credibility of research are posed and examined in the context of four quality standards that are deemed important to evaluate the worthiness of unitary appreciative inquiry for the advancement of nursing science and practice.

Key words: *appreciative inquiry, method, nursing science, Rogers' science of unitary human beings, unitary inquiry, unitary theory*

Unitary appreciative inquiry was developed as a method for uncovering the wholeness, uniqueness, and essence of human existence to inform the development of nursing science and to guide the practice of nursing.[1-5] It is grounded in the concepts, assumptions, and perspectives of the broad conceptual and theoretic frame of ref-

Advances in Nursing Science *2001;23(4):32–48*

About the Author

WILLIAM RICHARD COWLING III was born at Clark Air Force Base, Manila, Philippines, on December 10, 1948, where his mother and father were stationed after World War II. He received a diploma in nursing (1969) and then a BS from the University of Virginia (1972), an MS in psychiatric mental health nursing from Virginia Commonwealth University (1979), and a PhD in Nursing from New York University (1983). His hobbies and interests include gardening, feeding birds, reading, and watching movies that are unique in their presentation of life, and some of his other interests focus on his partner, daughter, 2 granddaughters, and animal companions Nina and V-tab. He is employed as a faculty member and teaches nursing concepts, theory development, and holistic and unitary perspectives and approaches applied to mental health issues and concerns. The focus of his scholarship is on unitary praxis related to the phenomena of despair and the life patterns of women living with despair. Key contributions made to the discipline are creating scholarship that provokes new and deepened understandings of despair in women, developing methods of inquiry specific to unitary research and practice, participating in promoting healing possibilities within women in despair, and supporting the development of students and others in learning about and using the unitary perspective in their work.

erence known as the science of unitary human beings developed and refined by Rogers.[6] Unitary appreciative inquiry was created, in part, on the premise that nursing needs, in addition to its current methods of inquiry, approaches that avoid the neglect of important facets of human life that are not fully accounted for when human phenomena are "clinicalized" with an over-emphasis on diagnostic representations.[1]

The development of unitary appreciative inquiry is in line with the pleas for the development of methods that are suited to answering questions that will advance nursing science and theory.[7,8] In particular, Thorne and her colleagues have called for the use of noncategorical qualitative alternatives to traditional methods responding to nursing's unique knowledge mandate that "has gradually shifted the priorities within our research enterprise to the point that we can begin to build methods that are grounded in our own epistemological foundations, adhere to systematic reasoning of our own discipline, and yield legitimate knowledge for our practice."[8(p172)] Of particular importance to these authors is the species of knowledge requisite for nursing practice, most notably general knowledge of the type that enhances particularization in practice as suggested by Dzurec.[9]

Although unitary appreciative inquiry is grounded in the science of unitary human beings, it responds to common disciplinary challenges for knowledge creation expressed in a number of critical dimensions. These dimensions are the dialectics between the general and particular or the universal and unique, action and theory, empirics and aesthetics, stories and numbers, sense and soul, and interpretation and emancipation. This article serves to explicate what unitary pattern appreciation is, how it may inform the knowledge dialectics of nursing science and practice, and to what extent it can be counted on as legitimate and credible.

Unitary Appreciative Inquiry: What is it?

Unitary appreciative inquiry has a primary focus on seeking to know the wholeness, uniqueness, and essence of human life as a context for understanding phenomena and conditions of concern to nursing and guiding action in practice. It has an orientation, involves a process, and uses a set of approaches or practices that serve to actualize ontologic and epistemologic assumptions of a unitary-transformative paradigm.[1-5,10]

Unitary appreciative inquiry originally was designed as a method of research and later as a method of practice. Subsequently it was combined into a unitary appreciative endeavor blending research and practice elements toward a potential praxis. It generates theory that is both general and particular, serving the parties engaged in the endeavor, the inquirer-participants. It was designed for inquiry related to individuals, groups, families, communities, or societies, but it has been used primarily with individuals and with a community.

Orientation

The orientation of appreciative inquiry arises from the assumptions, principles, and concepts of unitary science.[6] It is a conscious choice freely made and openly acknowledged by the researcher/practitioner to use the metaphysics of the unitary perspective as a means of viewing, seeking, and envisioning human life and possibilities. This orientation requires taking a stance toward inquiry that extends the vision of possibility for all participants. The basic referent of inquiry is the underlying pattern of human life that is reflected in one's experience, perceptions, and expressions.[3] The goal is the appreciation of wholeness, uniqueness, and essence manifested as a singular pattern, a process termed "pattern appreciation."[1-3] Whether the inquiry pertains to an individual, group, family, community, or society, the referent point is the field pattern of that entity. This form of inquiry requires an inclusive view of what counts as pattern information and involves multiple modes of awareness. The field pattern reflects the environment as all aspects of the context of human life. By seeking to know the pattern in its fullness, one comes to know environment; for example, when discussing despair with women, I have come to know context or environment through their experiences. A construction process of synopsis and synthesis is used for understanding information that emerges from unitary appreciative inquiry encounters.

The format for conveying and presenting pattern appreciation is dependent on what is meaningful for the participants and what best captures the fullness of the pattern as experienced by the participants. Actions of practice and design of inquiry emerge from the knowing participation in change inherent in the appreciative process. Concepts and theories of unitary nursing science and practice emerge that are specific to the case but may inform broader theory development. Examination across cases yields knowledge of potential universals of human life patterning.

Process

The process of unitary appreciative inquiry involves four essential aspects. The process is guided by the overarching ideal of appreciative knowing and is fundamentally participatory, synoptic, and transformative.[1,3] Although unitary appreciative inquiry was developed independently from the appreciative inquiry in organizational life proposed by Cooperrider and Srivastva,[11] there are striking similarities. In particular, the conceptualization of appreciation as a way of knowing is consistent with a unitary perspective. Appreciative inquiry in organizational life is portrayed by its developers as "a viable complement to conventional forms of action research"[11(p129)] and its potential target for knowing is organizational life. Unitary appreciative inquiry evolved from an intellectual commitment to the unitary view of existence as relevant to nursing and from a desire to develop a method that would be suited to exploring the fullness and richness of human life to inform nursing science and art. The potential target of unitary appreciative inquiry is individual, group, family, or societal life. Rather than being grounded in organizational conceptualizations and being concerned with organizational life, unitary appreciative inquiry is grounded in unitary conceptualizations and is concerned with human life. In spite of these contrasts, the language of appreciative inquiry in organizational life is consistent with a unitary perspective in many instances.

Appreciative Knowing

The ideal of appreciative knowing is best described as going beyond questions of epistemology and having as its basis a metaphysical concern positing that human life is a miracle that never can be comprehended fully.[11,12] Using the language of Cooperrider and Srivastva and replacing the words "social," "organization," and "organizing" with the words "human," "existence," and "living," respectively, as noted in brackets, for a unitary slant, "more than a method or technique, the appreciative mode of inquiry is a way of living with, being with, and directly participating in the varieties of [*human existence*] we are compelled to study."[11(p131)] Further, "serious consideration and reflection on the ultimate mystery of being engenders a reverence for life that draws the researcher to inquire beyond the superficial appearances to deeper . . . life generating essentials and potentials of [*human*] existence."[11(p131)] The unitary appreciative inquirer is "drawn to affirm, and thereby illuminate, the factors and forces involved in [*living*] that serve to nourish the human spirit."[11(p131)] Again, the focal points of organizational appreciative inquiry and unitary appreciative inquiry ideals are distinct, but the conceptualization is metaphysically consistent.

Appreciative inquiry, whether organizational or unitary, embraces the notion of a type of knowing that is different from critical knowing. Human life is viewed as a miracle of a variety of ordinary and extraordinary forces and is characterized by relatively unknowable mystery. This means that appreciative knowing seeks for something it can never fully know, and can probably never accurately and completely represent, particularly with language or diagnostic boxes. The power and possibility of appreciative knowing is the realization of the inquirer/participant that I/we have chosen, in spite of the unverifiability of the miracle and mystery of life, not to become "tranquilized by the trivial."[11(p163)] As an inquirer-participant, I come to be with another or other inquirer-participants, to reach to see a pattern that reflects the wholeness, uniqueness, and essence of the individual or group. That pattern, when represented and reflected on, provides a way of understanding human life conditions and situations that has potential to go beyond fragmentation, normative thinking, and superficial comprehension. As was pointed out by Marcel[12] and noted by Cooperrider and Srivastva,[11] a problem is something that bars my passage, whereas a mystery

is something I find myself caught up in. Further, according to Kolb[13] and also noted by Cooperrider and Srivastva,[11] unlike criticism that is based on skepticism, appreciation is a process of affirmation based on belief, trust, and conviction. "This act of affirmation forms the foundation from which vital comprehension can develop . . . .Appreciative apprehension and critical comprehension are thus fundamentally different processes of knowing."[13(pp104-105)]

Participatory

The metaphysical idea of human life as miracle and mystery gives rise to a "participatory consciousness," whereby there is a personal stake or partnership with the universe.[14] It implies that the inquirer-participant is not an alienated observer of what is happening in the world, in this case the intersection of human living with nursing, but rather is a direct participant in this process. In this sense unitary appreciative inquiry is dependent on the willingness of parties involved to come together freely and openly. Mutual understanding of the appreciative process is of extreme importance. This means being clear about "the egalitarian ideal inherent in the relationship, the openness to emergent discovery in the work, the potential for negotiation, and that potential outcomes are not predicted or prescribed."[1(p21)]

The capacity of humans to participate knowingly in change and in patterning is one of the central tenets of the science of unitary human beings. Opportunities for mutual discovery by inquirer-participants create possible avenues of action. Chosen actions emerge from appreciative knowing in exploration of unitary pattern. Although there is a partnership between a nurse and participants, all seen as inquirer-participants, "the participant is viewed as an expert on his or her own life and the source of his or her own power and knowledge."[1(p21)] Acausality and unpredictability are notions of a unitary perspective that are inconsistent with the ideal of control and imposed expectations or outcomes. Change is an emergent of knowing participation, and thus participatory relating is a cornerstone of unitary appreciative inquiry.

Synoptic

The process used for considering information from the appreciative encounters is synoptic. It is derived from the idea of synoptic empiricism[15] employed by Murphy[16] in his research on transformation. "Synopsis is the deliberate viewing together of aspects of human experience which for one reason or another, are generally kept apart by the plain man and even by the professional scientist or scholar."[15(p8)] The object of synopsis in unitary appreciative inquiry is on sensing an emerging pattern that reflects the wholeness, uniqueness, and essence of human life. "Thus, aspects of human life, namely the experiences, perceptions, and expressions associated with living are viewed together in an inclusive way to reveal the fullest picture of the inherent wholeness."[1(p20)] Inquirer-participants seek for themes, commonalities, connections, and relationships among the data of experience, perception, and expressions. An assortment of ways of knowing may be employed. The intent is to "reveal a compelling sense of wholeness amidst the variety of phenomena of life"[1(p20)] inherent in a unitary pattern or, to use a weaving analogy, to see beyond threads to the tapestry.

All forms of information are important to the inquirer-participants, and synopsis implies an inclusive view of what counts as pattern information. Although focus is on experience, perceptions, and expressions associated with living, phenomena, regardless of category or label such as physical, emotional, mental, social, and spiritual, are included as pattern information.[1,3] This encompasses information from inquirer-participants about the environmental and social context of living, including the experience and perception of barriers and forces that inhibit full expression of life. Unitary appreciative knowing does not strip environment or context from the synopsis, rather, appreciating a unitary pattern involves appreciating environment and context. Everything that emerges as information from the appreciative engagement and encounters is viewed and understood contextually as arising from wholeness and reflecting pattern, not parts that do not exist in the unitary perspective. "The multiple, and sometimes seemingly disparate, manifestations of the field pattern form an ensemble of information that conveys a singularity of expression."[6(p140)] Developing one's synoptic ability to sense life pattern and wholeness is one of the goals of appreciative inquiry.

Transformative

There are three ways in which the unitary appreciative process is potentially transformative:

1. the way in which it seeks to understand a condition of existence
2. the use of pandimensional or unitive consciousness
3. the development of one's self as an instrument of appreciation

The phenomena associated with human living are seen in a new light and a new context when attention is given to the wholeness, uniqueness, and essence of human existence through appreciative knowing. An example of this transforming potential occurred when working with women in appreciating the condition of living in despair. Revelations emerge "that go beyond the tendency to treat and/or understand the despair as a symptom of a disease or single condition."[1(p22)] Emphasis is placed in the unitary appreciative process on the essentials, potentials, and possibilities that exist within the wholeness of life and that reflect the uniqueness of each being.[1]

Unitary appreciative inquiry also offers inquirer-participants the possibility of looking at one's life situation and change within the perspective of pandimensional awareness or unitive consciousness, which is a concept of the unitary framework. This view is not imposed on the process but is offered by the nurse participant as a way of seeing time, space, and movement that may or may not be useful. It is critical to consider both unitary and nonunitary ways of understanding change in alignment with respect for all participants. Ultimately, the choice of viewing change is acknowledged and embraced as an aspect of the participatory and exploratory nature of unitary appreciative inquiry. Pandimensional awareness is congruent with the spiritual concept of "unitive consciousness,"[17] when individuals become referent to infinity, meaning that they realize infinite potential and infinite time-space-movement-change. It has been described as a state where sensing, thinking, and feeling become a unified continuum not limited by bodily boundaries, and time is experienced as "a new birth and what is being born is not merely the product of the past, not merely the cause of some earlier effect, but rather part of a ceaseless cosmos of revelation."[17(p66)] This means that we cease locating ourselves as finite. "We are movement and flow. Our careers, our health, our families and possessions may temporarily represent a harbor of our sense of self, but ultimately we are always far more."[17(p67)] It is this sense of revelation and possibility that offers the potential for transformation.

Finally, the transformative potential for inquirer-participants is in the development of one's self as an instrument for unitary appreciative knowing. The quest in appreciative knowing requires attention to all realms of data, and, consequently, one must develop data acquisition skills that allow for the data to reveal themselves. This can be likened to spiritual practices such as Zen. In Zen practices, injunctive tools are used for developing an ability to sense data disclosure.[18] The injunctive tools are developing in the quest for unitary appreciative knowing and need to be specified, honed, refined, and clarified. In essence, the inquirer-participant possesses a willingness to use injunctive devices that will open one to the revelation of unitary pattern data. Likewise, this inquiry process calls for using data in ways that respond to the wholeness, uniqueness, and essence of the individuals or the group involved. Inquiry design choices and action-practice strategies evolve from effectively using the injunctive tools of appreciative inquiry. This process requires at least a relative transformation toward being a more sensitive instrument of awareness. The aim is toward "appreciating an inherent wholeness that illuminates potentials of understanding and possibilities of action."[1(p23)]

Approach

Unitary appreciative inquiry is an approach that actualizes the ontologic and epistemologic assumptions of a unitary worldview and addresses the metaphysical concerns of an appreciating orientation toward human life.

It is important to emphasize that the set of practices that comprise the approach emerge from appreciative knowing and are individualized consistent with the particular situation and inquiry endeavor. The elements of the approach outlined are *suggestions* for implementing a plan of unitary appreciative inquiry.

The scientist/practitioner seeks or is sought out for the purposes of exploration of a life situation, phenomenon, or concern from a unitary perspective. The scientist/practitioner describes the inquiry endeavor, including its focus on unitary field pattern, emphasizing that the approach is aimed at appreciating the wholeness, uniqueness, and essence of the particular situation, phenomenon, or concern. The unitary appreciative inquiry is approved as a research project through the typical human subjects review, and an informed consent for participants is provided. A partnership is suggested that embraces all involved as coequal participants in the appreciative inquiry endeavor. The term "inquirer-participants" is used for both the scientist/practitioner and all other participants. Specific intentions of the inquirer-participants are made explicit with one another, and a form and structure for the unitary appreciative endeavor are agreed upon. This can take the form of dialogue, discussion, interview, observation, or any practice or practices that illuminate the underlying human life pattern. Storytelling, poetry, photography, drawing, and music have been used creatively for this purpose in appreciative inquiries. Other modes of inquiry and ways of knowing may be integrated into the approach consistent with achieving the deepest and fullest picture of the pattern.

Documentation of experience, perceptions, and expressions are accomplished through journaling, audiotaping and/or videotaping, photographing (including the photographing of meaningful artifacts), recording music, and actual creative products. The choice for documentation is based on what best reflects pattern information that is meaningful to participants. Journaling for the scientist/practitioner may involve theoretic notes, methodologic notes, peer review notes, and general reflective notes. All documentation is shared among participants if requested. The appreciative inquiry lasts for a period of time agreed upon by participants to meet their shared expectations and desires. The scientist/practitioner sees the other participants as the experts and honors and respects their wishes for determining the nature and length of the appreciative engagement. Some engagements have lasted for more than a year and others for only several weeks.

Synopsis is used to create a pattern profile that is a construction based on the information that emerges from the appreciative inquiry. The form of the profile is determined by the participants according to what meaningfully represents the underlying pattern as reflected in experience, perceptions, and expressions of participants and captures the wholeness, uniqueness, and essence of life. The profile can be constructed by the scientist/practitioner, by the other participant or participants, or it can be a joint venture. In some cases the scientist/practitioner may facilitate the construction. In cases where I have developed the profile, I have shared it with a participant who reviews it to assess whether it conveys the richness and fullness of the participant's life experience. It is altered depending on that assessment. The primary voice in the process and content of the profile construction is always that of participants other than the scientist practitioner. That voice is used to determine if the profile portrays life as lived by the participants. In all cases in which I created a profile and shared it with a participant, it was viewed as a gift, and I experienced the creation as an opportunity to acknowledge and honor the person's experience as perceived and expressed. However, the ideal profile would be created by the participant himself or herself. The profiles that have been developed in the praxis are primarily in the form of stories that integrate metaphor, images, and music.

The pattern profile becomes a referent point for knowledge development that serves practice aims and for the development of unitary theory. Because the knowledge is specific to the individual case, the concepts and theory generated reflect the uniqueness of the particular pattern. The scientist/practitioner may use the appreciative knowledge of the pattern profile as a context for exploration for participant-centered change.

The scientist/practitioner also may generate a theoretic synthesis from the unitary appreciative knowledge to posit further unitary theory, a kind of situation-specific theorizing. It is also possible to look for universals that may exist across cases as long as the individual differences are acknowledged while seeking the commonalties. This could be considered a group profile in the case of individuals with relatively similar situations. A report may be generated and shared with professional audiences through publications or presentations with the same respect for confidentiality and anonymity as any other formal research report and with the permission of participants.

Unitary Pattern Appreciation and Critical Dialectic Dimensions

Nursing scientists and practitioners are faced with an array of disciplinary tensions or dialectics that influence the course and content of the advancement of nursing knowledge that supports a practice discipline. Significant tensions create dialectics, namely of the general and the particular, action and theory, sense and soul, stories and numbers, aesthetics and empirics, and interpretation and emancipation. Unitary appreciative inquiry creates a potential dialectic bridge or conversation between these tensions.

General and Particular

The general and the particular dialectic centers around the need for practice knowledge that is shared by persons in similar situations and that is particular to the individual case.[8] Thorne and colleagues cited the work of Dzurec,[9] who described "a practice and scholarship climate within nursing that is clamoring for general knowledge of the sort that enhances particularization in practice."[8(p171)] Pointing to the work of Mitchell and Cody,[7] they claim that nursing theory has been one device facilitating the need by nurses for "forms of inquiry that reveal processes for applying aggregated knowledge to individual cases."[8(p170)]

In the 1960s, Allport[19] addressed the issue of the general and unique in psychologic science, describing research methods that provided two equally indispensable types of differentiated information. This holds true as well in nursing; we require information for practice of the varieties of general/universal *and* particular/unique. Allport described the information as dimensional for the general form and morphogenic or idiographic for the unique. "Dimensional information is derived from the commonalties that run through all individuals"[20(p57)] and "morphogenic information is derived from the unique world and experience of the particular individual."[20(p57)] Using a similar type of case scenario as that of Allport, if we were working with a person, Mary, who is depressed, and we used dimensional information based on research and clinical standards that are evidence based, we would have normative knowledge of what we might anticipate will occur and what strategies have been effective in large samples of individuals like Mary. We could use this information in helping Mary, and it probably would be useful. What we do not know from this information are the specifics of Mary's situation. We do not know from dimensional information that Mary has had experiences that lend themselves to her recovery, that she has a strong belief that helps her transcend some of her pain, and that she has a commitment not to use medications to treat her illness. This is a form of morphogenic information that complements dimensional information. It may be argued that nursing has become overly dependent on dimensional information in its endeavor to have a sound theoretic and scientific base. At the same time, nursing has a history of sensitivity to the individual receiving care. The general/universal and particular/unique dialectic in nursing is a dialectic of dimensional and morphogenic information and ways of knowing.

Unitary appreciative inquiry is a bridge between the general and particular, creating dialogue between the two. It starts with a premise of wholeness and uniqueness in each human life while it simultaneously comes from a theoretic base that encompasses principles about the nature of change, including human trends. Engaging appreciative inquiry allows for the generation of morphogenic information that comes from the intense focus on the case. At the same time, appreciative inquiry allows for the generation of dimensional information when the inquirer-participants look across cases or notice similarities or commonalties in other cases. In addition, the scientist/practitioner engaged in a broader program of inquiry guided by the overarching framework of unitary science may be doing a form of theory testing of the general type by comparing findings from the case or cases with other scientific and theoretic work in the field. This is not the same as traditional theory testing research driven by experimental and quasiexperimental designs, and the contribution of unitary appreciative inquiry is clearly more of the morphogenic variety. It offers the scientist/practitioner a tool for complementing dimensional information.

Action and Theory

Theory has been viewed as central to the formulation of reality, and the theoretic contributions of science as among the most powerful resources that humans have for contributing to change and development. However, nurses who deliver care are bound to be skeptical of theory that does not inform action in practice. Experience with graduate students suggests that the link between theory and action is rather tenuous at best. "When theories are viewed as relevant, rarely are those theories specific to nursing."[21(p132)]

The disconnection between theory and action is exemplified in two major stances taken in nursing by many academicians and practitioners. Practitioners are not likely to see theory as relevant to practice, given the multiplicity of contingencies they face in practice on a day-to-day basis. Academicians are fairly removed from action in practice because of the contingencies they face in academia. It could be that practitioners facing priorities of patient care delivery, economic considerations, immediacy of action requirements, and institutional priorities require action to take precedence over knowledge generated from theory. Academic scholars, on the other hand, unintentionally undermine the development of useful theory because of educational bias and expectations for credible scholarship grounded in detachment, unilateral control, rigor, and operational precision.[22] In a sense, creative theorizing is beleaguered by practitioners and academicians alike.[11]

It is warranted that practitioners and educators would reject theory derived without attention to pragmatics. Likewise, it is reasonable to call for actions in practice that speak to the wholeness and uniqueness of the person, group, family, community, or society, given nursing's espoused commitment to holistic and individualized care. The dialectic of theory and action is mediated most readily by the notion of "theory in action."

Unitary appreciative inquiry offers a bridge for the dialectic of theory and action in its ability to be action-oriented and theory-generative. The process of appreciative inquiry is one of participatory action and of theory emerging from action. This represents what Cooperrider and Srivastva refer to as a "bold shift in attention whereby theoretical accounts are no longer judged in terms of their predictive capacity, but instead on their generative capacity."[11(p137)] Rather than ameliorating the dialectic of theory and action, generative theorizing nourishes the dialectic. It brings about a dialogue between what is taken for granted and what is possible in generating new alternatives for action. In unitary appreciative inquiry, the test of the theory is not its correspondence with observed facts, but its ability to offer provocative possibilities for action.[11]

Sense and Soul

The rise of modernity in the West was the context for the creation of modern science with a differentiation of it from the cultural value spheres of art and morals. According to Wilber,[23] there was both dignity and disaster in this differentiation. Wilber's disaster was the invasion of scientific materialism and imperialism, which dominated the other value spheres. What accompanied this invasion was the pronouncement that "the Great Nest of matter, body, mind, soul, and spirit could be thoroughly reduced to matter alone."[23(p13)] Although nursing scholarship reflects the reductionism of modernity, there are many scholars of nursing who theorize about and research matter, body, mind, soul, and spirit connections in an integrative way. The vast amount of support for research is arguably within the domains of matter, mind,

and body. There is minor support for spiritual inquiries in spite of nursing's avowed embrace of diverse domains of inquiry.[21] Thus, the dialectic of sense and soul is evident in the work of nursing knowledge development.

Unitary appreciative inquiry requires attention to all realms of data, sensory and soul, in order to be truly unitary. Disregarding or denying the existence of physical, mental, or spiritual data diminishes the capacity of the scientist/practitioner to fully appreciate the wholeness of human existence. The goal is to create within a profile the richest representative tapestry reaching across the realms of matter and body and soul and spirit to the inherent pattern of unity that is human life and the fullness of human experience.[1,3]

Stories and Numbers

There have been considerable debates in nursing about what constitutes legitimate forms of knowledge and how knowledge should be generated.[24] However, it also can be argued that nursing has come quite some distance in embracing the credibility of both qualitative and quantitative methods and the accompanying roles of stories and numbers, depending on the aims of the research project.[24,25] A more sophisticated line of argumentative exposition, in juxtaposition to dichotomizing stories and numbers, has evolved that makes the case for distinctions between methodology and methods and the role of paradigm in methods choices.[24] The argument is that method "refers to the particular procedures used to gather evidence" and methodology "pertains to a theory of how research is carried out, or the general principles about how to conduct research and how theory is applied."[24(p19)] Paradigms do not constrain the methods being used, particularly not on the grounds of the way they have been used historically. More important than the selection of methods is "the way in which methods are used, the ways in which researchers interact with participants, and the ways in which researchers attempt to represent the experience of research participants."[24(p19)] It has been argued that stories and numbers may be useful in discovering knowledge in any of nursing's paradigms,[24] and that in the critical theory paradigm, the fundamental consideration is whether stories and numbers provide persuasive evidence to bring about personal empowerment and social and political change.[25]

In terms of unitary appreciative inquiry, the assumptions of a unitary perspective and the ideals of an appreciative stance toward knowledge are critical to methodologic concerns but do not constrain scientist/practitioners to either stories or numbers as sources of evidence. Some of the important method choice questions for the unitary appreciative inquirer are:

- In what ways might numbers or stories illuminate the wholeness, uniqueness, and essence of the unitary pattern of human life?
- Are there ways in which the scientist/practitioner might be informed by stories and numbers to evaluate whether a practice is fragmentary or responsive to personal wholeness?
- In what ways, if any, might stories and numbers be used to highlight unitary changes associated with actions in practice?
- Are there ways in which a combination of stories and numbers might more fully reflect manifestations of a unitary field and of the mutual environment/human process?
- In what ways are stories and numbers useful to the participants in shedding light on what is and what might be possible?

Aesthetics and Empirics

The complementary yet distinctive benefits for nursing of aesthetics and empirics as ways of knowing have been elucidated in the literature.[26,27] However, there is some tension between the aims of the science and art of nursing knowledge development similar to that of the general and particular tension. The practitioner needs to have practice-oriented knowledge of an aesthetic variety to provide nursing care while at the same time there is a need for normative-oriented knowledge of an empiric variety to guide clinical decisions and meet professional standards for sound practice. The nursing

scientist who lives in the academic world understands that the primary mode for advancement arises from research of an empiric variety generating normative-oriented knowledge, even though there may be a high regard for aesthetic knowledge.

One of the goals of many unitary scholars, consistent with the founding mother of unitary science, is to develop theory testing knowledge, including description and explanation, but perhaps not prediction because of the unitary tenet of acausality.[6] Certainly the conceptual, theoretic, and empiric representations of phenomena from a unitary paradigm perspective are desired. Moreover, if unitary science is a science, it would need its own kind of empirics.[21]

Comparatively, an examination of aesthetic knowing reveals descriptions engendering images of the unitary and the appreciative. Chinn and Kramer[26] define aesthetics as a noun for "the perceptual ability to appreciate artistically valid form" and as an adjective for identifying an object or experience as valid, being coherent in form and substance, conveying a sense of a whole beyond the formative and substantive elements, and evoking a response. The expression of aesthetic knowing is emergent and artistic in art/act or experience-action. Art is the process of creating an aesthetic object or experience and involves the ability to work with elements in creating a form, as in the pattern profile of unitary appreciative inquiry. It also involves "inner capacities to imagine the whole before it becomes an expression and intuitively brings into being the elements as an integral whole."[26(p185)] This is the essence of the process of unitary appreciative inquiry.

Rogers[28] was clear about the relationship of art and science and defined the art of nursing specifically within a unitary context, claiming that nursing art is the creative use of knowledge based on unitary theory in practice. The emphasis of unitary scientists primarily has been on the development of unitary empirics, and it may be time to consider the need for unitary aesthetics.[21] Unitary appreciative inquiry brings empiric and aesthetic aspects into complementary relationships serving dual purposes. The empirical aspects are mainly its theory-generative capacity, and the aesthetics aspects are its orientation toward action in practice.

Interpretation and Emancipation

There is an ongoing debate among some nursing scholars about whether the interpretive paradigm in nursing science can be emancipatory.[29] Specifically, the debate has centered on the issue of praxis, that is, the challenge that interpretive research is not praxis because it does not meet the critical paradigm standard of explaining and critiquing hegemony, which coincides with emancipation.[29] The unitary-transformative paradigm,[10] of which unitary science is an exemplar, has been described as falling within the domain of interpretation. Unitary appreciative inquiry is not precisely hermeneutic inquiry, which is clearly the exemplar of the interpretive paradigm. The unitary appreciative inquiry perspective does share in common with the interpretive paradigm "the ontological assumptions that reality is complex, holistic, and context dependent."[30(p71)] However, unitary appreciative inquiry does not have as its goal to "understand and derive meaning from the human experience,"[30(p71)] but rather to illuminate wholeness, uniqueness, and essence of human life, or what is conceptually labeled "unitary pattern" in theoretic terms, as a referent point for nursing knowledge development, both theoretical and practical.

Likewise, unitary appreciative inquiry is not precisely a form of critical social theory inquiry, which is exemplified by praxis and emancipation. However, unitary appreciative inquiry can be praxic and has emancipation as one of its potentials. Critical theory inquiry effectively uses the device of critique of the institutions and structures that oppress and exploit humans to accomplish social change and praxis accompanied by emancipation of participants.[29] Like the appreciative inquiry of organizational life,[11] the unitary appreciative inquiry of human life is both pragmatic and visionary as it seeks to expand the universe of exploration, kindle a perception of new possibilities, and foster innovations in human life arrangements and processes. The processes of unitary appreciative inquiry, including the creation of a pattern profile, provide the context for potential emancipation. The profile captures what liberates, as well as what oppresses, as it reaches for wholeness, uniqueness, and essence.

Unitary Appreciative Inquiry: Is It Legitimate and Credible?

Returning to the call by Thorne and her colleagues[8] for the building of methods that are grounded in nursing's uniqueness, it is important to note that it was also a call for "legitimate" knowledge and for "credible" research. Although the development of unitary appreciative inquiry is in its infancy, having been used over the past few years with some refinements, the questions of legitimacy and credibility must be answered in order for this method to be taken seriously as a tool for advancing nursing science and practice. It has been used by one team of researchers to address the pattern of a community and is being used or considered for use in several dissertations.

The issues of legitimacy and credibility were considered from the very beginning and were addressed by a set of approaches based on general tenets of qualitative research credibility, namely member checking, auditing, and peer review.[3] These were written with the intent of being beginning ways of achieving credibility and legitimacy, knowing that further development of standards might be necessary. A peer review system is encouraged to assist the scientist/practitioner in ensuring logical consistency in the process. It is desirable to engage a peer reviewer who is familiar with the conceptual system and method, a major challenge given the newness of the method. A peer reviewer's goal would be to enhance the reflective aspects of the process. Member checking is built into the process of unitary appreciative inquiry because of the high priority given to participation, the notion of "inquirer-participants" in an egalitarian relationship, and the primary emphasis on a pattern profile reflecting the voice of the participants. Audit procedures enable review of documentation for grounds for making unitary knowledge claims of the participants. The auditor should be an expert in the unitary conceptual system and understand the method. The case study report can be scrutinized for legitimacy by participants, peer reviewers, and auditors.

Standards of legitimacy and credibility have not been addressed fully by scholars of the unitary-transformative paradigm, generally, or of the unitary conceptual system, specifically. This is in part because of the evolving nature of and diversity within the paradigm and its openness to a variety of perspectives in its current state of development.

In order to address the issues of legitimacy and credibility, a perspective on the quality of inquiry is employed. This more general perspective of quality with its standards was chosen because it encompasses both legitimacy of knowledge and credibility of research that are intertwined, and because the standards "transcend paradigm boundaries."[24(p23)] The standards are those of Ford-Gilboe and her colleagues, who contend that there are four basic issues to be considered in evaluating the quality of any research: "(1) quality of the data, (2) investigator bias, (3) quality of the research process, and (4) usefulness of the study findings."[24(p23)]

The quality of data is related to trustworthiness in the interpretive paradigm,[31] and given the interpretive dimension of unitary appreciative inquiry, the same standards may apply. The gold standard for yielding higher quality data, as it is in interpretive inquiry, may be the diversity of data sources and theoretic schemes used by the researcher, as well as designs that uncover patterns of commonality and uniqueness.[24] Unitary appreciative inquiry accomplishes this standard by having an orientation toward inclusiveness of data sources through use of synopsis and synthesis for creating theoretic schemes, and by incorporating approaches that are designed to uncover unitary pattern, which would include uniqueness within cases and commonality across cases.

Again, because there is no current agreed upon standard for handling investigator bias in the unitary perspective, both the standards of interpretive inquiry and critical inquiry are used for the reasons of the interpretive quality, the praxic potential, and the emancipatory goals of unitary appreciative inquiry. Investigator bias relates to the interactivity of the researcher and

participant.[24] The interpretive position is one of acknowledging interactivity, and even capitalizing on it for gaining data, while strategizing to minimize it "so as not to impose the researcher's viewpoint."[24(p24)] The critical position is to view interactivity as a powerful force that can be used to benefit the research enterprise, and, therefore, a dialogic interview is the strategy of choice for inquiry.[24] The unitary appreciative position is one that creates a blend of these two positions. It attempts to acknowledge interactivity through a plan of documentation and audit that may uncover instances of imposition of the researcher's voice over the voices of inquirer-participants. However, being unitary in orientation, it acknowledges the mutuality of human existence that may make it difficult to separate voices. Likewise, being appreciative in orientation, it seeks to illuminate factors and forces that contribute to the human condition using the interactivity quality. Further, it is dependent on interactivity to create the potentials for praxis and emancipation.

Once again, because of the nature of unitary appreciative inquiry as interpretive, emancipatory, and having the potential of praxis, the quality of the research process is addressed within the interpretive and critical positions. The principle of confirmability associated with the interpretive paradigm is satisfied by "the use of audit procedures and validation of the findings of the study with research participants."[24(p24)] The critical position that "the degree of change brought about as part of the research is of primary importance"[24(p24)] is satisfied also within the unitary appreciative inquiry process. The quality of the research process standard from the appreciative and unitary positions is extended to include the generative-theory capacity of the study[11] and the capacity of the study to provide a context for knowing participation in change.

In unitary appreciative inquiry, the quality standard of the usefulness of study findings veers somewhat from the interpretive and critical positions. As in the interpretive paradigm, there is a desire to obtain transferability to other contexts by seeking rich descriptions of context and sample participants. In addition, the usefulness of the study findings rests in their ability to make a positive difference in the lives of the participants. It also rests in their ability to inform the use of process skills derived from the inquiry that might be applied to other areas of one's personal life or to facilitate broader knowledgeable change. In other words, the unitary appreciative stance concerning usefulness of findings might include the question: To what extent do the study findings illuminate the wholeness, uniqueness, and essence of these human lives that would inform knowing participation in change? The critical position on usefulness of study findings relates to applicability to other forms of oppression, and critical inquiry incorporates strategies that ensure this, including sample composition, design of the study, and interpretation of the data.[24] Unitary appreciative inquiry clearly is not targeted to the kind of oppression that critical theory addresses. Perhaps unitary appreciative inquiry might be judged on the usefulness of its research findings in understanding the potential for personal oppression that may occur when humans are subjected to nursing practices that do not account for important facets of human life.

Conclusion

Unitary appreciative inquiry responds to the call for developing new paradigm-directed methodologies[24] and the building of methods grounded in nursing's epistemologic foundations.[8] It provides an orientation, process, and approach that guide the inquiry endeavor aiming to uncover the wholeness, uniqueness, and essence of human life that is unitary pattern, and to mobilize the capacity for knowing participation in change to the benefit of participants. Unitary appreciative inquiry brings the scientist/practitioner together with others to mutually explore a focus of inquiry related to human conditions of concern, with everyone involved becoming inquirer-participants in an egalitarian relationship. The unitary appreciative enterprise is guided by knowledge that comes forth from a unitary understanding of human life. It has both a theory-generative aspect as well as a situation-specific aspect that provide theoretic and practical knowledge. The work of unitary appreciative inquiry considers

and embraces critical dimensions of nursing knowledge development, including the general and particular, action and theory, stories and numbers, sense and soul, aesthetics and empirics, and interpretation and emancipation. As part of the development and evolving application of unitary appreciative inquiry, there has been attention to the need for standards of quality, including legitimacy and credibility. These will be crucial in determining whether unitary appreciative inquiry will be considered a method worthy of advancing the aims of nursing science and practice.

REFERENCES

1. Cowling WR. Healing as appreciating wholeness. *Adv Nurs Sci.* 2000;22(3):16–32.
2. Cowling WR. Unitary case inquiry. *Nurs Sci Q.* 1998;11:139–141.
3. Cowling WR. Unitary pattern appreciation: the unitary science/practice of reaching for essence. In: Madrid M, ed. *Patterns of Rogerian Knowing.* New York: National League for Nursing; 1997.
4. Cowling WR. Unitary practice: revisionary assumptions. In: Parker MS, ed. *Nursing Theories in Practice.* Vol 2. New York: National League for Nursing; 1993.
5. Cowling WR. Unitary knowing in nursing practice. *Nurs Sci Q.* 1993;6:201–207.
6. Rogers ME. Nursing science and the space age. *Nurs Sci Q.* 1992;5:27–33.
7. Mitchell GJ, Cody WK. Nursing knowledge and human science: ontological and epistemological considerations. *Nurs Sci Q.* 1992;6:54–61.
8. Thorne S, Kirkham SR, MacDonald-Emes J. Interpretive description: a noncategorical qualitative alternative for developing nursing knowledge. *Res Nurs Health.* 1997;20:169–177, Review
9. Dzurec LC. The necessity for and evolution of multiple paradigms for nursing research: a poststructuralist perspective. *Adv Nurs Sci.* 1989;11(4):69–77.
10. Newman MA, Sime AM, Corcoran-Perry SA. The focus of the discipline of nursing. *Adv Nurs Sci.* 1991;14(1):1–6.
11. Cooperrider DL, Srivastva S. Appreciative inquiry in organizational life. *Res Org Chg Dev.* 1987;1:129–169.
12. Marcel G. *The Existential Background of Human Dialogue.* Cambridge, MA: Harvard University Press; 1963.
13. Kolb DA. *Experiential Learning: Experience as the Source of Learning and Development.* Englewood Cliffs, NJ: Prentice-Hall; 1984.
14. Berman H, Ford-Gilboe M, Campbell JC. Combining stories and numbers: a methodologic approach for a critical nursing science. *Adv Nurs Sci.* 1998;21(1):1–15.
15. Broad CD. *Religion, Philosophy and Psychical Research.* New York: Harcourt, Brace; 1953.

16. Murphy M. *The Future of the Body: Explorations into the Further Evolution of Human Consciousness.* San Francisco: Tarcher Press; 1992.

17. Moss R. *The Second Miracle: Intimacy, Spirituality, and Consciousness.* Berkeley, CA: Celestial Arts; 1995.

18. Wilber K. The problem of proof. *Revision J Consciousness Change.* 1982;5(1):80–100.

19. Allport GW. The general and unique in psychological science. *J Pers.* 1962;30(3):405–422.

20. Cowling WR. A template for unitary pattern-based nursing practice. In: Barrett EA, ed. *Visions of Rogers' Science-Based Nursing.* New York: National League for Nursing; 1990.

21. Cowling WR. A unitary-transformative nursing science: potentials for transcending dichotomies. *Nurs Sci Q.* 1999;12(2):132–135.

22. Argyris C. Action science and intervention. *J App Beh Sci.* 1973;19:115–140.

23. Wilber K. *The Marriage of Sense and Soul: Integrating Science and Religion.* New York: Random House; 1998.

24. Ford-Gilboe M, Campbell JC, Berman H. Stories and numbers: coexistence without compromise. *Adv Nurs Sci.* 1995;18(1):14–26.

25. Berman H, Ford-Gilboe M, Campbell JC. Combining stories and numbers: a methodologic approach for a critical nursing science. *Adv Nurs Sci.* 1998;21(1):1–15.

26. Chinn PL, Kramer MK. *Theory and Nursing: A Systematic Approach.* St. Louis, MO: Mosby; 1999.

27. Carper BA. Fundamental patterns of knowing in nursing. *Adv Nurs Sci.* 1978;1(1):13–23.

28. Rogers ME. Nursing science evolves. In: Madrid M, Barrett EAM, eds. *Rogers' Scientific Art of Nursing Practice.* New York: National League for Nursing; 1994.

29. Lutz KF, Jones KD, Kendall J. Expanding the praxis debate: contributions to clinical inquiry. *Adv Nurs Sci.* 1997;20(2): 23–31.

30. Monti EJ, Tingen MS. Multiple paradigms of nursing science. *Adv Nurs Sci.* 1999;21(4):64–80.

31. Lincoln YS, Guba EG. *Naturalistic Inquiry.* Beverly Hills, CA: Sage; 1985.

The Author Comments

Unitary Appreciative Inquiry

I was inspired to write this article because I wanted to share my work on developing a praxis inquiry approach that attends to the wholeness and uniqueness of human life pattern from a unitary perspective. I wished to articulate in detail the nature and process of this approach and to offer an example of how this approach was applied and could be applied in research and practice. I believe this article contributes to the development of nursing theory because it offers an example of the evolution of a praxis approach generated from a nursing theory that is consistent with concepts, tenets, and values congruent with a science and art of wholeness. In addition, it addresses issues of legitimacy of knowledge and credibility of research using proposed standards.

—WILLIAM RICHARD COWLING, III

CHAPTER 30

On Nursing Theories and Evidence

Jacqueline Fawcett
Jean Watson
Betty Neuman
Patricia H. Walker
Joyce J. Fitzpatrick

Purpose: *To expand the understanding of what constitutes evidence for theory-guided, evidence-based nursing practice from a narrow focus on empirics to a more comprehensive focus on diverse patterns of knowing.*

   Organizing construct: *Carper's four fundamental patterns of knowing in nursing—empirical, ethical, personal, and aesthetic—are required for nursing practice. A different mode of inquiry is required to develop knowledge about and evidence for each pattern.*

   Conclusions: *Theory, inquiry, and evidence are inextricably linked. Each pattern of knowing can be considered a type of theory, and the modes of inquiry appropriate to the generation and testing of each type of theory provide diverse sources of data for evidence-based nursing practice. Different kinds of nursing theories provide different lenses for critiquing and interpreting the different kinds of evidence essential for theory-guided, evidence-based holistic nursing practice.*

Key words: nursing theory, patterns of knowing, evidence-based practice

Evidence-based practice is in the forefront of many contemporary discussions of nursing research and nursing practice. Indeed, the term "seems to be the up-and-coming buzzword for the decade" (Ingersoll, 2000, p. 151).

The current call for evidence-based nursing practice has set the debate in a conventional, atheoretical, medically dominated, empirical model of evidence, which threatens the foundation of nursing's disciplinary perspective

JOURNAL OF NURSING SCHOLARSHIP, 2001;33:2, 115–119. Copyright © 2001 Sigma Theta Tau International.

About the Authors

JACQUELINE FAWCETT received her Bachelor of Science degree from Boston University in 1964, her master's degree in parent-child nursing from New York University in 1970, and her PhD in nursing from New York University in 1976. Dr. Fawcett is currently Professor, College of Nursing and Health Sciences, University of Massachusetts-Boston. She is Professor Emerita at the University of Pennsylvania. Starting with her dissertation, Dr. Fawcett conducted a program of research dealing with wives' and husbands' pregnancy-related experiences that was derived from Martha Rogers' conceptual system. Subsequently, she undertook a program of research dealing with responses to cesarean birth derived from the Roy Adaptation Model of Nursing. A third program of research, also derived from the Roy Adaptation Model, focuses on function during normal life transitions and serious illness. Dr. Fawcett is perhaps best known for her metatheoretical work, including many journal articles and several books. Since 1996, Dr. Fawcett has lived in the midcoast region of Maine with her husband John; two Maine Coon cats, Matinicus and Acadia; and a now-tame feral cat, Lydia Dasher. She and her husband own Fawcett's Art, Antiques, and Toy Museum. She swims laps and walks on a treadmill at a fitness center for exercise and relaxation and sails on a windjammer off the Maine coast during the summer.

JEAN WATSON is Distinguished Professor of Nursing and holds the Murchinson-Scolville Chair in Caring Science at the University of Colorado Health Sciences Center (HSC). She is founder of the original Center for Human Caring and previously served as Dean of the University of Colorado HSC School of Nursing. She is a Past President of the National League for Nursing. Born in West Virginia, July 21, 1940, Dr. Watson earned undergraduate and graduate degrees in nursing and psychiatric-mental health nursing and holds her PhD in educational psychology and counseling. Dr. Watson is known for her theoretical work on the art and science of human caring. Her latest books and articles address empirical measurements of caring and new postmodern philosophies of caring and healing that bridge paradigms and point toward transformative models for the 21st century. Dr. Watson is the recipient of many awards and honors, including an international Kellogg Fellowship in Australia, a Fulbright Research Award in Sweden, five honorary doctoral degrees, the National League for Nursing's Martha E. Rogers Award, New York University's Distinguished Nurse Scholar Award, and the Fetzer Institute's Norman Cousins Award. Her hobbies include international travel, skiing, hiking, biking, and writing.

BETTY M. NEUMAN was born September 11, 1924, on a 100-acre farm near Lowell, OH. She received her nursing diploma in 1947 from what is now the Akron General Hospital; her BSN in 1957 and MS (major in mental health and community health) in 1966, both from University of California, Los Angeles. In 1985, she obtained her PhD degree in Clinical Psychology from the Pacific Western University School of Psychology in Los Angeles. Her most significant contribution is her theoretical model, the Neuman Systems Model, first published in 1972. Despite its widespread significance and application, Dr. Neuman regards her model as a work in progress. Her model has helped enhance the scientific perspective and basis of nursing and provides theoretic grounding for nursing education, research, and practice throughout the world. Dr. Neuman's hobbies include participating in the holistic health movement through her own primary prevention health regimen of walking and weight training. She is also a licensed real estate agent and continues to travel for consultations and speaking engagements.

PATRICIA HINTON WALKER is Dean and Professor of the Graduate School of Nursing at the Uniformed Services University of the Health Sciences in Bethesda, MD. Born in Kansas, she graduated with a BSN from the University of Kansas and subsequently received her master's and doctorate degrees from the University of Mississippi. Dr. Walker is a recognized scholar who has continually tried to integrate education, practice, and research through faculty practice and practice-based research. She influenced the development of faculty practices as a business and nationally focused many of her presentations and publications on the link between practice and research, particularly cost and quality outcomes research. Her focus on outcomes is exemplified through the promotion of cost and quality outcomes research linked to the practice environment and her leadership with faculties nationally and internationally for competency-based education. For recreation and fulfillment outside nursing, she plays golf, plays the piano, and enjoys creative cooking.

JOYCE J. FITZPATRICK is the Elizabeth Brooks Ford Professor of Nursing, Case Western Reserve University, Frances Payne Bolton School of Nursing, where she served as Dean from 1982 to1997. Her educational background includes a BSN from Georgetown University, an MS from The Ohio State University (psychiatric nursing), a PhD from New York University, an MBA from Case Western Reserve University, and an honorary doctorate (Doctor of Humane Letters) from Georgetown University. She has a strong and continuing interest in nursing science development, including both theory and research. She is author of more that 250 scholarly publications and author/editor of more than 30 books (having won the *American Journal of Nursing* Book of the Year award 18 times in the past 20 years), editor of the *Annual Review of Nursing Research* series (now in its 20th volume), and editor of the journal that she launched in 1989, *Applied Nursing Research*.

on theory-guided practice (Walker & Redmond, 1999). More specifically, as Ingersoll (2000) pointed out, almost all discussions of evidence-based practice are focused on the primacy of the randomized clinical trial as the only legitimate source of evidence. Furthermore, most discussions of evidence-based practice treat evidence as an atheoretical entity, which only widens the theory-practice gap (Upton, 1999). Moreover, although multiple patterns of knowing in nursing have been acknowledged at least since the publication of Carper's work in 1978, nurses have ignored this disciplinary perspective and reverted to a medical perspective of evidence when discussing evidence-based nursing practice.

The purpose of this paper is to invite readers to join in a dialogue about what constitutes the evidence for theory-guided, evidence-based nursing practice. We are initiating the dialogue by offering a comprehensive description of theoretical evidence that encompasses diverse patterns of knowing in nursing. We advance the argument that each pattern of knowing can be considered a type of theory and that the different forms of inquiry used to develop the diverse kinds of theories yield different kinds of evidence, all of which are needed for evidence-based nursing practice.

On Nursing Theories

Diverse patterns of knowing were identified by Carper (1978), who expanded the historical view of nursing as an art and a science in her classic paper, "Fundamental Patterns of Knowing in Nursing." She identified four ways or patterns of knowing in nursing: empirics, ethics, personal, and aesthetics. Carper's work is significant in that it "not only highlighted the centrality of empirically derived theoretical knowledge, but [also] recognized with equal importance and weight, knowledge gained through clinical practice" (Stein, Corte, Colling, & Whall, 1998, p. 43). Chinn and Kramer (1999) expanded Carper's work by identifying processes associated with each pattern of knowing. Their work has enhanced understanding of each pattern of knowing and has brought Carper's ideas to the attention of a wide audience of nurses.

The pattern of empirical knowing (Table 30-1) encompasses publicly verifiable, factual descriptions, explanations, and predictions based on subjective or objective group data. In other words, empirical knowing is about "averages." This pattern of knowing, which constitutes the science of nursing, is well established in nursing epistemology and methods. Empirical knowing is generated and tested by means of empirical research. The next section of this paper extends the common focus on empirics as the primary focus of evidence, and offers a new lens for considering theory-guided evidence and diverse ways of knowing that can and should be integrated into nurses' evidence-based practice initiatives.

Diverse Patterns of Knowing

In contrast to empirics, the other patterns of knowing are less established, but they are of increasing interest for the discipline of nursing in particular and for science in general. Ethical knowing, personal knowing, and aesthetic knowing are required for moral, humane, and personalized nursing practice (Stein et al., 1998). The pattern of ethical knowing (Table 30-1) encompasses descriptions of moral obligations, moral and nonmoral values, and desired ends. Ethical knowing, which constitutes the ethics of nursing, is generated by means of ethical inquiries that are focused on identification and analysis of the beliefs and values held by individuals and groups and the clarification of those beliefs and values. Ethical knowing is tested by means of ethical inquiries that focus on dialogue about beliefs and values and establishing justification for those beliefs and values.

Table 30-1
Patterns of Knowing: Types of Nursing Theories, Modes of Inquiry, and Evidence

Pattern of Knowing: Type of Nursing Theory	Description	Mode of Inquiry	Examples of Evidence
Empirics	Publicly verifiable, factual descriptions, explanations, or predictions based on subjective or objective group data; the science of nursing	Empirical research	Scientific data
Ethics	Descriptions of moral obligations, moral and nonmoral values, and desired ends; the ethics of nursing	Identification, analysis, and clarification of beliefs and values; dialogue about and justification of beliefs and values	Standards of practice, codes of ethics, philosophies of nursing
Personal	Expressions of the quality and authenticity of the interpersonal process between each nurse and each patient; the interpersonal relationships of nursing	Opening, centering, thinking, listening, and reflecting	Autobiographical stories
Aesthetics	Expressions of the nurse's perception of what is significant in an individual patient's behavior; the art and act of nursing	Envisioning possibilities, rehearsing nursing art and acts	Aesthetic criticism and works of art

The pattern of personal knowing refers to the quality and authenticity of the interpersonal process between each nurse and each patient (Table 30-1). This pattern is concerned with the knowing, encountering, and actualizing of the authentic self; it is focused on how nurses come to know how to be authentic in relationships with patients, and how nurses come to know how to express their concern and caring for other people. Personal knowing is not "knowing one's self" but rather knowing how to be authentic with others, knowing one's own "personal style" of "being with" another person. Personal knowing is what is meant by "therapeutic nurse-patient relationships." Personal knowing is developed by means of opening and centering the self to thinking about how one is or can be authentic, by listening to responses from others, and by reflecting on those thoughts and responses.

The pattern of aesthetic knowing shows the nurse's perception of what is significant in the individual patient's behavior (Table 30-1). Thus, this pattern is focused on particulars rather than universals. Aesthetic knowing also addresses the "artful" performance of manual and technical skills. Aesthetic knowing is developed by envisioning possibilities and rehearsing the art and acts of nursing, with emphasis on developing appreciation of aesthetic meanings in practice and inspiration for developing the art of nursing.

Carper (1978) and Chinn and Kramer (1999) pointed out that each pattern of knowing is an essential component of the integrated knowledge base for professional practice, and that no one pattern of knowing should be used in isolation from the others. Carper (1978) maintained that "Nursing . . . depends on the scientific knowledge of human behavior in health and in illness, the aesthetic perception of significant human experiences, a personal understanding of the unique individuality of the self and the capacity to make choices within concrete situations involving particular moral judgments" (p. 22). Elaborating, Chinn and Kramer (1999) pointed out the danger of using any one pattern exclusively. They said:

> When knowledge within any one pattern is not critically examined and integrated with the whole of

knowing, distortion instead of understanding is produced. Failure to develop knowledge integrated within all of the patterns of knowing leads to uncritical acceptance, narrow interpretation, and partial utilization of knowledge. We call this "the patterns gone wild." When this occurs, the patterns are used in isolation from one another, and the potential for synthesis of the whole is lost. (p. 12)

The current emphasis on empirical knowing as the only basis for evidence-based nursing practice is an outstanding example of a "pattern gone wild."

Patterns of Knowing as Theories

The question arises as to whether the multiple, diverse patterns of knowing can be considered sets of theories. The answer to that question depends, in part, on one's view of a pattern of knowing and a theory. A pattern of knowing can be thought of as a way of seeing a phenomenon. The English word "theory" comes from the Greek word, "theoria," which means "to see," that is, to reveal phenomena previously hidden from our awareness and attention (Watson, 1999). For the purposes of this paper, a theory is defined as a way of seeing through "a set of relatively concrete and specific concepts and the propositions that describe or link those concepts" (Fawcett, 1999, p. 4). Theories constitute much of the knowledge of a discipline. Moreover, theory and inquiry are inextricably linked. That is, theories of various phenomena are the lenses through which inquiry is conducted. The results of inquiry constitute the evidence that determines whether the theory is adequate or must be refined.

Collectively, the diverse patterns of knowing constitute the ontological and epistemological foundations of the discipline of nursing. Inasmuch as both patterns of knowing and theories represent knowledge, and are generated and tested by means of congruent, yet diverse processes of inquiry (Table 30-1), we maintain that each pattern of knowing may be regarded as a type of theory. These four types of theories are subject to different types of inquiry. Henceforth, then, we will refer to the patterns of knowing as empirical theories, ethical theories, personal theories, and aesthetic theories. Our decision to regard the patterns of knowing as types of theories is supported by Chinn and Kramer's (1999) reference to ethical theories and Chinn's (2001) articulation of a theory of the art of nursing. Other global perspectives indicate the direction of diverse patterns of knowing as types of theories. For example, Scandinavian nurses view nursing within a caring science model, and they acknowledge personal knowing, personal characteristics, and moral and aesthetic knowing of caring practices as theoretical ways of knowing that elicit diverse forms of evidence (Dahlberg, 1995, Fagerstrom & Bergdom Engberg, 1998; Kyle, 1995; Snyder, Brandt, & Tseng, 2000; von Post & Eriksson, 2000).

Furthermore, we, like some of our international colleagues, maintain that the content of ethical, personal, and aesthetic theories can be formalized as sets of concepts and propositions, just as the content of many empirical theories has been so formalized (Fawcett, 1999; von Post & Eriksson, 2000). Moreover, regarding all four patterns of knowing as types of theories reintroduces the notions of uncertainty and tentativeness that typically are associated with empirical theories (Fagerstrom & Bergdom Engberg, 1998; Morse, 1996; Polit & Hungler, 1995).

The four types of theories constitute much, if not all, of the knowledge needed for nursing practice. A potentially informative analysis, which follows from the conclusion that the patterns of knowing can be regarded as sets of theories, is the examination of extant theories to determine in which pattern of knowing each is located. That analysis is, however, beyond the scope of this paper and will not be pursued here. Rather, we are attempting to make connections between the four types of theories, representing the four patterns of knowing, and what constitutes evidence for nursing practice.

On Evidence

These four types of theories underlie all methodological decisions, and they are the basis for generating multiple forms of evidence. The question of what constitutes evidence depends, in part, on what one regards as the basis of the evidence. We maintain that theory is the reason for and the value of the evidence. In other words, evidence itself refers to evidence about theories. Similarly, theory determines what counts as evidence. Thus, theory and evidence become inextricably linked, just as theory and inquiry are inextricably linked.

Any form of evidence has to be interpreted and critiqued by each person who is considering whether the theory can be applied in a particular practice situation. This view indicates acknowledgement of diverse forms of knowing as inherent in any global or cultural interpretation of knowledge or theory (Zoucha & Reeves, 1999). The four types of theories are diverse ontological and epistemological lenses through which evidence is both interpreted and critiqued. The current emphasis on the technical-rational model of empirical evidence denies or ignores the existence of a theory lens. In contrast, our theory-guided model of evidence requires and acknowledges interpretation and critique of diverse forms of evidence. As shown in the Table, we regard the scientific data produced by empirical research as the evidence for empirical theories. We count as scientific both qualitative and quantitative data and we support the call for qualitative outcome analysis (Kyle, 1995; Morse, Penrod, & Hupcey, 2000; Snyder et al., 2000). The evidence for ethical theories is illustrated in formalized statements of nurses' values, such as standards of practice, codes of ethics, and philosophies of nursing. The evidence for personal theories is found in autobiographical stories about the genuine, authentic self. The evidence for aesthetic theories is manifested or expressed as aesthetic criticism of the art and act of nursing and through works of art, such as paintings, drawings, sculpture, poetry, fiction and nonfiction, dance, and others.

Our view of the reason for evidence differs from the prevailing discussion in the literature. In current literature, typically a procedure or intervention is presented in isolation from the theory that undergirds that procedure or intervention, and in isolation from the value of the evidence. Hence the term, "evidence-based practice." We maintain that the more appropriate term is "theory-guided, evidence-based practice" (Walker & Redmond, 1999). Given the diversity of kinds of theories needed for nursing practice (See Table 30-1), evidence must extend beyond the current emphasis on empirical research and randomized clinical trials, to the kinds of evidence also generated from ethical theories, personal theories, and aesthetic theories.

Our view of the diversity of types of theories and the type of evidence needed for each type of theory addresses, at least in part, current criticisms of the evidence-based practice movement. We agree with Mitchell (1999) that the "proponents of evidence-based practice have . . . grossly oversimplified and misrepresented the process of nursing" (p. 34). Mitchell was particularly concerned that "The notion of evidence-based practice is not only a barren possibility but also that evidence-based practice obstructs nursing process, human care, and professional accountability" (p. 30). We respond to Mitchell's concern by including evidence about personal theories, which include authenticity in nurse-patient interpersonal relationships. Moreover, Mitchell (1999) maintained that "Evidence-based practice does not support the shift to patient-centered care, and it is inconsistent with the values and interests of consumers" (p. 34). Here, we respond to Mitchell's concerns by including evidence about ethical theories, which include the values of nurses. Mitchell (1999) also was concerned that "Evidence-based practice, if taken seriously, may restrain some nurses from defining the values and theories that guide the nurse-person process" (p. 31) and relationship. This point relates to our view that the art of nursing is expressed through the nurse-person process and the evidence derived from interpretations of tests of aesthetic theories and ethical theories.

Furthermore, our view of the diversity of types of theories and corresponding types of evidence needed for theory-guided, evidence-based nursing practice elaborates Ingersoll's (2000) definition of evidence-based nursing practice. Her definition is as follows: "Evidence-based nursing practice is the conscientious, explicit, and judicious use of theory-derived, research-based information in making decisions about care delivery to individuals or groups of patients and in consideration of individual needs and preferences" (p. 152). Our view makes explicit the multiple kinds of theories—ethical, personal, aesthetic, and empirical—

whereas Ingersoll's reference to theory could easily be construed to mean only empirical theory or, perhaps, because of the reference to individual needs and preferences, to include empirical and aesthetic theories.

We maintain the appropriateness of recognizing and appreciating empirical, ethical, personal, and aesthetic theories and the corresponding critique and interpretation of the evidence about each kind of theory. Such critique and interpretation of evidence is crucial for nursing practice because it is embedded in the values and phenomena located within a broad array of nursing theories. Moreover, by recognizing the four types of theories, more nurses and other health professionals may appreciate and use theories. They may agree with us that theories and values are the starting point for the critique and interpretation of any evidence needed to support clinical practices that may enhance the quality of life of the public we serve.

Conclusions

We invite readers to expand the dialogue about theory-guided, evidence-based practice. We urge nurses everywhere to consider the implications and consequences of the current virtually exclusive emphasis on empirical theories and empirical evidence-based nursing practice. We urge our nurse colleagues throughout the world to join us and those who have accurately pointed to the limitations of viewing nursing as a strictly empirical endeavor (Bolton, 2000; Dahlberg, 1995; Fagerstrom & Bergdom Engberg, 1998; Hall, 1997; Zocha & Reeves, 1999) to consider what might be gained by recognition and development of ethical, personal, and aesthetic theories and by formalization of those kinds of theories. Accordingly, we encourage all nurses to actualize their claim of a holistic approach to practice by adopting a more comprehensive description of evidence-based nursing practice, a descriptive that allows for critique and interpretation of evidence obtained from inquiry guided by ethical, personal, aesthetic, and empirical theories, as well as by any other kinds theories that may emerge from new understandings of nursing as a human science and a professional practice discipline.

REFERENCES

Bolton, S. C. (2000). Who cares? Offering emotional work as a "gift" in the nursing labor process. *Journal of Advanced Nursing, 32,* 580–586.

Carper, B. A. (1978). Fundamental patterns of knowing in nursing. *Advances in Nursing Science, 1*(1), 13–23.

Chinn, P. L. (2001). Toward a theory of nursing art. In N. L. Chaska (Ed.), *The nursing profession: Tomorrow and beyond* (287–297). Thousand Oaks, CA: Sage.

Chinn, P. L., & Kramer, M. K. (1999). *Theory and nursing: Integrated knowledge development* (5th ed.). St. Louis, MO: Mosby.

Dahlberg, K. (1995) Qualitative methodology as Caring Science Methodology. *Scandinavian Journal of Caring Science, 9,* 187–191.

Fagerstrom, L., & Bergdom Engberg, I. (1998) Measuring the unmeasurable: A caring science perspective on patient classification. *Journal of Nursing Management, 6,* 165–172.

Fawcett, J. (1999). *The relationship of theory and research* (3rd ed.). Philadelphia: F. A. Davis.

Hall, E. O. C. (1997). Four generations of nurse theorists in the U.S.: An overview of their questions and answers. *Vard i Norden: Nursing Science and Research in the Nordic Countries, 17*(2), 15–23.

Ingersoll, G. L. (2000). Evidence-based nursing: What it is and what it isn't. *Nursing Outlook, 48,* 151–152.

Kyle, T. V. (1995) The concept of caring: A review of the literature. *Journal of Advanced Nursing, 21,* 506–514.

Mitchell, G. J. (1999). Evidence-based practice: Critique and alternative view. *Nursing Science Quarterly, 12,* 30–35.

Morse, J. M. (1996). Nursing scholarship: Sense and sensibility. *Nursing Inquiry, 3,* 74–82.

Morse, J. M., Penrod, J., & Hupcey, J. E. (2000). Qualitative outcome analysis: Evaluating nursing interventions for complex clinical phenomena. *Journal of Nursing Scholarship, 32,* 125–130.

Polit, D. F., & Hungler, B. P. (1995). *Nursing research: Principles and methods* (5th ed.). Philadelphia: Lippincott.

Snyder, M., Brandt, C. L., & Tseng, Y. (2000). Measuring intervention outcomes: Impact of nurse characteristics. *International Journal of Human Caring, 5*(3), 36–42.

Stein, K. F., Corte, C., Colling, K. B., & Whall, A. (1998). A theoretical analysis of Carper's ways of knowing using a model of social cognition. *Scholarly Inquiry for Nursing Practice, 12,* 43–60.

Upton, D. J. (1999). How can we achieve evidence-based practice if we have theory-practice gap in nursing today? *Journal of Advanced Nursing, 29,* 549–555.

von Post, I., & Eriksson, K. (2000). The ideal and practice concepts of "Professional Nursing Care." *International Journal for Human Caring, 5*(3), 14–22.

Walker, P. H., & Redmond, R. (1999). Theory-guided, evidence-based reflective practice. *Nursing Science Quarterly, 12,* 298–303.

Watson, J. (1999). *Postmodern nursing and beyond.* New York: Churchill Livingstone.

Zoucha, R., & Reeves, J. (1999). A view of professional caring as personal for Mexican Americans. *International Journal of Human Caring, 3*(3), 14–20.

The Authors Comment

On Nursing Theories and Evidence

This article was the result of a meeting convened by Patricia Hinton Walker, then Dean of the University of Colorado School of Nursing, with Jean Watson, Betty Neuman, Joyce Fitzpatrick, and me. Our task was to identify the major issues in nursing theory development. I took the lead in writing a paper that addressed the need for a comprehensive view of evidence-based nursing practice. The result was this article, the content of which we drew from the seminal work by Carper on patterns of knowing in nursing and the expansion of that work by Chinn and Kramer. If the discipline of nursing is to advance in the 21st century, nurses must acknowledge multiple types of theories and sources of evidence for theory-guided evidence-based nursing rather than rely solely on empiric theory and evidence from only controlled clinical trials.

—JACQUELINE FAWCETT
—JEAN WATSON
—BETTY M. NEUMAN
—PATRICIA HINTON WALKER
—JOYCE J. FITZPATRICK

The Discipline of Nursing

Sue K. Donaldson
Dorothy M. Crowley

When one considers the gamut of research that nurses are undertaking, all of it is clearly important to the nursing profession, but the knowledge represented by the research problems and methodologies appears to be global. By definition, however, a discipline is not global; it is characterized by a unique perspective, a distinct way of viewing all phenomena, which ultimately defines the limits and nature of its inquiry.

This is the problem that plagues all of us: identification of the essence of nursing research and of the common elements and threads that give coherence to an identifiable body of knowledge. As nurse researchers, we seem to function primarily with tacit rather than explicit knowledge of the broad conceptualizations unique to nursing. We take for granted the nursing perspective as generally accepted and understood, until explanation of the particulars is required. Moreover, nursing authors tend to emphasize speculative formulations and theoretical reflections aimed at deriving the nature of nursing rather than explicating the structure of the body of knowledge that constitutes the discipline of nursing.

Rather than expanding a disproportionate amount of effort in the quest for *the* definition of the nature of nursing, it might behoove us—at least at this time—to seek relationships and commonalities in the ideas of writers whose work has influenced (and continues to influence) tacit knowledge of the scope of the field. At least since the time of Nightingale, there has been a remarkable consistency in the recurrent themes that

About the Authors

SUE KAREN DONALDSON (nee Bolitho) was born September 16, 1943, in Detroit, MI, where she earned her baccalaureate (BSN, 1965) and master's (MSN, 1966) degrees from Wayne State University. She received her PhD in physiology and biophysics in 1973 from the University of Washington, Seattle. While a doctoral student, she participated in graduate courses offered by the School of Nursing at the University of Washington, which were a part of the federally funded Nurse Scientist Program. Dr. Donaldson is currently Professor of Physiology, School of Medicine, and Professor of Nursing, School of Nursing, Johns Hopkins University, Baltimore, MD, where she served as Dean of the School of Nursing from 1994 to 2001. Before going to Hopkins, she served on the faculties of medicine and nursing at the University of Washington (from 1973 to 1978), Rush University in Chicago (from 1978 to 1984), and the University of Minnesota in Minneapolis (from 1984 to 1994). Dr. Donaldson is internationally known for her biologic research in cardiac and skeletal muscle and as a pioneer in nursing research demonstrating the relevance of basic science to clinical care. Her accomplishments are recognized by her election to the American Academy of Nursing (FAAN) and the Institute of Medicine, National Academy of Science. She continues to publish on the progress and conceptual evolution of the discipline of and research in nursing and to mentor others in the development and conduct of programs of research.

DOROTHY M. CROWLEY was born and reared in Mitchell, SD, and received a diploma in nursing from Presentation School of Nursing in McKennan Hospital in Sioux Falls. She continued her education at St. Louis University, receiving a BS in nursing education (magna cum laude) in 1950. She then earned two graduate degrees at the Catholic University of America, an MS in nursing education (1953), and a PhD in sociology (1961). At the time of her death in 1983, Dr. Crowley was on the faculty of the University of Washington, where she had been teaching since 1965.

nurse scholars use to explain what they conceive to be the essence or the core of nursing. Three general themes for enquiry emerge:

1. *Concern with principles and laws that govern the life processes, well-being, and optimum functioning of human beings—sick or well.* For example, a concern with the discovery of laws that govern health, knowledge of reparative processes, and prevention was manifest in the late nineteenth or early twentieth century in Nightingale's writings and certainly in Rogers' concern with laws principles governing life processes in the past two decades.
2. *Concern with the patterning of human behavior in interaction with the environment in critical life situations.* As evidence of this theme, Rogers' writings reflect a concern with life rhythms and their relationship to environmental rhythms. Similarly, Johnson's writings in the 1960s focused attention on systems of behavior, pattern-maintenance, and pattern-disruption. The conceptual frames for most nursing curricula today include coping processes, adaptation, and supportive and nonsupportive environments.
3. *Concern with the processes by which positive changes in health status are affected.* Peplau addressed herself to nursing as an interpersonal process, an educative and maturing force; whereas, Kreuter as well as Leininger and others addressed the particular type of process of support system seen as nursing's unique contribution.

These themes suggest boundaries of an area for systematic enquiry and theory development with potential for making the nature of the discipline of nursing more explicit than it is at present.

Integration of nursing research from the level of a conceptual framework for a particular study to the level of more general theories and ultimately to that of a unified body of nursing knowledge has not been pursued to any large extent. Nor have there been widespread efforts on the part of those doing research in nursing to relate individual studies to one another and, thereby, build a larger context for reference. This has contributed to fragmentation of knowledge and confusion about a perspective for nursing research.

As was the case in considering different ideas about the nature and themes of nursing, however, the goal is not to identify a single theory of nursing—rather, we would advocate pluralism. Nevertheless, it would seem desirable to be able to place such theories within the context of a discipline of nursing. More explicit identification of what we are doing in nursing research is imperative if we are to truly function as nurse researchers, rather than as nurses conducting research in other disciplines, and if we are to have nursing theories for the professional practice of nursing. There is also a crucial need for identification of the structure of the discipline of nursing in our educational program. How can we justify doctoral programs in nursing if the discipline of nursing is not defined? Perhaps of even greater importance is the content of these doctoral programs. In fact, the very survival of the profession may be at risk unless the discipline is defined. As Armiger noted "there exists today an unprecedented need for identification of the uniqueness of nursing science and practice, lest overriding forces in contemporary society lead to disintegration of nursing as a distinct profession" (Arminger, 1974, pp. 160–164).

What is needed is the thinking of nurse philosophers and also some philosophizing on the part of the nurse researchers. The problem is not to devise the structure of the discipline of nursing, but to make this structure explicit. Our purpose is to make a beginning along these lines. Throughout this paper, the term "nursing" will refer to the discipline, unless otherwise clarified, and "structure" will refer to the broad conceptualizations and syntax of the discipline, rather than the theories generated within this structure.

Classification of Human Knowledge: Discipline

Traditionally, human knowledge and enquiry have been considered in the context of disciplines. Disciplines reflect true distinctions between bodies of knowledge per se and, as such, become the realm of learning. The Oxford dictionary defines disciplines as "a branch of instruction or education, a department of learning or knowledge." Institutions of higher education are organized around these branches of knowledge into colleges, schools, and departments. Typically, disciplines have evolved as a consequence of a distinct perspective and syntax, which determine what phenomena or abstractions are of interest, in what context such phenomena are to be viewed, what questions are to be raised, what methods of study are to be used, and what canons of evidence and proof are to be required.

As a result of the complex way in which disciplines evolve, disciplines can be and have been identified and organized around a variety of characteristics and combinations of characteristics. Mathematics, for example, has been viewed as distinct from all other disciplines in that its subject matter appears to have no material existence; logic has been set apart because it is concerned with the development of canons of reasoning and evidence, which are utilized in the other disciplines. Thus, it is the unique relationship of logic to the other disciplines that sets it apart, rather than a peculiarity of its subject matter, as was the case for mathematics.

In identifying disciplines and classifying them, we are dealing with the nature and structure of the whole of human knowledge. It should be kept in mind that the number and membership of the disciplines are not agreed and that there is no single accepted organization of even the well accepted disciplines. This is reflected in the diversity of organization of branches of learning in universities and colleges. The broadest classifications of disciplines depend upon a view of the inherent nature of all phenomena. A distinction on the part of the philosophers between the generality of natural phenomena and the particularity of human events leads to a distinction between such sciences as physics and sociology, which seek general laws for repeating behavior, and such disciplines as history, which focuses on unique events, or ethics, which deals with human choices and value orientations (as shown in Figure 31-1). Among the sciences themselves, the biological sciences become distinct from physics and chemistry because they deal with the recognition of the phenomena of life and with living as opposed to nonliving things.

Nursing has both scientific aspects and aspects akin to the arts. For example, human health is considered within nursing in terms of political issues and history as well as in terms of inexorable laws of health. Therefore, nursing as a discipline is broader than nursing science and its uniqueness stems from its perspective rather than its object of enquiry or methodology.

You might well ask: Why bother with pursuing this discussion, especially since there is no agreement as to a single structure of human knowledge? There are at least two reasons: First, the discipline of nursing was not created *per se solum,* but emerged within the context of the other disciplines. Therefore, we must know its relationship to other disciplines in addition to its structure. Secondly, it must be remembered that the family of disciplines, because each of its members represents knowledge derived within a particular conceptual structure, is subject to revision in the form of fu-

sion, extinction, and multiplication of its members as new conceptualizations emerge. Nursing as a discipline is also subject to change based upon changes in its structural conceptual base; in fact, nurse researchers and scholars have the responsibility of questioning and revising nursing's structure.

According to Shermis (1962), the accepted academic disciplines are all characterized by an impressive body of enduring works, suitable techniques, concerns which are significant and relevant to humans, unifying and inspiring traditions, and considerable scholarly achievements. Although these are not criteria for distinguishing disciplines from nondisciplines, they do provide a basis for acceptance of a branch of learning as a discipline.

But what of emerging disciplines? In the professional field, there typically is an evolutionary process that occurs as the field moves from a vocational level, in which the art and technology are preeminent, to the rationalization of practice and the establishment of a cognitive base for professional practice. It is important to recognize that a discipline emerges as a result of creative thinking related to significant issues. Because of the vital significance of nursing's perspective, its concern with human health and well-being, and its growth through research and scholarly work, nursing will gain full acceptance in time.

For purposes of this discussion, a distinction between academic disciplines and professional disciplines will be utilized (as illustrated in Figure 31-2). The academic disciplines include sciences such as physics, physiology, and sociology, as well as liberal arts disciplines such as mathematics, history, and philosophy. The aim of academic disciplines is to know, and their theories are descriptive in nature. In contrast, professional disciplines such as law, medicine, and nursing are directed toward practical aims and thus generate prescriptive as well as descriptive theories.

For academic disciplines, the goal is to know, regardless of whether the research is basic or applied. In fact, the distinction between applied and basic research seems appropriate only in relation to descriptive theories, since applied research answers questions

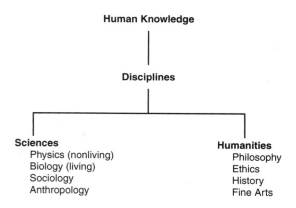

Figure 31-1 *Structuring of human knowledge.*

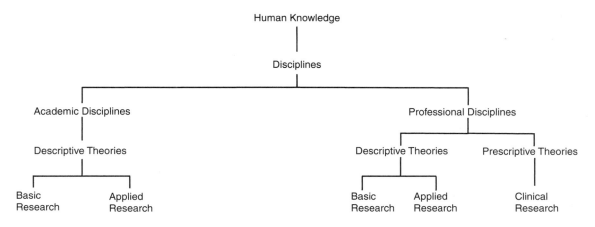

Figure 31-2 *Theories and research characteristics of academic and professional disciplines.*

related to the applicability of basic theories in practical situations, rather than questions related to *how* basic theories are to be applied. Thus, applied physicists test the practical limits of theories of physics but would not derive information as to the best design for a bridge, for example.

Fields that emphasize applied research would be more correctly termed applied disciplines, or applied branches of academic disciplines, rather than professional disciplines, which have prescriptive theories in addition to descriptive ones. The prescriptive theories characteristic of professional disciplines deal with the actual implementation of knowledge in a practical sense. As Johnson has stated " . . . professional knowledge does not consist of basic science theory which has been validated in practice" (Johnson, 1974, p. 373). In this regard, it is not correct to view professional disciplines simply as applied sciences.

Within the professional discipline there is a need "to know" and to work from descriptive theories in addition to prescriptive ones. As Gortner has pointed out, "some of the work is basic, in that it is applicable to a general understanding of human behavior or responses to illness" (Gortner, 1974, p. 765), and other studies of nursing are applied. Basic and applied re-

search are both needed in a professional discipline because each discipline has a different practical aim which influences the perspective of that field, the way it conceptualizes the relevant world, and the questions it poses for investigation. Therefore, because of the uniqueness of each discipline's perspective and the context in which knowledge from each discipline fits, it is not possible to simply "borrow" theory or knowledge from other disciplines.

Schwab (1964a) has noted that in general the statements of a given discipline are like single words of a sentence; their meanings derive more from their context than from their dictionary sense. In other words, statements of disciplines, their conclusions, are properly understood only in the context of the enquiry that produced them. They are true only in that they fit the criteria for truth in the given discipline. From this standpoint, nurse scientists may help in utilization of information from other disciplines, but this will not eliminate the need for undertaking basic research in nursing from nursing's perspective. Viewing phenomena from the perspective of healthy function of individuals in interaction with their environments will generate distinctive research at all levels and a defined, structured body of knowledge.

Even when useful information might be derived from the research of another discipline, the studies are not pursued, either because of lack of interest or because the conditions used invalidate the results for nursing's purpose. For example, a physiologist studying mechanisms underlying a given cellular process may work with intact cells but at a very low temperature, say 0°C, to slow the process down to allow measurement of its kinetic properties. The low temperature does not invalidate the physiologist's conclusions, but may make the data inappropriate in terms of knowing exact rates characteristic of the process at in vivo temperatures. Furthermore, animal and suborganismal, even subcellular, research is valid in its own right in physiology, whereas in nursing the information is ultimately being sought in relation to intact human beings.

Nursing cannot rely upon the academic disciplines to supply its requirement for knowledge of laws and processes. Rather, appropriately prepared nurse researchers must generate and test descriptive theories as necessary and develop their own technology, as has been recommended for other professionals.

Another very important issue is the extent to which each discipline is dependent upon the development of the others. The Comtian view of the sciences, which is a hierarchical one, is noteworthy in this regard, since it has influenced curricula; in turn, these curricula can lead to unwarranted views of the dependence of some disciplines on the others.

Comte held that not only human knowledge in general but also each branch of knowledge passes through states or stages of progress on its way to becoming scientific. He also conceived of the branches of knowledge as evolving in an increasingly complex organizational hierarchy ranging from the physical to the social. As a result of an arbitrary interpretation of Comte's hierarchy in curricula, physics and chemistry have been required, for example, for the mastery of biology, and so on. Although there may be increased efficiency of instruction following this plan, it should be remembered that learners influenced by such curricula may come to view all knowledge as hierarchical.

Yet hierarchical nature of knowledge has not been demonstrated; in fact acceptance of hierarchical structuring of knowledge can be very limiting and should be questioned.

In the first place, there is the danger that one conceive all knowledge of scientific quality as being encompassed by the academic disciplines, with the professions resting on these disciplines for their cognitive base. Secondly, if even the potential for professional disciplines is conceded, it is difficult for proponents of the hierarchical view to envision how professional disciplines could expand their respective bodies of knowledge independently. In contrast, professional disciplines can be viewed as emerging *along with* rather than *from* academic disciplines.

This is not to imply that disciplines are totally independent of each other. Certainly, logical formulations in one discipline cannot ignore the "truths" of the others. The quality of theories and research designs and the validity of conclusions drawn within one discipline are dependent upon their congruence with all of knowledge. Therefore, knowledge in one discipline may set constraints on or enhance the process of enquiry in another. Perhaps the most obvious interrelationship of disciplines is in their associated practice realm.

Every discipline exists in part to provide knowledge which is to be utilized and thus has an associated practice realm (Figure 31-3). Accordingly, every discipline has educators and researchers who function in this realm to impart the knowledge base to others and expand the knowledge base through research. In addition, professional disciplines have practitioners who deliver a service by engaging in professional practice in the form of clinical service, education, and research.

Sharing of knowledge from many disciplines occurs in the realm of practice associated with each discipline. For example, researchers affiliated with academic disciplines may borrow relevance or reality orientation from observations of professional practitioners and use prescriptive or practice theories from professional disciplines and practice. Similarly, professional disciplines derive knowledge from academic disciplines.

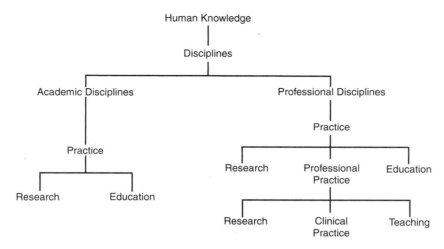

Figure 31-3 *Practice realms of disciplines.*

Relationship of the Discipline to Practice

Although the discipline and the profession are inextricably linked and greatly influence each other's substance, they must be distinguished from each other. Failure to recognize the existence of the discipline as a body of knowledge that is separate from the activities of practitioners has contributed to the fact that nursing has been viewed as a vocation rather than a profession. In turn, this has led to confusion as to whether the discipline of nursing exists.

Part of the problem in viewing a professional discipline as distinct from professional practice stems from the fact that both the discipline and practice evolved interdependently in response to societal needs; as a result, both possess a common practical aim related to these needs (Figure 31-4). Professions evolved because the service they provided was valued. Given the emphasis placed upon science and rationality in the postindustrial age, it is not surprising that there was a strong impetus for establishing a scientific and theoretical base for professional practice. The process of upgrading professional practice also entailed the establishment of closer relations between knowledge serving as the basis of professional practice and knowledge in the academic disciplines. Since the university traditionally has been the locus of development of theoretical knowledge, the professional disciplines were eventually housed there along with the academic disciplines.

The location of professional disciplines such as nursing in institutions such as universities, which are primarily concerned with human knowledge as a product rather than service, does not change the accountability of these disciplines for societal needs and the practical aim of their associated professions. As Johnson has noted, the decisions of what to study and what questions to ask necessarily have stemmed from social decisions about the profession's realm of responsibility in giving services or in clinical practice.

Florence Nightingale (1860) defined the discipline in terms of the responsibility of nursing's practitioners to promote human health based on systematic enquiry into nature's "laws of health." Part of the reason for nursing's struggle in evolving stems from the slow emergence of the recognition of its social relevance. Nurses give service related to the quality of human life; this service is only recently being valued. After all, why should quality of life be considered before biological survival can be assured?

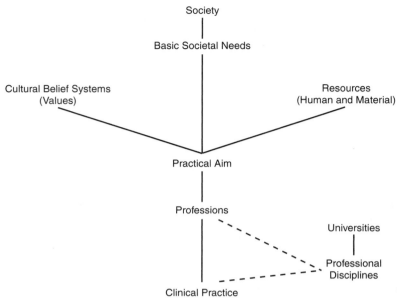

Figure 31-4 *Interdependent evolution of discipline and practice of a profession.*

Ethical and moral values inherent in clinical practice have profoundly influenced the perspective and value orientation of the discipline. Thus, nursing has traditionally valued humanitarian service. But in addition, the self-respect and self-determination of clients are to be preserved. The goal of nursing service is to foster self-caring behavior that leads to individual health and well-being. These values and goals, which are intrinsic to professional practice, have shaped the value orientation of the discipline. As a result of this value orientation, knowledge of the basis of human choices and of methods for fostering individual independence are sought, rather than knowledge of interventions that control and directly manipulate the person per se into a societally determined state of health.

The clinical practice of nursing requires the development of prescriptive theories on the part of the discipline. Much of the early research related to the nursing profession consisted of investigations about nurses, their characteristics and behavior, but these investigations could not actually be considered nursing research. In recent years, the amount of research concerned with theories fundamental to clinical practice has increased.

A key point, however, is that the discipline of nursing should be *governing* clinical practice rather than being defined by it. Of necessity, clinical practice focuses on the individual in the here and now who has a problem requiring relevant and appropriate action. The discipline, in contrast, embodies a knowledge base relevant to all realms of professional practice and which links the past, present and future. Its scope goes far beyond that required for current clinical practice. If the discipline were so narrowly defined, professional nursing could be limited to functioning in the realm of disaster relief rather than serving as a force in the promotion of world health. This is not meant to diminish the importance of problems encountered by nurses in current clinical practice. These problems deserve attention, but they are not the only concern of the discipline.

Part of the problem is that "clinical practice" is too often used synonymously with "professional practice," and clinical practice is narrowly defined. Professional competency goes beyond that required for delivery of health care to individuals, preparation of future practitioners, and conduct of systematic enquiry. For example McGlothlin (1960) believes that competency includes the need on the part of professionals for social understanding of sufficient breadth to place the practice in the context of society and the need for leadership skills.

Some of the knowledge required for achieving these competencies can only come from the discipline of nursing. Prescriptive theories essential to clinical practice and the appropriate design of nursing research can only be derived from the discipline of nursing. Similarly, although knowledge from political science, history, philosophy, and other disciplines is very important for social understanding, the professional nurse cannot put nursing into a societal context without knowledge derived from the discipline of nursing. This knowledge is obtained in part from nurse philosophers and nurse historians who view nursing as it relates to other disciplines and can articulate how nursing's heritage relates to its perspective. The discipline of nursing must also provide essential components of the knowledge base for preparation of world leaders in the field of health.

The need for philosophical, historical, and similar types of enquiry within the discipline of nursing is crucial not only in terms of providing the knowledge base for professional preparation but also for the development of the discipline. It must be remembered that the discipline is defined by social relevance and value orientations rather than by empirical truths. Thus, the discipline and profession must be continually reevaluated in terms of societal needs and scientific discoveries. Similarly, the entire structure of the discipline may need to be revamped in time, and this should be done by nurse researchers.

For this reason we have been very careful not to equate the discipline of nursing with the science of nursing. As mentioned earlier, only part of nursing employs scientific method. We need doctoral preparation for nurse historians as well as nurse scientists. As Schlotfeldt has pointed out "nursing faculties rarely have among their members scholars who are concerned with establishing the history of nursing science and with identifying the philosophies or conceptualizations of nursing that have influenced the structure of that knowledge at various times in nursing's history"

(Schlotfeldt, 1977, p. 8). Once again, the purpose in having nurse philosophers and historians is not to duplicate the efforts of other disciplines, but rather to provide these approaches from the perspective of nursing.

It should be remembered that although nursing requires researchers and scholars who utilize a variety of approaches, all research that is important to the profession of nursing is not derived from the discipline of nursing. Only information and theories stemming from nursing's perspective come from nursing per se. Nursing educators utilize information and theories from education. Even clinical practice should not be viewed as being grounded solely in the discipline of nursing.

In delivering health care, practitioners must in fact draw from many disciplines, such as business administration, medicine, education, and basic sciences. Rarely, if ever, does the skilled clinician rely only on knowledge from one discipline or even rely solely on scientific knowledge. Clinical practice is always to some extent empirical, pragmatic, intuitive, and artistic.

Once we agree that the discipline of nursing does not have to embody all, the entire whole, of knowledge utilized by the profession of nursing, then we can begin to define the discipline. Nursing is not global in its subject matter and therefore does not subsume part of any other disciplines—for example, education—just because practitioners are educated. Similarly, studies of higher education in nursing that deal with the educational process are not nursing research but educational research. In contrast, a study of the effects of educational techniques on clients' achievement of self-care is within nursing per se. Even though nursing care delivery is greatly affected by attitudes of nurses administration policies, such problems may be studied appropriately in other disciplines.

The purpose in excluding some research from nursing is not to create a ranking of importance or prestige, but rather to make the essence of nursing explicit. Nurses who conduct administrative or educational research may contribute as much to the professional practice of nursing as nurses who conduct nursing research.

In summary, the discipline and clinical practice of nursing share a common social relevance and practical aim. However, the discipline, which is a body of knowledge, must not be confused with its associated practice realm, which embodies the processes of conducting research, giving service, and educating. Furthermore, some members of the profession must engage in enquiry that is not immediately applicable to current clinical practice. As a branch of knowledge, the discipline embodies more than the science of nursing and requires researchers who employ a variety of approaches from nursing's perspective. Although the discipline provides crucial and unique content for nurse researchers, clinicians, and educators, these practitioners draw on many disciplines. Appropriately prepared nurses may elect to conduct research within other disciplines because of the critical importance of this non-nursing research to professional practice or the growth of the discipline.

Structure of the Discipline of Nursing

We are now at the point of examining the structure of the discipline. According to Schwab (1964a), disciplines have both substantive and syntactical structures. The substantive structure is composed of conceptualizations which are borrowed or invented, but their inclusion is always based on their fit with the perspective of the discipline. The syntax of a discipline refers to the research methodologies and criteria used to justify the acceptance of statements as true within the discipline (See Figure 31-5).

We have incorporated the syntax of nursing as value systems (both of science and of professional ethics) and research constraints. Such constraints include consideration of accessibility of controls, congruity with existing knowledge, manifest and latent consequences, and technological feasibility. Both values and constraints influence theory generation and actual research design. In effect, they function to ensure that enquiry will result in conclusions and statements that are appropriate, reliable, and valid for the purpose of the discipline.

Thus, the substantive structure determines primarily the scope and subject of enquiry (what is of interest), and the syntactical structure determines primarily the procedure for conducting research and criteria for acceptability of findings as truth. The findings generated by enquiry are then incorporated into the structure as concepts, theories, and facts—the statements of the discipline. In this paper, we have focused upon the structural conceptualizations, but it should be remembered that the syntax of the discipline is also important, since the syntax determines the extent to which the truth of

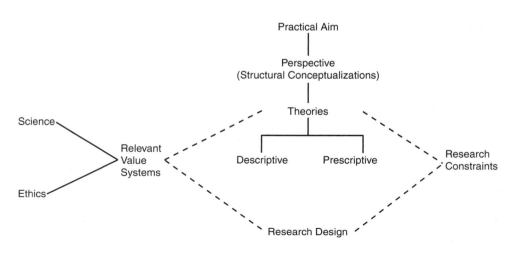

Figure 31-5 *Structure of a professional discipline.*

statements of the discipline is warranted. In contrast, the substantive structure relates to the subject matter of the enquiry. The structural conceptualizations are selected for inclusion in a given discipline with its perspective as a screen.

From its perspective, nursing studies the wholeness or health of humans, recognizing that humans are in continuous interaction with their environments. Nursing's perspective evolves from the practical aim of optimizing of human environments for health. Examples of major conceptualizations in nursing deal with:

1. Distinctions between human and nonhuman beings
2. Distinctions between living and nonliving
3. Nature of environments and humans-environmental interactions from cellular to societal levels
4. Illness versus health and well-being
5. Functioning of the whole human organism versus functioning of the parts
6. Levels of functioning of whole organisms
7. Human characteristics and natural processes, such as consciousness; abstraction; adaptation and healing; growth; change; self-determination; development; aging; dying; reproducing; drive satisfaction; and relating.

The structural conceptions are being utilized, but they are usually not identified or clarified, and rarely questioned. It is important, for example, to know whether health is viewed, in the context of a given theory or design, as a specific state, or as it is defined by each individual.

Depending upon the particular structural conceptualizations utilized, or combinations of them, widely different theories are proposed for testing. Such variation in theories does not lead to different bodies of knowledge, but to different aspects of a single body.

Pluralism of theories promotes productivity; in fact, without testing of a wide variety of theories, progress towards "truth" cannot be made. In physiology, for example, where knowledge of the functions and nature of vital processes of living organisms is sought, a pluralism of theories exists. Many physiologists conceive the functioning of the organism as explainable in

terms of the functioning of its parts, whereas others propose an explanation utilizing a conception that the whole is more than the sum of its parts. This dual approach is very useful, regardless of the correctness of the theories, since testable theories are generated that yield empirical evidence related to knowledge of the nature of and mechanisms underlying behavior of living systems. The goal in generating theories is not just to propose an all encompassing theory but to provide testable theories.

Research designed to test hypotheses stemming from theories is very important to the discipline and practitioners when the relationship of nursing theories to the structure of the discipline is explicit. This is the type of research that is easily identified as nursing research. Schwab (1964b) calls this stable enquiry, in that there is no hesitation about what questions to ask or what structural conceptualizations to employ. For example if the current principles of physiology are organ and function, the researcher engaged in stable enquiry discovers the function of one organ after another.

This type of stable research tends to be the most rewarded, but there is another very important realm of enquiry which must be expanded. We refer to questions relating to the structural conceptualizations and value orientations of the discipline. For example, what is the nature of health? Is health on a continuum with illness? Is health for every person a reasonable goal for society?

At least two major benefits are derived from this second type of research. First the structural conceptualizations are clarified or altered to make them consistent with reality. They should not be accepted as givens. Secondly, the discipline will be continually shaped according to significant themes, those which are of vital significance to man. If nurse researchers are to provide the knowledge base for societal directions in relation to health, they must engage in this type of research.

For the continued growth, significance, and utility of the discipline of nursing, researchers must place their research within the context of the discipline. Theories must also be viewed in terms of the basic structural conceptualizations of the discipline. The responsibility for revising and clarifying the structural conceptions, the very framework, of the discipline of nursing rests with nurse researchers. This means lessening our preoccupation with the process of nursing and pedagogy and placing emphasis on content as substance.

REFERENCES

Armiger, B. (1974). Scholarship in nursing. *Nursing Outlook, 22,* 160–164.

Gortner, S. R. (1974). Scientific accountability in nursing. *Nursing Outlook, 22,* 764–768.

Johnson, D. E. (1974). Development of theory: A requisite for nursing as a primary health profession. *Nursing Research, 23,* 372–377.

McGlothlin, W. J. (1960). *Patterns of professional education.* New York: G. P. Putnam's Sons.

Nightingale, F. (1860). *Notes on nursing: What it is and what it is not.* London: Harrison.

Schlotfeldt, R. M. (1977). Nursing research: Reflection of values. *Nursing Research, 26,* 4–9.

Schwab, J. (1964a). Structure of the disciplines: Meanings and significances. In G. W. Ford & L. Pugno (Eds.), *The structure of knowledge and the curriculum.* Chicago: Rand McNally.

Schwab, J. (1964b). The structure of the natural sciences. In G. W. Ford & L. Pugno (Eds.), *The structure of knowledge and the curriculum.* Chicago: Rand McNally.

Shermis, S. (1962). On becoming an intellectual discipline. *Phi Delta Kappan, 44,* 84–86.

The Author Comments

The Discipline of Nursing

Dr. Dorothy Crowley and I began having philosophic discussions about the nature of science and research in nursing when I was a doctoral student. These discourses continued after I joined her as a faculty member of the School of Nursing at the University of Washington. Our intellectual work at that time was primarily to inform each other, sharing our biologic and behavioral science perspectives. It was distinct from our work on the task force that was planning the PhD Program in Nursing. At the point in our discussions at which we had reached a broad definition of the discipline and science of nursing, I was invited to participate in the organization of the research abstracts for the 1977 Western Council on Higher Education for Nursing (WCHEN) Tenth Communicating Nursing Research Conference, where I "tested" our conceptualization by using it to organize the meeting sessions. The planning committee for the 1977 WCHEN conference was sufficiently impressed and invited Dr. Crowley and me to present the keynote address for the meeting entitled "Discipline of Nursing: Structure and Relationship to Practice." The article is almost the same as the keynote address that I delivered, coauthored with Dr. Crowley, and published first in *Communicating Nursing Research* (1977) and then in *Nursing Outlook* (1978). The article presented the first conceptualization of the discipline of nursing as distinct from the profession and practice, which identified its boundaries and placed it among the other established disciplines. Central to this conceptualization were the identification of three themes of inquiry and the research perspective, which can be applied to the study of health of individual humans or groups. Nursing theories are formulated within the discipline of nursing. Because the three themes of inquiry identified in this article have endured, evolving theories in nursing are expected to relate directly to one or more of them.

—SUE KAREN DONALDSON

CHAPTER 32

Philosophical Sources of Nursing Theory

Barbara Sarter

This article analyzes the philosophical roots of four contemporary nursing theories: Rogers' science of unitary human beings, Newman's theory of expanding consciousness, Watson's theory of caring, and Parse's theory of man-living-health. It is shown that these theories share many common philosophical views, but also maintain some significant differences. With the purpose of contributing to the development of a single metaparadigm for nursing, the following commonly shared themes are identified as forming an appropriate philosophical foundation for the discipline: process, evolution of consciousness, self-transcendence, open systems, harmony, relativity of space-time, pattern, and holism. Views of causality show some divergence between Watson and the other three theorists. Also of particular interest is the finding that Eastern philosophy has provided an important influence, both direct and indirect, on nursing theory. It is recommended that further philosophical exploration of Indian and Chinese world views be conducted and that the above metaparadigmatic themes be more fully developed in future nursing theory development.

As nursing begins to establish its power as a human science, it becomes increasingly important that its philosophical foundation be firmly established. The purpose of this article is to examine the philosophical roots of four contemporary nursing theories and frameworks, to describe their common philosophical themes, and to suggest future lines for theory development on the basis of these themes. The theories and frameworks to be analyzed are Rogers' science of unitary human beings, Newman's theory of expanding consciousness, Watson's

About the Author

BARBARA SARTER was born at Moses Lake Air Force Base near Soap Lake, WA, 1 of 7 children. A passion for synthesis of the humanities and sciences has characterized her education and scholarship. She took honors English and honors chemistry in high school, began college as a premedicine/biology major, then switched her major to English literature because she could not thrive away from the humanities. At New York University, she was thrilled to find that she could pursue philosophic research for her doctorate in nursing. For the last 20 years at the University of Southern California, she has pursued a scholarship of synthesis; this culminated in 2000 with the publication of her book *Evolutionary Healing*, which she considers to be her key contribution to the nursing discipline. She has lived for nearly 30 years with a family of friends who share the same teacher and path of spiritual evolution, and her hobbies include reading biographies of great scientists and listening to classical music.

theory of human care, and Parse's theory of man-living-health. These theories share many common themes and perspectives, yet also maintain some significant differences, both of which will help to clarify their philosophical stances.

The distinction between philosophy and theory is one that has been blurred in the theoretical works of nursing scholars. In fact, some nursing scholars have argued that many of nursing's "theories" are actually "philosophies" (Uys, 1987). It is true that nursing theories are laden with philosophical assumptions which are not always explicitly acknowledged. Hutchison (1977) describes the difference between scientific theory and philosophy as involving the scope of intellectual activity. Whereas scientific theory involves a definite, delineated domain, philosophical thinking deals with unlimited totality, the entire universe. With this distinction in mind, one can argue that nursing's intellectual activity is not only the development of scientific theories, but also the development of a philosophical foundation to place its theories within a larger context.

As part of the structure of a discipline, a philosophical foundation forms the *metaparadigm* of the discipline and ideally should be shared by all its members (Donaldson & Crowley, 1978; Fawcett, 1984). Nursing scholars must develop a metaparadigm that can support a variety of nursing theories, while maintaining a coherent and common philosophical orientation. In the following analysis of the philosophical sources of four major nursing theories, one of the ultimate goals will be to contribute to the development of this metaparadigm for nursing.

Rogers's Science

Rogers's (1970, 1980, 1983, 1986) science of unitary human beings, the oldest and most influential of the four theories to be examined, is an appropriate starting point. Perhaps one of the reasons why Rogers's theory has drawn so much attention and stimulated so much debate is because it appears to be nursing's first attempt to philosophize on a grand scale. Rogerian science attempts to describe the entire universe, while focusing in depth on unitary man within that universe.

A review of Rogers's references and bibliographies is an inspiration to proponents of liberal education. A number of philosophers and scientists have provided important influences on her theoretical formulations. Among the most dominant of the philosophical influences are Ludwig von Bertalanffy, Pierre Teilhard de Chardin, Bertrand Russell, and Michael Polanyi. Scientific theorists have also had a significant influence on Rogers' work. Although they will not be included in this discussion, the ideas of Kurt Lewin, Theodosius Dobzhansky, and Albert Einstein should be acknowledged in this regard.

Ludwig Von Bertalanffy's (1968) rejection of reductionism in favor of a systems view of the world provides an important foundation for Rogerian science. The holistic approach espoused by von Bertalanffy was one of the earliest to receive wide recognition. Von Bertalanffy maintains that macroscopic organizational laws occur and need explanation. He also proposes an evolutionary view of living systems, arguing that there is a negentropic trend in nature, due to the fact that nature consists of open systems. This trend implies that there are innate principles of self-organization in the evolutionary process.

The Rogerian view of open systems in a process of negentropic unfolding is virtually identical with Von Bertalanffy's. Although the language of negentropy has decreased in her later writings, the concept still holds a pivotal place in the theory, since openness remains one of the foundational concepts of the theory. Open systems, by definition, are negentropic (Sarter, 1987). Von Bertalanffy is not the only theorist to have proposed the concept of open systems and in fact is relatively cautious in his use of the term, limiting it to living organisms, whereas Rogers maintains that there are only open systems and that the universe itself is an open system.

Bertrand Russell, one of the great modern empiricists, appears to also have had a significant influence on Rogers, specifically in the development of her view of noncausality. Russell points out that modern science does not support a law of causality; it merely makes an assumption regarding the uniformity of nature. "The principle 'same cause, same effect,' which philosophers imagine to be vital to science, is therefore utterly otiose" (Russell, 1964, p. 182). Russell identifies a number of philosophical fallacies about causation:

- Cause and effect must more or less resemble each other.
- Cause is analogous to volition.
- The cause compels the effect (but not vice versa).
- A cause cannot operate when it has ceased to exist.
- A cause cannot operate except where it is (Russell, 1964, p. 183).

He also explains that the traditional view of cause and effect is based on a simplified version of an isolated system, not on naturally occurring systems. Russell's careful analysis of causality is not duplicated in Rogers's work, but she accepts his conclusion that traditional views of causation are invalid, maintaining that change is continuously innovative.

Pierre Teilhard de Chardin's view of evolution supports a number of central themes in Rogerian theory. This philosopher is cited by Rogers repeatedly (Rogers, 1970). Teilhard de Chardin views human beings, as well as other evolutes, as centers of conscious energy that are organized into ever more complex and integrated wholes. Energy being inherently conscious at all levels of existence, the evolutionary process consists of an increasing personalization that is ultimately self-transcending into a mystical unity with all. Human self-awareness is a critical point in evolution, when complexity and consciousness become so centered that an entirely new order of experience and understanding emerges (Teilhard de Chardin, 1965, 1969, 1970).

Clearly, Rogers's early theme of an evolutionary trend toward increasing complexity, differentiation, and heterogeneity must have been influenced by Teilhard de Chardin's philosophy. Although she has dropped her characterization of evolution as moving toward increasing complexity and heterogeneity, this trend is implicit in the concept of an open system, as discussed above. Teilhard de Chardin's holism is another important aspect of his work that may have had an influence on Roger's early theoretical formulations. Teilhard de Chardin's holism is epistemological as well as metaphysical, as is Rogers's. All forms of experience, from sensory to mystical, objective and subjective, are accepted as legitimate sources of knowledge. This is what is meant by epistemological holism. Metaphysically, the primary units of existence are irreducible wholes; consciousness is not a separate aspect but innate in the very substance of the universe, and each evolving unit is coextensive with the entire universe, all knit into one grand unity. Such a view is virtually identical to that presented by Rogers, although she avoids use of the word *consciousness* in favor of *sentience*.

Michael Polanyi's discussion of personal knowledge was also a significant force in the development of Rogers's framework. Polanyi explores the "tacit coefficient" of scientific knowledge, which involves the elements of personal judgment, decision making, intuition, and discerning the Gestalt of a phenomenon or theory. In emphasizing the role of the tacit coefficient or personal knowledge in the development of scientific theory, Polanyi comments that "apart from meaningless sense-impressions there is no experience that abides as a 'fact' without an element of valid interpretation of events . . . " (Polanyi, 1946, p. 89). In turn, the interpretation of objective experience involves a weighing of alternative theories that is dependent on the mental satisfaction of the theorist. Verification of theory, then, involves intuition.

Rogers quotes Polanyi when commenting on the relationship between theory and practice: "Almost every major systematic error which has deluded men for thousands of years relied on practical experience" (Polanyi, 1958, p. 183). Her discussion of an epistemology for nursing science emphasizes the synthesis of objective and subjective data. One can also speculate that Polanyi's influence may have been operating in the development of Rogers's view of four-dimensionality, in which the importance of subjective awareness is held paramount. In summarizing the influence of Russell and Polanyi on Rogerian science, it may be said that they appear to have been important resources for the development of Rogers's epistemological views. In contrast, Teilhard de Chardin and von Bertalanffy contributed more directly to the actual content of the framework in relation to concepts, propositions, and world view.

Although a complete synopsis of each of the theories under consideration is beyond the scope of this article, it will be appropriate to summarize the key philosophical themes of each theory and the philosophers who influenced these themes. Holism, process, four-dimensionality, evolution, energy fields, openness, non-causality, and pattern are the major philosophical threads of Rogers' theory, and the above discussion has pointed to their probable sources. Von Bertalanffy has discussed extensively the concept of openness. Teilhard de Chardin's work shows links to Rogers's conceptions of evolution, holism, process, and energy fields. Polanyi appears to have directly contributed to the concept of four-dimensionality, and Russell played an important and acknowledged role in the perspective on non-causality.

The key concept of pattern has received increasing emphasis in Rogers's later writings. There does not appear to be a single philosopher who had a particular influence on the development of this concept, although, at the same time that Rogers's thinking was focusing on pattern, there were a number of scientist-philosophers who were developing similar perspectives, such as Capra, Bohm, Pribram, Prigogine, and Bateson (Malinski, 1986). Rogers is familiar with all of these thinkers, and undoubtedly their influence has been important.

Newman's Theory

Newman's (1986) theory of expanding consciousness has strong connections with Rogers's science of unitary human beings. Newman was a graduate student at New York University and acknowledges openly the strong influence of Rogerian science on the development of her own theory of health. Rather than describing the individual as a human energy field, Newman defines a person as a unique pattern of consciousness within a field of absolute consciousness. The critical change from Rogerian science to Newman's theory is the attribution of consciousness to all matter/energy. This is an implied assumption in Rogers's theory (Sarter, 1987), but Newman has made it the foundation of her work. Evolution, then, becomes a process of expanding consciousness.

Newman explicitly acknowledges the direct influence of Teilhard de Chardin, Bentov, Bohm, Young, and Moss on the development of her theory. Of these, the contributions of philosophers Teilhard de Chardin, Bohm, and Young will be examined here. In Newman's theory, Teilhard de Chardin's view of an evolution of complexity/consciousness remains intact, as well as Teilhard de Chardin's belief that the higher stages of evolution involve an expansion of consciousness toward unity with the entire universe. Newman sounds remarkably like Teilhard de Chardin when she explains that evolution is toward higher levels of consciousness and that persons are centers of energy within an overall pattern of expanding consciousness. The continuation of consciousness after death as part of a universal consciousness is explicitly identified as an idea from the work of Teilhard de Chardin, which confirmed Newman's own personal belief and became incorporated into her theory.

Physicist-philosopher Bohm's theory of the implicate order has contributed to the development of Newman's conception of pattern in the universe as a whole. According to Bohm (1980), the metaphysical ground of being is a multidimensional pattern, unseen, yet generating the explicate, or seen, world. Bohm also rejects mind/matter dualism, viewing them as different aspects of a higher dimensional, implicate order. From this theory is derived Newman's view of health as the visible manifestation of the unseen pattern of person-environment. Bohm's philosophy also supports Newman's holism. The implicate order is a total undivided pattern. Pattern recognition, the basis of nursing intervention, is "moving from looking at parts to looking at patterns. The pattern is information that depicts the whole, understanding of the meaning of all the relationships at once" (Newman, 1986, p. 13). Newman speaks of a holism similar to Rogers's in which not only the individual is an irreducible whole, but ultimately, the entire universe is an indivisible unity. Newman also attributes her view of movement as a manifestation of consciousness to Bohm's description of movement as the immediate experience of the implicate order.

Arthur Young (1976a, 1976b) has had perhaps the most significant influence on the development of Newman's theory, in the sense that Newman's specific delineation of the process of evolution is derived from Young's complex and creative synthesis of science and philosophy. Young's work has the stated purpose of developing a theory of the evolution of the universe that can accommodate and explain the numerous examples of higher consciousness documented in human history. Young maintains that the universe is a process that is put in motion by purpose, developing in seven stages, each of which manifests a new power. A diagram of the arc of process illustrates that the emergence of life marks a turning point. The early stages of evolution are characterized by increasing constraint as light becomes substance. From the emergence of life onward, the process is marked by the conquest of constraint and the development of controlled freedom, as opposed to the random freedom of atomic particles. Einstein's theory of relativity, Bertrand Russell's mythic cosmology, Plato, Pythagoras, and Eastern mystical philosophy are Young's acknowledged sources.

Newman applies the principles of Young's arc of process to develop her theory of expanding consciousness. This is an attempt to synthesize her insights regarding movement as an integrating force and the transcendence of space and time through the expansion of consciousness. Young's seven substages of human evolution are incorporated into Newman's theory of expanding consciousness. Her summary statement of this theory is as follows: "We come into being from a state of potential consciousness, are bound in time, find our identity in space, and through movement learn the 'law' of the way things work and make choices that ultimately take us beyond space and time to a state of absolute consciousness" (Newman, 1986, p. 46). Newman equates absolute consciousness with love.

Moss (1981) is also credited by Newman as having been influential in the development of her theory. Moss is a physician, not a philosopher, but his work can be placed within the same tradition as Young and Teilhard de Chardin, process philosophy and mysticism. Moss's focus as a physician is on the personal transformation of consciousness that can occur during illness.

To summarize, the key themes of Newman's theory are pattern, expanding consciousness, movement, process, evolution, space, and time. The concept of pattern was influenced primarily by Bohm. Teilhard de Chardin was influential in the conceptualizations of expanding consciousness, process, and evolution. Young was an especially strong force in the integration of the concepts of space, time, and movement into a theory of the evolution of consciousness. The roots of these philosophers, in turn, are in relative and quantum theory, mysticism, and early Greek and Eastern philosophy.

Watson's Theory

Watson (1985) presents perhaps the most philosophically complex of current nursing theories. She is the only nursing theorist to explicitly support the concept of soul and to emphasize the spiritual dimension of human existence. Watson states that her philosophical orientation is existential-phenomenological, spiritual, and based in part upon Eastern philosophy. Watson also draws substantially from the schools of humanistic, existential, and transpersonal psychology. Specific philosophers acknowledged as sources by Watson are Hegel, Marcel, Whitehead, Kierkegaard, and Teilhard de Chardin.

At several points, Watson lists her assumptions, basic beliefs, and value. She assigns special importance in human existence to the soul. Synonyms such as spirit, inner self, and essence are also used for soul. The characteristics of the soul that she identifies are self-awareness, higher and greater degrees of consciousness, inner strength, power, intuitive and mystical experience, and continuation beyond physical death. This conception of soul is characteristic of certain Eastern philosophies, although to generically name the East as a source is meaningless, as Eastern philosophy encompasses the entire range of human thought from materialism to spiritualism. The only specific reference to Eastern philosophy is a book on the *Abhidhamma,* one of the three original Canons of Buddhist thought, which does not uphold the soul or the self as "real" entity (Robinson & Johnson, 1977). Watson's view of soul is actually more similar to Hindu philosophy, in which the inner self (atman), or soul, endures through thousands of incarnations and merges into the Divine when liberation is attained. Teilhard de Chardin may also have been an influence on these ideas, although his view is less dualistic than Watson's appears to be.

The issue of Watson's dualism is an important one, for it sets her apart philosophically from the other three theorists under consideration. Body, mind, and soul are clearly distinguished from each other and assigned different functions and qualities. Soul is held to be the most powerful force in human existence, being the source of each individual's innate striving toward self-transcendence, or actualization of one's spiritual essence. This separation of soul and mind from body seems to create a dualistic stance. However, Watson would undoubtedly describe herself as holistic in the sense that harmony among the three spheres of body, mind, and soul is held to be the highest form of health and the goal of nursing care.

Another form of dualistic expression occurs in Watson's distinction between subjective and objective experience. In fact, whenever Watson speaks of harmony among various aspects of human life, there is an implicit dualism. The harmony that is identified as desirable includes person/world, perceived self/actual experience of self, actual self/ideal self, person/other, and person/nature. Another particularly significant dichotomy is that between health and illness. Health is harmony; illness is turmoil, or disharmony. Illness may lead to disease in the traditional sense of the word.

Watson's view of time differs from that of Rogers. Rather than rejecting the reality of past, present, and future, that is, rejecting the concept of time altogether, Watson describes them as different modes of being that merge and fuse in human subjective experience. Watson acknowledges the reality of time when describing how each person's causal past and presentational immediacy has the potential to influence the future. Time, however, is transcended in subjective experience. Causality is implicitly accepted as a relational mode in Watson's theory, as can be seen in the expression causal past and in the proposition that a troubled inner soul can lead to illness, which can produce disease.

A strong theme in Watson's theory is that of spiritual evolution, at both the individual and societal levels. Self-transcendence and transcendence of space and time in higher consciousness and mystical experience are held to be indicators of spiritual evolution. The basic inner striving of each person is to fulfill one's evolutionary potential "and in the highest sense, to become more Godlike" (Watson, 1985, p. 57). The evolution of civilizations is not characterized, but is referred to in statements describing the East as more spiritually evolved than the West. Of the philosophical sources acknowledged by Watson, Teilhard de Chardin appears to be the closest to Watson's view of evolution. Hegel as well as Whitehead also deal with the evolution of consciousness, but Hegel views self-consciousness and reason as the highest manifestations of consciousness. Again, it appears that Vedic and Hindu philosophy are indirect sources of Watson's view of evolution, through their influence on popular holistic views.

From the writings of Whitehead (1960), Watson has made an interesting adaptation of the concept of an actual occasion. An actual occasion is the fundamental ontological unit of Whitehead's metaphysics. An individual person or object is a succession of actual occasions, which are characterized by emotion, purpose, valuation, and causation. Every actual occasion is a process of becoming, which perishes once its subjective aim is accomplished. When it perishes, it becomes a datum of consciousness for successive actual occasions. Watson defines her concept of an actual caring occasion (or "event") as "two persons together with their unique life histories and phenomenal field in a human care transaction" (Watson, 1985, p. 58). Although Watson does not further develop this concept along Whitehead's metaphysical lines, her use of the term appears to be an attempt to capture the immediacy and subjectivity of a caring interaction.

Additional key concepts in Watson's theory are person, self, and phenomenal field. Here the influence of Buddhist psychology can be seen. Although there are several distinctive schools of Buddhist thought, some common beliefs are the doctrine of momentariness and the illusion of a permanent self (Hiriyanna, 1949). The person is a being-in-the-world, the experiencing and perceiving organism consisting of three spheres, body, mind, and soul. The self is a process, a perceptual/conceptual Gestalt. The phenomenal field is the subjective reality or individual frame of reference of the person. Implicit in all of these concepts is the idea of process, change, and impermanence. Watson does support the idea of a (more or less) permanent soul. In this her

views come closest to those expressed in the *Bhagavadgita,* the most eloquent expression of Upanishadic and early Hindu thought and the most widely read spiritual treatise in the world. The influence of existentialist philosophers can be seen in connection with the ideas of being-in-the-world and phenomenal field.

To summarize, the key philosophical elements of the theory are soul, dualism, harmony, causality and time, spiritual evolution and self-transcendence, actual caring occasion, and self. Watson's conception of soul appears to be most similar to Teilhard de Chardin's and even more similar to that of Hindu philosophy (Sankhya-Yoga) as expressed in the *Bhagavadgita.* Her dualism of soul and body as well as mind and body, again, is most similar to that expressed in the *Bhagavadgita* and texts of the Sankhya-Yoga system of Indian philosophy (Hiriyanna, 1949). The concept of harmony among body, mind, and soul is not attributable to any of the philosophies that serve as sources for Watson; however, it is a commonly used term in popular holistic health views and may be indirectly derived from some Eastern source such as Taoism. Watson's view of causality and time is not traceable to a particular source but appears to be consistent with her stated influence from existentialist philosophy. The perspective on spiritual evolution and self-transcendence, as stated above, appears to be derived from Teilhard de Chardin and Hindu philosophy, which in turn have influenced the transpersonal psychology movement in the West. And, again as indicated above, the concepts of actual caring occasion and self are derived from Whitehead and Buddhist philosophy, respectively.

Parse's Theory

Parse (1981) has constructed a theory of nursing that is probably most explicit in acknowledging its philosophical sources. Parse shows how she has derived her work from her sources. Her creative synthesis of concepts justifies the characterization of her theory for nursing as unique. Parse's acknowledged sources are Rogers and existentialist philosophers Martin Heidegger, Jean-Paul Sartre, and Maurice Merleau-Ponty.

From Rogers, Parse has drawn from the principles of helicy, integrality, and resonancy and the four concepts of energy field, openness, pattern, and four-dimensionality. All nine of Parse's listed assumptions incorporate at least one of the elements from Rogerian theory in a synthesis with at least one of the existential tenets or concepts. It is assumed that the reader is familiar enough with the elements of Roger's theory that the focus here may turn to existentialism.

The primary concern of the existentialist philosophers is human existence. The human situation is the source of their basic metaphysical categories, the rationale being that this is the aspect of reality that can be understood most fully. The basic question to be answered by the existentialist is "Who am I?" Kierkegaard and Nietzsche were the most influential sources of existentialist thought, which in turn become a fully developed philosophy through the works of Heidegger, Karl Jaspers, Sartre, Albert Camus, Martin Buber, and Paul Tillich. Edmund Husserl has been closely associated with existentialist philosophy through his development of phenomenological philosophy. Husserl focused on the nature of human consciousness, which he characterized as exhibiting intentionality, or objective reference; in other words, the mind is always actively encountering the world. Parse explicitly refers to Husserl's contribution to her work (Parse, 1981, p. 5).

Hutchison (1977) identifies the common themes that are expressed by existentialist writers. The distinction between essence and existence is the defining feature of this philosophy. In man, existence precedes essence; in other words, he knows *that* he is, but not *what* he is. In exploring the nature of man, the qualities of freedom, self-awareness, and self-transcendence are emphasized. Freedom means here man's self-determination, which is realized through the selection of and commitment to values. Closely related to human freedom is anxiety, another theme of existentialist writing. Alienation and nothingness are the result of anxiety in its pathological form. Authentic existence, living fully in the awareness of freedom and its accompanying responsibility, is the cure for alienation. A concern with ethics and human values is another dominant theme of existentialism. Finally, time and history are important foci of concern, for to be human means to have a history.

The tenets that Parse has drawn from existentialism-phenomenology are intentionality, human subjectivity, coconstitution, coexistence, and situated freedom. Although Parse's terminology and definitions are not exact renditions of those to be found in her citations, a careful reading will show her to be true to the meanings of the original sources. The tenets from existentialism and from Rogers are synthesized in the following summary statement of her assumptions: "Man is postulated as a unitary being simultaneously and mutually cocreating with environment rhythmical patterns of relating. As an open being, man freely chooses meaning in situation and bears responsibility for the choices. Man transcends with possibles in negentropically unfolding health" (Parse, 1981, p. 39). The phenomenon of human consciousness dominates this theory, in keeping with its existentialist roots. This becomes even more evident in the three principles of Parse's theory: structuring meaning multidimensionally, cocreating rhythmical patterns of relating, and cotranscending with the possibles. Utilizing a tripartite analysis of consciousness, the three aspects of knowing, feeling, and willing are respectively represented by each of these principles.

Parse's view of health and illness is nondichotomous. As in Newman's theory, health is a process, one of ongoing participation with the world, a synthesis of values, a way of living. Disease is a pattern of man's interrelationship with the world. There is no clear distinction made between health and illness or disease and nondisease. Certain parameters of health are implied by the theory, however. For example, it is maintained that the individual grows more diverse and more complex, chooses values, and molds his or her own ways of living. These behaviors may be viewed as aspects of health. Parse's multiple meanings of health may be grasped by viewing the three principles stated above as principles of health or, more accurately, principles of "man-living-health."

Assumption number four of the theory deals with Parse's philosophy of *space-time*. Absolute space and time are rejected, replaced by the view that these form a unified and multi-dimensional web within which probabilistic patterns of interrelationships unfold. Possibilities and potentialities are active forces in the present; thus, past, present, and future merge, as in Watson's theory.

To summarize, Parse has explicitly derived her assumptions and principles from Rogerian theory and existentialism, producing a creative synthesis that is logically constructed and organized. The rhythmical patterns of human-environment (or person-world) interaction and man's negentropic unfolding are concepts taken from Rogers but interpreted in a new way. The free choosing of meaning and values in life, its attendant self-responsibility and self-transcendence through fulfillment of the potentialities of one's being are aspects of human health that Parse has developed through an application of existentialist thought to the domain of nursing.

Common Philosophical Themes

In reviewing the specific philosophical themes of these four theories and frameworks, a pattern of its own emerges to describe the overall Gestalt. Process is one of the most striking overall themes. There is a view of constant change, but not of random change. The change is evolutionary in a predictable (though never certain) direction. The evolutionary process described by these theorists is not one of physical evolution, but of the evolution of human consciousness. The ways in which this evolution is characterized vary, but one consistent term that appears is self-transcendence. The implications of the view of human evolution as an evolution of consciousness are seen in the definitions of health. Health is this evolution. Human beings as open systems is another dominant view. The interaction between the person and the world is dynamic, continuous, and essential for the evolution described above. Harmony is a related theme that is seen in the writings of the theorists, either harmony within the person or between person and world. Views of space and time are nonlinear, fluid, and relative. Space-time forms a matrix in which past and future merge into present. Another key theme is that of pattern. This is one expression of the holism, both epistemological and metaphysical, of the theories.

Keeping in mind the opening comments in this article about the need for a common metaparadigm or world view for the discipline of nursing, it is now clear that in these four theories and frameworks there are consistent philosophical themes that address nursing's metaparadigmatic domain. The themes together form a potentially powerful and coherent metaphysical and epistemological foundation for the further development of a variety of nursing theories. Of particular significance is the impact, both direct and indirect, that Eastern philosophy has had upon the development of nursing theory. Virtually all of the philosophical themes shared in common by these theories have been fully explored by several systems of Indian and Chinese philosophy. It is time that serious attention be paid to the formal systems of thought of the East, both ancient and modern, so that accurate interpretation and application, rather than vague references, can be made. A significant philosophical foundation has been laid for the development of a distinctive and commonly shared disciplinary world view. Nurse scholars should feel proud of the work done to date and commit themselves to further development of this world view. What is needed is nurse philosophers who can deal with philosophically complex issues, drawing upon past tradition as well as their own insights to develop a unique philosophy of and for nursing.

REFERENCES

Bohm, D. (1980). *Wholeness and the implicate order.* London: Routledge & Kegan Paul.

Donaldson, S., & Crowley, D. (1978). The discipline of nursing. *Nursing Outlook, 26,* 113–120.

Fawcett, J. (1984). *Analysis and evaluation of conceptual models of nursing.* Philadelphia: F. A. Davis.

Hiriyanna, M. (1949). *Essentials of Indian philosophy.* London: George Allen & Unwin.

Hutchison, J. (1977). *Living options in world philosophy.* Honolulu: University Press of Hawaii.

Malinski, V. (1986). Contemporary science and nursing: Parallels with Rogers. In V. Malinski (Ed.). *Explorations on Martha Rogers's science of unitary human beings* (pp. 15–23). Norwalk, CT: Appleton-Century-Crofts.

Moss, R. (1981). *The I that is we.* Berkeley, CA: Celestial Arts.

Newman, M. (1986). *Health as expanding consciousness.* St. Louis: C. V. Mosby.

Parse, R. R. (1981). *Man-living-health: A theory of nursing.* New York: John Wiley & Sons.

Polanyi, M. (1946). *Science, faith and society.* Chicago: University of Chicago Press.

Polanyi, M. (1958). *Personal knowledge.* Chicago: University of Chicago Press.

Robinson, R., & Johnson, W. (1977). *The Buddhist religion* (2nd ed.). Encino, CA: Dickenson.

Rogers, M. (1970). *An introduction to the theoretical basis of nursing.* Philadelphia: F. A. Davis.

Rogers, M. (1980). Nursing: A science of unitary man. In J. Riehl & C. Roy (Eds.). *Conceptual models for nursing practice* (2nd ed.) (pp. 329–337). Norwalk, CT: Appleton-Century-Crofts.

Rogers, M. (1983). Science of unitary human beings: A paradigm for nursing. In I. Clements & F. Roberts (Eds.). *Family health: A theoretical approach to nursing care.* New York: John Wiley & Sons.

Rogers, M. (1986). Science of unitary human beings. In V. Malinski (Ed.). *Explorations on Martha Rogers's science of unitary human beings.* Norwalk, CT: Appleton-Century-Crofts.

Russell, B. (1964). *Mysticism and logic.* Garden City, NY: Doubleday Anchor (Original work published 1917).

Sarter, B. (1987). *The stream of becoming: Metaphysical foundations of nursing science.* New York: National League for Nursing.

Teilhard de Chardin, P. (1965). *The phenomenon of man* (B. Wall, Trans.). New York: Harper.

Teilhard de Chardin, P. (1969). *Human energy* (R. Hague, Trans.). New York: Harcourt Brace Jovanovich.

Teilhard de Chardin, P. (1970). *Activation of energy* (R. Hague, Trans.). London: Collins.

Uys, L. (1987). Foundational studies in nursing. *Journal of Advanced Nursing, 12,* 275–280.

Von Bertalanffy, L. (1968). *General system theory: Foundations, development, applications.* New York: Braziller.

Watson, J. (1985). *Nursing: Human science and human care: A theory of nursing.* Norwalk, CT: Appleton-Century-Crofts.

Whitehead, A. (1960). *Process and reality.* New York: Harper (Original work published 1929).

Young, A. (1976a). *The geometry of meaning.* San Francisco: Robert Briggs.

Young, A. (1976b). *The reflexive universe: Evolution of consciousness.* San Francisco: Robert Briggs.

The Author Comments

Philosophical Sources of Nursing Theory

Rosemarie Parse asked me to write this article in 1987 for publication in her new journal *Nursing Science Quarterly.* I had recently published a philosophic analysis of Rogers' *Science of Unitary Human Beings,* based on my doctoral thesis. I used a similar approach in my doctoral research for this article: examine the reference list of each theorist, identify from it the primary sources of inspiration for the theorists' key ideas and themes, go to the primary sources and thoroughly study them, compare one theorist's philosophic roots to another, and place them within a spectrum of philosophical schools. I believe that this approach to philosophic analysis can be applied to emerging and future nursing theories, and that it should be an essential element for analysis of all conceptual work in our discipline. This article offers, then, a model for 21st-century nursing scholars as they engage in philosophic theory analysis.

—BARBARA SARTER

CHAPTER 33

The Focus of the Discipline of Nursing

Margaret A. Newman

A. Marilyn Sime

Sheila A. Corcoran-Perry

The focus of nursing as a discipline has not been clearly defined but is emergent in the centrality of the concepts of caring and health. The authors propose a focus for nursing as a professional discipline in the form of a statement that identifies a domain of inquiry that reflects the social relevance and nature of its service. Several perspectives from which the focus can be studied are described. The authors assert that a unitary-transformative perspective is essential for the full explication of nursing knowledge.

A discipline is distinguished by a domain of inquiry that represents a shared belief among its members regarding its reason for being. A discipline can be identified by a focus statement in the form of a simple sentence that specifies the area of study. For example, physiology is the study of the function of living systems; sociology is the study of principles and processes governing human society.

A professional discipline, in addition, is defined by social relevance and value orientations.[1,2] The focus is de-

rived from a belief and value system about the profession's social commitment, nature of its service, and area of responsibility for knowledge development. These requisites need expression in the focus statement. For exam-

Discussions in the School of Nursing Curriculum Coordinating Committee stimulated ideas for this article. The authors acknowledge the contributions of other members of the committee: Monica Bossenmaier, Dorothy Fairbanks, Carol Reese, Mariah Snyder, and Patricia Tomlinson. The authors also thank Ellen Egan and Kathleen Sodergren for manuscript critiques.

About the Authors

MARGARET A. NEWMAN was born in Memphis, TN, on October 10, 1933. She received her first degree (BSHE, 1954) in home economics at Baylor University. She entered nursing at the University of Tennessee, Memphis, in 1959 and received a BSN in 1962. Her graduate study included an emphasis on medical-surgical nursing at the University of California, San Francisco (MS, 1964) and a further emphasis on rehabilitation nursing and nursing science at New York University (PhD, 1971). Except for a short tenure as director of nursing for the clinical research center at the University of Tennessee, the emphasis of her work has been in education (at New York University, Penn State University, and the University of Minnesota). The focus of her scholarship has been on theory development in nursing. The books *Health as Expanding Consciousness* (1986, 1994) and *A Developing Discipline* (1995) represent her major contribution to nursing theory. She is an avid fan of live theater and music, with subscriptions to two local theater groups' offerings and the St. Paul Chamber Orchestra.

A. MARILYN SIME was born and raised in North Dakota, and received degrees from the University of Minnesota (BS and PhD) and Boston University (MS). Most of her academic career was spent at the University of Minnesota, where she is now Professor Emerita. Her research has focused on testing interventions that enhance patients' and families' abilities to cope with stressful health situations. Her didactic interests include research design, theoretical foundations of nursing, and the structure of professional bodies of knowledge. Now retired, she enjoys spending time with her family and friends, reading, listening to music, and walking in the woods with her dogs.

SHEILA A. CORCORAN-PERRY was born and educated in Minnesota. She received her baccalaureate degree from the College of St. Catherine in St. Paul, MN, and her master's and doctoral degrees from the University of Minnesota. Currently, Dr. Corcoran-Perry is Professor Emerita at the University of Minnesota School of Nursing, where she served on the faculty for 30 years. Before her positions at the University of Minnesota, she served on the faculties at the College of St. Catherine and Edinboro State College in Edinboro, PA. Dr. Corcoran-Perry has been recognized for her pioneering research on the cognitive processes used by nurses and family caregivers when making decisions about health care. She and her husband Jim enjoy spending time with family and friends, volunteering in the community, reading, taking liberal arts courses, and traveling extensively.

ple, medicine is the study of the diagnosis and treatment of human disease. The social relevance and value orientation of medicine as a professional discipline is conveyed by the commitment to alleviate disease.

Knowledge development within a discipline may proceed from several philosophic and scientific perspectives (worldviews). From this standpoint, the focus of a discipline could be considered paradigm free. The purpose of this article is to present a focus for the discipline of nursing and to discuss the implications of differing paradigmatic perspectives for the nature of nursing knowledge.

Concepts Relevant to the Focus of Nursing

The focus of nursing as a professional discipline has emerged most prominently over the past decade. A number of concepts have been identified as central to the study of nursing. An example is the frequently cited tetralogy: person, environment, nursing, and health.[3,4] While identification of these concepts begins to narrow the focus of nursing, there remains the need for more explicit connectedness and social relevance to describe the field of study that constitutes nursing. Such unconnected concepts do not raise the philosophic issues or scientific questions that stimulate inquiry.

Recently, there has been concentrated emphasis on two concepts as central to nursing: health and caring. Health has been heralded as the centerpiece of nursing knowledge since the days of Florence Nightingale and continues to be discussed by many theorists and researchers.[5-8] The concept of caring also has occupied a prominent position in nursing literature and has been touted as the essence of nursing.[9-11] The accelerated emphasis on health and caring within the past decade has been accentuated by recent Wingspread Conferences[12,13] and the devotion of entire issues of nursing scholarly journals to these concepts.[14,15] These efforts raise questions about nursing's domain of inquiry. Does health or caring represent the focus of the discipline of nursing? Is knowledge gained from research on caring or health specifically identified as nursing knowledge? Although caring and health are indeed central to nursing, no one has developed a unifying focus statement that includes these concepts, and neither concept alone meets the criteria for the focus of a professional discipline. A synthesis of current knowledge development regarding caring and health suggests a focus that meets these criteria.

Caring has generally been linked with the concept of health. In Leininger's historical review of care and caring, she consistently links caring with health and states that "caring is the . . . explanadum for health and well-being."[16(p19)] Watson combines caring and healing in a causal connection and refers repeatedly to "caring-healing."[17] Benner's tenets, as well, specifically link caring with health and well-being.[18]

In a similar fashion, the concept of health is often linked with actions. Pender questions what interventions assist clients in achieving health.[19] Newman submits that the essential question of the discipline of nursing "has something to do with how nurses facilitate the health of human beings" and poses the question, "What is the quality of relationship that makes it possible for the nurse and patient to connect in a transforming way?"[20(p234)]

Further, in nursing, health means *human* health and, most significantly, human health *experience*.

Phillips states that "research should focus on . . . the study of people's *experiencing of their health,* their sense of interconnectedness with others, and specifically how health emerges from a mutual process" (emphasis added).[21(p103)] Pender uses the term "health experience" throughout her recent article on health patterns; she points out that "when illness occurs, it is synthesized as part of the on-going *health experience*" (emphasis added).[19(p116)] Parse has been explicit in her emphasis on human experience as the basis of her theory of man-living-health,[22] which might be rephrased as human health experience.

Considerable evidence exists that caring, health, and health experience are concepts central to the discipline of nursing. These concepts can be related to each other to identify the domain of inquiry for nursing.

A Focus Statement for Nursing

We submit that nursing is the study of *caring in the human health experience*. This focus integrates into a single statement concepts commonly identified with nursing at the metaparadigm level. This focus implies a social mandate and service identity and specifies a domain for knowledge development. The social mandate and service identity are conveyed by a commitment to caring as a moral imperative. It is important to note that at this level, the concepts are not associated with any particular theory.

The domain of inquiry is caring in the human health experience. This focus dictates that nursing's body of knowledge includes caring and human health experience. A body of knowledge that does not include caring and human health experience is not nursing knowledge. For example, knowledge about health without consideration of caring would be knowledge of a discipline of health. Nursing theories would link caring to the human health experience.

The tasks of nursing inquiry will be to examine and explicate the meaning of caring in the human health experience to ascertain the adequacy of this focus for the discipline, and to examine the philosophic and scientific questions provoked by the focus statement.

Differing Paradigmatic Perspectives

What may appear to be confusing and inconsistent meanings of concepts in the proposed focus may actually be a reflection of the use of different paradigms for knowledge explication.[20,23] Nursing research has been conducted from an orientation consistent with at least two, and possibly three, paradigms. Each paradigm specifies a point of view from which the field of study is conceptualized, the assumptions that are inherent in that view, and the basis upon which knowledge claims are accepted. These differing paradigms reflect the shift in focus from physical to social to human science. The three perspectives extant in nursing literature could be described as: particulate-deterministic, interactive-integrative, and unitary-transformative. To explain the effect of a paradigm on the development of nursing knowledge, each perspective will be addressed briefly.

From the particulate-deterministic perspective, phenomena can be viewed as isolatable, reducible entities having definable properties that can be measured. These entities have orderly and predictable connectedness to each other. Change is assumed to be a consequence of antecedent conditions—conditions that, if sufficiently identified and understood, could be used to predict and control change in the phenomena. Relationships within and among entities are viewed as linear and causal. Kinds of knowledge sought include facts and universal laws. Knowledge claims that cannot be refuted are admitted to the body of knowledge. From the perspective of this paradigm, caring in the human health experience could be studied by examining the concepts that comprise the focus. For example, caring could be isolated for study as a human trait having definable and measurable characteristics. Similarly, health could be reduced and dichotomized in terms of characteristics considered healthy versus those considered unhealthy. Caring also could be studied as a therapeutic intervention affecting patients' health in terms of measurable responses.[23]

From the interactive-integrative perspective (an extension of the particulate-deterministic perspective that takes into account context and experience and legit-imized subjective data), phenomena are viewed as having multiple, interrelated parts in relation to a specific context. To explain a phenomenon, the interrelationships of parts and the influence of the context are taken into consideration. Thus, reality is assumed to be multidimensional and contextual. Change in a phenomenon is a function of multiple antecedent factors and probabilistic relationships. Relationships among phenomena may be reciprocal. Knowledge claims may be context dependent and relative. From this perspective, caring in the human health experience would be studied as interactive-integrative phenomena within specific contexts, but still with probabilistic predictability.

The unitary-transformative perspective represents a significant paradigm shift. From this perspective, a phenomenon is viewed as a unitary, self-organizing field embedded in a larger self-organizing field. It is identified by pattern and by interaction with the larger whole. There is interpenetration of fields within fields and diversity within a unified field. Change is unidirectional and unpredictable as systems move through stages of organization and disorganization to more complex organization. Knowledge is personal, involves pattern recognition, and is a function of both viewer and the phenomenon viewed. The subject matter includes thoughts, values, feelings, choices and purpose.[24] Inner reality depicts the reality of the whole. From this perspective, caring in the human health experience would be studied as a unitary-transformative process of mutuality and creative unfolding.

Relationship of Focus to Paradigmatic Perspective

The explication of knowledge relevant to caring in the human health experience is affected by the paradigmatic perspective. As described earlier, concepts in the focus statement could be isolated for study within the first two perspectives, while the unitary-transformative perspective requires the focus to be studied as an indivisible whole. For example, knowledge generated from the particulate-deterministic perspective includes behaviors that characterize caring, physiologic and psychologic aspects of human health, and acontextual rules that relate observable caring behaviors with measurable health outcomes. Examples of knowledge generated from the interactive-integrative perspective include the reciprocal nature of nurse-client interactions, culture-specific caring responses to life process events that are disruptive to health, and rules regarding the influence of specific caring behaviors on the health-related behaviors of particular groups of clients. Knowledge from a unitary-transformative perspective is more difficult to characterize. An example generated from this perspective might be an understanding of the synchrony and mutuality of nurse–client encounters that transcend the time and space limitations of a present situation.

Although multiple perspectives are appropriate for knowledge development in nursing, we are convinced that a unitary-transformative perspective is essential for full explication of the discipline. This position is consistent with a changing world view of the conduct of inquiry into human experience[25-27] and with other nurse scholars who recognize the value of a unitary perspective to nursing inquiry.[22,28-30] Insights from our research and practice reveal a rich and fertile glimpse into caring in the human health experience.

The focus of a professional discipline is an area of study defined by the profession's shared social and service commitment. We conclude that the focus of nursing is the study of caring in the human health experience. The explication of nursing knowledge based on this focus takes different forms depending on the perspective of the scientist. We conclude that a unitary perspective is essential for full elaboration of caring in the human health experience. A unified focus derived from the coalescing of theory on caring and health has the potential for claiming the shared vision of nursing.

REFERENCES

1. Johnson DE. Development of theory: A requisite for nursing as a primary health profession. *Nurs Res.* 1974;23(5):372-377.
2. Donaldson SK, Crowley DM. The discipline of nursing. *Nurs Outlook.* 1978;26(2):113-120.
3. Torres G, Yura H. *Today's Conceptual Framework: Its Relationship to the Curriculum Development Process.* New York, NY: National League for Nursing, 1974.
4. Fawcett J. The metaparadigm of nursing: Present status and future refinements. *Image.* 1984;16(3):84-87.
5. Newman MA. *Health as Expanding Consciousness.* St. Louis, Mo: Mosby, 1986.
6. Meleis AI. Being and becoming healthy: The core of nursing knowledge. *Nurs Sci Q.* 1990;3(3):107-114.
7. Pender NJ. *Health Promotion in Nursing Practice.* Norwalk, Conn: Appleton & Lange, 1987.
8. Newman MA. Health conceptualizations and related research. *Ann Rev Nurs Res.* 1991;9.
9. Leininger M, ed. *Care: The Essence of Nursing and Health.* Thorofare, NJ.: Slack, 1984.
10. Watson J. *Nursing: The Philosophy and Science of Caring.* Boulder, Col: Colorado Associated University Press, 1985.
11. Benner P, Wrubel J. *The Primacy of Caring.* Menlo Park, Calif: Addison-Wesley, 1989.
12. Stevenson JS, Tripp-Reimer T, eds. *Knowledge About Care and Caring.* Proceedings of a Wingspread Conference, February 1-3, 1989. Kansas City, Mo: American Academy of Nursing, 1990.
13. Duffy ME, Pender NJ, eds. *Conceptual Issues in Health Promotion.* Proceedings of a Wingspread Conference, April 13-15, 1987. Indianapolis, In: Sigma Theta Tau, 1987.
14. *ANS.* 1981:3(2); 1984:6(3); 1988:11(1); 1990:12(2); 1990:13(1).
15. *Nurs Sci Q.* 1990:3(3).
16. Leininger M. Historic and epistemologic dimensions of care and caring with future directions. In: Stevenson JS, Tripp-Reimer T, eds. *Knowledge About Care and Caring.* Proceedings of a Wingspread Conference, February 1-3, 1989. Kansas City, Mo: American Academy of Nursing, 1990.
17. Watson MJ. New dimensions of human caring theory. *Nurs Sci Q.* 1988;1(4):175-181.
18. Benner P. *Nursing as a caring profession.* Presented at meeting of the American Academy of Nursing: October 16, 1988; Kansas City, MO.
19. Pender NJ. Expressing health through lifestyle patterns. *Nurs Sci Q.* 1990;3(3):115-122.
20. Newman MA. Nursing paradigms and realities. In: Chaska NL, ed. *The Nursing Profession: Turning Points.* St. Louis, Mo: Mosby, 1990.
21. Phillips JR. The different views of health. *Nurs Sci Q.* 1990;3(3):103-104.
22. Parse RR. *Man-Living-Health: A Theory of Nursing.* New York, NY: Wiley, 1981.
23. Morse JM, Solberg SM, Neander WL, Bottorff JL, Johnson JL. Concepts of caring and caring as a concept. *ANS.* 1990;13(1):1-14.
24. Manen MV. *Researching Lived Experience: Human Science for an Action Sensitive Pedagogy.* Albany, NY: State University of New York Press, 1990.

25. Bohm D. *Wholeness and the Implicate Order.* London, England: Routledge & Kegan Paul, 1980.

26. Prigogine I. Order through fluctuation: Self-organization and social system. In: Jantsch E, Waddington CH, eds. *Evolution and Consciousness.* Reading, Mass: Addison-Wesley, 1976.

27. Briggs J, Peat FD. *Turbulent Mirror.* New York, NY: Harper & Row, 1989.

28. Rogers ME. *An Introduction to the Theoretical Basis of Nursing.* Philadelphia, Pa: FA Davis, 1970.

29. Munhall PL. Nursing philosophy and nursing research: In apposition or opposition? *Nurs Res.* 1982;31(3):176-177, 181.

30. Sarter B. Philosophical sources of nursing theory. *Nurs Sci Q.* 1988;1(2):52-59.

The Authors Comment

The Focus of the Discipline of Nursing

This article came about as I listened to the ongoing harangue of nursing scientists regarding the validity of different modes of research. The answer, I believed, was "all a matter of paradigm." Concurrently, colleagues at the University of Minnesota (Marilyn Sime and Sheila Corcoran-Perry) and I were involved in curriculum development and recognized that the focus and methods of the research of our faculty colleagues varied considerably. How could all these viewpoints be reconciled in nursing? Hence, this article emphasizes the different paradigms that prevailed in nursing and suggests an overarching focus to define the discipline.

—Margaret A. Newman
—A. Marilyn Sime
—Sheila A. Corcoran-Perry

CHAPTER 34

Nursing: The Ontology of the Discipline

Pamela G. Reed

The purpose of this article is to contribute to clarifying the ontology of the discipline by extending exist-ing meanings of the term nursing *to propose a substantive definition. In this definition, nursing is viewed as an inherent human process of well-being, manifested by complexity and integration in human sys-tems. The nature of this process and theoretical implications of the new nursing are presented. Nurses are invited to continue the dialogue about the meaning of the term and explore the implications of nurs-ing, substantively defined, for their practice and science.*

Keywords: *Deconstruction, Knowledge Development, Metaparadigm, Ontology, Postmodernism*

Distinguishing the term *nursing* as a noun from its use as a verb was put forth most profoundly by Rogers (1970), whose vision extended the scholarship of ear-lier nursing theorists to thrust nursing forward to be recognized as both a scientific discipline as well as a professional practice. It is time, however, to push back the frontier once again, beyond these two important un-derstandings of nursing, by proposing a new meaning of nursing. With this new meaning, the term itself repre-sents the nature and substance of the discipline. In other words, *nursing* is the ontology of the discipline.

The ideas put forth here are done so in the spirit of accepting Watson's (1995) "postmodern challenge" to exploit the climate of deconstruction of nursing (see

About the Author

PAMELA G. REED was born in Detroit, MI, in June 1952 and grew up in an environment enriched by the sociopolitical and musical events of Motown. She is a three-time graduate of Wayne State University in Detroit, receiving a BSN in 1974, an MSN in 1976 (with a double major in child-adolescent psychiatric mental health nursing and teaching), and her PhD, with a major in nursing (focus on lifespan development and aging, nursing theory) in 1982. She worked as a psychiatric-mental health clinical nurse specialist and was an Instructor in Nursing at Oakland University, Rochester, MI, from 1976 to 1979. From 1983 to the present, she has been on the faculty at the University of Arizona College of Nursing in Tucson, including 7 years serving as Associate Dean for Academic Affairs. With her doctoral work, she pioneered nursing research into spirituality and its role in well-being. Dr. Reed has developed a theory of self-transcendence and two widely used research instruments, the *Spiritual Perspective Scale* and the *Self-Transcendence Scale*. Her publications reflect her three main passions and contributions to nursing: the conceptual and empirical bases of the significance of spirituality in health experiences, a lifespan developmental perspective of well-being in aging and end of life, and the philosophic dimensions of the development of the discipline. Dr. Reed also enjoys classical music, hiking in the Grand Canyon, swimming, and raising her two daughters, Regina and Rebecca, with her husband, Gary.

Rampragus, 1995; Reed, 1995) to extend and, by some degree, reconstruct current understandings of nursing. Smith's (1988a) article outlined the ongoing dialogue about two meanings of nursing, as a verb and a noun. This dialogue is revisited here for the purpose of further clarifying what is the ontology of the discipline, long considered a crucial question by seminal thinkers in nursing (Ellis, 1982; Rogers, 1970; Roy, 1995).

Continuing the Dialogue: Nursing as a Process of Well-Being

It is proposed here that there exists a third and perhaps most basic definition of nursing in which nursing represents the *substantive* focus of the discipline. Disciplines are characterized by their substantive focus: archaeology is the study of the archaeo, or what is ancient and primitive; astronomy is the study of the astro, astronomical phenomena such as the motion and constitution of celestial bodies; biology is a branch of knowledge about biol, or living matter; chemistry deals with the processes and properties of chemical substances;

physics is the study of physical properties and processes; psychology is the study of the psyche, referring to mental processes and activities associated with human behavior; and nursing, the discipline, is proposed here to be the study of nursing processes of well-being, inherent among human systems.

This meaning of nursing, as an inherent process of well-being, derives in part from the root word, nurse, defined as a process of nourishing, of promoting the development or progress of something. The meaning also derives from synonyms of nurse meaning to heal, to foster, to sustain (Laird, 1971; *Webster's New Collegiate Dictionary,* 1979). These descriptions signify that nursing involves a process that is developmental, progressive, and sustaining, and by which well-being occurs.

The Inherent Nursing Process

The theme of human beings' inherent nursing processes as the substantive focus of the discipline is supported in nursing theorists' works from Nightingale in 1859, to the mid-20th century writings of Henderson, to the contemporary turn-of-the-century ideas of Schlotfeldt. Nightingale (1859/1969) wrote about the person's "innate power" and the inner "reparative process." Henderson (1964) eloquently symbolized the power of the nurse within, describing nursing as "the consciousness of the unconscious, the love of life of the suicidal, . . . the eyes of the newly blind, a means of locomotion for the infant, . . . the voice for those too weak or withdrawn to speak" (p. 63). Watson (1985) referred to "self-healing processes," and Schlotfeldt (1994) stressed human beings' "inherent ability and propensity to seek and attain health." In addition, this nursing process is not necessarily based upon a reversal of a disease process, but more upon a moving forward, to gain a sense of well-being in the absence or presence of disease.

The discipline's understanding of how a nursing process is manifested is shifting away from the mid-20th century mechanistic conception of nursing as a process external to patients and conducted by the nurse, that is, the old nursing process. The process of nursing is viewed now more from a relational perspective, congruent with contextual and transformative conceptions of the world (see Newman, 1992; Pepper, 1942). Nursing is a participatory process that transcends the boundary between patient and nurse and derives from a valuing of what Rogers (1980, 1992) described as human systems' inherent propensity for "innovation and creative change."

"Human systems" refers to an individual or a group of human beings (Rogers, 1992, p. 30). As such, human systems, whether in the form of individuals, dyads, groups, or communities, emanate and participate in nursing processes. Nursing processes may be manifested, for example, in the grieving that an individual experiences, in the caring that occurs among people and their families and nurses, in the healing practices shared by a culture, or in many other as yet undiscovered patterns of nursing. Today, these patterns may be described as intentional or unconscious, automatic or contemplative, relational or chemical, or simply unknown. Nevertheless, with continued nursing research, education, and practice, nursing processes can be learned and knowingly deployed to facilitate well-being. Murphy's (1992) visionary book, for example,

addresses some of these possibilities. He proposes a future wherein people are more aware of their innate healing potential and employ it to more purposefully enhance health.

Nightingale did not invent nursing, described here in terms of an inherent propensity for well-being. Just as earthquakes existed before geologists and photosynthesis before botanists, nursing processes existed in human beings, ultimately described by Nightingale (1859/1969) as that which nurses were to facilitate by placing the patient in the best situation possible. It follows, then, that nursing does not belong exclusively to certain groups of people, such as "well" persons or professional nurses; it belongs to human nature.

Defining the substance of the discipline of nursing in terms of a well-being process inherent among human beings does not negate the importance of knowledge of factors that interface with nursing to influence well-being and healing. Examples of these factors, often the focus of study in ancillary professions and disciplines, include the environmental, financial, cultural, surgical, and pharmacological. However, any sense of well-being involves, most basically, a nursing process. The quest for nursing is to understand the nature of and to facilitate nursing processes in diverse contexts of health experiences.

The Nature of Nursing Processes

What is the nature of nursing processes that distinguishes them from other human processes? It is proposed that the intersection of at least three characteristics—complexity, integration, well-being—distinguishes human processes as nursing; specifically, nursing processes are manifested by changes in complexity and integration that generate well-being. Importantly, other distinguishing characteristics of nursing processes may be identified as the dialogue continues beyond this article.

This new understanding of the nature of nursing processes derived from various theorists' work, such as von Bertalanffy's (1981) systems view of human beings; Rogers' (1970, 1992) science of unitary human beings; Lerner's (1986) developmental contextualism; and complexity theory (see Kauffman, 1995; Waldrop, 1992). While the translation of these theorists' ideas may not be entirely congruent with those presented here, their ideas nonetheless can help inform development of a new nursing ontology.

Human beings are viewed as open, living systems and not as passive but intrinsically active and innovative. As an open system, human systems are capable of self-organizing, where *self* refers to the system as a whole. Self-organization is an inherent capacity for generating qualitative change out of ongoing events in the life of a system and its environment.

In his seminal work on development, Werner (1957) explained this process of qualitative change as his "orthogenetic principle," which posits that living organisms change over time from lower to higher levels of differentiation and integration. Werner (1957) called this change "development," in contrast to mechanistic processes of change, which are not developmental.

Similarly, Rogers' (1980) principles of homeodynamics describe the inherent innovative patterning of change that occurs in open systems, both environmental and human. Her three principles of helicy, resonancy, and integrality together depict the nature of qualitative change in human beings in terms of ongoing movement from lower to higher levels of diversity. Complexity theorists (for example, Kauffman, 1995; Waldrop, 1992), and developmentalists (for example, Lerner, 1986; Werner, 1957) in particular have clarified a distinction between quantitative and qualitative change, both of which are necessary for development; contrasting terms such as complexity and order, and differentiation and organization, depict this distinction. Similarly, two distinct forms of change can be identified in Rogers' (1980, 1992) works, namely diversity and innovation (Reed, 1997).

Because of the articulation between quantitative and qualitative change, human systems are not simply complex systems (SCS) but rather are complex innovative systems (CIS) (see Stites, 1994). In the context of nursing, then, nursing processes entail at least two forms of change, complexity and integration.

Complexity. Complexity refers to the number of different types of variables that can be identified in a given situation. A variable is simply something that varies (*Webster's,* 1979). Complexity occurs when human systems experience or express variables (for example, life events, physiologic events) as parts, separated from the whole, rather than as patterns of the whole. So, for example, complexity is evident when loss of a loved one or chronic illness introduces many new and seemingly disconnected variables into an individual's life, on various levels of awareness. Increasing complexity means change in quantity (size or number) not change in quality of the whole; this would become chaotic were it not accompanied by corresponding changes in integration.

Integration. Integration refers to a synthesizing and organizing of variables such that there is a change in form, not just change in size or number of events. A certain level of complexity is needed for integration to occur. Integration is evident, for example, when people construct meaning or identify a pattern in the variables or events experienced. Integration may also occur on levels of awareness that are not yet so readily apparent. Integration is trans*form*ative, involving qualitative change in form.

Well-Being

While changes in complexity and integration may be used to explain many facets of human development and systems' changes, this process may also be used to understand health, healing, and well-being. The rhythm between complexity and integration is proposed here to be a means by which innovative change occurs, as a manifestation of the underlying process called nursing. Thus, well-being may be explained in part by changes in complexity that are tempered by changes in integration. Complexity provides life with diversity, specialization, and depth in experiences, whereas integration provides organization, coherence, and breadth.

Examples of nursing processes are abundant. For example, groups incorporate new attachments or children into an organization called family. Persons with spinal cord injuries develop different pathways that link together shattered parts of life and bodily functions. Premature infants' behaviors become more innovative as they organize the complexity of their environment. Adults reminisce to integrate past life events and inevitable death. Healing after the loss of a loved one or the occurrence of chronic illness requires an integration of what seem like disjointed events and experiences, including memories of the past, future dreams, altered rhythms and routines, physical pain and other bodily symptoms, sadness, anguish, and self-doubt. Further, Sachs (1995) depicted what can be called nursing processes, through his stories about people with various maladies, such as a colorblind painter and a surgeon with Tourette's syndrome. These people were able to create a new organization that fit with their altered needs and world. These health events, in all their initial complexity and heartbreak, gave way to metamorphoses and innovation. Regardless of whether there is a "cure" that can reverse a particular ailment, well-being occurs when the particulars of a life experience are brought together and synthesized in a coherent way. Any less, and people risk feeling dis-integrated, dis-associated, dis-organized.

While the centrality of well-being as a focus in nursing has been established, other disciplines also may be concerned with well-being and its correlates. However, promoting well-being based upon a perspective of the inherent process of complexity and integration is distinctly nursing.

Challenging the Status Quo: Nursing Reconstructed

The definition of nursing proposed here is that of an inherent process of well-being, characterized by manifestations of complexity and integration in human systems. The substantive focus of the discipline, then, is not how *nurses* per se facilitate well-being but, rather, how *nursing processes* function in human systems to facilitate well-being. The focus is, in a very basic sense, how nurses can facilitate nursing.

Refocusing the Lens

This new construction of nursing provides another lens of focus for nursing researchers and practitioners. Smith (1988b) wrote metaphorically about three different camera lenses used to view human wholeness. One in particular, the motion lens, focuses on process and rhythmic flow, and requires a "creative leap" to identify this process. Nurses typically encounter people in motion, in dynamic flow with their environment, whether in life-threatening experiences or perceived memory loss, chronic illness or acute pain.

The creative leap necessary for formulating the motion lens of nursing inquiry may be to address the rhythmic processes of complexity and integration that enhance well-being across these health experiences. From premature infants to dying adults and their families and communities, it is proposed that human systems have nursing processes, that is, inherent resources for well-being based on a capacity to integrate their complexities.

Debates on holism and on what represents the critical focus of nursing may be enlivened by including a new ontology of nursing—an ontology that transcends debates about part versus whole, person versus environment. Nursing processes are not necessarily bound by dimensions such as biologic, environmental, or social. Instead, the lens is focused on any human process that manifests complexity and integration related to well-being. Looking through this new lens, researchers and practitioners may identify a myriad of human manifestations of wholeness, whether they be labeled physiologic, phylogenic, or philosophic, that are integral to well-being.

Nursing as a Metaparadigm Concept

Given this reconstructed view of nursing, as a substantive focus of the discipline, the term *nursing* should be a central concept in the nursing metaparadigm. In the past, for good reason, some have suggested the elimination of the term nursing from the metaparadigm (Conway, 1985). However, rather than remove the term nursing from the metaparadigm, this fin-de-siècle may be the time in nursing history to consider renaming the discipline to something other than a verb, to better distinguish the disciplinary label from the substantive focus of the science and practice.

To help clarify this distinction, a term such as Paterson and Zderad's (1976) "nursology," or another disciplinary label with the "nurs" prefix could be developed, while reserving the term nursing as the *process* word and verb that it is, for the metaparadigm. By identifying nursing as a substantive, metaparadigm concept, nurses can better claim their unique focus and clarify the ontology of their discipline.

Approaching the Frontier

Rogers (1992) explained that one could not push back the frontier of knowledge until one approached it. This article has not been about maintaining the status quo, but about approaching a frontier so that others might join in a dialogue that pushes back the frontier a bit more. In this era of healthcare reform, the discipline must define nursing as nurses truly envision it and not necessarily as others would have it be defined. Nurses may decide against renaming the discipline as was suggested here. Nevertheless, within a broadened and partially reconstructed view of the discipline that embraces nursing at its most fundamental meaning, new understandings that blend with the old can emerge to present a fuller picture of the discipline.

Nursing (as practice and praxis) is a way of doing that creates good actions that facilitate well-being. Nursing (as syntax and science) is a way of knowing that creates goods in the form of knowledge. And nursing (the substance and ontology) is a way of being that creates patterns of changing complexity and integration experienced as well-being in human systems.

Nurses are invited to try on the substantive definition of nursing to see how it fits within the context of their practice and science. Ongoing philosophic dialogue about the ontology of the discipline will help ensure that nurse theorists are theorists of nursing in its fullest sense, and likewise, that nurse researchers are researchers of nursing, and nurse practitioners are practitioners of nursing.

REFERENCES

Conway, M. E. (1985). Toward greater specificity in defining nursing's metaparadigm. *Advances in Nursing Science, 7*(4), 73–81.

Ellis, R. (1982). Conceptual issues in nursing. *Nursing Outlook, 30*(7), 406–410.

Henderson, V. (1964). The nature of nursing. *American Journal of Nursing, 64*(8), 62–68.

Kauffman, S. (1995). *At home in the universe: The search for laws of self-organization and complexity.* New York: Oxford University Press.

Laird, C. (1971). *Webster's new world thesaurus* (rev. ed.). New York: Simon and Schuster.

Lerner, R. M. (1986). *Concepts and theories of human development* (2nd ed.). New York: Random House.

Murphy, M. (1992). *The future of the body: Explorations into the further evolution of human nature.* New York: J. P. Tarcher.

Newman, M. (1992). Prevailing paradigms in nursing. *Nursing Outlook, 40,* 10–13.

Nightingale, F. (1969). *Notes on nursing: What it is and what it is not.* New York: Dover (Original work published 1859)

Paterson, J. G., & Zderad, L. T. (1976). *Humanistic nursing.* New York: Wiley.

Pepper, S. P. (1942). *World hypotheses: A study in evidence.* Berkeley: University of California Press.

Rampragus, V. (1995). *The deconstruction of nursing.* Brookfield, VT: Ashgate.

Reed, P. G. (1995). A treatise on nursing knowledge development for the 21st century: Beyond postmodernism. *Advances in Nursing Science, 17*(3), 70–84.

Reed, P. G. (1997). The place of transcendence in nursing's science of unitary human beings. In M. Madrid (Ed.), *Patterns of Rogerian knowing* (pp. 187–196). New York: National League for Nursing Press.

Rogers, M. E. (1970). *Introduction to the theoretical basis of nursing.* Philadelphia: F. A. Davis.

Rogers, M. E. (1980). A science of unitary man. In J. P. Riehl & C. Roy (Eds.), *Conceptual models for nursing practice* (2nd ed., pp. 329–337). New York: Appleton-Century-Crofts.

Rogers, M. E. (1992). Nursing science and the space age. *Nursing Science Quarterly, 5,* 27–34.

Roy, C. L. (1995). Developing nursing knowledge: Practice issues raised from four philosophical perspectives. *Nursing Science Quarterly, 8,* 79–85.

Sachs, O. (1995). *An anthropologist on Mars: Seven paradoxical tales.* New York: A. Knopf.

Schlotfeldt, R. (1994). Resolving opposing viewpoints: Is it desirable? Is it practicable? In J. F. Kikuchi & H. Simmons (Eds.), *Developing a philosophy of nursing* (pp. 67–74). Thousand Oaks: Sage.

Smith, M. J. (1988a). Nursing: What's in a name? *Nursing Science Quarterly, 1,* 142–143.

Smith, M. J. (1988b). Perspectives of wholeness: The lens makes a difference. *Nursing Science Quarterly, 1,* 94–95.

Stites, J. (1994). Complexity research on complex systems and complex adaptive systems. *Omni, 16*(8), 42–50.

von Bertalanffy, L. (1981). *A systems view of man* (P. A. LaViolette, Ed.). Boulder: Westview Press.

Waldrop, M. M. (1992). *Complexity: The emerging science at the edge of order and chaos.* New York: Simon and Schuster.

Watson, J. (1985). *Nursing: Human science and human care.* Norwalk, CT: Appleton-Century-Crofts.

Watson, J. (1995). Postmodernism and knowledge development in nursing. *Nursing Science Quarterly, 8,* 60–64.

Webster's new collegiate dictionary. (1979). Springfield, MA: G. & C. Merriam Co.

Werner, H. (1957). The concept of development from a comparative and organismic point of view. In D. B. Harris (Ed.), *The concept of development* (pp. 125–148). Minneapolis: University of Minnesota Press.

The Author Comments

Nursing: The Ontology of the Discipline

The focus of this article is based on an epiphany I had when preparing a presentation for the 1993 National Forum on Doctoral Education. It struck me that nursing is so much more than we typically assume it to be—more than the practice we observe by people called "nurses" and more than a disciplinary body of knowledge. I proposed that nursing is a basic human process of healing that has evolved within and among human beings. This substantive focus (ie, ontology) of the discipline extends beyond the cell or the human field. Like any natural processes (eg, biologic or geologic) that define a disciplinary focus, understanding nursing processes requires the attention of educated practitioners and researchers who can study, appreciate, and facilitate nursing for human betterment.

—Pamela G. Reed

CHAPTER 35

Nursing as a Practice Rather Than an Art or a Science

Anne H. Bishop
John R. Scudder

The uncritical designation of nursing as a science and an art creates vague images of nursing that suggest that the identity of nursing is not to be found in practice. Thinking and talking about nursing as a practice more adequately articulates the meaning of nursing as nurses encounter it.

Nurses have often assigned meaning to nursing by designating nursing as an art and a science. Some nurses have uncritically accepted the assertion that nursing is a science, confident that this designation assures academic and professional respectability. However, because experience tells them that important aspects of nursing cannot be captured by the term science, they add the qualification that nursing is also an art. In this article we will show why nursing as it is practiced cannot be adequately articulated either as an art or as a science. Attempts to do so in both common and scholarly literature lead nursing away from seeking its identity in practice. Articulating nursing as a practice more adequately interprets the meaning of nursing than articulating it as either an art or a science.

We will first consider an example from common literature, because such literature often informs the initial image of nursing. An example of this literature is evident in the recruitment material entitled "What is Nursing?" in *Nurse Recruitment Magazine.*[1] In this

Nurs Outlook *1997;45:82–5.*

About the Authors

ANNE H. BISHOP is Professor of Nursing Emerita, Lynchburg College, VA. She was born on June 27, 1935, and obtained her BSN from the University of Virginia in 1958. In 1968, she received her MEd in guidance and counseling from Lynchburg College. Dr. Bishop obtained her MSN, majoring in psychosocial nursing, in 1986 and her EdD in higher education administration in 1980 from the University of Virginia.

JOHN R. SCUDDER is Professor of Philosophy, Emeritus, at Lynchburg College. He was born on March 9, 1926. Dr. Scudder received a BA from Vanderbilt University in 1950, his MA from the University of Alabama in 1952, and his EdD from Duke University in 1961.

The focus of Dr. Bishop's and Dr. Scudder's scholarship has been to develop a philosophic interpretation of nursing. The results of their research have appeared more in books than journal articles. Their broader interests have been the philosophy of human science, especially those that explore caring. Their latest books concern how personal and social relationships are distorted by society's obsession with sexuality.

material, nursing is said to be a science when nurses "give injections in the correct muscle," "know what to do and why, when a patient collapses," and "are able to identify and report symptoms being shown by a patient."[1] Nursing is said to be an art when nurses "soothe a crying mother whose child is ill," "comfort an elderly person whose family never visits" and "be with a frightened patient going into surgery."[1] The relationships referred to as art could be those of any person who has cared for the ill. The knowledge of the cause of a patient collapse or of the meaning of a symptom could come from science, but it also could come from the knowledge nurses have secured through many years of practice. We have chosen this example from a nonscholarly publication to illustrate how the uncritical designation of nursing as a science and an art creates vague images of nursing that suggest that the identity of nursing is not to be found in practice.

Nursing as a Science

Nursing cannot be a science in the traditional sense of science in the West. In this tradition, the purpose of science has been to disclose the truth about some aspect of the world. Sciences in this tradition seek theoretical explanation of the natural world. This approach to science originated with the classical Greek philosophers, who believed in the existence of a rational order behind all appearances. The Greeks called this rational order *logos,* a term that appears in contemporary sciences as "ology." Modern sciences, following this way of thinking, seek theoretical explanations for the way the world is. For example, biology is a science that seeks to discover the rational order of all living things. Darwin attempted to account for this order with the theory of evolution. Newton sought explanation for natural phenomena in the theory of gravitation and Einstein in the theory of relativity. Traditional science begins with theoretical explanation and attempts to expand knowledge by using, testing, and expanding theoretical explanation.

Nursing is not primarily a quest for truth through theoretical explanation. Rather than seeking theoretical truth, nurses attempt to foster healing and the well-being of patients. For this reason, nursing cannot be a science in the traditional sense, but it might be a technology. The term *technology* originated from combining two Greek concepts: *logos,* the rational order behind things, and *techne,* the know-how of making things. Technology applies scientific knowledge of the rational order of things to make changes in the world.

Nurses do use knowledge obtained from scientific inquiry in caring for patients. Recognition that nursing involves applied science, however, does not mean that nursing itself can be constituted as a science or a technology. The inadequacy of using either traditional science or technology as a designation for the complex practice called nursing has led nursing scholars to seek a definition of science more appropriate to nursing than the traditional rationalist approach.

One author who contends that traditional science does not adequately describe nursing science is Donaldson.[2] She believes that nursing science must include empirical and pragmatic science as well as traditional science. Rather than contending that nursing practice itself is a science, Donaldson maintains that nursing uses various scientific interpretations in carrying out nursing practice. Both Sandra Weiss,[3] who is wedded to an empiricist approach to science, and Christine Kasper,[4] who takes a pragmatic approach, agree with Donaldson. Weise stated this position well when she said that in nursing science, "Scientific inquiry must produce tangible concrete knowledge that promotes health, prevents illness, or increases the potential for recovery from illness."[3] All of these authors are concerned with the role of science in the study of nursing and believe that the purpose of that scientific study is to improve practice. Sara Fry states clearly why the practice of nursing itself cannot be a science: She contends that nursing "is a practical discipline" that has the moral end of fostering the well-being of the client.[5]

Nursing as an Artful Practice

If nursing practice cannot be a science because it is a practical discipline with a moral end, can it appropriately be called an art? The traditional purpose of art in the West has been to create beauty, whereas the purpose of nursing is to foster healing and wellness. Nurses do foster healing and wellness in ways that can legitimately be called artistic. However, regardless of how "aesthetically" a nurse cares for a patient, he/she would not be said to be engaged in the art of nursing if that care caused unneeded pain, inhibited healing, or enhanced

the possibility of death. Because the purpose of the art of nursing is to foster health and healing, nursing at best could be called an artful practice.

The inadequacy of seeking the identity of nursing by labeling it as an art is evident in an article by Johnson[6] on the art of nursing. Johnson divides scholars who attempt to identify nursing as art into two groups: those who interpret the art of nursing as rational and those who oppose this definition of the art of nursing. She contends that those who define art as rational believe that "the artful nurse solves problems by selecting the intervention best suited to the intended end: Instrumental problem solving is said to be a thorough consideration of the facts of the situation, and is made rigorous by the application of scientific theory."[6] It is unclear from the article whether the many nursing scholars that she cites call this definition a definition of art or whether she has classified their work in this way. However, this definition describes well the position of Donaldson,[2] Weiss,[3] Kasper,[4] and Fry,[5] whose works appear not in a book on art but in a book entitled *In Search of Nursing Science.*

When the rationalistic interpretation of nursing, described by Johnson, is accurately labeled as science rather than art, the opponents of that interpretation would seem to favor nursing as an art, especially since they stress sensitivity and creativity. Johnson acknowledges that they do not call nursing an art, but she fails to recognize why. One leading opponent, Benner,[7] does not identify nursing as art because she believes that nursing is a practice that is appropriately studied as a human science. Johnson's treatment of the conflict between those who study nursing as an applied science and those who study nursing as a human science is confused by her attempt to treat this conflict as one concerning the art of nursing rather than the study of nursing. The conflict Johnson attempts to place in the art of nursing is identical to the one that is central to the book, *In Search of Nursing Science.* This struggle concerning the definition of nursing itself is being contested between those who believe that the meaning and direction of nursing should come from applied science and those who believe that nursing is a caring practice that can be best articulated and developed with enlightenment from the human sciences. Johnson discusses this struggle ably, but her attempt to treat it as an art suggests the inadequacy of trying to force nursing into the mold of an art or a science rather than interpreting nursing as a practice.

Nursing as a Practice

Nursing, as well as medicine, has traditionally called itself a practice. One physician, when asked to define practice, said, "It is the care that I give to my patients." His wife, who is a nurse, could make the same claim. Note that their ways of caring are necessarily different, not just because they are different persons but because they are engaged in different practices. The philosopher Hans Georg Gadamer[8] defines practice in a way that could include not only medicine and nursing but many other practices; he defines a practice as communally developed ways of being that promote human good. A practice is concerned not only with how to bring about the good, but what good or value is worth pursuing. In a practice the goods or values of a people become concretely instantiated in the world in which they live. The ways of being, doing, and the ends sought are integrally related to each other, unlike in an applied science, which is value neutral and detachable from the end sought. (For a more extensive treatment of nursing as a practice and the study of nursing as a human science, see Bishop and Scudder.[9,10])

One indication that nursing is a practice is that it has an essential moral sense. Neither an art nor a science has an essential moral sense in the way that nursing does. A study of fulfillment in nursing indicated that nurses recognize this moral sense.[9] We asked 40 practicing nurses at a community hospital and at a university medical center to describe their most fulfilling experience of nursing. On the basis of nursing literature, we expected that a large number of the fulfilling events would be ones in which nurses demonstrated great professional or technical proficiency. In actuality, all but one of the participants described experiences in which the moral sense of nursing was fulfilled. Even the nurse whose greatest fulfillment

came from technical competence said that without the moral sense, she would not be a nurse.

The dominance of the moral sense in nursing as reported by nurses should not have surprised us; after all, nursing is caring for the well-being of others by fostering healing and wellness. Even when the description of fulfillment contained much technical and professional language, the moral sense was evident in this language. For example, a nurse who described a patient who had undergone an aneurysm clipping as "a GCS5T, E4, M1, VT [who] opened his eyes but [had] no movement and was trached," concluded her description by saying, "I can't describe the sensation I felt; but to see him follow a command for the first time—moving his thumb made me feel wonderful inside. All of our diligent nursing care, positioning, ROM, stimulation, etc., was working, and it felt good." Interestingly, in a follow-up interview with this nurse, she stated that although this work was very technical, she would not remain in nursing if it were not for personal and moral fulfillment.[9]

This example shows how the moral sense of practice is fulfilled when the technical is integrally incorporated into practice. Labeling a patient as a "GCS5T, E4, M1, VT" is beyond our (i.e., the authors') technical competence, and understanding the meaning of ROM requires an involvement in nursing practice that one of us (Scudder) lacks. Noting that ROM means range of motion is hardly adequate for understanding what the term means. Grasping the meaning of ROM involves understanding that the purpose of ROM is to assure the continued flexibility of the joint and to maintain muscle strength. This requires applying scientific understanding in nursing practice. However, the way that a nurse performs ROM for a patient requires experience in feeling muscles as they move in response to various movements by the nurse—an example of how nursing practice is artful. Nurses learn the meaning of ROM initially by appropriating it from other nurses, which is an example of why novice nurses rely on clinical experience rather than theory. The knowledge of the muscle movement cannot be acquired from a scientific treatment of muscles in a book; it has to be felt and recognized in the body. Sensitivity to the tension, relaxation, and strengthening of the muscle cannot be gained by reading a multi-step procedure in a textbook. Obtaining such sensitivity requires first working with an experienced practitioner and gradually appropriating the communally developed ways of nursing practice.

When a nurse appropriates the practice of nursing, she/he becomes a competent nurse. The practice of nursing includes many practical skills and understandings that cannot be called an art or an applied science. Skillfully bathing a patient would not generally be considered an art. It could, however, be called artful practice, as the following example will illustrate.

> "It was after breakfast. I did not eat as much as I wanted to. I felt surprised, because I couldn't mobilize my will. I leaned back, as if I had used my body for hours. Suddenly she was there again, a nurse who had spent a lot of time with me the day before. She was smiling, full of energy. She went straight to the point, leaned onto the table and offered to help me have a shower in the bathroom. It seemed like climbing a mountain, but she was so convincing that I agreed. She explained the whole procedure, how she would cover the wound with plastic, etc. It began sounding like heaven. I had confidence in her; she seemed to have been doing this for a hundred years. And it was heaven. Never had I thought that I would appreciate water running slowly down my body as I did that morning. I was sitting on a chair, and the nurse was next to me. I relaxed. She had a special way of offering her help in concrete ways like washing my back and my feet, which I literally could not reach that morning. 'I suggest that you . . . ,' and 'what you could do is turn your body . . . '. Yes, she was assisting me, never taking over. I was in command, I felt. I mattered. Even though the only thing I could manage was steering the shower handle."[11]

Nursing is often called an art in recognition of the integral relationship of practical know-how with artistry that fulfills the moral sense of nursing by promoting healing and well-being.

Another reason that nurses call nursing an art is that they move from competency to excellence through creative action and interaction, as Benner[7] has shown. For Benner, nursing is a practice in which the highest level of practice is highly creative. A nurse becomes an excellent practitioner when she/he can draw on the resources of the practice in creative ways that foster healing and well-being.

Mary Cucci, a critical care unit nurse, described her experience of helping a patient learn to live his body once again after the removal of a misfiring defibrillator. The pain from the defibrillator misfiring plus the uncertainty in his life from his previous heart attacks had led this former well-ordered, self-directed businessman to retreat in fear from engagement with the world. He had become a prisoner in an alien body. Cucci creatively helped him learn to trust and live in his body again. "I teased him, cajoled him, and danced with him as he transferred to the chair. I challenged him more each day and ignored his fake whine when he half-heartedly pleaded abuse. It became a joke. He learned to monitor his pulse to guide his activity progression. This was a long, slow process of building belief in himself."[12] Cucci's artful practice is directed at fostering the healing and well-being of her patient. She uses the practice in ways that creatively express her way of being and that are sensitive and appropriate to her patient's way of being in his current circumstances.

A practice is a communally developed human way of being that fosters human good. A practice exists only in practitioners who appropriate these ways of being in ways that are appropriate to their own being and those of the persons for whom they care. Practices are continually being developed both by creative individual care and communal care. To account for this creative aspect of nursing practice, nurses have defined nursing as art. We believe it is more appropriately called an artful practice.

Conclusion

Although nursing cannot strictly be called a science or an art, the tendency of nursing to use these terms stems from recognition that nurses apply science in their care and that excellent care involves creativity and sensitivity. However, the involvement of science and art in nursing care does not mean that nursing itself is constituted as either an art or a science. The attempt to constitute nursing as an art or a science leads nursing scholars away from the issues of the day, such as applied science versus human science, and from seeking the identity of nursing in the practice itself. Nursing cannot be an art or a science because, rather than creating beauty or pursuing truth, nursing seeks to foster healing, health, and well-being. Having a dominant moral sense is the primary characteristic of a practice. Nursing is a practice in that it seeks to foster healing and wellness through communally developed ways of being with patients that sometimes involve applying science and other times artistic, creative care. At all times, artful practice and applied science are integrally woven into the fabric of the practice of caring called nursing.

REFERENCES

1. What is nursing? Nurse Recruitment Magazine 1992;7(6):A2.
2. Donaldson SK. Nursing science for nursing practice. In: Omery A, Kasper CE, Page GG, eds. In search of nursing science. Thousands Oaks (CA): Sage, 1995:3–12.
3. Weiss SJ. Contemporary empiricism. In: Omery A, Kasper CE, Page GG, eds. In search of nursing science. Thousand Oaks (CA): Sage, 1995:13–26.
4. Kasper CE. Pragmatism: the problem with the bottom line. In: Omery A, Kasper CE, Page GG, eds. In search of nursing science. Thousand Oaks (CA): Sage, 1995:27–39.
5. Fry ST. Science as problem solving. In: Omery A, Kasper CE, Page GG, eds. In search of nursing science. Thousand Oaks (CA): Sage, 1995:72–80.
6. Johnson JL. The art of nursing. Image 1996;28:169–75.
7. Benner P. From novice to expert: excellence and power in clinical nursing practice. Menlo Park (CA): Addison-Wesley, 1984.
8. Gadamer HG, Lawrence FG, trans. Reason in the age of science. Cambridge (MA): MIT Press, 1991.
9. Bishop AH, Scudder JR Jr. The practical, moral, and personal sense of nursing: a phenomenological philosophy of practice. Albany (NY): State University of New York Press, 1990.
10. Bishop AH, Scudder JR Jr. Nursing: the practice of caring. New York: The National League for Nursing Press, 1991.
11. Bishop AH, Scudder JR Jr. Nursing ethics: therapeutic caring presence. Boston: Jones & Bartlett, 1996.
12. Benner P, Wrubel J. The primacy of caring: stress and coping in health and disease. Menlo Park (CA): Addison-Wesley, 1989.

The Authors Comment

Nursing as a Practice Rather Than an Art or a Science

Many nurses believe that nursing is often regarded as a mere collection of techniques and procedures for the care of the ill. Unfortunately, they have often tried to remedy this misconception by uncritically defining nursing as a science and an art. We believe this is the wrong approach because the worth of nursing should be found in nursing as practiced. We attempt to show that although nursing uses science and practices artfully, nursing is best conceived as a practice in the sense of the great philosopher Hans Georg Gadamer. Interpreting nursing as a practice shows the worth of nursing itself and suggests possibilities for future development of nursing out of its past achievements. (Please note that reference 11 in this article should read: Harder, I. [1993]. *The world of the hospital nurse: Nurse patient interactions—body nursing and health promotion. Illustrated by use of combined phenomenological/grounded theory approach.* Aarhus, Denmark: Sygeplejerskehojskole ved Aarhus Universitet, Skrift-serie fra Danmarks Sygeplejerskehojskole.)

—Anne H. Bishop
—John R. Scudder

CHAPTER 36

Nursing as Means of Governmentality

Dave Holmes
Denise Gastaldo

Background. *This paper conceptualizes nursing as a health profession in transformation at the beginning of the 21st century. We frame our analysis using Michel Foucault's concept of governmentality. While extensively quoted and used in other disciplines, the work of the late French philosopher has been cited infrequently in the nursing literature. Yet a closer look at his work reveals how Foucault offers a relevant entry point for revisiting nursing theory and nursing practice.*

Aim of paper. *The aim of this paper is to reflect on nursing practice as it is inscribed within the state's modus operandi. We discuss the prevalent notion that nurses are powerless and suggest they do exercise power in many ways and that they are a powerful group.*

Results. *In this paper we show how nursing is a means of governmentality of individuals and of the population because its practices contribute to the management of society through a vast range of power techniques. These techniques range from disciplining individuals to promoting discourses that construct desirable subjectivities. Within this perspective, the emergence of political aspects of nursing theory and nursing practice are made explicit.*

Conclusion. *We explore the limits and potentials of the concept of governmentality to the understanding of nursing as a health profession. This concept can generate a form of critical immobilism, but also promotes a more politically complex understanding of nursing practice.*

Keywords: Foucault, governmentality, nursing practice, nursing theory, poststructuralism, power, powerlessness.

Holmes D. & Gastaldo D. Copyright © 2002. Journal of Advanced Nursing 38(6), 557–565.
Permission from Blackwell Science Pub.

About the Authors

DAVE HOLMES currently lives in Montreal, Canada. He received his BScN from the University of Ottawa, Canada, and his MSc and PhD (nursing) from the Faculté des Sciences Infirmières, Université de Montréal, Canada. He currently holds a position as Assistant Professor at the University of Ottawa, Faculty of Health Sciences, School of Nursing, where he teaches at the undergraduate and graduate levels. He is also a nurse researcher at the Douglas Hospital Research Centre in Montreal, a teaching psychiatric hospital affiliated with McGill University. He is completing his postdoctoral studies at the University of Toronto, Canada. His main contributions to nursing are poststructuralist analysis of nursing practice in forensic psychiatry and public health.

DENISE GASTALDO is an Assistant Professor at the Faculty of Nursing and Centre for International Health, University of Toronto, Canada. She was born in Brazil, where she obtained her BScN and MA degrees. Dr. Gastaldo completed her PhD in the United Kingdom, where she studied health promotion and sociology of health at the University of London. Subsequently, she completed postdoctoral studies at the Faculté des Sciences Infirmières, Université de Montréal, Canada. Her main contributions to nursing are international capacity building for research, critical analysis of nursing and health promotion from a poststructuralist perspective, and exploration of interdisciplinary perspectives on gender and health.

Nursing and Health Care in the 21st Century

Traditionally, nurses have described themselves, and have been depicted by others, as a powerless professional group, which lacks social prestige, is poorly paid, and experiences very limited professional autonomy because of physicians' socially dominant role in providing health care to the population (Lunardi Filho, 2000). In this paper, however, we adopt a different perspective. Employing a Foucauldian notion of power, we draw on the concept of *governmentality* to reconceptualize nursing as an internationally recognized profession of fundamental importance to the provision of health care in the Western world. In many countries, nurses are the largest professional group working in the health field. In qualitative terms, preceding decades witnessed nursing's consolidating higher education degrees and offering more alternatives to graduate studies at master's and doctoral levels (Arruda & Silva, 2000). Increasing numbers of graduate programs are producing more knowledge, and efforts towards providing evidence-based care are being made in many countries (MacGuire 1990, Martin & Forchuk 1994, Francke *et al.* 1995, Gastaldo 2000). Concurrently, nurses have achieved more management positions and political roles, which lead to political influence.

In advanced liberal societies, neoliberal policies have attempted to downsize governmental provision of health care services. For example, in the last decade in Canada length of stay in hospitals has been reduced and family caregivers have been involved in home care activities that were previously provided by health care professionals. Meanwhile, in countries like Brazil that are under the influence of the International Monetary Fund, relying on private health insurance has become a common practice among the middle class. The concentration of resources in the private sector and the globalization of the economy have been reshaping the health field. In some countries, health care has become a commodity that one should be able to afford through insurance [in the United States of America (USA), for example], while in others [such as Australia, Canada, United Kingdom (UK) and Sweden], access to health care is still perceived as a basic right for all citizens. Presently, globalized markets do not translate into global rights for workers regarding salaries or working conditions. Shortages in the nursing workforce in some countries have generated migration trends between countries, such as nurses from the Philippines and Spain applying for jobs in UK or Canadian nurses moving to the USA Nurses, among others, have been struggling with cuts in the health care system and are directly involved in maintaining the quality of care provided. Despite the cuts, they remain accountable for the provision of 'good' nursing care.

In this complex context, nurses may see their practices strongly shaped by economic and health care reforms. Their powerlessness would be even more evident when they chose to provide quality services (spending time on patient education, keeping a certain number of working hours for revising practices according to new scientific evidence or engaging in long-term healthy community development), but they are compelled to be loyal to urgent patient needs and employers' strategic plans, and keep the system running under almost any circumstances. In doing so, nurses experience nonegalitarian, historically situated nonpriviledged positions within society, the health care system and even within nursing. Nurses' powerlessness is the internationally prevalent account for the profession's current situation; yet, what is also inherent to this discourse is the fact that nurses constitute and make feasible the institutions and systems that they believe are the source of their oppression.

Therefore, rather than having our analysis restricted by the myth of the powerless nurse, dependent on medical knowledge and lacking autonomy, we will discuss how nursing takes an active role in the health care system disseminating knowledge and promoting health practices and, thereby, engages in the politics of health. The aim of this article is to discuss the theoretical possibilities and limits of a concept known as governmentality in the analysis of nursing's influence on individual and population governance through caring practices, health policies, and knowledge production. We will explore how nursing professionals, being located at the interface of political rationalities and the provision of care, participate in the government of human conduct both at the individual and collective levels.

Before Governmentality: The Issue of Power

Power is a well-studied concept that has been examined from various theoretical perspectives. Well known works from Lukes (1974), Marx (1946), Weber (1986), and Arendt (1995) were particularly useful for understanding recent and current socio-political issues. Michel Foucault, the late French philosopher, offered an original way to look at power that differed from many theories which address power as it deals with the state, the legitimacy of power, the notion of ideology, and questions regarding the possession and source of power (Dean 1999).

Foucault maintained that we must look at power not only as a repressive exercise (a dimension which of course exists); we must also concentrate upon its constructive aspects. For Foucault, power 'seems to include everything from overt forms of coercion and manipulation to the subtle exercise of authority and influence' (Weberman 1995, p. 193). This understanding of power is innovative because power has been conceived of traditionally as only a negative and repressive force. Power has been linked to prohibition, punishment, and imposition of laws, but Foucault also explored the notion of constructive (or productive) power, arguing that there are ways to exercise power that generate little conflict or frustration; power relations that are more difficult to resist (Weberman 1995). In summary, we distance ourselves from the traditional 'jurico-discursive' point of view (McHoul & Grace 1993, Weberman 1995), which tends to state that:

> Power takes the form of openly articulated (hence discursive) prohibition, coercion, threats and punishment (hence juridical) and has the effect of restricting the activities of the ruled by preventing them from doing what they want to do (Weberman 1995, p. 191).

According to Foucault, we must overcome this obsession with repressive and sovereign power if we want to offer a more comprehensive understanding of how power is exercised in society. We must investigate, through research, how power produces subjectivities. Foucault observed that the construction of self (subjectivity) is linked to established forms of knowledge and institutionalized practices. Self is not an essence; it is created by the influence of multiple forms of power. Foucault also emphasized the idea of studying power where it produces effects, locally and often in subtle forms. For Foucault, power is to be seen as:

> The multiplicity of force relations immanent in the sphere in which they operate and which constitute their own organization; as the process which, through ceaseless struggles and confrontations, transforms, strengthens, or reverses them, as the support which these force relations find in one another, thus forming a chain of system . . . power is not an institution, and not a structure, neither is it a certain strength we are endowed with; it is the name that one attributes to a complex strategical situation in a particular society (1990, pp. 92–93).

Power does not function only on the basis of law, but also through techniques related to discipline and normalization (Foucault 1980a). Nor is power based on violence, but on control and productive exercises in ways that surpass the state and its institutions (Foucault 1994a). Moreover, power relations are not one-sided, and any particular group does not hold power. In fact, power is fluid and circulates among and through bodies (McHoul & Grace 1993). Power is employed and exercised through a net-like organization; it is not the property of someone or a group. Power acts upon individuals as they, in turn, act upon others. Therefore, power is relational. Foucault insisted that 'power is everywhere; not because it embraces everything, but because it comes from everywhere' (Foucault 1990, p. 93).

Governing Life to Govern Society: The Concept of Governmentality

From his later work on disciplinary power (Foucault [1975] 1995) and, subsequently, on bio-power (Foucault 1990), Foucault further developed his analysis of

power, and defined his concept of 'governmentality'. Foucault's writings on bio-power, or power over life, situated biological life as a political event and explored the global character of power in economic, social and historical terms (Gastaldo 1997, Moss 1998). Through his historical research on sexuality, and while articulating the concept of bio-power, Foucault (1990) progressively manifested an interest in government (Hindess 1996). Exploring both the local and the general levels involved in the exercise of power, Foucault expanded the notion of governance and explained more successfully how power functions (Moss 1998).

Governmentality, a term Foucault (1979) coined, describes the general mechanisms of society's governance and does not refer specifically to the term, *government*, as commonly used. As Gordon (1991) explained:

> Government as an activity could concern the relation between self and self, private interpersonal relations involving some form of control or guidance, relations within social institutions and communities and, finally, relations concerned with the exercise of political sovereignty. (pp. 2–3)

According to McNay (1994), Foucault considered governmentality as a complex system of power relations that binds sovereignty-discipline-government in a tripartite manner. Governing involves these three forms of power. This conception allows us to appreciate how Foucault integrated the states of domination (sovereignty), disciplinary power (discipline) and the government of others and self (government). Governmentality involves domination and disciplinary techniques, as well as self-governing ethics (Deflem 1998). In his own terms, Foucault defined governmentality as:

> The ensemble formed by the institutions, procedures, analyses and reflections, the calculations and tactics that allow the exercise of this very specific albeit complex form of power, which has as its target population, as its principal form of knowledge political economy, and as its essential technical means apparatuses of security. (1979, p. 20)

In short, government means to conduct others and oneself, and governmentality is about how to govern. 'The concept of government implies all those tactics, strategies, techniques, programmes, dreams and aspirations of those authorities that shape beliefs and the conduct of population' (Nettleton 1991, p. 99). Hence, government is an activity that aims to shape, mould or affect the conduct of an individual or a group, that is, to conduct the conducts of people (Gordon 1991). According to Foucault, this *governmentalization* of the state relies on a specific security apparatus that links all together in a very specific complex of procedures and techniques: diplomatic-military techniques, the police, and pastoral power, such as the care of others.

Diplomatic-military techniques, the first dimension of the security apparatus, allows the state to protect itself against external threats and to preserve its territorial integrity through diplomatic representations, a permanent armed force, and established war policies (Gros 1996). In addition, to protect itself against internal threats, the state is endowed with a police force. Finally, pastoral power achieves care of others through various therapeutic regimes while ultimately helping to shape the self so that it fits within an appropriate, 'normalized' way of living (Dean 1999). The normalized way of living refers to a conformity to a set of social rules and ways of concerning oneself and others. The power of normalization imposes homogeneity by setting standards and ideals for human beings (Rose 1998).

Governing is as much about practices of government as it is about practices of the self because the concept of governmentality deals with those practices that try to shape, mould, mobilize and work through the choices, desires, aspirations and needs of individuals and populations (Rose & Miller 1992). Governmentality connects the question of government and politics to the self (Dean 1999). In our discussion, we will explore how nursing is a constitutive element of governmentality by looking at power over life as the governance of populations and individuals (Gastaldo 1997, Gastaldo & Holmes 1999).

Nursing and the Governance of the Population

Nursing as a profession and a discipline is inherently political because it deals with biological existence and generates knowledge about it. Shaping the population for economic and social purposes demands supervision and intervention over biological processes (Foucault 1990). Hence, nursing is a constitutive element of governmentality because it takes part in this management. Currently, nursing's role in managing the population is centred on promoting life and recuperation from illness. Life is governed in a variety of ways, but we will explore two particular methods in this section—knowledge production and social policy.

As one of the largest professional groups in the health field in many countries, nursing plays a major role in the population's health education. Nursing's academic gains and political development have meant that many professionals now serve as professors, researchers, policy makers, consultants and evaluators. These positions give them opportunities to gather information and create policies to be implemented from the local to the international level (Gastaldo et al. 2001).

Acknowledging nursing's influence in managing the population does not mean that nurses work in unison, or that they share a Machiavellian plan to rule society. Nursing, like any other profession, is divided by distinct philosophical and political positions, and it is often motivated by members' self-interests and personal agendas. Any attempt at producing a discourse to promote health is challenged by other discourses, and the governance of society occurs within a constant struggle of conflicting interests. As with any other exercise of power, dominant discourses in nursing face resistance (Gastaldo 1997). As power is the multiplicity of force relations extant within the social body, one specific manifestation of power will encounter another one resisting it. According to Foucault, we are continuously involved in struggles, because struggle for power is pervasive in every society:

> Power is not something that is acquired, seized, or shared, something that one holds to or allows to slip away; power is exercised from innumerable

points, in the interplay of nonegalitarian and mobile relations . . . there is no binary and all encompassing opposition between rulers and ruled at the root of power relations . . . (1990, p. 94)

Social policy constitutes its objects; it helps to give meaning to abstract concepts, such as health and caring. Policies about health generate new understandings of health. As Hewitt (1991) pointed out:

> Social policy plays a co-ordinating role in forming 'the social.' It promotes and organizes knowledge, norms and social practices to regulate the quality of life of the population, its health, security and stability. (p. 225)

Health is considered a desirable asset in most societies and health policies tend to involve measures designed to promote health and recuperation from illness. Therefore, nursing is a profession that is well perceived (even though not prestigious), and its interventions are generally well accepted by the public. Since the 1980s, the health promotion movement has linked health to most aspects of public and private life. Moreover, healthy public policy may include issues such as housing, pollution, and violence, among others (Gastaldo 1997).

Two examples illustrate how nurses create policies and knowledge. In Canada, nurses have been instrumental in advancing the health promotion and home care movements during the last decades (McKeever 1996, Stewart 2000). Through research and political action, nurses have helped to de-institutionalize long-term care and to reframe health as a socially determined construct. While claiming to promote a humane and socially grounded care, these movements also reinforced the importance of self-care and self-responsibility for health, and they produced norms for the good citizen, the caring mother, and the acquiescent chronically ill or disabled person. The expectation created by these discourses fosters comparisons between individuals and groups. "The comparisons allow nurses to establish 'normality.'" As a consequence, the "deviant individual becomes a target for surveillance and intervention" (Gastaldo & Holmes 1999, p. 21).

Governmentality also depends on access to knowledge. Those governing society need to understand the politics of everyday life. Epidemics, fertility, and life expectancy are at the core of the rationalities of government (Foucault 1990). Nursing research provides knowledge about the population and helps to decide priorities in funding. "Research findings have provided scientific authority to justify policies that have saved huge amounts of public money by minimizing institutional costs and shifting many of the costs of long-term care to family caregivers" (McKeever 1996, p. 203).

In the case of the home care movement, McKeever (1996) argued that policies also reflect a particular notion of family and home. The home has become the most important site for health care and health promotion in our society, and women the main producers of such services. But this place and worker remain rarely conceptualized in research (McKeever 1996). What prevail in research are samples of 'white' and nuclear families, where the psychological burden of caregivers is stressed over social and economic issues, such as social class, ethnicity, occupational history, and power relations between family caregivers, care recipients, and professionals (McKeever 1996). The home care movement naturalized the home as the optimal site for long-term care (institutional care is now seen as impersonal) and as a private space, where family provision of care is free and therefore saves public funds. As a consequence, long-term care recipients who do not have a family become a burden to society and families that do not provide care according to standards usually proposed by nurses are a problem—somehow they challenge the norm. These situations require management as difficult cases (McKeever 1996).

In the case of health promotion, the discourse of risk reduction for society, once again, takes women's work for granted as free labour. The genderless health promotion discourse assumes that healthy diets will be cooked and served to families without asking by whom. Currently, 'good women' not only provide physical and emotional care, but also promote the health of their families. Furthermore, many of the changes in lifestyle proposed by the health promotion movement will take place at home. The stimulus, the surveillance, and the punishments and rewards for adopting, or not adopting, a healthier lifestyle are constituents of power relations among the members of the household. Knowing that the family is a privileged site for the regulation of individuals where power is capillary, as it reaches the core of its members, one could see that what is achieved in the household serves society at large, where power continues to operate at a macro-level, in order to govern the population.

Nursing and the Governance of Individuals

Throughout history, nurses have been involved in the governance of individual bodies by using an array of power techniques whose effects construct subjectivities such as establishing standards for 'good patient,' 'healthy citizen,' and 'caring mother.' For the purpose of this paper, we will concentrate on how disciplining and caring are used as strategies to govern individual bodies. The limits of disciplinary and pastoral power, however, are often blurry, and nurses frequently use the two types of power at the same time.

Disciplinary Power

For Foucault, disciplinary power is a very important form of power that emerged in 17th century Europe and gained ground quickly in the modern Western world. He reminded us that despite its often being seen as repressive in nature, this kind of power is also productive in character (Hindess 1996):

> If power were never anything but repression, if it never did anything but to say no, do you really think one would be brought to obey it? What makes power hold good, what makes it accepted, is simply the fact it doesn't only weigh on us as a force that says no, but that it traverses and produces things, it induces pleasures, forces knowledge, produces discourses (Foucault 1980a, p. 119).

Disciplinary power is one form of power exercised over an individual or many persons to produce effects on

their conduct, habits, and attitudes in order to help them achieve particular skills and new ways of thinking or to render them ready for instruction (Hindess 1996). It is subtle and does not need violence to be effective. McHoul and Grace (1993) argued that modern bodies are not physically constrained; rather, they have legal rights and brutal forms of control, like coercion, are not easily acceptable. Disciplinary power trains and enhances individuals, utilizes people's productive potential, and makes optimal use of their capacities. It operates through an impressive set of tools such as hierarchical observation (unrelenting surveillance of captive patients, patients at risk, and communities); normalizing judgement (creation of norms, micro penalties, and rewards); and examination (clinical gaze, use of time and space, creation of individual cases) (Foucault [1975] 1995).

When Clinton and Nelson (1999) employed Foucault's perspective to study mental health, they focused on the construction of subjectivity through nursing care. They showed that discipline and surveillance can also occur through noncoercive approaches. The authors suggested that discourses about empowering psychiatric patients, currently perceived as 'consumers' of mental health services, do not necessarily overcome discipline and surveillance, but replace them. Instead of being 'externally' driven, patients are 'internally' directed:

> For by engaging in self-care, people with a mental illness not only seek to recover themselves, but also to regulate themselves and their behaviours in more deeply penetrating ways than was possible when psychiatric practice was at its most coercive. (p. 270)

These authors suggested that self-regulation is a dominant form of social control and that nurses' therapeutic practice is currently based on the principles of self-care, which foster patient self-regulation (Gastaldo & Holmes 1999). Individuals could reach self-regulation by being involved in a therapeutic enterprise where, through pastoral care, nurses would promote processes of self-surveillance and self-awareness, among others.

Therefore, pastoral power plays a major role along with disciplinary power in the governance of individuals and populations.

Pastoral Power

Pastoral power, developed in Christian societies around the 3rd century AD, has become an important form of power. It requires a person to serve as a guide for another. Through this benevolent power, 'the guide' cares for others (Lunardi 1999): 'The pastoral model is adopted and vastly elaborated by Christianity, as the care of souls' (Gordon 1991, p. 8). Introduced in the Western world along with Christianity, pastoral power is an individualizing form of power (Foucault 1994b), which knows its subjects in detail. It lies in a power technique that must penetrate souls, decode hearts, and reveal the most intimate secrets. Pastoral power seeks disclosure of consciousness; it penetrates the soul and acts upon it to ultimately direct it (Foucault 1994b).

Nursing staff regularly use pastoral power as part of a control mechanism that produces a *savoir* (knowledge) regarding the patients (governed subject). This acquired *savoir,* through its main tool, the confession, is codified and integrated within, but not exclusive to, the specialized discourses of medicine, psychiatry, psychology, sexology, criminology, and nursing care. The strange secrets of the individual, exposed to professional scrutiny, are incorporated in expert professional discourses (Foucault 1990). This process is often the starting point for labelling the patient as normal or deviant. Professional intervention is likely to take place in these circumstances (Moss 1998).

If detailed knowledge about individuals is required for this form of power to be effective, the therapist can count on the therapeutic notion of confession to uncover these secrets (Foucault 1994b). Patients must open themselves up to the other and are in part subjugated to avowal. Therefore, this trustful, unconditioned obedience, as well as the unrelenting examination and the confession, form a powerful combination where these three elements are linked together. Knowledge about patients, hidden until now in their souls, constitutes an important element in the governance of others (Foucault 1994a).

Confession, an essential element of pastoral power, provokes an intensification of regulatory controls over citizens. Moreover, 'professions investigating psychic states could be extremely useful to a bio-power construct intent on managing the variables associated with population' (Ransom 1997, p. 65). Power always questions, inquires, records, and institutionalizes truth. Furthermore, it does it in a professional way (Foucault 1997). Today, the pastoral use of confession, introspection, and self-examination is found not only in churches or sects, but in the day-to-day work of health care professionals, including nurses. These techniques are part of the therapeutic tools used for counselling, personality modification, personal development, health education and, of course, psychiatric care. 'This exercise of self-government serves as an instrument of the government of their conduct' (Hindess 1996, p. 122). In short, pastoral power is a form of power 'which makes individuals subject, subject of someone else by control and dependence, and tied to his own identity by a conscience of self-knowledge' (Ransom 1997, p. 67). 'There is no need for arms, physical violence, material constraints. Just a gaze. An inspecting gaze, a gaze . . . which each individual thus exercises this surveillance over and against himself' (Foucault 1980b, p. 155).

The productive effect of pastoral power is often obtained despite the objectives formulated by the therapist. Even when the therapist's goal is to help patients to find out more about themselves, this process is mediated by the therapist's agenda for normalcy and adequate modes of functioning in society. Sometimes patients come to believe that their thinking arises from their own concerns and not from others (the therapist). They begin to work on themselves as if they desired to change a particular behaviour or attitude. When they share their secrets with a professional, a self-examination process takes place. They are becoming aware of certain phenomena that they are experiencing. But patients become aware through the lens and evaluation of someone else, the therapist: 'Is it not the supreme exercise of power to get another or others to have the desires you want them to have, that is, to secure their compliance by controlling their thought and desire' (Lukes

1974, p. 23). For example, in psychiatric care, nurses are actively involved in this form of power through therapeutic communication in individual therapy.

Data from a grounded theory research study showed that nurses working in a correctional psychiatric setting used both types of power to govern inmates with psychiatric problems (Holmes 2001). On a daily basis nurses, accompanied by correctional officers, participated in rounds where they inspected inmates' cells in order to evaluate their degree of conformity to rules regarding hygiene and allowed content. Nurses working in this setting met inmates/patients once a week for a formal evaluation of their mental health status. It is through this 'therapeutic encounter' that nurses obtained information about the inmates they cared for. But for nurses to know, inmates have to share information about themselves. Confession constitutes the major tool of pastoral power that allows nurses to gather information. The therapeutic encounter is also a privileged moment where inmates/patients can share their feelings, fears and suffering. Pastoral power is also effective because it raises inmates' awareness regarding their condition and thus constitutes the first step to self-regulation.

So, although nurses are using disciplinary techniques such as surveillance, control of activities, punishments, and rewards in order to achieve obedience from inmates, they are also caring for them through pastoral care. In nursing theories, caring traditionally is viewed as being apart from disciplinary regimes in which social control is pervasive (Gastaldo & Holmes 1999). These research findings, on the contrary, confront us with the fact that there is no such paradox between disciplining and caring. To punish and forbid do not exclude treatment, care, reform, rehabilitation and transformation. Indeed, in this correctional psychiatric setting, disciplinary techniques rely on nursing care, while the latter relies simultaneously on the former.

As we can see, nurses use and often combine these two forms of power in their clinical practice. The previous examples illustrate how nurses are directly involved in the governance of individuals through disciplinary and pastoral power.

Governmentality and its Implications for Nursing

As Foucault stated, the concept of governmentality creates a new way of regarding the conduct of humankind; its aim is directed at 'the domains of ethics, government, and politics, of the government of self, others, and the state, of practices of government and practices of the self, of self-formation and political subjectification, that weaves them together *without a reduction of one to the other* (emphasis added)' (Dean 1994, p. 158).

Governing now implies going beyond the state and its official institutions or figures. Based on Foucault's idea, government can be understood as 'an active process which joins political rationalities . . . with governmental technologies' (Curtis 1995, p. 575); a process in which some ideals of social life set the conditions and create fields for intervention in most aspects of everyday living (Simon 1993, Curtis 1995). The articulation of political rationalities with technologies of government is ensured by a specific form of knowledge (scientific *savoir*) and the presence of an expert (nurse) who mediates between the political objectives and the object of intervention (population and individual). The state should now be considered as a 'network of institutions, deeply embedded within a constellation of ancillary institutions associated with society and the economic system' (Hall 1986, p. 17). Power operates within tiny, subtle and complex ramifications established by competent authorities. In an era of governmentality, power is pervasive and it relies on agents who can ensure the optimal functioning of this new art of government (Curtis 1995).

Nurses are health care professionals who are in direct contact with individuals, groups, communities, and populations. They are a powerful group of experts upon whom the state and its institutions rely. Working at the junction of the individual and collective body within power relations that promote and recuperate life, nurses are able, through their interventions, to mould, conduct or affect people as well as to construct, with the help of other health care professionals, people's subjectivities. This is accomplished through a vast range of techniques such as gathering information, producing and disseminating knowledge, and engaging in therapeutic encounters. Similar practices are undertaken by physicians, psychologists and social workers, to name a few. However, nurses are the biggest professional group of the Western world health care systems and the ones who are frequently made invisible, feel unimportant and victims of the organizations and groups that they help to create, sustain, and manage. The traditional framework used by nurses to analyse their practices helps to perpetuate the impression of a powerless profession.

According to Foucault's definition of governmentality, we believe that nurses constitute an important group that helps the state to govern at a distance. Nurses also form a critical group that challenges the status quo and works for a more equitable society. However, we believe that nurses predominantly conceive of health care as a neutral and apolitical practice (Meyer 1998, Freed 1999). Yet nurses' privileged position close to patients and communities allows them to act upon these individuals and groups. Through education, they normalize and discipline; through care, they alleviate the suffering of vulnerable individuals and communities and participate in the construction of patient identities as sick bodies or healthy bodies. They possess a scientific *savoir* that is generally accepted as true knowledge and are able to influence patient behaviours regarding their health, illness, and well-being. Nurses, as good translators of sophisticated medical and nursing terminology, are close to the public's needs and have their confidence.

Indeed, nurses are a group able to exercise power as health care providers, despite the fact that they seldom reflect about their own ways of exercising power or rarely perceive health care as a political activity. Nurses operate within a web of power relations defined by a society (also constituted by nurses) ruled by disciplinary and pastoral power strategies which are the main tools to govern conduct in our contemporary era. Despite the well known rhetoric regarding nurses' powerlessness, we believe that nurses constitute a powerful group of health care professionals located at the crossroad of the state's rationalities and patients' bodies and souls. This understanding situates them as an agency of governmentality.

Final Remarks: Exploring the Limits and Potential of Governmentality

Rethinking nursing through the concept of governmentality could be perceived by many as a threatening experience. We have commented previously that the use of Foucauldian concepts 'can generate a form of critical immobilism' (Gastaldo & Holmes 1999, p. 23) because governmentality links together repressive and constructive ways of exercising power. The deterministic nature of 'power everywhere' and the sense of being governed, even through our freedom, generate strong and emotive responses such as a need to escape, especially because moral attributes traditionally have been attached to different ways of governing. We are used to searching for "the right way' of practising nursing care and of being ethical in our interpersonal relationships or when governing society. For instance, compliance through disciplinary power becomes an imperative for patients suffering from life-threatening diseases, which can be managed by medication. However, the concept of governmentality challenges many assumptions taken for granted in nursing: ethics becomes politics, patient empowerment becomes a call for self-regulation, and in many ways nursing research serves the economic elites to the detriment of social equity.

The concept of governmentality should be seen as a valuable tool for deconstructing nursing as an apolitical practice and a powerless profession. However, it should also help us to envision alternative ways of practising nursing. To insist on a single unified identity as powerless professionals means many times that no criticism can be raised against nurses; it represents the creation of an analytic shield that protects and explains the current arrangements of power. Critical perspectives are seen as unreasonable or victim blaming. To conceive nurses as professionals who exercise power serves a two-fold purpose: it allows for a more complex conceptualization of practice and it can potentially reveal some of the elements that perpetuate nurses' underprivileged position in society.

Being historically situated in a nonpriviledged position to negotiate working conditions or to benefit from social prestige does not mean that nurses do not exercise power or that they are not powerful. The examples presented in this paper illustrate some of the ways in which nurses exercise power in their everyday practices. What remains is the need to articulate power exercises with political rationalities to which groups of nurses subscribe and to analyse the governmental technologies we develop and support. This process should be guided by critiques that emerge from considerations of governmentality because this concept reminds us that competing discourses, even among nurses, are constantly reshaping ideas and practices regarding nursing and health in the social, economic, and political arenas. Personally and as professionals, we have been exploring the potential of combining ideas about governmentality with critical social theories such as emancipatory feminism (Manias & Street 2000). To understand power without being able to identify 'possible transformations' (Meyer 1998) derived from this Foucauldian perspective will not lead nursing into critical political action. However, the concept of governmentality sheds light on the impossibility of a single strategy to achieve more social recognition for nurses and reminds us that we are powerful at the same time that we are situated historically in a nonpriviledged position.

Acknowledgments

The authors would like to thank our colleague Dagmar Meyer from the Faculty of Education, Federal University of Rio Grande do Sul, Brazil, for many discussions on the subject of the paper and the scholars from the St Bartholomew School of Nursing and Midwifery, City University, UK, for their comments on this paper, which were shared after a presentation in November 2000. The authors are also grateful to the anonymous reviewers for their comments.

REFERENCES

Arendt H. (1995) Idéologie et terreur: un nouveau type de régime. *Les Origines Du Totalitarisme—Le Système Totalitaire*. Seuil, Paris.

Arruda E. & Silva A. (2000) Perspectiva internacional cerca de indicadores de qualidade em cursos de doutorado em enfermagem. *Revista Basileira de Enfermagem* **53**, 63–73.

Clinton M. & Nelson S. (1999) Recovery and mental illness. In *Advanced Practice in Mental Health Nursing* (Clinton M. & Nelson S. eds), Blackwell Science, Oxford, pp. 260–278.

Curtis B. (1995) Taking the state back out: Rose and Miller on political power. *British Journal of Sociology* **46**, 575–589.

Dean M. (1994) A social structure of many souls: moral regulation, government, and self-formation. *Canadian Journal of Sociology* **19**, 145–168.

Dean M. (1999) *Governmentality*. Sage, Thousand Oaks, CA.

Deflem M. (1998) Surveillance and criminal statistics: historical foundation of governmentality. *Studies in Law, Politics and Society* **17**, 1–28.

Foucault M., ([1975] 1995) *Surveiller et Punir: Naissance de la Prison*. Tel/Gallimard, St-Amand.

Foucault M. (1979) Governmentality. *Ideology and Consciousness* **6**, 5–21.

Foucault M. (1980a) Truth and power. In *Power/Knowledge and Selected Interviews and Other Writings 1972–1977 by Michel Foucault* (Gordon C. ed.), Pantheon Books, New York, pp. 109–133.

Foucault M. (1980b) The eye of power. In *Power/Knowledge and Selected Interviews and Other Writings 1972–1977 by Michel Foucault* (Gordon C. ed.), Pantheon Books, New York, pp. 146–165.

Foucault M. (1990) *History of Sexuality 1: An Introduction*. Penguin Books, London.

Foucault M. (1994a) *Dits et Écrits, tome 4*. Editions Gallimard, Paris.

Foucault M. (1994b) *Dits et Écrits, tome 3*. Editions Gallimard, Paris.

Foucault M. (1997) *Il Faut Défendre la Société*. Seuil/Gallimard, Paris.

Francke A., Garssen B. & Huijer Abu-Saad H. (1995) Determinants of changes in nurses' behaviour after continuing education: a literature review. *Journal of Advanced Nursing* **21**, 371–377.

Freed L. A. (1999) Power, politics and public policy. In *Community Health Nursing: Caring in Action* (Hitchcock J., Schubett P. & Thomas S. eds), Delmar Publishers, Boston, pp. 745–764.

Gastaldo D. (1997) Is health education good for you? Re-thinking health education through the concept of bio-power. In *Foucault, Health and Medicine* (Petersen A. & Bunton R. eds), Routlege, London, pp. 113–133.

Gastaldo D. (2000) Caring beyond nursing: politics from the South—Editorial. *Nursing Inquiry* **7**, 73.

Gastaldo D., De Pedro J. & Bover A. (2001) El reto de investigar en enfermería: una reflexión sobre las universidades españolas y el contexto internacional. *Enfermería Clínica* **11**, 220–229.

Gastaldo D. & Holmes D. (1999) Foucault and nursing: a history of the present. *Nursing Inquiry* **6**, 17–25.

Gordon C. (1991) Governmental rationality: an introduction. In *The Foucault Effect* (Burchell G., Gordon C. & Miller P. eds), The University of Chicago Press, Chicago, pp. 1–51.

Gros F. (1996) *Que Sais-Je? Michel Foucault*. Presses Universitaires de France, Paris.

Hail P. (1986) *Governing the Economy: The Politics of State Intervention in Britain and France*. Cambridge Polity Press, Cambridge.

Hewitt M. (1991) Biopolitics and social policy: Foucault's account of welfare. In *The Body: Social Processes and Cultural Theory* (Featherstone M., Hepworth M. & Turner B. eds), Sage, London, pp. 225–255.

Hindess B. (1996) *Discourses of Power: From Hobbes to Foucault*. Blackwell Publishers, Oxford.

Holmes D. (2001) Articulation du contrôle social et des soins infirmiers dans un contexte de psychiatrie penitentiaire. Thèse de doctorat, Université de Montréal, Montréal.

Lukes S. (1974) *Power: A Radical View*. Macmillan, London.

Lunardi V. (1999) *A Ética Como O Cuidado de Si E O Poder Pastoral Na Enfermagem*. Editoras Universitárias UFSC/UFPel, Florianópolis.

Lunardi Filho W. (2000) *O Mito Da Subalternidade Do Trabalho Da Enfermagem Á Medicina*. Editoras Universitárias UFSC/UFPel, Florianópolis.

MacGuire J. (1990) Putting nursing research findings into practice: research utilization as an aspect of the management of change. *Journal of Advanced Nursing* **15**, 614–620.

Manias E. & Street A. (2000) Possibilities for critical social theory and Foucault's work: a tool box approach. *Nursing Inquiry* **7**, 50–60.

Martin M. & Forchuk C. (1994) Linking research and practice. *International Nursing Review* **41**, 184–187.

Marx K. (1946) *Capital-Volume 1*. George Allan & Unwin, London.

McHoul A. & Grace W. (1993) *A Foucault Primer: Discourse, Power and the Subject*. New York University Press, New York.

McKeever P. (1996) The family: long-term care research and policy formulation. *Nursing Inquiry* **3**, 200–206.

McNay L. (1994) *Foucault: A Critical Introduction*. Continuum Publishing, New York.

Meyer D. (1998) Espaços de sombra e luz: reflex?es em torno da dimens?o educativa da enfermagem. In *Marcas Da Diversidade: Saberes E Fazeres Da Enfermagem Contemporânea* (Meyer D., Waldow V. & Lopes M. eds), Artes Médicas, Porto Alegre, pp. 27–42.

Moss J. (1998) *The Later Foucault*. Sage, Thousand Oaks, CA.

Nettleton S. (1991) Wisdom, diligence and teeth: discursive practices and the creation of mothers. *Sociology of Health & Illness* **13**, 98–111.

Ransom J. S. (1997) *Foucault's Discipline: The Politics of Subjectivities*. Duke University Press, Durham, NC.

Rose N. (1998) *Inventing Ourselves: Psychology, Power and Personhood*. Cambridge University Press, Cambridge.

Rose N. & Miller P. (1992) Political power beyond the state: problematics of government. *British Journal of Sociology* **42**, 173–205.

Simon J. (1993) *Poor Discipline: Parole and the Social Control of the Underclass, 1890–1990*. University of Chicago Press, Chicago.

Stewart M. (2000) *Community Nursing: Promoting Canadians' Health*, 2nd edn. W. B. Saunders, Toronto, ON.

Weber M. (1986) Domination by economic power and by authority. In *Power* (Lukes S. ed.), New York University Press, New York.

Weberman D. (1995) Foucault's reconception of power. *The Philosophical Forum* **26**, 189–217.

The Authors Comment

Nursing as Means of Governmentality

We have entered the 21st century, a time of global markets and fast information flow, and nurses are probably the most important group of health care providers in the world. Despite this assertion, nurses often describe themselves as powerless. Intrigued by this issue, we decided to write two articles (the first one, published in *Nursing Inquiry*, in 1999, was entitled "Foucault & nursing: A history of the present") to illustrate an alternative way to conceptualize power and demonstrate how nurses exercise power, even though they are frequently viewed as a group of professionals in an underprivileged position.

—Dave Holmes
—Denise Gastaldo

Nursing Theorizing as an Ethical Endeavor

Pamela G. Reed

This article addresses the ethical dimensions of nursing theorizing. Nursing theorizing, whether it occurs primarily at the outset or emerges during the process of inquiry, is inescapably linked to the theorist's value choices and beliefs about human beings, the environment, and health. These choices are reflected in the conceptual frame of one's research. The normative commitment of the conceptual frame is explored using examples from nursing and nonnursing research. Elements of critical ethical reflection are outlined. It is suggested that the discipline's understanding of what constitutes health and how best to promote health, as well as solutions to ethical dilemmas posed by research, may be enhanced by purposeful ethical inquiry that occurs as an integral component of theorizing activities.

Nurses and other scientists who are embracing the postpositivist tradition in science recognize the historical evolution of knowledge: that knowledge is not absolute but changes in interaction with the culture as a whole and with the scientists, theologians, practitioners, philosophers, and others who contribute to perceptions of truth. There is no one truth about the pathway to health that allows theorists, once it is discovered and described, to sit back, content in knowing that they had laid out the facts and cannot be held accountable for the consequences of their theories. No one dominant paradigm exists as a guide for nursing inquiry in the selection of the right worldview, the right perspective on human health and nursing, the right questions and goals, the right method, or the right answers. Instead, development of nursing knowledge seems to be flour-

About the Author

PAMELA G. REED was born in Detroit, MI, in June 1952 and grew up in an environment enriched by the sociopolitical and musical events of Motown. She is a three-time graduate of Wayne State University in Detroit, receiving a BSN in 1974, an MSN in 1976 (with a double major in child-adolescent psychiatric mental health nursing and teaching), and her PhD, with a major in nursing (focus on lifespan development and aging, nursing theory) in 1982. She worked as a psychiatric-mental health clinical nurse specialist and was an Instructor in Nursing at Oakland University, Rochester, MI, from 1976 to 1979. From 1983 to the present, she has been on the faculty at the University of Arizona College of Nursing in Tucson, including 7 years serving as Associate Dean for Academic Affairs. With her doctoral work, she pioneered nursing research into spirituality and its role in well-being. Dr. Reed has developed a theory of self-transcendence and two widely used research instruments, the *Spiritual Perspective Scale* and the *Self-Transcendence Scale*. Her publications reflect her three main passions and contributions to nursing: the conceptual and empirical bases of the significance of spirituality in health experiences, a lifespan developmental perspective of well-being in aging and end of life, and the philosophic dimensions of the development of the discipline. Dr. Reed also enjoys classical music, hiking in the Grand Canyon, swimming, and raising her two daughters, Regina and Rebecca, with her husband Gary.

ishing in what Laudan (1984) described as a "dissensus" rather than consensus among nursing paradigms. Philosophical aims of nursing are changing toward a focus on "continuing a conversation rather than discovering truth" (Rorty, 1979, p. 373).

The nature of the discipline of nursing is such that the ethical implications of nursing science in general and the ethical implications of the selected conceptual perspective of the individual's research in particular are enormous. This is so not only because the consequences of nursing conceptualizations are intimately linked to promotion of a good of society—health—but also because of the shifting axiology of the discipline. Criteria for what characterizes essential knowledge and for making value choices and judgments in conceptualizing the phenomena of nursing vary across extant nursing paradigms. The indeterminate nature of nursing phenomena is such that these criteria may never, and perhaps should never, be definitively described. Nevertheless, the "assumptions, value choices, and judgments" (Chinn & Jacobs, 1987, p. 80) on which theory is based are ultimately translated into nursing knowledge for actions that directly affect human health. Ac-

cording to Bellah, "what [our theories] say human beings [and health] fundamentally are has inevitable implications about what they ought to be" (Bellah, 1981, p. 15).

Nursing theorizing, then, is an ethical endeavor. Theorizing refers here to the reasoning processes involved in constructing what Kaplan (1964) has termed the "conceptual frame," or the framework or theory in scientific inquiry. Choices made in theory have ethical consequences in practice. In addition, the act of theorizing alone constitutes a "moral situation" (Dewey, 1948) in that it entails reflective choice and deliberate consideration of what may be better or worse. Thus, both the purpose of nursing inquiry and the nature of the phenomena studied render nursing theorizing its ethical dimension.

Nursing theorizing, whether it occurs at the outset or emerges during the process of inquiry, is inescapably linked to the theorist's value choices and beliefs about human beings, the environment, and health. The message in Nietzsche's "dogma of immaculate perception" (Nietzsche, 1966) extends to qualitative and quantitative methodologies alike. No observation is free from conceptual contamination; observation is already cognition, valuing, and believing (Kaplan, 1965). More precisely, there is no such thing as immaculate conceptualization in theorizing. Regardless of the methodology by which theories are advanced, theorizing likely entails value choices made by the nursing theorist or researcher that ultimately influence the good of society. Kaplan's thesis "that not all value concerns are unscientific, that indeed some of them are called for by the scientific enterprise itself" (Kaplan, 1965, p. 373) is an understatement for nursing science where value-laden terms such as health are the prime focus of inquiry.

The Normative Commitment of the Conceptual Frame

All phases of scientific inquiry in nursing are embedded in "normative commitments" (Bellah, 1981). Deontological judgments of moral value and obligation occur in nursing theorizing, evidenced for example in the theorist's speculations about what may be good for health or well-being, why it may be good, and what ought to be done to promote that good. The distinction between cognitive and normative knowledge is hazy at best and, because of this, ethical inquiry must accompany inquiry into human processes (Bellah, 1981).

Critical ethical reflection is important not only in the testing and application of knowledge, but also in the conceptualization of knowledge. Ethical knowing has been put forth as an essential component of nursing knowledge (Carper, 1978) and fundamental to the development of theory (Chinn & Jacobs, 1987). However, the ethical dimension of selecting or developing a conceptual frame for research has been addressed in the literature by only a few, such as Archbold (1987) or mentioned only in passing (White, 1983).

Ethical issues continues to be addressed in nursing research most characteristically in reference to methodology (Connors, 1988; Moccia, 1988; Munhall, 1988), but also in reference to health care policy (Hinshaw, 1988) and allocation of resources for research (Fowler, 1987). Conspicuous references to the ethical aspects of research methodology and overall purpose of

research are found in the American Nurses' Association's *Code of Ethics* (ANA, 1985) and *Human Rights Guidelines* (ANA, 1984). However, selection of a research strategy, generally recognized as a value-laden decision, is often so because the conceptual frame out of which this decision flows is value laden. Careful attention to the values and assumptions operant in the conceptual perspective of a study could facilitate solutions to ethical dilemmas encountered at other points in the research process. Ethical inquiry into the components of an individual's conceptual frame, as prerequisite to the ethical inquiry into the methodology suggested by Munhall (1988) and others, could further enhance the likelihood that the means and ends of research will be morally justified.

The ethical responsibilities associated with scientific knowledge cannot be relegated entirely to the implementors of the research design nor to those who translate the findings in clinical practice. Normative commitments are made in the earliest efforts in theorizing. Dewey (1928) rejected the positivist, continental European image of the scientist as one whose dedication to reason and truth sets him or her apart from the ethical concerns related to the products of science. Dewey denied any dualism between scientific and moral thinking and proclaimed that scientific activity is inherently moralistic in its concern with understanding natural processes and their relationship to the welfare of humankind.

Laudan's (1977, 1981) historicist view on scientific progress reinforces the normative commitment of the conceptual frame in research. Scientific progress is evaluated, according to Laudan, in terms of the problem-solving effectiveness of the discipline's theories. A major problem of interest in nursing is the facilitation of health as a good of society. The nature of nursing is such that, if nurses are to contribute to the scientific progress of their discipline, their theorizing must incorporate a moral dimension that includes logical reasoning and creative reflection on what may be considered good or best vis-à-vis the health of individuals and groups. If nursing theories are to have problem-solving effectiveness, clarification of an individual's ontology, values, and goals must occur not only in reference to implementing the research design as pointed out by Moccia (1988), but also in reference to the act of conceptualizing.

Value-based choices about the sorts of conceptualizations or theories invoked in research influence decisions regarding the problems deemed worthy of study, the perceived societal benefits, definition and measurement of concepts, the types of participant risks worth taking, acceptable threats to internal and external validity, the interpretation and significance of the findings, and most importantly the knowledge offered for use in effecting health in human beings. It is not inconceivable that the conceptual nets (Popper, 1968) cast out by scientists could be used for catching fish only for their liking and not necessarily for the good of society. .

So powerful is the conceptual frame of a study that Kaplan (1964) noted one could more easily dispense with the physical operations of a study than with the framework that gives meaning to all of the research activities. The same methodology can constitute a different study and result in different outcomes if the conceptual framework changes. Secondary analysis is an example of this. Moreover, Laudan (1981) explained that changes in scientific knowledge occur more often due to conceptual issues rather than questions of empirical support.

Ethical Implications of Selected Conceptual Frameworks

The ethical implications of theorizing can be illustrated in examples from nursing and nonnursing literature. In the nonnursing literature, examples of the ethical significance of conceptual frameworks can be found in classic studies of human development. Human development, like health, is a value-laden concept and not easily defined. Personal biases have entered into conceptualizations of development with moral consequences.

Developmental Psychology Literature
The late 17th-century conceptualization of the tabula rasa view of people held moral implications related to the potential for human development and well-being.

Neither the environment nor the person was perceived as having an active role in development. The infant, in particular, was viewed as insignificant in terms of his or her value in effecting change in the environment; infants were perceived as ineffectual, empty vessels waiting to be filled with information. Research hypotheses derived from this conceptual stance were directed toward the study of maturity in terms of the acquisition of a quantity of information using the adult white male as the standard. This framework limited the scope of study about sources of human potential and ways in which development could be enhanced from early life onward. Primary intervention for the emotional development of infants, for example, was unheard of, since the infant was not conceptualized as a unique and dynamic being.

The nature vs. nurture controversy was brought to public scrutiny with Jensen's (1973) well-known conclusions about genetically based racial differences in intelligence. Jensen was proclaimed as having hoodwinked large segments of government and society into believing that IQ was genetically based, and as having an oppressive effect on disadvantaged, primarily black individuals (Jensen, 1973; Kamin, 1974). The ethical implications of Jensen's work relate to provision of educational opportunities, hiring practices, and to the self-concept and self-expectations of certain ethnic groups. The debate about the heritability of intelligence continues to be fueled by contrasting views about the development of intelligence, particularly by conceptual frameworks such as Jensen's, which dichotomize the contributions of heredity and environment in development and do not account for the possibility of interaction between the two factors.

The decrement model of human aging provides an example of the influences that a conceptual frame may have on human welfare. This model was most popular 15 years ago, although its influences can still be felt today. The decrement model emphasized quantitative biological changes that occur with age, such as cardiovascular and perceptual losses (Botwinick, 1973; Horn, 1976). These losses were generalized to the overall process of aging; regression of capabilities was regarded as a normal process. Young adulthood marked the time of maximal level of development, after which linear and irreversible decrement occurred.

Aging was conceptualized as a first in, last out process, whereby the most recent and complex abilities are lost first and the earliest and simplest are retained (Labouvie-Vief & Schell, 1983). The older adult was conceived of as becoming more childlike with development. In addition, the environmental context was not valued as significant in the process of aging. Research based on this model focused solely on ontogenetic rather than contextual factors in development (Labouvie-Vief, 1977). Thus, for example, plasticity, the ability to learn from the environment (now recognized as a characteristic ability of the elderly), was not identified as an issue of aging worthy of study.

The decrement model, in which developmental changes were conceptualized primarily as losses rather than as adaptive or progressive, did little to facilitate means to improve health care, educational programs, and career opportunities of the elderly, not to mention promotion of self-esteem among older adults and a basic societal value for the elderly persons. Research efforts guided by this conceptual frame and directed toward its support could be regarded as unethical, particularly in view of the theorizing and scientific evidence to the contrary that were emerging at the time (Baltes & Baltes, 1977; Labouvie-Vief, 1980; Schaie, 1973).

Nursing Literature

Examples of ethical issues in theorizing exist in current nursing literature, although perhaps they are not yet viewed as being as dramatic as the historical accounts from the developmental psychology literature. A research report on social support by Ellison (1985) increases awareness of the potential dangers in conceptualizing social support as a purely positive phenomenon. Her findings suggest that social support is most health promotive only during certain phases of the lifespan and that social support in other developmental phases may be detrimental to individuals. Personal biases about the desirability of social support that enter the research framework unchecked can have costly effects on well-being when applied in clinical practice.

Boyd's (1985) analysis of the concept of "identification" demonstrates the different meanings the term acquires within various theoretical frameworks. A key point presented was that identification in the parent-child relationship typically has been conceptualized as a one-way, time-limited process in which the child is influenced by the parent. This view contrasts sharply with the mutually interactive and dynamic view of interpersonal relationships depicted in some nursing conceptual frameworks. Research and intervention approaches stemming from a one-sided framework have neglected the potential influence of the child on the parent, including influences on fulfillment of the parental role and the parent's well-being as parent and as a human being.

Narayan and Joslin's (1980) critique of the medical conceptual model of human crisis and their proposal of a nursing model of crisis illustrate the striking difference that a conceptual perspective could make in terms of clinical intervention. In one model, pathogenic risks of crisis are emphasized and a return to the pre-crisis level of functioning is the treatment goal; in the other model, opportunities for growth enhancement are emphasized and treatment goals acknowledge the human potential for change and further development. Because the definitions of health and goals for intervention differ markedly between the medical and nursing models, it is likely that different outcomes in the client's health and well-being would occur as well. Explicating a conceptual framework of crisis is an ethical endeavor, requiring reflection on one's beliefs about human potential, the level of functioning of which the client is perceived capable, and the ideals the clinician may envision for the client.

There are many nursing phenomena that, when conceptualized for research, stimulate if not demand ethical reflection by the theorist. Personal biases and assumptions about emotional illness, adolescent development, and female sexuality, for example, which typically elicit presumptive notions about the value of time, independence, and other assumed goods, can have moral influences on the types of conceptualizations constructed in the study of these phenomena as they relate to health.

Ethical Reflection— Response to a Calling

In the spirit of Nightingale's ideas, Kaplan stated that science is a "calling" and "cannot flourish if it is always an occupation only" (Kaplan, 1964, p. 379). He explains further that, while one chooses an occupation, a calling chooses the individual and commits him or her to the professional ethic of science—values that guide the conduct of inquiry. The professional ethic of scientific inquiry extends beyond basic moral principles such as beneficence, nonmaleficence, and justice. This ethic is also evident in theorizing about nursing phenomena in a manner unwavered by "habit, by tradition, by the Academy, or by the powers that be" (Kaplan, 1964, p. 380). Normative commitments made in theorizing must not be limited by traditions that exist, either in practice or theory, in hospitals or schools of nursing. The potential for human health is not static, but is ever expanding. Ideas put forth in the conceptual frame must not compromise or constrain this human potential.

Theorists are morally obligated to deliberately examine their motives and values as reflected in their conceptualizations about health and health-related issues. Propositions implicit and explicit to the conceptual frame should be judged not only in reference to what they state but also in reference to what they make more likely (Kaplan, 1964).

Ethical inquiry into one's conceptual frame requires examination of both intrapersonal factors (e.g., worldview, personal and professional experiences) and eonal factors (e.g., historical context, influential others) (DeGroot, 1988) as they influence the motives and purposes underlying one's conceptual frame. Ethical reflection also entails:

- assessment of the moral ideals underlying the concepts of health, human being, environment, and nursing practice that may be represented in the framework;
- creative imagining of the consequences of one's framework;
- depth of personal knowledge;

- moral vision, described by McInerny (1987) as awareness of the deepest beliefs about such things as the value of life and death, and the nature and worth of the environment; and
- an openness to undergo a "transformation of values" (Chinn, 1985) when it is determined that concepts need redefining or theories need reformulating.

An ethical framework in nursing reflects not only a basic concern for human welfare, but also a moral commitment to the discipline. The theorizer must refrain from being lured into conceptualizations "framed in the unique perspective of other disciplines" (Smoth, 1988, p. 3) that offer more certainty or specificity for the theorists but make little contribution to the aims of nursing. Smith (1988) admonishes nurses to stay tough during the process of theorizing. Moral timidity creates trivial theory. Bellah was highly critical of those who lacked moral vision in their inquiry, who misrepresented human processes with reductionistic and deterministic conceptualizations, and who hid behind the excuse that "our science is still young" (Bellah, 1981, p. 17).

Toward Boldness in Nursing Theorizing

There is movement underfoot to become more deliberate in exploring the philosophical bases of nursing theorizing. Evidence for this can be found not only in the nursing literature over the past decade, but also among graduate students' requests for more courses and course content on the history and philosophy of science, in lunch-hour seminars in which various philosophical views are debated, and in conference proceedings that address philosophical issues as integral to theory development. Doctoral students are embracing a new philosophy of their science, a philosophy that thrives on the indeterminate nature of nursing phenomena, entertains radically new hypotheses, welcomes diversity among paradigms, and values independent thought. At the same time, it is a philosophy that challenges scientists to examine the ethical questions associated with their value choices, judgments, and patterns of reasoning. As nursing turns toward a greater focus on substance rather than structure in the science (Downs, 1988; Fitzpatrick, 1987), increased attention may be given to the ethical dimensions of conceptual processes in research as has been given to the ethical dimensions of the methodological processes in research.

The discipline's understanding of what constitutes health and how best to promote optimal well-being, quality of life, and other values may be clarified by purposeful ethical reflection as a routine occurrence in theorizing. Carper, in explaining the importance of the ethical pattern of knowing, stated that differences in normative judgments may have more to do with disagreements over conceptualizations of health than with a lack of empirical evidence (Carper, 1978). Ethical knowledge about the underpinnings of the conceptual frame may also facilitate solutions to ethical dilemmas encountered in other stages of the research process and in the eventual clinical applications of knowledge.

Nursing scientists today are being challenged to make choices in their theorizing—choices that touch their own identity as well as affect the good of society. Tensions between theory and practice, the conceptual and the operational, help bring into focus the variety of philosophical views and values inherent among nursing paradigms, and the choices one makes in explicating a framework. Is human health best measured and promoted from a reductionistic or holistic perspective or is there yet another perspective? Is the environment best conceptualized as integral or external to human functioning? Is the human cell or human field, or some other human dimension, the fundamental unit of study in nursing?

In nursing's present phase of development as a science, scientists need to explicate the value choices underlying their frameworks in a bold, self-informed manner. Knowledge can be used as sociopolitical power to enforce a theorized good and to affect human health in unforeseeable ways. Ethical inquiry into one's conceptual frame can provide needed constraints on the human tendency to blur the distinction between a researcher's beliefs and societal needs and can also provide the moral vision needed to effectively and humanely solve nursing problems.

REFERENCES

American Nurses' Association (1985). *Code of ethics.* Kansas City: Author.

American Nurses' Association (1984). *Human rights guidelines.* Kansas City: Author.

Archbold, P. G. (1981). Ethical issues in the selection of a theoretical framework for gerontological nursing research. *Journal of Gerontologic Nursing, 7,* 408–411.

Baltes, M. M., & Baltes, P. B. (1977). The ecopsychological reactivity and plasticity of psychological aging: Convergent perspectives of cohort effects and operant psychology. *Psychology, 24,* 179–197.

Bellah, R. N. (1981). The ethical aims of social inquiry. *Teachers College Record, 83*(1), 1–18.

Botwinick, J. (1973). *Aging and behavior.* New York: Springer.

Boyd, C. (1985). Toward an understanding of mother-daughter identification using concept analysis. *Advances in Nursing Science, 7*(3), 78–86.

Carper, B. A. (1978). Fundamental patterns of knowing in nursing. *Advances in Nursing Science, 1*(1), 13–24.

Chinn, P. L. (1985). Quality of life: A values transformation. *Advances in Nursing Science, 8*(1), vii–ix.

Chinn, P. L., & Jacobs, M. K. (1987). *Theory and nursing* (2nd ed.). St. Louis: C. V. Mosby.

Connors, D. D. (1988). A continuum of research-participant relationships: An analysis and critique. *Advances in Nursing Science, 10*(4), 32–42.

DeGroot, H. A. (1988). Scientific inquiry in nursing: A model for a new age. *Advances in Nursing Science, 10*(3), 1–21.

Dewey, J. (1928). In J. Rather (Ed.). *The philosophy of John Dewey.* New York: Holt, Rinehart & Winston.

Dewey, J. (1948). *Reconstruction in philosophy.* Boston: Beacon Press.

Downs, F. (1988). Doctoral education: Our claim to the future. *Nursing Outlook, 36*(1), 18–20.

Ellison, E. S. (1985). Social support and the constructive-developmental model. *Western Journal of Nursing Research, 9,* 19–28.

Fitzpatrick, J. J. (1987). Philosophical approach: Empiricism. In C. Bridges & N. Wells (Eds.). *Proceedings of the Fourth Nursing Science Colloquium: Strategies for Nursing Theory Development.* Boston: Boston University School of Nursing.

Fowler, M. D. (1987). Ethical issues in nursing research. *Western Journal of Nursing Research, 9,* 269–271.

Hinshaw, A. S. (1988). Using research to shape health policy. *Nursing Outlook, 36*(1), 21–24.

Hirsch, J. (1975). Jensenism: The bankruptcy of "science" without scholarship. *Educational Theory, 25,* 3–28.

Horn, J. L. (1976). Human abilities: A review of research and theory in the early 1970s. *Annual Review of Psychology, 27,* 437–485.

Jensen, A. R. (1973). Race, intelligence, and genetics: The differences are real. *Psychology Today, 12,* 80–86.

Kamin, L. J. (1974). *The science and politics of IQ.* New York: Halstead.

Kaplan, A. (1964). *The logic of scientific discovery.* New York: Thomas Y. Crowell.

Labouvie-Vief, G. (1977). Adult cognitive development: In search of alternative interpretations. *Merrill-Palmer Quarterly of Behavior and Development, 23*(4), 227–263.

Labouvie-Vief, G. (1980). Adaptive dimensions of adult cognition. In N. Datan & N. Lohmann (Eds.). Transitions in aging. New York: Academic Press.

Labouvie-Vief, G., & Schell, D. A. (1983). Learning and memory in later life: A developmental view. In B. Wolman & G. Striker (Eds.). *Handbook of developmental psychology.* Englewood Cliffs, NJ: Prentice-Hall.

Laudan, L. (1977). *Progress and its problems: Toward a theory of scientific growth.* Berkeley, CA: University of California Press.

Laudan, L. (1981). A problem-solving approach to scientific progress. In I. Hacking (Ed.). *Scientific revolutions.* New York: Oxford University Press.

Laudan, L. (1984). *Science and values.* Berkeley, CA: University of California Press.

McInerny, W. F. (1987). Understanding moral issues in health care: Seven essential ideas. *Journal of Professional Nursing, 3,* 268–277.

Moccia, P. (1988). A critique of compromise: Beyond the methods debate. *Advances in Nursing Science, 10*(4), 1–9.

Munhall, P. L. (1988). Ethical considerations in qualitative research. *Western Journal of Nursing Research, 10,* 150–162.

Narayan, S. M., & Joslin, D. J. (1980). Crisis theory and intervention: A critique of the medical model and proposal of a holistic nursing model. *Advances in Nursing Science, 2*(4), 27–40.

Nietzche, F. (1966). *Beyond good and evil* (W. Kaufmann, trans). New York: Vintage.

Popper, K. R. (1968). *The logic of scientific discovery.* New York: Harper & Row.

Rorty, R. (1979). *Philosophy and the mirror of nature.* Princeton, NJ: Princeton University Press.

Schaie, K. W. (1973). Methodological problems in research on adulthood and aging. In J. R. Nesselroade & H. W. Reese (Eds.). *Life-span developmental psychology: Methodological issues.* New York: Academic Press.

Smith, M. J. (1988). Wallowing while waiting, *Nursing Science Quarterly, 1*(1), 3.

White, G. B. (1983). Philosophical ethics and nursing—a word of caution. In P. L. Chinn (Ed.). *Advances in nursing theory development.* Rockville, MD: Aspen.

The Author Comments

Nursing Theorizing as an Ethical Endeavor

This article was written to address a gap in the ethics literature and course content that I noticed early in my teaching career. Ethics was depicted as an important component of practice and research but not theory. This was so despite the links professed to exist between theory, research, and practice. Theorizing is a powerful tool in knowledge building, affecting the focus and outcomes of research. It calls for ethical reflection on the variables we choose to study, how we define them, and how they fit into a theoretic framework to influence the nursing that is practiced. I anticipate that ethics will move into the center of nursing theory development as the 21st century progresses.

—PAMELA G. REED

CHAPTER 38

Integration of Nursing Theory and Nursing Ethics*

Michael Yeo

Nursing theory and nursing ethics are two main areas of inquiry in nursing scholarship today. Each addresses common themes and each, in its own way, speaks not only about but for nursing. In spite of this commonality there is remarkably little dialogue between them. Both theory and ethics shall benefit from increased integration.

Nursing today is a profession in flux and a profession profoundly self-critical and self-examining. This self-examination is primarily taking place in two proliferating areas of scholarship, nursing theory and nursing ethics. A rich dialogue exists within each of these areas but remarkably little communication occurs between them.

One important shared factor behind the rapid growth of scholarship both in nursing theory and nursing ethics is the ascending importance of professionalism in nursing. Although the rhetoric of professionalism has been around for some time—as early as 1900 Nightingale[1] was proclaiming that nursing had become a profession—developments in the 1950s marked a decisive turning point.[2,3] This is evidenced by increased emphasis on fundamental questions having to do with the education, role, and responsibility unique and proper to nursing. A more radical questioning has occurred about the nurse's role and responsibility in relation to patients, other health care professionals, and society in general. Both nursing theory and nursing ethics attempt to come to terms with such issues and define a distinct professional identity for nursing.

*This article was supported by a grant from Associated Medical Services and the Richard and Jean Ivey Fund.

About the Author

MICHAEL YEO is a philosopher who specializes in ethics, particularly professional ethics. He received his PhD in philosophy from McMaster University. He was a researcher at the Westminster Institute for Ethics and Human Values for 5 years, during which time he wrote this article. He subsequently worked as an ethicist for the Canadian Medical Association for 5 years, during which time his primary area of research was (and remains) health privacy. He is a Visiting Professor in the Department of Philosophy at Carleton University and consultant on ethics to various professions and organizations, including the Canadian Nurses Association. He is currently working on a third edition of his book *Concepts and Cases in Nursing Ethics* (Broadview Press).

Dispute about the necessary requirements for a profession exists, but there is some consensus on at least two demarcating criteria: a profession must possess a distinct knowledge base and it also must possess some ethical standards to which its practitioners can be held accountable.[4,5] Nursing theory addresses the first requirement, nursing ethics the second.

There is a remarkable lack of communication between nursing theory and nursing ethics. They address common questions and themes but, judging from the scant cross-referencing, each does so independently of the other. For example, Roy,[6] in her most recent account of the adaptation model, does not cite any works in the nursing ethics literature. Conversely, Muyskens,[7] in a major investigation of the philosophical and ethical foundations of nursing, cites none of the major theorists. Although nursing theory and nursing ethics are mutually relevant, for the most part this has gone unremarked.

Relevance of Nursing Ethics to Nursing Theory

In order to disclose the relevance of nursing ethics to nursing theory, it is important to call into question what might appear to be a fundamental difference separating the two. This difference centers on the idea, or better, the ideal of science. Science is highly valued in the nursing theory literature. To be sure, the sense in which a nursing theory could be said to be scientific, and the sense in which nursing science is science, has been much debated. This debate has taken into account the discussions among philosophers of science about the nature of science and of scientific method.[8,9] Nevertheless, the requirement much in evidence is that theory, if it is to be legitimate, must meet some criteria for being scientific.

This valuation of science is largely a response to the search for a legitimate knowledge base for nursing, which in turn is part of nursing's general drive for professionalism.[10] Science commands authority and power in this society, and was bound to appeal to nursing theorists as a sure route to professional legitimacy and status. Even while attempting to define a professional identity distinct from medicine, nursing theory chose the same proven path to professional legitimacy.

Nursing ethics, on the other hand, has not conferred such value on science. It has not, and in the nature of the discipline, could not have, aspired to being scientific. Ethics is almost by definition a nonexact discipline, although a discipline nonetheless. Ethics, and nursing ethics in particular, make use of science where appropriate, but with an awareness that science only goes so far in sorting out value questions by helping us to better understand their empirical dimension, for nursing ethics is above all concerned with values and value conflicts arising out of nursing practice and research. Ultimately questions of value must necessarily escape the scientist's probing forceps.

This difference between nursing theory and nursing ethics conceals more than it reveals. Nursing theories, some more explicitly than others, invariably have assumptions about the kind of value issues under discussion in the nursing ethics literature, although too often these are not identified or explicitly thematized as ethical issues. The rhetoric of science, and especially the pretense to objectivity characteristic of the received view, has had the effect of obscuring the values dimension of nursing theory.[11] An argument could be made that other views of science might not have this effect and this may be so, but the fact is that until recently it has been a more or less standard view of science that has dominated nursing theory.

Roy's[6] model is a good example of how overvaluing science can obscure decisive ethical issues in nursing theory. The adaptation model is thick with values and value choices, but they are concealed in the shadows cast by Roy's overt commitment to the ideology of science. Questions of value extend even to her choice of language. The vernacular is quite self-consciously borrowed from physiology and behavioral science, a decision already subject to ethical scrutiny. Terms like stimulus, response, and adaptation are not value neutral. They come from and yield a certain view of man (there is valuation in gender too), and are in marked contrast to terms employed in more humanistic language games.

The term managing stimuli, for example, which Roy[6] has lately adopted for describing nursing intervention, is not without important value assumptions and implications. The management metaphor conceptualizes the nurse as in some sense having a superior role in the nurse-patient relationship: the nurse manages, the patient adapts. This is reinforced by carving up the patient's life-world into stimuli, a conceptualization somewhat removed from the terms in which patients conceptualize their own experience. The language itself creates an epistemic barrier between patient and nurse and is less than conducive to dialogue or partnership, as nurses have learned from experience with the scientific but user-unfriendly vernacular of medicine.

There is also a values dimension to the definition of men as adaptive systems. Roy herself has come to see problems here. She claims that she "adds humanistic values to this scientific concept [the person as an adap-

tive system]" and admits that "these values received little attention in the earlier writings."[6(p25)] However, this is misleading. Rather than saying that she later adds humanistic values, it would be more accurate to say that she earlier subtracted them.

Related to the above point, there is valuation in the idea or ideal of adaptation. How does one distinguish adaptation from ineffective responses? By what norms? More importantly, by whose norms, the nurse's or the patient's? Who decides? To be sure, Roy does expressly endorse "the humanistic approach of valuing other person's opinions and viewpoints."[6(p36)] Indeed, in another writing, Roy and Roberts go even further, maintaining that according to their model, "the person is to be respected as an active participant in his care. . . . The goal arrived at is one of mutual agreement between the nurse and patient. Interventions are the options that the nurse provides for the patient."[12(p47)] This rhetoric is not congruent with the rest of Roy's model, however, and especially the sections of *Introduction to Nursing*[6] entitled *"Criteria for Setting Priorities," "Goal Setting,"* and *"Intervention,"* in which the patient maintains virtually no voice at all. The humanistic values are appended virtually as an afterthought, and are not integrated throughout the model. If these values are to be taken seriously, it is not enough to add them to a scientific base—the model needs to be reconstructed from the ground up.

Notwithstanding certain explicit statements to the contrary, Roy's adaptation model is heavily biased toward paternalism. The nurse is in a privileged position to set goals and plan interventions mandated by his or her guiding science. Since the patient does not have such knowledge and since this knowledge is expressed in a language that is difficult for the uninitiated to comprehend, the patient is on very unequal footing concerning setting goals, planning care, and so forth. It is difficult to achieve mutual agreement between partners who speak different languages, especially when one of the languages is highly abstract and bears the authoritative ring of science.

It is telling that in *Introduction to Nursing* (no less than 500 pages), Roy[6] does not speak expressly about patient autonomy. Given the considerable advocacy movement in nursing, this is quite remarkable. It is, however, understandable, given Roy's scientific orientation. When the person is defined as an adaptive system (a definition mainly fleshed out in physiologic terms) there is not much room for autonomy (or for the person to be humanistically understood). Roy may be an extreme example, but it is generally true that questions having to do with autonomy and paternalism, questions that reach to the core of the nursing profession, are seldom tackled directly by nursing theorists.

Nursing theory is rife with value dimensions—only a few have been touched here—but too often these are not brought to the fore and made the theme of analysis. There is a tendency for nursing theory to obscure its own operative norms. Typically, theorists present their work as if it were merely descriptive (science is not supposed to be normative), as if they were merely stating what nursing is. In fact, all of them, directly or indirectly, are also taking a stand on what nursing should be, and offering recommendations for the future direction of the profession—recommendations that cannot be evaluated on scientific grounds alone.

Thus, it is conceptually muddled and highly misleading to divide nursing theories into those that are valuational (normative) and those that are descriptive (scientific) as does Walker,[13] positing different standards of evaluation for each. All nursing theories, however scientific, are in some considerable measure normative or valuational, although some more self-consciously than others. They are structurally cemented with values throughout. The key definitions of nursing theory—human beings, nurse, health, environment (society)—are thickly laden with value. Disputes about them, for the most part, are not of a sort that science alone can be expected to resolve. As Gadow writes, "the very definition of nursing is an ethical problem—moreover the most fundamental and pressing ethical problem facing nursing today."[14(p93)]

One should not have to decipher the ethical face of a nursing theory behind the mask of science. The values dimension of nursing theories should be brought more out into the open and tackled more directly. Ethical issues should be identified as such and confronted head on. Here nursing theorists would stand to benefit from increased dialogue with those working in nursing ethics, who have taken as their focus the values dimension of nursing. This dimension has been somewhat obscured in nursing theory owing to the value it places on science, or perhaps even on a narrow view of science, it being an open question whether other views of science might not be more congruent with ethical interests.

Evaluation of Nursing Theories

The potential for overenthusiasm about science to eclipse ethical considerations in nursing theory is even more evident at the level of theory evaluation. To pick a somewhat early example, King,[15] placing a great deal of value on the scientificity of nursing theories, lists ten criteria for theory evaluation, none of which explicitly addresses the ethical dimension of nursing theories. Theory evaluation has become much more sophisticated since then, but the scientific paradigm (and frequently a very narrow interpretation of it) continues to dominate at the expense of sensitivity to ethical dimensions of nursing theory.

Parse,[16] a theorist who is more explicit about values than most, nevertheless sacrifices ethical concerns at the altar of science when it comes to speaking about theory evaluation. Following Kaplan,[17] she distinguishes between structure and process criteria for evaluation. Value considerations are implicit in the detailed analysis she gives of these criteria, but nowhere are they explicitly stated. This omission is telling, but all the more so given that she deems esthetic criteria significant enough to warrant special reference.[16] Surely if esthetics is worthy of honorable mention, ethics is all the more so, especially given nursing's traditional sensitivity to ethical matters.

Even Chinn and Jacobs,[18] who are otherwise refreshingly open-eyed about the limitations of the scientific ideal, do not escape its allure when it comes to theory evaluation. They are certainly to be lauded for acknowledging that there are other patterns of knowing besides the scientific one, and for assigning a legitimate place to moral knowledge or ethics in nursing as distinct from empirics. They call for the "integration of all patterns."[18(p17)] of knowing, and this *holistic* ideal approximates what this article advocates. Furthermore, they point out that "the assumptions and purposes of scientific theory form the template against which nursing theories have been judged, although many traits of theories in general and nursing theories in particular both draw on and reflect other patterns of knowing besides empirics."[18(p7)] Nevertheless, when it comes to presenting their criteria for evaluation, the guidelines they offer, although broader than many, remain dominated by the scientific ideal and concentrated on empirics. They list clarity, simplicity, generality, empirical applicability, and consequences (more or less a rehash of the familiar scientific standards), and neglect to include an evaluative category addressing the values dimension of theory in a direct manner.[18] Presumably, the value assumptions of nursing theory with respect to such matters as patient autonomy, nursing autonomy, advocacy, and so on, do not count. If, as the authors state, the integration of the various patterns of knowledge is desirable, what better place to start than in the evaluation of nursing theory?

Nursing theorists and those writing about nursing theory evaluation need to become more reflective about the fact that evaluation is valuation. More scrutiny needs to be given to the various elements that are valued and why this is so. Why are ethical (value) considerations typically overlooked or even excluded in theory evaluation? Why should simplicity be valued or evaluated while something like the moral basis of the theory is not valued at all? Could it be that, dazzled by the allure of science and obsessed with being scientific, evaluators have been somewhat blinded to questions of ethics and values?

Relevance of Nursing Theory to Nursing Ethics

If nursing theory stands to benefit from the kind of questioning that takes place in nursing ethics, so too nursing ethics stands to benefit from the not inconsid-erable achievements of nursing theory. Just as nursing theorists have sought to carve an identity for nursing distinct from the medical model, there is also growing concern to develop nursing ethics as a unique field of enquiry, and something "more than a footnote to medical ethics,"[19(p72)] as Yarling and McElmurry have put it:

Nursing theorists and those writing about nursing theory evaluation need to become more reflective about the fact that evaluation is valuation.

Nursing ethics today is reaching to find its own voice, an endeavor in which nursing theory, even if overly concerned about sounding scientific, is qualified to furnish some guidance. Gadow comments that in framing ethical problems, "nursing regrettably has retained medicine as its referent in an area of concern where nurses most need to engage in independent, critically reflective self-examination."[14(p92)] Gadow's remark should be qualified, since it would not apply to everyone working in nursing ethics, but overall her characterization of the state of affairs is insightful. The general tendency has been to adopt a ready-made ethics and bring it to bear on the nursing profession.

Scholarship in nursing ethics can be divided roughly into two streams, each borrowing its conceptual paradigm from a different source. On the one side, the ethical theory approach borrows heavily from moral philosophy. On the other the moral development approach borrows heavily from developmental psychology.

The Ethical Theory Approach

What James and Dickoff[20] have claimed about Beckstrand[21] could be applied to the ethical theory approach. They charge that "Beckstrand takes some selected version of what is ethics,"[20(p58)] as being authoritative, seemingly unaware that ethics is itself a contentious discipline, embracing a broad diversity of often conflicting opinions. To be sure, nursing ethicists do acknowledge some diversity. Almost everyone makes the standard distinction between deontologic and teleologic theories. However, the scope of this diversity is narrowly circumscribed.

Nursing ethics primarily borrows its framework for ordering ethical theories from medical ethics. By itself, this would not be so significant were it not that medical ethics has been very selective in circumscribing the discipline of ethics. The focus is placed almost exclusively on Kant and Mill, while other legitimate contenders are buried in the background. A list of neglected or even excluded voices would include names like Aristotle, Plato, Spinoza, Kierkegaard, and Nietzsche, all of whom wrote substantial works in ethics. Why has nursing ethics uncritically subscribed to the same canon as medical ethics? How different might the ethical landscape of nursing appear if existentialism, for example, enjoyed the same privilege accorded to utilitarianism in the nursing ethics literature?

Nursing ethics has borrowed from medical ethics not only its list of canonical authors, but also certain ways of relating to ethical issues. What White[22] calls formula ethics is a case in point. Formula ethics "involves applying ethical theories to specific situations and suggesting, for instance, what the contractarian versus the utilitarian position might be."[22(p42)] Carroll and Humphrey's[23] *Moral Problems in Nursing* is typical: "I feel I used Kant's theory when I refused to call the police and have Ms B committed for I was respecting her autonomy."[23(p82)] It is a mistake to think that Kant's theory can be used like a cookie cutter to shape the moral situation of nursing into tidy resolutions. Moreover, if one has to derive one's respect for autonomy from an ethical theory, one is in deep trouble. Nurses have practiced respect for autonomy long before Kant was brought into the hospital setting.

Formula ethics is misguided for several reasons, and not least of all because it simplifies ethical positions almost to the point of caricature. More importantly, however, it reduces ethical practice to correct technique, and promotes an overly mechanical (and therefore insensitive) comportment to ethical problems. The moral situation of nursing is squeezed into imported categories that are applied in a top-down fashion. The danger is that the experience of nursing will be distorted or otherwise denied.

While it would be folly to ignore the rich untapped resources of ethical theory, it is important to be critical in bringing them to bear on the moral situation of nursing. Those working in nursing ethics are becoming increasingly critical of the ethical theory approach. There is a growing desire for an ethic that issues from nursing itself, rather than one borrowed from elsewhere and applied from the top down. Bishop and Scudder exemplify this in urging that nursing ethics should begin "with the moral sense of nursing rather than with ethical theory."[24(p42)] This sentiment is echoed by Packard and Ferrara, who maintain that "the moral foundation of nursing will have to derive from bold excursions into the meaning of nursing."[25(p63)] What does it mean to speak of the "meaning of nursing," however? Where would one look to find such a thing?

Nursing theory would be a good place to start. If nursing ethics must borrow, why not borrow from the rich tradition of nursing theory, which at least has the advantage over ethical theory of being derived from nursing experience? Nursing theory could play an important role in a bottom-up approach to nursing ethics. It offers an alternative made-in-nursing framework (or rather several) in which to think about humans, health, environment, society, and the meaning of nursing. Nursing theory tackles these fundamentals at the very outset, whereas nursing ethics has tended to be somewhat more narrow in its focus. The tendency has been to focus on cases, which are analyzed along the traditional lines of autonomy, paternalism, and beneficence. Nursing theory can teach nursing ethics to think more profoundly about the meaning of nursing and help to broaden the frame of reference in which ethical questions are being examined. It may be illuminating in ways hardly imaginable to rethink the stock ethical terms—autonomy, justice, beneficence—in light of nursing theory.

The Moral Development Approach

The moral development approach in nursing ethics differs from the ethical theory approach by being more empirical. It looks at the moral situation of nursing with an eye to how nurses actually respond to ethical issues, and analyzes the moral behavior of nurses in light of models of moral development. At one level, one could contrast the ethical theory approach to the moral development approach as the normative to the descriptive, but this would be misleading. Models of moral development are not value neutral, and norms come into play in describing moral behavior in the framework of a given model.

> The moral development approach in nursing ethics shares with the ethical theory approach the habit of borrowing uncritically.

The moral development approach in nursing ethics shares with the ethical theory approach the habit of borrowing uncritically. In particular, the work of Kohlberg[26] has exerted a profound influence on research on the moral development of nurses. Ketefian[27-31] has been a major catalyst in this area. Without negating the value of her work, it is fair to say that she has not been very critical in her acceptance of the paradigm for moral development laid out by Kohlberg. For the most part, she has accepted it as being authoritative without interrogating its fundamental norms. This is ironic, since the model's overarching norm is autonomy, which calls for such interrogation. Kohlberg has always had his detractors, but recent work by Gilligan[32] has cast his model in a critical light that is particularly illuminating for nursing. Gilligan found that, as a group, women score differently than men on Kohlberg's moral development scale. If one accepted Kohlberg's value premises, one would have to say that women score lower than men. Gilligan's innovation was to interpret this difference in a positive way. Rather than accepting the norms supporting Kohlberg's scale and interpreting this difference as deficiency, she made a virtue of it, and used it to call into question the fundamental values of Kohlberg's theory. Women do indeed define moral issues differently, but this difference is not a minus. Gilligan calls this difference the ethic of care, which is different from, but not subordinate to, the ethic of justice presupposed as norm in Kohlberg's theory. She cele-

brates the ethic of care as being the different voice of women.[32] Interestingly, Gilligan's work converges with that of James and Dickoff,[20] who, inspired by the French feminist Helene Cixous,[33] advanced a new ethic for nursing based on reciprocal nurturance.

The moral lesson to be drawn from Gilligan's critique of Kohlberg is a profound one: rather than trying to speak the language that happens to be authoritative, one should learn to speak unashamedly in one's own voice and to celebrate one's difference rather than apologize for it. This lesson has special relevance for nursing. Applying Gilligan's work to nursing, Huggins and Scalzi write, "If an ethical base for nursing practice is built on the ethics of justice, and the nurse's orientation is the ethic of care of another model, there will continue to be a denial of the nurse's own voice."[34(p46)] Uncritical borrowing can lead to the denial of the unique experience of nursing and to the disvaluation of the ethic of care to which Gilligan,[32] turning Kohlberg upside down, assigns a positive evaluation.

Directing their concerns specifically to Ketefian,[27-31] Huggins and Scalzi caution, "A theory of ethical practice, as is sought by Ketefian, is essential to the maturation of the nursing profession, but it must be carefully built to speak to the true voice and experience of nursing."[34(p44)] This is a very important point, but it raises a difficult question: What is the true voice and experience of nursing? Perhaps there is no one true voice, but there are several voices, the voices of nursing theorists speaking about the experience of nursing. Anyone undertaking to develop an ethic for nursing based on the experience of nursing would do well to begin by listening carefully to those voices.

Nursing theory and nursing ethics speak about and for nursing, an onerous challenge and responsibility for a profession so self-conscious and self-examining. Each, in its own way, is searching to find its own voice. To this end, would it not be desirable for each to broaden the parameters of its conversation and listen to the voice of the other? Only by joining together can the voices of nursing theory and nursing ethics hope to lay legitimate claim to be the voice of nursing.

REFERENCES

1. Nightingale, F., cited in Palmer IS.: From whence we came, in Chaska NL. (ed): The *Nursing Profession: A Time to Speak.* New York, McGraw-Hill, 1983.
2. Crowley, D. M.: Perspectives of pure science. Nurs Res 1968;17:497–499.
3. Aydelotte M. K.: Issues of professional nursing: The need for clinical excellence. *Nurs Forum* 1968;7(1):73675.
4. Conway, M. E.: Prescription for professionalization, in Chaska NL (ed): *The Nursing Profession: A Time to Speak.* New York, McGraw-Hill, 1983.
5. Greenwood, E.: Attributes of a profession, in Baumrin B., Freedman B. (eds): *Moral Responsibility and the Professions.* New York, Haven, 1983.
6. Roy, C.: Introduction to Nursing: An Adaptation Model, ed. 2. Englewood Cliffs, NJ, Prentice-Hall, 1984.
7. Muyskens, J. L. *Moral Problems in Nursing: A Philosophical Investigation.* Totowa, NJ, Rowman and Littlefield, 1982.
8. Meleis, A. I.: *Theoretical Nursing: Development and Progress.* New York, Lippincott, 1985.
9. Watson, J.: Nursing's scientific quest. *Nurs Outlook* 1981;29:413–416.
10. Johnson, D. E.: The nature of a science of nursing. *Nurs Outlook* 1959;7:291–294.
11. Tucker, R. W.: The value decisions we know as science. *Adv Nurs Sci* 1979;1(2):1–12.
12. Roy, C., Roberts, S. L.: *Theory Construction in Nursing: An Adaptation Model.* Englewood Cliffs, NJ, Prentice-Hall, 1981.
13. Walker, L. O.: Theory and research in the development of nursing as a discipline: Retrospect and prospect, in Chaska, N. L. (ed): *The Nursing Profession: A Time to Speak.* New York, McGraw-Hill, 1983.
14. Gadow, S.: ANS open forum. *Adv Nurs Sci* 1979;1(3):92–95.
15. King, I.: *Toward a Theory for Nursing: General Concepts of Human Behaviour.* New York, Wiley, 1971.
16. Parse, R. R.: Paradigms and theories, in Parse, R. R. (ed): *Nursing Science: Major Paradigms, Theories and Critiques.* Philadelphia, Saunders, 1987.
17. Kaplan, A.: *The Conduct of Scientific Inquiry.* Scranton, Penn, Chandlisher, 1964.
18. Chinn, P. L., Jacobs, M. K.: *Theory and Nursing: A systematic Approach,* St. Louis, Mosby, 1983.
19. Yarling, R. R., McElmurry, B. J.: The moral foundation of nursing. *Adv Nurs Sci* 1986;8(2):63–73.
20. James, P., Dickoff, J.: Toward a cultivated but decisive pluralism for nursing, in McGee (ed): *Theoretical Pluralism in Nursing.* Ottawa, University of Ottawa Press, 1982.
21. Beckstrand, J.: The notion of practise theory and the relationship of scientific and ethical knowledge to practise. *Res Nurs Health* 1978;1(3):131–136.
22. White, G. B.: Philosophical ethics and nursing—a word of caution, in Chinn, P. L. (ed): *Advances in Nursing Theory and Development.* Rockville, Md, Aspen, 1983.
23. Carroll, M. A., Humphrey, R. A.: *Moral Problems in Nursing: Case Studies.* Washington, University Press of America, 1979.
24. Bishop, A. H., Scudder, J. R.: Nursing ethics in an age of controversy. *Adv Nurs Sci* 1987;9(3):34–43.
25. Packard, J. S., Ferrara, M. S. N.: In search of the moral foundation of nursing. *Adv Nurs Sci* 1988;10(4):60–71.
26. Kohlberg, L.: The cognitive developmental approach to moral education, in Scharf, P. (ed): *Readings on Moral Education.* Minneapolis, Minn: Winston Press, 1978.
27. Ketefian, S.: Critical thinking, educational preparation, and development of moral judgment among selected groups of practising nurses. *Nurs Res* 1981;30:98–103.
28. Ketefian, S.: Moral reasoning and moral behavior among selected groups of practising nurses. *Nurs Res* 1981;30:171–176.
29. Ketefian, S.: Tool development in nursing: Construction of a scale to measure moral behavior. *J NY State Nurs Assoc* 1982;13:13–18.
30. Ketefian, S.: Professional and bureaucratic role conceptions and moral behavior in nursing. *Nurs Res* 1985;34:248–253.
31. Ketefian, S.: A case study of theory development: Moral behavior in nursing. *Adv Nurs Sci* 1987;9(2):10–19.
32. Gilligan, C.: *In a Different Voice: Psychological Theory and Women's Development.* Cambridge, Harvard University Press, 1982.
33. Marks, E., de Courtivron, I. (eds): *New French Feminisms, an Anthology.* New York, Schocken Press, 1981.
34. Huggins, E. A., Scalzi, C. C.: Limitations and alternatives: Ethical practice theory in nursing. *Adv Nurs Sci* 1988;10(4):43–47.

The Author Comments

Integration of Nursing Theory and Nursing Ethics

Professor Marguerite Warner, who was then on the Faculty of Nursing at the University of Western Ontario, first introduced me to nursing theory. Her passion for the subject was infectious, and I learned much from her (and miss our conversations). As I worked through the nursing theory literature, I was struck by what I believed to be an uncritical and unwise deference to science and lack of attention to ethics, which was surprising to me, given nursing's rich tradition of ethical reflection. I believe that nursing theory should be grounded primarily not in science but in ethics. The articulation of this viewpoint in this article is my modest contribution to dialogue in and about nursing theory.

—MICHAEL YEO

CHAPTER 39

Caring Knowledge and Informed Moral Passion*

Jean Watson

This article is based on an invited challenge address at the 1989 National Doctoral Forum related to future directions for substantive knowledge development. The focus is on the inclusion of caring knowledge into nursing's metaparadigm. Art and metaphor are used to make a case for caring knowledge and caring ontology as a metaphorical landscape for diverse epistemological "set pieces," all converging on a Commons Room of caring knowledge within a broader human and natural landscape. Such a framework links ontology and epistemology as both substance and form, and allows matter and spirit to be of a piece, but distinguishable; human caring knowledge then becomes Annie Dillard's "Absolute base" and "Holy the Firm."

Future Directions for Caring Knowledge Development

In Margaret Mead's reflective book, *Blackberry Winter,*[1] the author ponders a paper that her first husband

Luther had written. As demonstrated in the following excerpt, the paper contains a metaphor relevant to the issue of caring knowledge and nursing science. Perhaps I can best illustrate the meaning of my thoughts by going back to Oppenheimer's felicitous metaphor of the house

*This article is based on the Challenge Address given at the 1989 National Forum on Doctoral Education in Nursing, Indianapolis, Indiana, June 7–9, 1989. The author thanks Douglas Watson for his assistance with literary metaphors and Diane Lenfest for her assistance with references and preparation of this article. Special permission for quotations has been granted from the following sources: Blackberry Winter, by Margaret Mead, copyright

1972 by Margaret Mead. Reprinted by permission of William Morrow & Company, Inc.; Holy the Firm, by Annie Dillard, copyright 1977, excerpt reprinted by permission of Harper & Row, Publishers, Inc; and adaptation of Upward Causation Model of Science, by Willis Harman, reprinted from Noetic Sciences Review, courtesy of The Institute of Noetic Sciences, Sausalito, California, copyright 1987, all rights reserved.

About the Author

JEAN WATSON is Distinguished Professor of Nursing and holds the Murchinson-Scolville Chair in Caring Science at the University of Colorado Health Sciences Center (HSC). She is founder of the original Center for Human Caring and previously served as Dean of the University of Colorado HSC School of Nursing. She is a Past President of the National League for Nursing. Born in West Virginia, July 21, 1940, Dr. Watson earned undergraduate and graduate degrees in nursing and psychiatric-mental health nursing and holds her PhD in educational psychology and counseling. Dr. Watson is known for her theoretical work on the art and science of human caring. Her latest books and articles address empirical measurements of caring and new postmodern philosophies of caring and healing that bridge paradigms and point toward transformative models for the 21st century. Dr. Watson is the recipient of many awards and honors, including an international Kellogg Fellowship in Australia, a Fulbright Research Award in Sweden, five honorary doctoral degrees, the National League for Nursing's Martha E. Rogers Award, New York University's Distinguished Nurse Scholar Award, and the Fetzer Institute's Norman Cousins Award. Her hobbies include international travel, skiing, hiking, biking, and writing.

called 'science.' I would like to see us build a NEW room in that vast and rambling structure. This room, like the others, would have no door and over the entrance would be the words, THOUGHT, REFLECTION, CONTEMPLATION. It would have no tables with instruments, no whirring machinery. There would be no sound except the soft murmur of words carrying the thought of men [and women] in the room. It would be a Commons Room to which men [and women] would drift in from those rooms marked geology, anthropology, taxonomy, technology, biology, paleontology, logic, mathematics, psychology, linguistics, and many others. Indeed, from without the walls of the House would come poets and artists. All these would drop in and linger. This room would have great windows; the vistas our studies have opened. Men [and women] singly or together would from time to time walk to those windows to gaze out on the landscape beyond. This landscape in all its beauty, sometimes gentle, sometimes terrible, cannot be seen fully by any one of the occupants of the room. Indeed, it cannot be known fully by a whole generation of men [and women]. Explorers of each generation travel into its unknown recesses and, with luck, return to share their discoveries with us. So the life of the NEW room would go on—thought, reflection, contemplation—as the explorers bring back their discoveries to share with the room's occupants. This landscape that we gaze on and try to understand is an epic portion of the human experience.[1(pp289-290)]

This metaphoric introduction sets an appropriate stage for nursing science, now into its fourth generation of knowledge development, or into what Stevenson[2] calls era II. As we continue to question what room we will build for caring knowledge, we challenge ourselves with how we will furnish this room. What sounds or noise will fill the space, for current and future generations of nurse scientists?

In framing some of the key issues about future directions for knowledge of caring, let us be reminded that the boundaries, furnishings, and set pieces for the rooms that we propose have the power, as do science and doctoral education, to establish the nature and standards of reality, to fashion *how* we see. We must be careful with the choices we make.

Commons Room vs "Set Pieces"

In developing caring knowledge for nursing science, perhaps we can create a commons room. Commons room features that are explicitly included in contemporary nursing knowledge are concepts of person, health, environment, and nursing. Thus a commons room epistemology is beginning to emerge for nursing science.

However, what is not generally addressed with nursing science knowledge and what needs more attention is a commons room ontology of caring in relation to person, environment, health, and nursing. Moreover, we must ask whether there is a metaphoric landscape connection between the ontology of caring and the epistemological rooms that we may propose for nursing science. In addition, we need to ask what kind of door or entrance there is for the rooms of nursing and caring knowledge. Would those currently outside the walls—for example, artists, poets, and musicians—be able to enter, linger, and assist with opening the windows onto the landscape? Is the landscape natural or artificial? Are horizons of landscape defined, or is the landscape continuous with the universe?

Perhaps we can metaphorically anchor the epistemological house, room, and furnishings to the ontological caring landscape. But first let us consider the commons room against different rooms or set pieces within the rooms. In drama and literature, the "set piece" provides each of the scenes with little plays within the novel.

Different views of the world generally result in different uses of set pieces. For example, the English novel makes great use of the technical set piece; it encloses the world, takes care of everything, and sees that everything is controlled and wrapped up into a neat package (including human conditions such as birth, death, marriage, and so forth). In Russian novels the drawing room serves as the technical set piece; however, the Russian novel uses the set piece to expand, to transcend, to free. In contrast to the enclosing set piece of the English novel, the Russian novel's set piece opens to the landscape: it looks out into the world and the universe.

In a metaphoric sense, English novels are about time, and Russian novels are about space. The former are fixed in time and space, the later depict human processes as transcending time and space and as being continuous with nature and the larger universe. Both convey different metaphysical assumptions about human nature and ontologies of being.[3]

The following quotes vividly illustrate these differences. The English novel *Vanity Fair* makes the point for Rebecca Sharp's world:

> The catastrophe came, and she was brought to the mall as to her home. The rigid formality of the place suffocated her; the prayers and the meals, the lessons, and the walks which were arranged with a conventual regularity oppressed her almost beyond endurance; and she looked back to the freedom and the beggary of the old studio in Soho with so much regret.[4(p17)]

The Russian short story "Streams Where Trout Play" makes the contrasting point:

> The marshall spent two days in the forester's house. We shall not speak about love, because to this day we do not know what it is. Perhaps it is the thick snow falling all night, or the wintry streams where trout play. Or perhaps it is laughter and singing and the smell of old pitch just before dawn when the candles burn down and the stars press against the window pane . . . . Who knows? . . . .how at times life becomes like music?[5(pp317,318)]

In considering nursing knowledge development in general and knowledge of caring in particular, it is tempting to avoid differences in ontologic and epistemic landscape assumptions about what constitutes knowledge, how knowledge is created, and what the ultimate aims of science and knowledge are. What, indeed, is substance and what is substantive knowledge? Is it restricting or liberating, enclosing or expanding? Is our epistemology (or are our rooms of science) linked to an ontological landscape, or is it (or are they) disconnected and distinctly separate?

> It is tempting to avoid differences in ontologic and epistemic landscape assumptions about what constitutes knowledge, how knowledge is created, and what the ultimate aims of science and knowledge are.

Clarifying the Assumptions

In spite of a backdrop of several eras of nursing science and development of nursing knowledge, it has been recently acknowledged that "approaches to knowledge development show an alarming absence of theoretical [and philosophical] consistency and relevance, and nursing theory displays wide divergence."[6(p2)] Allen[7] pointed out that there are several emerging and at times competing (or possibly incompatible) ideas about what kind of science or knowledge development nursing should consider. He highlighted the dominant analytic-empirical, the phenomenological-interpretive, and the critical social theory, emphasizing such concerns as understanding, free discourse, critical reflection, argumentation, and ultimate emancipation and liberation of the evolving human mind and spirit. Others, including this author, raise issues associated with the moral, the aesthetic, the relational, the spiritual, and the transcendent aspects of person, environment, caring, healing, and health.

Stevenson[2] indicated that since we are into era II of knowledge development (the first being dedicated to the educational preparation of nurse scholars for attainment of doctoral degrees, supporting research, etc), nursing will now be more concerned with knowledge per se, foci for knowledge development agenda, and new methods that overcome the Cartesian tradition of parts. Meleis,[8] however, pointed out that we need to go beyond the debate of holism and particularism in relation to knowledge development and method: and we must instead refocus debate on substance, on personal commitment to the phenomena of health care in general, and on the discipline of nursing in particular. Furthermore Meleis recommends revising our passion for methodology, for science, and for philosophy. "Let us have a similar *passion for substance*, for the *business* of nursing. A passion for knowledge itself and not how we get the knowledge."[8(p8)]

But I ask, *What is substance?* What is knowledge *qua* caring?

The Challenge for Caring Knowledge

From "Passion for Substance" to Wide Awakeness for Informed Moral Passion

I return to Mead's[1] concept of a new room for these rambling issues. My room also has thought, reflection, and contemplation over its entrance and has great open windows with a landscape into infinity. The room is set in the midst of an even greater, vaster, more mysterious landscape of nature, human nature, and the wider universe—a universe that is constantly changing and evolving, as is science, as is doctoral education, which we are cocreating at this moment.

In spite of the urgent and appropriate call from Meleis[8] and others[9] for a passion for substance and knowledge itself, we do not and cannot create nursing and caring knowledge in a void. The house, room, and furnishings we create either connect with the metaphoric landscape in a harmonious, human, and natural way, or we artificially, technically contrive the set and decor that is inhospitable and uncomfortable for those who live there, and for visitors, and which may be even more remote for future generations who will occupy the corridors.

My plea is for informed passion, passion that is informed by thought, reflection, and contemplation, giving rise to moral landscapes and contexts of human and nature relational concerns. If not thoughtful, reflective, and contemplative about our knowledge, we become accomplices in stifling freedom, staying behind. Then knowledge development takes a simplified approach; we reduce humans and caring-healing health processes to problems to diagnose. Problems become laws, and we begin to empower problems as foci for study and external intervention void of the human and natural landscape, which results in purely technical, mechanical nursing interventions.

Perhaps the greatest challenge with knowledge is preserving an absolute value and wisdom while breaking new ground into the metaphoric landscape.

Greene's[10] expansive book *Landscapes of Learning* has much relevance to the issues and questions nursing continues to ponder and to pursue as an evolving scientific discipline. Greene challenges us to develop "wide-awakeness," to become in touch with our human landscape as educators and scientists; to seek paradigm-shattering, emancipatory, self-reflective processes; to engage in futuring, going beyond to what is not yet but might be. Freire[11] calls for critical consciousness to acknowledge the void, to liberate and free the mind to reflect and to imagine how things might be.

The wide awakeness Greene advocates, consistent with the author's thinking, calls for aesthetic, moral, intellectual, and reflective encounters that disturb as well as confuse, that promote experiences and questions with an emancipatory, rather than a restrictive, function. As Pierre in Tolstoy's *War and Peace* confessed, most people study and become enlightened, but he studied and became confused.[12] Greene[10] states that even committed rationality rests on the capacity for self-reflection in a wide-awake landscape. Wide awakeness of our moral, ontological landscape informs the passion and the perceptions and frames the questions about substance, knowledge, and reality. If knowledge is void of informed passion, it can be used for domination, for manipulation, for control, for power, for *fixing* the vision for the next generation on a reality others have already predefined.

Nonawakeness leads to only one path for knowledge; a formula approach to people; objectifying, codifying, and reifying human experiences with "official" knowledge that takes on a life of its own—a life that is separate, decontextualized, rather than connected. Again, Tolstoy's approach is simple. There is nothing complicated about this syntax or message. By contrast, Jane Austen's work captures her society's restrictiveness in a style that is beautiful but regulated, like a fine watch. If our aim for caring knowledge in nursing is higher than achieving machinelike knowledge, if our aim is to express and to reflect life and life forces, it is not enough to be technically correct. Much of nursing contains caring knowledge that enriches the soul, that

connects with the landscape. How does any one way to knowledge development exemplify the wonder of humanity and human caring processes of nursing?

> If our aim for caring knowledge in nursing is to express and to reflect life and life forces, it is not enough to be technically correct.

Thus, knowledge structures of all sorts ought to be considered for their diverse expressions in relation to various communities of scholars and in terms of various commitments. Each perspective and each subject matter must be considered in relation to the human interest that gave rise to it—to the question it was invented to solve, in this instance, to human caring and to the human spirit in relation to healing, health, and illness experiences. According to conversations with N. Noddings (1990) and J. Quinn (1990), Figure 39-1 outlines the pressing epistemological, ontological, praxis, and methodologic structure that helps to organize the development of nursing's full range of knowledge.

Chinn reminds us that "when we begin to cease all forms of erosion of the human spirit, compassion, and caring and find approaches that yield not only knowledge, but also substantive [wide-awakeness] wisdom, we will be on the path to healing the great wounds of our present social and health care system."[13(p10)]

Opening the Windows and Doors: Surveying the Landscape

The human-science, human-caring lens proposed here is more like that of the Russian novels and seeks wide awakeness, even if we do not have all the answers, even if we do not always know what to say or how to say it, even if what we say disturbs and confuses. If we deal with human relational processes, the human wholeness of mindbodyspirit, and evolving human consciousness that is continuous with nature and the universe, we have to become part of the processes. We must be willing to enter into them, and we have no choice but wide awakeness and informed passion.

Like Tolstoy's characters, we may start to speak and not finish our sentences because it is now openly ac-

Epistemology

- (Knowing, Knowledge Generation), "Wide – Awakeness"

Knowledge of:

- Person – Life Spirit
- Caring
- Health – Illness Experience
- Healing
- Human Phenomena

Different Ways of Knowing

- Aesthetics
- Personal – Intuitive
- Empirical
- Ehtical – Moral
- Metaphysical–Spiritual

Ontology

- (Being – Meaning)

What Does it Mean to Be?

- Person
- Human
- Nurse

Caring as Special Way of Being

- Caring
- Healthy
- Healed, Ill

Praxis

- (Application of Learning to Practice – Study of Practice) "Informed Passion"

Caring Practices

- New Caring Modalities
- Practice of Knowing and Being and Doing in Caring Relationship
- Natural Healing Modalities

Methodology

- (Nature of Study – The Way One Pursues Knowledge)

Human Science Method

- Qualitative – Art and Science
- Combination of New Methods of Inquiry
- Quest for New Contextual Methodologies

Figure 39–1 *Four dimensions affecting advancement of the art and science of human caring. Adapted with permission from Watson J. Academic and clinical collaboration: Advancing the art and science of human caring.* Commun Nurs Res. *1987; 20:11.*

knowledged that all knowledge development is a distinctively human endeavor, not a technical activity. All knowledge is contextual, emotional, subjective, intersubjective, rational, passionate, controlled, evolving, and so forth.[2,14-18] Thus our technocratic knowledge is not the same as our lived human experiences and life processes.

In a knowledge-building sense, caring in nursing requires informed moral action, informed passion, which incorporates this changing, natural, and technical humanmade landscape. Nursing's knowledge of caring needs open windows and doors that will create harmonious and aesthetic decor and sounds—an ontological relational structure that clings to a distinct moral, passionate, and substantive position that adamantly resists reducing person to the moral status of object.[19]

Human Science and Human Caring as Substance

In integrating caring into our knowledge development to date, it is becoming increasingly obvious that caring is the foundational ontological substance of nursing and under-

pins nursing's epistemology. However, human caring needs to be explicitly incorporated into nursing's metaparadigm. Furthermore, specific theories of caring in relation to specific human conditions and specific health-illness experiences with identified populations calls for both micropsychoimmune system-level and macroglobal-level approaches. Approaches to knowledge that preserve human caring as the interface between technologic and biobehavioral sciences and ecosystems need urgent research. Finally, differing epistemological perspectives can still allow for diverse set pieces for organizing caring knowledge, for example, use of carative factors,[20] use of cultural-care concepts,[21] and considerable use of human-environment energy patterns,[22-24] all possible classifications of human caring during transpersonal caring occasions.[25] All of these approaches to knowledge development include human caring as substance within a metaphysical and ontological landscape.

To develop nursing knowledge that incorporates human caring within its metaparadigm, the most fundamental wide-awake landscape question is how we view person and caring.[6,18] Walker suggests that we "start with nursing's most pervasive phenomenon of concern—people."[26(p3)] To address the nature of being human calls for expanded views of person and phenomena.

Other considerations are whether being a nurse in a caring transaction is a special way of being-in-relation; whether we view caring as an inherent value; whether nursing and caring are a means to some broader end; or whether caring can be both a means and an end. Should we acknowledge moral ideals associated with caring in nursing practice as the highest form of commitment to person and society?[19]

Stevenson[2] noted that after 40 years of struggle, a consensus is developing about the nature of nursing knowledge, its philosophic and ethical bases, its content foci, and even the processes necessary to produce and to disseminate its knowledge. It is not clear whether such a view is accurate. However, once the issues are reframed into foundational assumptions that are central to knowledge development, once anomalies become evident, once we unveil underlying or implied epistemological assumptions and ontologies in our views of person and being and caring, we may more easily inform our passion. Our informed moral passion and caring ontology, in turn, becomes our substance.

Pulitzer prize-winning contemporary author Annie Dillard helps us to understand this issue and this quest for substance in her book *Holy the Firm:*

> I . . . posit a substance. It is a created substance, lower than metals and minerals on a "spiritual scale," and lower than salts and earths, occurring beneath salts and earths in the waxy deepness of planets, but never on the surface of planets where men could discern it; and it is in touch with the Absolute, at base. In touch with the Absolute! At base. The name of this substance is: Holy the Firm.

Holy the Firm: and is Holy the Firm in touch with metals and minerals? With salts and earths? Of course, and straight on up, till "up" ends by curving back . . . .

> But if Holy the Firm is "underneath salts," if Holy the Firm is matter at its dullest, Aristotle's *materia prima*, absolute zero, and since Holy the Firm is in

touch with the Absolute at base, then the circle is unbroken. . . . Thought advances, and the world creates itself, by the gradual positing of, and belief in, a series of bright ideas. Time and space are in touch with the Absolute at base. Eternity sockets twice into time and space curves, bound and bound by idea. Matter and spirit are of a piece but distinguishable.[27(pp68-71)]

The extended, upward-looking model of knowledge development can more fully and uniquely provide meaningful philosophic, ontological, and epistemological foundations for caring knowledge in nursing (Figure 39-2).[28] Figure 39-2 help to provide the full range of Dillard's[27] holy-the-firm, absolute-at-base landscape of human caring knowledge while still allowing movement upward and downward. Holy the Firm and the Upward Causation Model of Science can help us harmonize the whole and create an expansive landscape upon which to build our structures. Through them we can pursue wide awakeness for informed passion for substantive knowledge and for knowledge of human caring, healing, and health as a consciousness context wherein the human

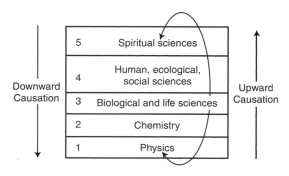

Figure 39–2 *"Holy the Firm," an upward causation model of science: "Absolute at Base; Matter and Spirit are of a piece but distinguished" (Dillard, 1977). Adapted with permission from Harman W. Upward causation model of science. Noetic Sci Rev. 1987;4:23. The table "Downward Causation/Upward Causation" appeared in the article "Further Comments on . . .an Extended Science" published in IONS Review, No. 4, Autumn, 1987 (p.23) and is reprinted by permission of the Institute of Noetic Sciences (website: www.noetic.org). Copyright © 1987 by IONS, all rights reserved.*

spirit is open to multiple ways of being, knowing, and doing.

The future landscape that advances toward us bears little resemblance to what we have known before. Process, transcendence, transformation, emergence, patterns of relationships, relativity of time and space, nonphysical phenomena, fluid, energy fields all have implications for a new room of nursing science—as we now seek new knowledge for new reasons.[29] As we more consciously choose informed moral passion and a relational caring ontology as context, as we seek to enfold ourselves into the human health, healing, caring landscape, we need Greene's[10] wide awakeness and Dillard's[27] Holy the Firm. These call for paradigm-shattering approaches for the set, the furnishings. We need windows and doors that embrace the humanity and the relational life processes of patients and nurses and ecology as part of the vast metaphysical landscape that is continuous with the universe into infinity: a landscape that is sometimes gentle, sometimes terrible, sometimes confusing. Let caring knowledge in nursing guide us into the freshness of this expanded landscape with an informed moral passion that leads to wide awakeness for this absolute substance at base.

REFERENCES

1. Mead M. *Blackberry Winter.* New York, NY: William Morrow; 1972.
2. Stevenson J. Nursing knowledge development: into era II. *J Prof Nurs.* 1988;4(3):152–162.
3. Forster EM. *Aspects of the Novel.* New York, NY: Harcourt, Brace Jovanovich; 1955.
4. Thackeray WM. *Vanity Fair.* New York, NY: Dell Publishing; 1961.
5. Paustovsky K. Streams where trout play. In: Richards D, ed, trans. *The Penguin Book of Russian Short Stories.* London, England: Penguin Books; 1981.
6. Sarter B. Philosophical sources of nursing theory. *Nurs Sci Q.* 1988;1(2):52–59.
7. Allen D. Nursing research and social control: alternate models of science that emphasize understanding and emancipation. *IMAGE.* 1985;17:58–64.
8. Meleis A. ReVisions in knowledge development: a passion for substance. *Scholar Inq Nurs Prac An Int J.* 1987;1(1):5–19.
9. Downs FS. Doctoral education: our claim to the future. *Nurs Outlook.* 1988;36:18–20.
10. Greene M. *Landscapes of Learning.* New York, NY: Teachers College Press, Columbia University; 1978.
11. Freire P. *Pedagogy of the Oppressed.* New York, NY: Continuum Publishing; 1988.
12. Tolstoy L; Edmonds R, trans. *War and Peace.* New York, NY: Viking Penguin; 1982.
13. Chinn P. Awake, awake. Editorial. *ANS.* 1989;11(2):10.
14. Moccia P. A critique of compromise; beyond the methods debate. *ANS.* 1988;10(4):1–9.
15. Belenky M, Clinchy B, Goldberger N, Tarule J. *Women's Ways of Knowing.* New York, NY: Basic Books; 1986.
16. Kidd P, Morrison E. The progress of knowledge in nursing: a search for meaning. *IMAGE.* 1988;20(4):222–224.
17. Schultz P, Meleis A. Nursing epistemology: traditions, insights, question. *IMAGE.* 1988;20(4):217–222.
18. Watson J. *Nursing: Human Science and Human Care.* Norwalk, Conn: Appleton-Century-Crofts; 1985.
19. Gadow S. Nurse and patient: the caring relationship. In: Bishop A, Scudder J, eds. *Caring, Curing, Coping: Nurse, Physician, Patient Relationships.* Tuscaloosa, Alabama: University of Alabama Press; 1985:31–43.
20. Watson J. *Nursing: The Philosophy and Science of Caring.* Boston, Mass: Little, Brown; 1979.
21. Leininger M. *Transcultural Nursing: Concepts, Theories and Practices.* New York, NY: Wiley; 1978.
22. Newman M. *Health as Expanding Consciousness.* St. Louis, MO: Mosby; 1986.
23. Parse R. *Man-Living-Health: A Theory of Nursing.* New York, NY: Wiley; 1981.
24. Fitzpatrick J. Conceptual basis for the organization and advancement of nursing knowledge: nursing diagnosis/taxonomy. Paper prepared for National Doctoral Forum; June 7–9, 1989; Indianapolis, Ind.
25. Watson J. New dimensions in human caring theory. *Nurs Sci Q.* 1988;1(4):175–181.
26. Walker L. Conceptual bases for the organization and advancement of nursing knowledge: clinical content. Paper prepared for National Doctoral Forum; June 7–9, 1989; Indianapolis, Ind.
27. Dillard A. *Holy the Firm.* New York, NY: Harper & Row; 1977.
28. Harman W. Further comments on an extended science. Commentary. *Noetic Sci Rev.* 1987;4:22–25.
29. Moccia P. Deciding to care. Presented at the 11th International Caring Conference; May 1989. Denver, Colo.

The Author Comments

Caring Knowledge and Informed Moral Passion

This article was written as part of a keynote address to the American Academy of Nursing meeting. I was attempting to once again make a place for caring as moral and epistemic foundation for nursing science and to make more explicit that caring belonged in the metaparadigm of nursing for its disciplinary focus.

—JEAN WATSON

CHAPTER 40

Relational Narrative:
The Postmodern Turn in Nursing Ethics

Sally Gadow

A philosophy of nursing requires an ethical cornerstone. I describe three dialectical layers of an ethical cornerstone: subjective immersion, objective detachment, and relational narrative. Dialectically, the move from immersion to detachment is the turn from communitarian to rational ethics, replacing traditions with universal principles. The move from universalism to engagement is the turn from rational to relational ethics, replacing detached reason with engagement between particular selves. Conceptually, the three layers correspond to premodern, modern, and postmodern ethics. I propose that the layers be viewed not as stages, but as elements that coexist in an ethically vital profession, and I conclude with an illustration of their coexistence in a clinical situation.

A philosophy of nursing requires an ethical cornerstone, because a profession is informed by moral ends. Discussions of ethics in nursing usually are framed in the categories of philosophical ethics, such as deontology, virtue, and consequentialism. While useful for locating nursing ethics within the disciplinary context of philosophy, the categories are not helpful because they manifest no internal relationship to each other, no connection within an encompassing framework. Without a coherent framework, ethics cannot provide the cornerstone for a philosophy of nursing.

In the hope that establishing philosophical connections among different ethical approaches will lead to the

Acknowledgement: *An early version of this article was presented at the conference "Philosophy in the Nurse's World: Practical Knowledge in Nursing," sponsored by the Institute for Philosophical Nursing Research, University of Alberta, Baoff, Alberta, Canada, May 1995.* Scholarly Inquiry for Nursing Practice: An International Journal, *1999, 13(1), 57–70. Copyright © 1999 Springer Publishing Company, Inc. New York, Used by permission.*

About the Author

SALLY GADOW was born in Boston. She received a baccalaureate degree in nursing from the University of Texas at Galveston; a master's degree in nursing from the University of California, San Francisco; and a PhD in philosophy from the University of Texas at Austin. Her academic career has included faculty positions at Johns Hopkins University, the University of Maryland, Georgetown University, the University of Florida, the University of Texas, and the University of Colorado. Her scholarship focuses on the philosophy of nursing, with emphasis on ethics and phenomenology. Her key contribution to the discipline is her philosophic examination of the nurse-patient relationship within a broad humanities framework. Her principal hobby is long-distance sailing.

construction of an ethical cornerstone, I offer a method for understanding different ethical views within a dialectical framework. The framework I describe is a triad of ethical layers: subjective immersion (ethical immediacy), objective detachment (ethical universalism), and intersubjective engagement (relational narrative)—corresponding, respectively, to premodern, modern, and postmodern ethics (see Figure 40-1). After a brief discussion of dialectic, I describe each of the three layers and conclude with an illustration of their coexistence in a clinical situation.

Dialectic

The method of developing a philosophical dialectic is adapted here from the work of Hegel (1807/1977). A brief elaboration of method is important to the thesis of this discussion, namely, that premodern, modern, and postmodern ethics represent a dialectical relationship among different ethical approaches in which none of the three can stand alone and only their coexistence constitutes a sound basis for practice.

The nature of dialectic can be expressed as mediation. Mediation is the negation of simplicity, resulting in increasing complexity as each new level of differentiation is in turn negated, producing further distinctions. At the same time, the opposition among distinctions is itself mediated. Negativity, in other words, becomes increasingly positive as the original opposition is qualified by a new relationship in which once antithetical elements are no longer mutually exclusive but become mutually enhancing.

A clinical example of dialectic is the experience of injury and rehabilitation (Bloom, 1992; Gadow, 1982). (1) Before injury, the body is experienced as a taken-for-granted immediacy that accomplishes the aims of a person, such as climbing stairs, without reflection or even awareness. (2) An injury negates that immediacy in two ways: the body opposes the aims of the self by its inability to climb, and the inability is itself the antithesis of the lost immediacy. (3) Rehabilitation negotiates a new relationship between body and self. While the body remains an other for the self (an otherness the injury produced), harmony between them is cultivated through attentiveness to the injured part. That cultivated unity based on care entails the possibility for climbing stairs as a cooperative, rather than an unconscious, activity of body and self.

A characteristic rhythm is associated with dialectic because of the three phases of simplicity, opposition, and reconciliation. The formulaic description of dialectic as thesis-antithesis-synthesis, however, can be deceptive; it masks the principle of ongoing *self*-negation at the heart of dialectic. No phase is exclusively thesis, antithesis, or synthesis. Each phase serves as antithesis of the one before, and each synthesis becomes a new thesis as its own unity is further differentiated. The rehabilitated body, for example, can train for a marathon, involving further cycles of immediacy, opposition, and reconciliation.

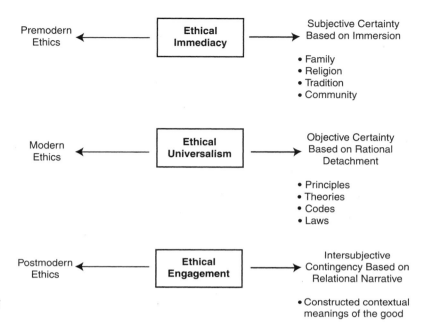

Figure 40–1. *Triad of Ethical Layers.*

If an inherent telos is assumed, a dialectic will move inexorably toward culmination. Hegel insisted on a telos, but I do not. Without a telos, the movement of mediation can proceed indefinitely. Without closure, a dialectic of ethical levels such as I propose can give rise to further cycles of differentiation. Ethics, in other words, need not culminate in the postmodern. Indeed, the most interesting question evoked by a dialectic of premodern-modern-postmodern ethics may be, "What now?" Given the nihilism sometimes associated (mistakenly, I believe) with postmodern ethics, treating it as the thesis for a new set of negations might be a fruitful sequel to the discussion that follows.

Premodern Immersion: Ethical Immediacy

In a dialectical framework the first level is immediacy. In ethical terms, immediacy is an unreflective and uncritical certainty about the good. A certainty powerful enough to resist reflection originates outside an individual in order to avoid being undermined by particularity.

Certainty about the good, if it is to be more than personal conviction, must derive from a source that transcends the individual, such as religion, family, customs, or the ethos of a profession.

Ethical immediacy is an experience of certainty that needs and allows no explication; it is nondiscursive. That, in fact, is its power. A discursive description of a morally good nurse can be argued and revised, requires consideration, and has to be consciously accepted in order to have power. In contrast, a nondiscursive portrayal—an image rendered in film, a virtue modeled by a mentor—bypasses deliberation to gain acceptance. With a cultural, professional, or religious basis for certainty, a nurse intuits the good directly, without recourse to reflection. That immediacy is the phenomenon I call immersion: a nurse is immersed in a tradition that provides an ethical appraisal of the situation, as well as immersed in the situation itself. Depending on the tradition, that appraisal may dictate, for example, that nurse-assisted suicide is wrong (or that it is right). Whatever the tradition, immersion offers a degree of certainty unavailable to the other ethical layers because it is nonreflective. It needs no defense.

The strength of immersion as an ethical approach is the solidarity it achieves. Nurses and patients sharing an unquestioned view of the good are united in their attempt to realize that good. Differences in interpretation may arise between individuals, but the foundational unity that grounds their values prevents differences from becoming divisive. Similarly, within an individual, ethical immediacy prevents fragmentation of the self that can result from self-questioning and critique. Immediacy serves to maintain the self—and the group—as a coherent, harmonious whole. Immersion and immediacy, in other words, describe community. "In community persons cease to be other, opaque, not understood, and instead become mutually sympathetic, understanding one another . . . , fused" (Young, 1990, p. 231).

Immediacy, like a spell, would be broken by the detachment needed to explain or defend it. Defense is unnecessary in a community characterized by a common tradition, but few nurses practice in such a community. One of the hallmarks of contemporary nursing is the decline of moral immediacy (Benjamin & Curtis, 1992). In place of actual groups united by a single worldview, there are diffuse disciplines (Foucault, 1975/1979) and discourses (Bordo, 1993). They invite a form of immersion, but they unite individuals through abstract ideology rather than community identity (Gouldner, 1978).

Community-based certainty is not obsolete, however. Its contemporary form is communitarian ethics. Communitarians regard individuals as situated within a natural community such as the family, neighborhood, or nation, a community of origin that anchors personal identity and guarantees moral certainty (MacIntyre, 1981). For communitarians, immersion is the ideal form of moral knowledge and the only basis for ethical certainty.

Because the likelihood of a shared community is low for contemporary nurses, ethical immediacy will be challenged in most settings. Merely identifying an ethical issue (Should we allow this person to die?) undermines immediacy, since ethical issues do not arise in a premodern approach. Once a question is posed, there are two choices. One is to reinforce certainty using force, such as shame or exclusion, against the questioner, thereby ending inquiry and reinstating immediacy. The other option is to answer the challenge by articulating the basis for certainty. That response, however, entails translating subjective certainty into objective forms (language and reasons) that another could understand, and, in so doing, immediacy is shattered. When a person surfaces from ethical immersion to defend a view of the good, certainty is compromised and immediacy is lost.

Modern Detachment: Ethical Universalism

Dialectically, the move away from immediacy produces its opposite, rational objectivity. Historically, the rational turn is symbolized by the Enlightenment celebration of reason as liberator from the Dark Ages of superstition, parochialism, and feudalism (Poole, 1991). In health care, too, an ethics based on rational principles has been heralded as a moral enlightenment following an era of professional feudalism known as paternalism (Beauchamp & Childress, 1994).

Because immersion in unquestioned certainty is an extreme form of ethical knowing, its antithesis too is uncompromising. Rationality counters subjectivity with principles that are categorical and unconditional. Detachment provides the distance needed for objectivity, for viewing from a vantage point outside, instead of inside, a situation. Freed from the limiting perspective of particularity, reason equals universality. The modern turn in ethics aims at overcoming the relativity of competing parochial certainties by producing one incontestable system of universal principles.

The strength of ethical universalism is epitomized by the principle of respecting individuals equally. Respect for individuals is based on the rational autonomy that each person possesses, the ability to transcend personal feelings in making universalistic choices. Formulated another way, ethical choices respect others as ends in themselves, affirming them as rationally autonomous and capable of transcendence; individuals are equivalent units of universality (Friedman, 1993). The principle is blind to actual identities of both the agent and the other, not unlike the double-blind design that assures objectivity in science. In nursing, the principle restrains us from discriminating against patients; prevents us from coercing, oppressing, or lying to them; and prevents our treating them as mere objects, material, or means to others' ends. In short, it commits us to a contract of reciprocity in which we respect the value that they and we share as universal, free persons.

Despite the appeal of rational principles, especially in health care, they provide less certainty than they promise. Three limitations of rational ethics can be identified. First, interpretations of a principle can conflict in clinical situations. A requirement to protect life can be interpreted as maintaining physiologic functioning or as alleviating suffering. One way to reconcile the conflict involves redefining terms so that life means quality of life, but for some nurses a life is more than its quality, while for others, suffering enhances the quality of a life. For still others, a nurse's view of life is irrelevant, because only the patient's view matters. Application of a principle, in other words, compromises its universality because interpretation is required, and interpretations differ according to the perspectives of the people involved.

A second limitation is the contradiction that universalism, alleged alternative to force, governs by force when it insists on the suppression of particularity, stripping from persons and situations their lived reality. Universal principles provide ethical knowledge in a situation only if all cases are alike but actual issues and the people involved are not identical. The only way a principle could provide solutions would be by force, that is, by requiring a nurse to suppress particular knowledge about a situation and blindly apply the principle; but that reduces a professional from an ethical agent to an automaton.

A feminist critique of universalism identifies a third limitation of rational ethics. That critique exposes the cultural hegemony of reason, specifically the oppressive authority of those whose status affords them the luxury of transcendence as long as others remain bound by conditions of hunger, exhaustion, or pain (Benhabib, 1992). Ethical universalism is founded on a dualist metaphysics in which reason is the essence of humanness, and other aspects (especially emotions and the body) are inessential, unruly, and, ideally, transcended. Because universalism values persons as transcendent, it devalues those experiences, already marginalized by dualism, that are not fully controllable, such as illness and suffering. The moral high ground of rationality becomes synonymous with privilege and power instead of the equality it promised.

The question raised by a critique of rationalism is whether nondualist respect is possible, valuing persons as irreducibly ambiguous: particular and universal, embodied and intellectual, emotional and rational. Dialectically, nondualist respect represents an ethical level beyond both immersion and detachment as sources of certainty, a third level characterized by uncertainty and engagement.

Postmodern Engagement: Relational Narrative

The move beyond rational objectivity in ethics can be considered an existential or postmodern turn. In existentialist ethics, the uniqueness of individuals is their essential feature. A self has a particular perspective as a situated subject. Transcendence is only the ability to imagine and appreciate different perspectives, not to assume a universal view from nowhere. The situated self encompasses not only rationality but emotion, imagination, memory, language, the body, and even other selves. Individuals are intrinsically relational; existential subjectivity is intersubjectivity.

Respect for persons as existential selves involves more than detached regard for abstract autonomy; it entails attentive discernment and valuing of an individual as unique. Dillon (1992) describes this discernment as care respect, because its valuing of particularity parallels that of care ethics. The valuing of persons requires perception of each one's uniqueness, and perception involves engagement. In contrast to rational ethics, which demands detachment in order not to perceive people concretely or respond to them personally, care respect conveys "cherishing, treasuring, profoundness of feeling" (p. 120).

The engagement of care respect is the opposite of ethical objectivity; it is personal responsiveness to the particular other, a relation between individuals that is grounded in the ambiguity of their being at once encumbered and free, situated and transcendent. Engagement cannot be regulated by principles; they would remove the relation from its grounding in actual persons and orient it toward external authority. Codes have no authority to command engagement. The only form that moral authority takes is authorization, the call from the other commanding concern simply by being the other. "The moral call is thoroughly personal, . . . the command is not universalizable" (Bauman, 1993, p. 51).

The move from rational principles to existential engagement is a postmodern turn. Postmodern ethics can be characterized as embracing contingency, refusing certainties, and resisting the modern drive for unity, order, and foundations (Bauman, 1995; Tester, 1993). Postmodernism expresses its resistance by dismantling the fixed meanings rationalism has constructed. Every form of order becomes a target for deconstruction, from the social, sexual, and political to the epistemological and metaphysical, but none is as inimical to postmodern ethics as the hermeneutic order, the modern hierarchy of meanings. In that hierarchy, rational meanings are authoritatively assigned, fixed rather than fluid, and ranked by their degree of objectivity. A diagnosis of HIV, for example, is assigned its correct meaning by clinical experts, the meaning remains constant among experts, and the assigned meaning ranks higher on the hermeneutic scale than an emotional or imaginative interpretation by a person with the diagnosis. Significantly, experiences that pose the greatest threat to rational control—dying, illness, pain, dementia— become objects of the strictest

hermeneutic control, often with disabling consequences. A social construction of aging, for example, as decline and deterioration can be more disabling than physical changes accompanying aging. From a postmodern perspective, the modern oppression through meanings represents hermeneutic terrorism in which experience is held hostage to authority.

Postmodernism destabilizes the hierarchy of meanings by displaying them as contingent, demonstrating that any interpretation of an experience can be revised because other meanings are always available. Moreover, no uninterpreted basis exists from which to decide objectively among meanings, "no neutral ground on which to stand and argue that either torture or kindness is preferable" (Rorty, 1989, p. 173). Our most trusted ethical certainties are our own creation. We may choose kindness rather than torture, but there is no authorization for our choice. Without a higher authority than ourselves, we have no certainty that our meanings are better than those of others. Ethically, we are on our own, without a metaphysical warrant from either religion or reason.

Meanings are contingent because they are human creations, but the most radical contingency is that of meaningfulness itself. The very enterprise of making meaning is conditional, never assured. It depends on our continuing acts of interpretation, always subject to the possibility that we may be overwhelmed into silence and incapable of interpretation. Scarry (1985) describes intense pain as world-destroying. Grief, fear, and despair also can unmake the meanings that comprise a person's world, including the central meaning of the person as meaning-maker. If disintegration of both world and self are possible, then meaningfulness itself, not just one or another meaning, is radically uncertain.

Radical contingency is not captured by the nihilist certainty that life is meaningless. That certainty in fact reassures us that there is no possibility of meaninglessness. Radical contingency is more serious. It lacks the comfortable universality of nihilism. It is the concrete possibility in each situation that meaning might not be created, a human interpretation might not be voiced in time to keep the world from ending. If I can say, at least, "this pain is meaningless," I am safe from meaninglessness. If I can say nothing because language is powerless or my voice is silenced, then my world ends.

Dismissing end-of-the-world talk is hubris, the modern certainty that there can be no gap in the plenum of meanings, no abyss into which one could fall. Nurses rarely indulge in that hubris. Most have glimpsed the abyss through a patient's eyes. At the edge of the abyss ethical certainties fail, and nothing remains except possible engagement between nurse and patient; but engagement is enough (without it a patient is alone, no matter how many nurses are present). The ethical narrative a nurse and patient compose through their engagement interprets the situation, saving it, for the moment, from meaninglessness.

Narrative meaning is communicative, the saying of something another can understand; it represents a "moral party of two" (Bauman, 1993, p. 82). Beyond that, it requires that at least one of the two is not silenced by their situation, remaining able to imagine and voice an interpretation: one of the two serves as their poet. "In times of strangeness, . . . by being strangers together, people and poet reconstitute an internal homeland" (Cixous, 1993, p. 26). That homeland for nurse and patient is the narrative they compose together, the words of their engagement.

Engagement includes the danger that the poet too will fall silent. By joining another in vulnerability, I myself become vulnerable, and the other's pain may silence me. Wordless, I can only turn to the other for meanings, as did the poet Akhmatova (1983), waiting with the other mothers outside Leningrad prisons, writing her poems with their words. In engagement, even authorship is contingent; "if Akhmatova, mother among mothers, writes with the mothers' meager words, then the mothers are also poets among poets" (Cixous, 1993, p. 27). In composing a narrative between nurse and patient, it does not matter who is author, because each is poet; it matters only that there are enough words between them to make a story.

The attempt to compose meanings, given their contingency, is flawed from a modern standpoint. The ethical knowledge created through a relational narrative is particular, contextual, and nongeneralizable; even its authorship is ambiguous when one person speaks with the other's words. An ethical narrative fails all criteria for objective knowledge, and terms like poem or story only further demean it in the rationalist view.

Dialectically, however, rationalism is flawed by its suppression of engagement as avenue to ethical knowledge. From a postmodern standpoint, modern ethics fails to grasp a significant feature of human experience, its narrative nature (Carr, 1986). To claim that "we lead storied lives" (Connelly & Clandinin, 1990, p. 2) is not only to point out that crafting stories is an important human activity, but, more fundamentally, to assert that an experience, in order to be my experience, has narrative form; it has to be fitted into the rest of my experience with a connecting meaning, a thread of sense, even if sensible only for me. To make sense of experience is to make the narrative connection, to relate otherwise inchoate events to my story, the life I am living as mine (LeGuin, 1989).

Nursing has (re)discovered narrative as a form of coherence in the absence of encompassing certainties. Through narrative intervention patients can be helped to create emancipatory narratives, that is, to revise disabling into enabling views that allow movement toward a self with possibilities (Sandelowski, 1994). Ethical narratives are emancipatory in their portrayal of a good toward which a person can move. Because individuals are particular, situated, and self-interpreting, the most faithful way to know the good they seek is through their own accounts, their personal ethical narratives. At times of vulnerability, however, personal narratives can fail, just as ethical certainties fail in the face of radical contingency. In those moments a new narrative is needed, and help may be needed to compose it. Ethical narratives created by patient and nurse from the homeland of their engagement are thus more than individual accounts: they are relational narratives.

Because a relational narrative expresses engagement, it extends beyond the particularity of either person alone but does not extend beyond their relationship; it is more than personal but not universal (Gadow, 1994, 1995). It embodies intersubjectivity, an alternative to both the subjectivity of immersion and the objectivity of detachment. The paradox of a relational narrative is that it narrates uncertainty, but in so doing can offer a safer home, existentially, than would be found in subjective or objective certainty. Either of those would cost the nurse and patient their relationship. Their lived reality together would be displaced. The aim of relational narrative is to provide a place of shared, and therefore safer, contingency. By combining contingencies through engagement, persons are able to coauthor an interpretation that may be more inhabitable than either of their individual narratives as they seek a new form of the good.

A Dialectical Framework in Practice

I have proposed that the philosophical cornerstone of nursing is dialectically layered rather than unitary. The question now emerges: What would the dialectic among different ethical layers look like in practice?

A dialectic can be reduced to ideology by theorizing a telos that draws the movement toward a final level. To avoid that reduction and its coerciveness, I suggest that the three ethical approaches be regarded not as successive stages in the profession's advance, but as possibilities coexisting in an ethically vital practice. Dialectic offers a way of envisioning contradictory approaches as intrinsically related. None of the three is fully intelligible without its connection to the others. Each complements the limitations of the other two.

Dialectic as a philosophical framework is more than a heuristic device for conceptualizing nursing. It is a also a framework for the continuing development of the discipline. If otherwise opposing approaches can be appreciated as inseparable, they may then be acknowledged in practice as being mutually enhanc-

ing instead of oppositional. Nursing becomes more than a moral high ground from which difference is excluded. It becomes, instead, a region of existence large enough to accommodate, even encourage, diversity among those who live there.

Just as a geographic region cannot be conveyed in its totality by a map, an existential region cannot be captured in a theory, but something of its vitality can be rendered by images. In a beginning attempt to answer the question of how a dialectical framework might look in practice, I offer instead of theory a metaphor and a clinical example that may serve as an impetus to further exploration.

The flourishing of premodern, modern, and postmodern ethics in nursing can be imagined metaphorically as the biodiversity of a coral reef where different life forms integrate and where organisms even after their death provide a structure that supports life. At the level of immediacy, we are immersed in ethical currents that carry us safely through situations where reflection would be impossible. When crosscurrents require us to reflect and to hold a position, an edifice of ethical principles offers a structure for steadying ourselves. Finally, there are situations where no edifice can alleviate our vulnerability, and in those cases we can only turn to each other and together compose a fragile new form of the good.

To illustrate, I consider the reef-like situation described by Schroeder (1998) in which Carole (mother) and Morgan (daughter) found themselves while Morgan spent the first 3 months of life undergoing surgical heart repairs, inept and relentless technical procedures, and near-fatal nursing and medical errors. Schroeder's description does not indict professionals for being unethical, but displays instead the inevitable collisions when a mother's immersion in her daughter's danger meets the detachment of ethical objectivity.

"How can she be in congestive heart failure if I'm rooming-in?" He looked impatiently at me. "You're a nurse. Call the intensive care nursery if her respirations go over 60" (p. 14).

Instead of calling, Carole brought her baby into bed with her, pulled the blanket over them, and unplugged the phone, mutely sinking into the quicksand of isolation that immersion becomes when no hand is offered.

Hands eventually were offered from each of the three ethical layers. All of them were essential to the survival of both mother and child.

1. From the urgency of another mother's immersion in her own child's situation:

> "Get her out of here no matter what," she whispered, . . . "Get her out of here if she is getting better at all" (p. 13).

And from the same mother, the offer of community in an informal group where mothers' stories to each other kept them from drowning in the immediacy of their children's pain.

2. From the honesty of a nurse who countered institutional hierarchy with her own ethical autonomy:

> One day, Lea told me that the physicians at this hospital were unable to do anything further for Morgan . . . Although she merely confirmed what I had already been thinking, I was unable to summon the strength to act upon my thoughts without her support. I now know that Morgan would have died in that hospital cubicle if Lea had not risked angering the physicians and telling me the truth (p. 19).

3. From a nurse whose overtures opened the door to a different story, to engagement instead of isolation:

> Carolyn would ignore my hostile looks and sit with me at Morgan's bedside on work breaks . . . Her words and presence began to fill some of the emptiness inside me. Although I would never admit it to her, I began to look forward to her visits, and eventually we began to communicate on a level very foreign to our previous working relationship (p. 19).

And from a nurse who transcended moral duties:

Cathy came out of the ICU and said that they were trying to get her off the heart-lung machine now; "I'll be right back to let you know," she said, and walked back into the ICU. I stared at the door, awestruck at her bravery. She'll have to let me know, I marveled, now she can't just stay behind those doors and let someone else tell me the news. I felt ready to handle anything, almost exhilarated that someone would risk so much when it wasn't even required (p. 21).

The coral reef that I believe Schroeder describes is ethically layered. Modern, premodern, and postmodern elements alternately prevailed. The situation would have been ethically diminished by an absence of any of the elements. Philosophically, the dialectical nature of nursing entails the presence of all of them. Without a telos to drive the dialectic, there is no basis on which to insist that nursing limit itself to one. The postmodern turn only makes explicit an element that has been implicit; it does not establish a superior ground from which to dismiss the others. In the case of Carole and Morgan, no single element was decisive in determining the ethical course to pursue. They did escape, as the first mother urged, but not before a nurse had urged moving to a better hospital where surgery was successful, and not until other nurses had offered engagement as alternative to immersion.

A dialectical ethical narrative such as Schroeder provides is the equivalent of a relational narrative that a nurse and patient together create. Both narratives are layered with voices from immediacy and objectivity in a continuing tension that cannot be resolved in favor of either without destruction of the narrative's relational nature, its contingency and vitality. The postmodern turn is not an advance that dismisses immersion and detachment as ethical approaches. It is instead a turn toward the absurd, as Camus (1955) would call it, the cultivation of a life "without appeal" (p. 39) in which the longing for certainty and the impossibility of certainty are both embraced passionately. From a modern or premodern perspective, that contradiction is absurd in the sense of being hopeless. From the postmodern perspective, an absurd life is filled with "a wild kind of hope" (Schroeder, 1998, p. 20).

The practice of an absurd life, an absurd ethics, is dialectical because it grants at once the validity of subjective and objective ethics. In nursing the story of that practice can only be intersubjective, a relational narrative. The narrative is layered with voices of immersion and detachment like a medieval motet in which several voices simultaneously sing parts of the text that counter and complement one another (Gadow, 1999). Perhaps the fact that a philosophical cornerstone can be compared metaphorically to a phenomenon as ephemeral as a song is one more indication of the postmodern turn in nursing ethics.

REFERENCES

Akhmatova, A. (1983). *Poems.* New York: Norton.

Bauman, Z. (1993). *Postmodern ethics.* Oxford, England: Blackwell Publishers.

Bauman, Z. (1995). *Life in fragments: Essays in postmodern morality.* Oxford, England: Blackwell Publishers.

Beauchamp, T., & Childress, J. (1994). *Principles of biomedical ethics* (4th ed.). Oxford, England: Oxford University Press.

Benhabib, S. (1992). *Situating the self: Gender, community and postmodernism in contemporary ethics.* London: Routledge.

Benjamin, M., & Curtis, J. (1992). *Ethics in nursing* (3rd ed.). Oxford, England: Oxford University Press.

Bloom, L. R. (1992). How can we know the dancer from the dance?: Discourses of the self-body. *Human Studies, 15,* 313–334.

Bordo, S. (1993). *Unbearable weight: Feminism, western culture, and the body.* Los Angeles: University of California Press.

Camus, A. (1955). *The myth of Sisyphus and other essays.* New York: Vintage Books.

Carr, D. (1986). *Time, narrative, and history.* Bloomington, IN: Indiana University Press.

Cixous, H. (1993). We who are free, are we free? In B. Johnson (Ed.), *Freedom and interpretation: The Oxford Amnesty Lectures, 1992* (pp. 14–44). New York: HarperCollins.

Connelly, F., & Clandinin, D. (1990). Stories of experience and narrative inquiry. *Educational Researcher, 19*(5), 2–14.

Dillon, R. (1992). Respect and care: Toward moral integration. *Canadian Journal of Philosophy, 22,* 105–131.

Foucault, M. (1979). *Discipline and punish: The birth of the prison* (A. Sheridan, Trans.). New York: Vintage Books. (Original work published 1975)

Friedman, M. (1993). *What are friends for? Feminist perspectives on personal relationships and moral theory.* Ithaca, NY: Cornell University Press.

Gadow, S. (1982). Body and self: A dialectic. In V. Kestenbaum (Ed.), *The humanity of the ill: Phenomenological perspectives* (pp. 86–100). Knoxville, TN: University of Tennessee Press.

Gadow, S. (1994). Whose body? Whose story? The question about narrative in women's health care. *Soundings, 77,* 295–307.

Gadow, S. (1995). Clinical epistemology: A dialectic of nursing assessment. *Canadian Journal of Nursing Research, 27,* 25–34.

Gadow, S. (1999). *I felt an island rising: Interpretive inquiry as motet.* Manuscript submitted for publication.

Gouldner, A. (1978). *The dialectic of ideology and technology: The origins, grammar, and future of ideology.* Oxford, England: Oxford University Press.

Hegel, G. W. F. (1977). *The phenomenology of spirit* (A. V. Miller, Trans.). Oxford, England: Clarendon. (Original work published in 1807)

LeGuin, U. (1989). Some thoughts on narrative. In U. LeGuin (Ed.), *Dancing at the edge of the world: Thoughts on words, women, places* (pp. 37–45). New York: Harper & Row.

MacIntyre, A. (1981). *After virtue.* Notre Dame, IN: University of Notre Dame Press.

Poole, R. (1991). *Morality and modernity.* London: Routledge.

Rorty, R. (1989). *Contingency, irony, and solidarity.* Cambridge, England: Cambridge University Press.

Sandelowski, M. (1994). We are the stories we tell: Narrative knowing in nursing practice. *Journal of Holistic Nursing, 12,* 23–33.

Scarry, E. (1985). *The body in pain: The making and unmaking of the world.* Oxford, England: Oxford University Press.

Schroeder, C. (1998). So this is what it's like: Struggling to survive in pediatric intensive care. *Advances in Nursing Science, 20,* 13–22.

Tester, K. (1993). *The life and times of post-modernity.* London: Routledge.

Young, I. (1990). *Justice and the politics of difference.* Princeton, NJ: Princeton University Press.

Offprints. Requests for offprints should be directed to Professor Sally Gadow, RN, PhD, 4365 Snowberry Court, Boulder, CO 80304.

The Author Comments

Relational Narrative: The Postmodern Turn in Nursing Ethics

All my work reflects an appreciation for philosophic dialectic as described by Hegel. This article was my attempt to use a dialectic perspective to understand ethics as a whole and to integrate opposing ethical approaches that were, to me, incompatible. I wanted to demonstrate how relational ethics could evolve naturally in nursing as a response to the limitations of traditional and rational ethics. I hope the article contributes to an emerging view of not only ethical theory but also nursing theory as postmodern.

—SALLY GADOW

CHAPTER 41

Nursing Ethics in an Era of Globalization

Wendy Austin

We live in an era of globalization in which our essential interdependence is increasingly revealed. Transportation and communication technology plus worldwide health, environmental, and security risks and a world economy driven by transnational corporations are connecting us in a new kind of way. Incredible advances in biotechnology, the pressing demands of equity and justice in resource allocation, and the need for a universal perspective in health ethics are some of the issues challenging our moral imagination in significant ways. Nurses need to ask themselves: What changes for nursing ethics when the global—not the local—becomes the dominant frame of reference?

Key words: *biotechnology, globalization, nursing ethics, resource allocation, universalism*

Originally, the word "globe" referred to a ball created by winding thread together.[1] In this era of globalization, we are increasingly aware that we are intertwined. We need to reconsider, in a profound way, a foundational ethical question: How should we live together? Nurses are strategically placed—by our history, our education, and our experience in working across diversity and car- ing for all—to contribute to the discourse exploring this question. We might begin by asking ourselves: What does a shift to a global frame of reference mean to the ethical practice of the 11 million nurses providing health care around the world? Although nursing has had an international perspective for over a century (in 1870 nurses were serving with the International Red Cross),

The author acknowledges the Alberta Heritage Foundation for Medical Research's support of this work through a research fellowship.
Adv Nurs Sci 2001:24(2):1–18. Copyright © 2001 Aspen Publishers, Inc. Reproduced with permission
of Lippincott Williams & Wilkins.

About the Author

WENDY AUSTIN is an Associate Professor in the Faculty of Nursing and the John Dossetor Health Ethics Centre, University of Alberta. Her clinical expertise lies in psychiatric/mental health nursing, and she is Co-Director of the Faculty's Pan American Health Organization/World Health Organization Collaborating Centre in Nursing and Mental Health. Dr. Austin is a member of the Canadian Nurses Ethics Committee and of the Ethics Advisory Council of the Aboriginal Capacity for Development and Research Environments (ACADRE) at the University of Alberta. She has been an adviser in mental health to the International Council of Nurses and is a former President of the Canadian Federation of Mental Health Nurses.

an international outlook (one that exists "among nations") is different than a global one. What are the ethical concerns for nurses living and working in a global community? In this article, the argument is made that we are living in a global age, followed by the identification of three key health ethics issues on which we, as nurses, need to reflect and act. These issues are the advances in biotechnology and the business associated with it, the pressing demands of equity and justice in global resource allocation, and the challenge of devising a universal ethic that is respectful of diverse values to guide action in the area of health.

Living in a Global Village

It is said that you need to leave home to truly recognize who you are. Space travel has allowed us to see the Earth and to behold ourselves as we really are—beings living together on one small planet. The science and technology that made this vision possible also are connecting us to one another in a new kind of way. McLuhan's[2] "global village" has come to fruition. Technological advancement has changed the way we travel and communicate to such a degree that geographical space no longer defines "neighbor." We may not know the person living next door, but we may have a daily "over-the-fence" chat with someone thousands of miles away via e-mail. Contemporary images and icons are recognized worldwide. Satellite dishes bring *Star Trek* and *Bay Watch* into the lives of villagers in the far Arctic and along the shores of the upper Amazon River.

Mickey Mouse speaks nearly every language; children in Beijing are asking their parents for "Kentucky Fried Chicken." Whether or not things go better with Coca-Cola, everyone knows what you are talking about.

The conception of a nation as a place that has a language, culture, and literature distinct from the rest of the world is fading. The spread of the English language and American cultural products, as well as worldwide movements such as that for women's rights, has diminished that meaning and decreased the power of the nation state as our chief frame of reference.[3] Like the butterfly's wing of chaos theory, environmental, economic, or political events in one part of the world have effects thousands of miles away. Courtesy of Internet technology, anonymous stock, bond, currency, and transnational investors drive the marketplace, having become a force strong enough to affect national economies and bring down governments.[4] It seems, in fact, that a line between international and domestic issues can no longer be drawn.

We have instead what Jowitt[5] terms "intermestic situations," with political borders increasingly irrelevant. We watch war, famine, epidemics, and the sufferings of the poor a continent away "live" from our homes. With this immediacy, television takes us beyond family, local community, and nation in such a way that the scope of our moral concern is altered.[6] We see (or must actively refuse to see) distant human distress and anguish as they are happening. Our pressing problems are global ones: the effects of human activities on the environment, nuclear weaponry, chemical and biologic terrorism, and emergent and resurgent infectious diseases[3,6-8] Science, always a force moving beyond national boundaries, is increasingly a global influence. A striking example of this is the recent worldwide cooperation of scientists in deconstructing human biology in the Human Genome Project. The ultimate consequences of this discovery will be so immense that they are difficult for us to imagine. In fact, the magnitude of the changes currently affecting our world is almost too great for us to grasp.[9] What is becoming absolutely apparent, however, is our fundamental interdependence.

The shift to a global frame of reference signifies epochal change in the bases of our societal actions and organizations.[3] It is noteworthy that the term "globalization" is most often used in the economic sense, referring to the rise of a worldwide economy driven by transnational corporations and the spread of a free-market ideology. In *The Lexus and the Olive Tree*, Freidman[4] describes how economic globalization has come to replace the Cold War as the force that shapes all domestic policies and international relations. Rather than the world being divided into "friends" and "enemies" according to one's alignment in the politics of the Cold War, everyone now has become a "competitor." The imperatives of the marketplace are depicted as the sum and substance of daily life. At this point, it seems that the global village is foremost a consumer society, a society whose members' value is based on their capacity for and commitment to the consumer role.[10] The reality of the free market as the dominating paradigm can be illustrated with one chilling example: Russia's once top-secret missiles are up for sale via a 511-page catalogue, with weapon details listed on the Internet at www.tommax.military.com.[11]

In *Globalization: The Human Consequences*, Bauman[10] declares that this form of economic globalization is radically different from globalization as a hope of a universal order. The ideal of a universalism in which the life conditions of all people are made similar—so that life chances are more equable—is not shaping current forces. Bauman finds that the process of globalization is dividing even as it unites. A localizing phenomenon is occurring so that while those with resources are becoming "global" and literally or virtually mobile, those without resources are fixed in their localities. Being fixed locally in a globalized world means being separated and excluded. Separation, according to Bauman, is one of the major survival strategies in the new global order—there is no more loving or hating your neighbors; one just keeps them at a distance. In a free-market ideology, no one is responsible for anyone else. Collective action on social issues is not part of the discourse.

A potentially perilous element of globalization is the "free for all" fostered in world affairs.[3,4,10] We are not in control of the powerful forces, particularly the economic ones, that are shaping our lives and our futures. There is no sign "of a centre, of a controlling desk, of a board of directors, of a managerial office."[10(p59)] Freidman exhorts, *No one is in charge.*"[4(p93)] Not even in America is it different. Albrow[3] coined the term "globality" to replace "globalization" in an effort to eliminate the connotation of necessary outcomes that "-ization" suggests. In his book on the global age, he argues that the world is significantly transforming, but the change is nondirectional and with an open future (including the possibility of "deglobalization"). We can no longer have faith in the teleology of progress. In these postmodern times, there is no endpoint to which we are evolving.

As our technological power radically alters the human and the nonhuman world and ungoverned transnational economic forces shape our relations with one another, moral issues are being raised for which we have no real precedents. The global condition of human life and our new power to affect the very nature of existence (perhaps even to extinguish it) are demanding a reshaping of our moral horizons.[6,10,12] Hans Jonas,[12] the late American ethicist, warned us more than 20 years ago that the altered nature of human action calls for a radical change in ethics. The solidarity of our interest with one another, and with nature, must move us to a new kind of humility and an ethics with responsibility as the imperative. Jonas' words have even more significance today. In this era of globalization, new conceptions of rights, duties, and responsibilities are required.

We need an ethics that acknowledges the excess of our power over our wisdom and understanding. We need an ethics that addresses our essential interdependence.

What form would such an ethics take? Is a macro-ethic appropriate to global times? Is it even a possibility, given the diversity of values and beliefs in the world? What would it mean in the realm of health ethics? Before such questions can be answered, there must be dialogue around core issues. Nurses can contribute to such a dialogue and must, if we take our commitment to the health and well-being of our societies seriously. Following is a description of three particular issues that nurses will need to address as they consider what this era of globalization means to the substance of nursing ethics.

The Business of Biotechnology

On June 26, 2000 the Human Genome Project and a biotech company, Celera, jointly announced that the working draft of the DNA sequence was complete. This accomplishment is so profound that human evolution may be fundamentally and forever changed. With it, incredible possibilities for human health are opened, including opportunities for identifying individuals' predisposition to inheritable diseases (eg, diabetes and Alzheimer's disease), for revealing genetically oriented disease prevention and treatment strategies (eg, the breast cancer suppressor gene), for stimulating the development of new biologic therapeutics and vaccines, and for extending human longevity.

This new knowledge, however, has significant potential for abuse. Fearful images of what could occur have been portrayed for the public in movies. *Gattaca,* for example, is the story of a cold, segregated, controlled society based on genetic discrimination. Discrimination based on genetic makeup, however, is not science fiction. In 1998 Israeli scientists were said to be developing an "ethno-bomb," made from lethal viruses and bacteria designed to attack persons with particular DNA.[13] In the United States, federal agencies already are banned from using genetic testing in employee selection, or at least are banned from denying a promotion

or job to persons based on their genes. Privacy protection of medical information is increasingly a concern. In fact, the nefarious use to which information could be put, especially by insurance companies, is substantial.

With the race to identify the human genome finished, scientists are now competing to be the first to clone a human being. Professor Severino Antinori, an in vitro fertilization (IVF) specialist of the International Association for Human Reproduction Infertility Unit in Rome, and Professor Panayiotis Zavos of the Kentucky Center for Reproductive Medicine announced their human cloning project in March 2001.[14] They are going ahead despite strong warnings from researchers such as Ian Wilmut of the Roslin Institute in Edinburgh, the designer of that famous sheep, Dolly. Although Wilmut's scruples did not extend to the replication of an animal, he is against human cloning for social and ethical reasons, as well as for the practical reason that cloning technology is still limited. He believes that the inevitable failures in any human cloning attempt (such as birth defects) will arouse public concern and set back other research, such as the therapeutic cloning of embryonic stem cells for use in treating diseases such as Parkinson's.[15]

Genetically modified (GM) foods are already a reality in the global marketplace. Whereas consumers in some countries, such as those in the European Union, are resistive and hostile to the introduction of genetically engineered biologic products, other consumers, such as those in Canada, are largely unaware that they are using them. Canada does not require the labeling of engineered food unless it alters the nutrition of that food or poses a risk of allergy. More than 50% of the Canadian canola crop and 30% of its soybean crop are genetically modified to resist herbicides and pesticides, respectively.[16,17] Use of plants modified to resist drought or to contain higher amounts of essential nutrients could be vital in feeding the world, and fruits and vegetables could be modified to act as vaccines for diseases such as hepatitis B.[18] It may be too soon to know, however, whether GM foods can be harmful to human health, wildlife, or the environment, and some argue that they should not be grown outside research facilities until such knowledge is available.[19] One problem is that it is difficult to control GM plants' interaction with the rest of the environment. Another is that mistakes can be made. Canada, for instance, inadvertently provided Scottish farmers with GM rapeseeds that were sown over 11,000 acres of land.[17] Ultimately, getting people to accept GM foods may be a matter of marketing. If feeding the hungry and providing vaccines do not excite consumers and secure their support, the opportunity for products such as a GM potato that can make low-fat chips likely will.[17]

Vaccines and potent pharmaceuticals are other major contributions of the business of biotechnology. Powerful new weapons in the fight against disease are increasingly available, particularly for those living in the developed world. Access to new products in less developed areas, however, is a current problem surrounded by much controversy. Although the pharmaceutical industry is interested in expanding into emerging markets in developing countries, it is encountering political and regulatory constraints: failure to respect and enforce intellectual property rights, drug piracy, pricing restrictions, and lack of consistency in standards of regulation and enforcement.[8] As well, companies expect the manufacture of particular drugs to be profitable if the drugs are to be made widely available. For instance, Eflornithine, the cure for trypanosomiasis, the fatal sleeping sickness that infects an estimated 300,000 people a year in Africa, became available because it was discovered that it removes female facial hair, making it a more marketable product.[20]

The acquired immune deficiency syndrome (AIDS) pandemic is bringing the accessibility issue to a head. While life-extending drugs have made the human immunodeficiency virus (HIV) infection more a chronic illness than a death sentence in affluent regions, millions are dying in Sub-Saharan Africa from AIDS without access to the drugs. Pharmaceutical companies are under considerable international pressure to provide AIDS drugs at lower prices to these areas. South Africa is being taken to court by the pharmaceutical industry over its plans to promote the import or local manufacture of AIDS drugs. The industry argues that this in-

fringes on their intellectual property rights.[21] Proponents argue that it is imperative to protect these rights so that generated revenue can be used to support research. (This argument is usually countered by the fact that 30% to 60% of the research and development costs for antiretroviral drugs was funded by public money in the United States and Europe.[20]) Some countries nevertheless are producing generic AIDS drugs in the time lag before international patent laws apply to them or through a loophole in global trade rules that permits the breaching of patents during national emergencies. At a cost to Brazil of $3,000 a year (compared with the $10,000 to $15,000 cost in the United States), it offers the generic drugs free to its citizens with AIDS.[21] The bargaining between the drug conglomerates and desperate countries continues, but in the meantime, United Nations Secretary General Kofi Annan has reached an agreement with major corporations to accelerate substantially their reductions in the prices for AIDS treatment for the least developed countries (LDCs).[22]

The extraordinary advances made in biotechnology have enormous and unpredictable implications for the quality of life and the rights of humans and other living beings. Coupled with the open-ended pressures of the global free market, these "advances" may bring with them potentially devastating consequences for how we live together. How do we respond when embryos are put up for sale on the Internet ($500 each),[23] or when we learn that kidneys from prisoners executed in China can be bought for transplant in Taiwan,[24] or when a new life form is patented? Do we respond? In *The Enigma of Health* Gadamer cautions that our social-political consciousness has not evolved at a pace with our scientific and technological progress, that "the progress of technology encounters an unprepared humanity."[25]

In 1997, the United Nations Educational, Scientific and Cultural Organization adopted a Universal Declaration on the Human Genome and Human Rights. In it, human rights principles are applied to interventions affecting human genes, emphasizing particular concepts: the human genome as the heritage of humanity, the dignity of the human person, and the rejection of genetic reductionism. The protection of the individual and solidarity for vulnerable families and populations are stressed. Freedom for research development, however, also is an acknowledged priority.[26,27] There are now calls for an international advisory organization to oversee the genetic engineering of plants and animals.[19]

Will international declarations and advisory groups be sufficient mechanisms to address the significant and escalating changes brought about by our quest for biotechnological know-how? How do we answer questions never before raised, such as who owns particular genes and sequences of DNA or newly created life forms? Is it too late to ask whether limits should be placed on the extent of biotechnological research and development? Should we be tinkering with genes when, for many parts of the world, the most acute biotechnological problem is a safe water supply?

Justice, Solidarity, and Resource Allocation

The negotiations over lower pricing of AIDS cocktails seem moot when many of those with AIDS in LDCs are too poor to buy adequate amounts of food for themselves and their children. Poverty is the cause of much of the disease, disability, and death that are in our power to prevent.[28,29] Ninety percent of the global burden of disease is situated within the Third World, the area of the globe that has access to only 10% of the resources for health.[30] The World Health Organization (WHO) emphasizes that, if we are ever to achieve health for all, ways must be found to permit people to overcome poverty and to recover from disadvantage, rather than being permanently immobilized by them.[31] The globalization of the marketplace, however, is resulting in greater, not lesser, marginalization of the poor.

Although the rhetoric supporting a worldwide free-market economy creates a picture of more wealth for everyone, this is not happening. The shocking fact is that, according to the 1996 United Nations Human Development Report,[32] 358 people have more wealth than the combined incomes of 45% of the world population (ie, 358 rich people own more than 2.3 billion poor people). As marketplace values replace other ones, in

particular that of solidarity, there is a race to see which localities can give the highest productivity for the lowest wages. In their efforts to lure transnational investors, governments are privatizing former public services to meet corporate demands for lower taxes. The poorest countries, many with economies weakened by the structural reforms demanded by the World Bank in the 1980s, end up as the losers in global trade.[33] Furthermore, national governments, in this era of globalization, cannot control the fiscal fluctuations that affect the lives, and livelihoods, of their ordinary citizens.

There are some strategies being recommended that could reduce the enlarging disparities between the rich and the poor. Kapstein[34] believes that it is possible to reconcile globalization with a moral sense of social justice. Societies that accept a responsibility for the welfare of all citizens and that support health care and education will be able to increase productivity, wealth, and domestic peace if there is international cooperation to create just economic policy. He argues that the International Monetary Fund and the World Bank need to demand that official lending programs strengthen rather than slash social nets (as their structural adjustment programs have required in the past). A poor reputation in social policy should be a barrier, not a condition, for investment in a nation. It also has been suggested that a global tax, collected by transnational authorities (eg, a tax on particular natural products such as oil and gas), could be levied and the monies redistributed to the global poor. Such taxes would be something similar to the Islamic "zakat," a mandatory obligation on those of wealth and not considered "charity."[35]

How might economic policies and reforms affecting the quality of life (including the health) of a people be evaluated? Nobel Prize winner Amartya Sen proposed an alternative to the focus on measures of opulence (such as Gross National Product per capita) and on utility (opportunities for the satisfaction of subjective preferences, an approach in which deprivation can be accepted as normal), both of which ignore the distribution of resources. He recommended that a "capabilities" approach be taken. The prime question to be asked becomes: "What are the people of the country in question actually able to do and to be?"[36] With this approach, inquiries are made into the variable need for resources that would allow people to become capable of an equal level of functioning.

Examining the functioning of females in a region, for instance, can reveal "cooperative conflicts," situations in which interests of a cooperative body (such as a family) are divided. The well-being of some members may be at the expense of others, such as when there is an underlying assumption that women's work is an unlimited resource.[37]

In the past, in many regions of the world, women were absent when economic reforms were discussed and initiated, and they had little influence in the development of economic policy. This is beginning to change. For instance, the Gender and Economic Reforms in Africa (GERA) program has been formed in response to the lack of women's input during the structural adjustment and economic reforms imposed by the World Bank in many African countries, reforms that led to privatization of health care and education. Research sponsored by this program indicates that, although the international economic community holds up micro-credit initiatives as a cure for poverty, many women prefer improving health services over better access to credit.[38] Attention needs to be paid to the life situations of women in a community. We know that the education of women, particularly those of maternal age, is one of the strongest factors positively correlated with the health of a nation.[39]

In the last two decades there has been increasing recognition that more than good genetic endowment, personal health, coping practices, and health services are necessary for health. In 1997, building on previous work such as the Ottawa Charter for Health Promotion,[40] the Jakarta Declaration was drafted.[29] It calls for a global alliance on health promotion and inspired the WHO Resolution on Health Promotion, adopted at World Health Assembly in May 1998. The Jakarta Declaration delineates peace, shelter, education, social security, social relations, food; income, the empowerment of women, a stable ecosystem, sustainable resource use, social justice, respect for human rights, and equity as prerequisites for health. Any community, including a global one,

must attend to these factors and their complex interactions if health for its members is to be achieved and sustained.[41] Underlying the declaration is the assumption that health is a basic human right, as well as an essential for social and economic development.

Priorities change if we seriously embrace the perspective that every human being, regardless of economic and geographic situation, has a right to the opportunity for a healthy life. Health must then be considered within a broad social and political context with justice as a key ethical concern.[30,42] The criteria for the allotment of resources for health are then based on need rather than ability to pay. Although worldwide free-market forces are increasingly structuring health as a commodity rather than as an entitlement, this is a change from the international efforts of the past. Following the horrors of World War II and the Holocaust, efforts were made to create a more secure, peaceful world in which the dignity and rights of every individual were recognized and protected. WHO's constitution, adopted in 1946, outlined a fundamental right for all persons to "the enjoyment of the highest attainable standard of health." In 1948 health as a right was included in the Universal Declaration of Human Rights (UDHR).[43] Article 25 of the UDHR acknowledges that everyone has a "right to a standard of living adequate for the health and well-being of himself and of his family, including food, clothing, housing, and medical care and necessary social services, and the right to security in the event of unemployment, sickness, disability, widowhood, old age, or other lack of livelihood in circumstances beyond his control."[43] Aspects of the right to health have been included in many of the international rights documents that followed the UDHR, such as the International Covenant on Economic, Social and Cultural Rights, and UN Resolution 46/119 (Protection of Persons with Mental Illness and Improvement of Mental Health Care).

If health is conceived as a right of members of the global community, ways must be found to distribute health-related resources in a just way. Difficult questions need to be asked, questions such as: Should we be spending resources on lung transplants in one region while those in another lack the resources to fight tuberculosis? Health policies and practices, whether deliberately or through neglect, can affect human rights adversely.[44,45] How can we assess and monitor the impact of public health policies on human rights?[46] How can we respond to national policies that have global effects on the right to health?

This year, for instance, the United States withdrew from the 1997 Kyoto Treaty, an initiative to fight global warming, as "It is not in the United States' economic best interest."[47] Under the treaty, the United States, by 2001, would have had to reduce carbon dioxide, methane, and other pollutant emissions to 7% less than 1990 levels. This American decision has ramifications for the health of the entire planet. Is this the type of issue to which health professionals need to respond? If so, how? We need to clarify our role and responsibilities as health professionals in protecting rights and exposing rights violations. If we value equity and justice we need to consider how, as nurses, we will uphold them within the larger global community.

Reutter[18] believes that if nurses adopt a critical social perspective, they can act to reduce inequities. This would involve understanding the experience of the impoverished (eg, by asking critical questions), as well as facilitating collective strategies and community involvement in meeting community needs. Nurses need to understand the context of poverty in terms of the systemic forces that influence access to the prerequisites for health. If nurses decide to become politically active regarding health and public policy, they will need to develop the skills necessary to advocate for structural changes to alleviate poverty and its effects. Many already have the know-how and experience to help community groups with their own advocacy. Nurses and other health professionals who work in the trenches, so to speak, can provide first-hand evidence of the ramifications of economic, social, and political reforms on the health of individuals, families, and communities. Nurses working with disadvantaged groups are often less removed from them, socially and economically, than other professionals and may be able to understand and help them articulate their views. Nurses can, themselves, take positions on policy issues such as housing and its affordability, social welfare reform, employment policies, and environmental standards.[49]

Nursing academics and researchers could consider the activist role as well. Academics can help those challenging oppressive or detrimental practices by making theory accessible rather than obscure and by showing ways to question relevant political assumptions.[50] For instance, nurse researchers can raise issues of distributive justice in clinical research situations such as when research participants, exposed to the risks of experimental trials, are unlikely to be able to afford the resulting benefits. This is a major concern regarding research undertaken in developing countries by researchers based in developed nations. Nurses must be made aware of the international guidelines for research, such as the Council for International Organizations of Medical Sciences (CIOMS) guidelines and the Declaration of Helsinki. They need to secure a place on the committees conducting ethical reviews of research proposals and to help ensure that when persons consent to participate in research that such consent is freely given, not brought about by being too poor to reject proffered inducements.[51]

Reutter[48] urges nurses to "think upstream" to the broader societal contexts of health, to attend to the interrelationships between health and socioeconomic status and to the inequities that exist in access to the determinants of health. Health professionals need to work with those outside the health sector as well if significant improvements in the health of populations are to be secured.[52] Naeema Al-Gasser, Chief Nurse Scientist, WHO, in opening the year 2000 conference of the Global Network of WHO Collaborating Centers in Nursing, urged nurses to act to advance "health security." WHO identifies health security as universality in health care, access to education and information, right to food in sufficient quantity and good quality, and the right to decent housing and to live and work in an environment where known health risks are controlled.

Can we imagine how the need for health security translates into the everyday life of the less fortunate of the world's population? In the article "Death Stalks a

Continent,"[53] journalists reviewed the current situation of HIV/AIDS in Africa. They attempted to capture our moral imagination by beginning with a request for readers to picture living in the southern quadrant of Africa. Imagine a life, they ask, with a dying infant (one of your three children) and a husband rarely home because he must work away, whose promiscuity makes the marriage bed a deathtrap.

> You go to work past a house where a teenager lives alone tending young siblings without any source of income. . . Over there lies a man desperately sick without access to a doctor or clinic or medicine or food or blankets or even a kind word. At work you eat with colleagues and every third one is already fatally ill.[53(p28)]

Powerful images are evoked by this description of a life. Are we able, however, to imagine that it could be our own lives? Are we willing to see ourselves in such a situation of vulnerability and suffering? Is it too overwhelming to contemplate? Can we picture doing something to change the situation, to make a difference? These journalists conclude that the wealthy world must use both its zeal and its cash to help southern Africa if this "plague" is to be stopped.

Benner[54] argued that the starting point in health care ethics needs to be in recognition and relationship to such human reality. The principle of justice can provide us with "ethical moorings" but it is not sufficient: "The moral and emotional work of meeting the other and caring for the other in situations of need and vulnerability are hidden in the language of rights, autonomy and justice."[54(p160)] She suggests that we need to embrace more than justice—we need to strive for mercy, generosity, hope, and even love.

The American ethicist Arthur Caplan[55] decries the emphasis on autonomy and individual rights in Western societies. He believes an "obsession" with individualism has led to a denial of our mutual dependency and diminished our sense of brotherhood. He recalls an old Boys Town advertisement depicting a teenage boy carrying a younger boy on his back with the slogan. "He ain't heavy; he's my brother." He notes that today, to be real-

istic, the slogan would have to read: "He's pretty heavy but I got paid twenty bucks to carry him so I will for awhile."[55] Helping one another with the inevitable burdens of illness, death, and disability is not supererogatory, Caplan argues. It is the decent thing to do.

We do know that a factor common to ordinary men and women who have reached out to help others—to the extent that they risked their own lives—is "inclusiveness." These individuals have a tendency to regard all people as equals, without regard to social status or ethnicity.[56] At the 1996 UNESCO forum on moral universalism and economic triage, philosopher Richard Rorty maintained that the real question of our times is: "Who are we?" That is, who are the members of our moral community? To whom do we have responsibilities? Is it possible to form a meaningful moral community to which every human belongs?

The Possibility of a Universal Ethic

Can we conceive of a macro-ethic that could guide our moral actions in a global community? How might we create and support dialogue about what constitutes a "good life," about our relationships with one another, about our rights, our responsibilities? Is it even possible to articulate a universal ethical framework, given the diversity of cultures, values, and beliefs in the world? Can we hope to achieve cross-cultural understanding, let alone consensus about basic life assumptions?

There are those—"universalists"—who embrace a belief that all humans share an intrinsic human nature that connects us. It is on this assumption that human rights are based. There are others—"relativists"—who find this idea untenable. The American Anthropological Association, for instance, argued against the drafting of the UDHR on the basis that no common humanity existed.[57] Cultural relativists maintain that cultural differences are such that values in one culture, and therefore the persons living in that culture, cannot be comprehended by those living in another. The possibility of significant intercultural dialogue is denied, given that no single religious, moral, cultural, or philosophic perspective can be used to frame the discourse. The relativist viewpoint usually is grounded in tolerance and a respect for diversity, but it has serious implications for the viability of a global society. An inability to understand and communicate with one another seems like an insurmountable barrier to the development of a true community.

How do we manage our interdependence if our differences are so complete? In a discussion of peace and violence in Africa, Kaphagawani says that those who deny "that a Yoruba can understand a Luo or a Julu" are wrong.[58] All languages, he argues, share a small subset of universal concepts. He finds, for instance, that although what is considered normal or deviant varies between cultures, the ideas of normalcy and deviance are universal. Martha Nussbaum, a philosopher who takes an admittedly universalist and essentialist position, rejects the extreme relativist stance, quoting Aristotle's comment in *Nicomachean Ethics:* "One may also observe in one's travels to distant countries the feelings of recognition and affiliation that link every human being to every other human being."[59] She constructs an argument for a common humanity using a set of functional capacities basic to all humans, one that complements well Sen's idea of functional capabilities. This account of the shared capacities that distinguish human life from other forms includes our awareness of our mortality; our embodiment; our need for food, drink, and shelter; the fact that we experience sexual desire; are mobile; and have cognitive capacities (perceiving, imagining, thinking). Humans, she points out, are extremely dependent in early infancy, have a capacity for practical reason, and feel some sense of affiliation to other humans and a relatedness to other species and to nature. We can experience humor and play, and we have a separateness that gives each human life a unique context. Nussbaum[59] also delineates a second level of human functional capacities, those that she believes are fundamental to a good life. Among them are the capacities to have good health; to be adequately nourished; to use the senses; to imagine, think, and reason; and to have attachments. These, she argues, should be the goals of societies for their citizens. If Nussbaum and other universalists are right, humans do have enough in common to open a dialogue about collective human needs and problems, about hopes and expectations for the earthly community in which they have to live.

Such a dialogue seems crucial. The world has become too small; we are too intertwined for silence to be a sensible option. On the other hand, constructing a meaningful discourse on how we should be with one another will not be easy. All communities experience disagreement and plurality of viewpoints; argument and controversy will be nothing new. The real difficulty will be in opening up the space for other than the most powerful voices to be heard. We will need to determine what those who have been silent out of fear or ignorance need in order to speak, and what the rest need in order to listen.

Lane and Rubinstein[60] have some practical ideas about getting beyond the impasse between cultural relativism and universalism. They use as an illustration what is becoming the classic example of cultural differences: the practice of female circumcision. Their advice on how to structure a conversation about this issue is informative. They suggest that we first need to recognize one another's priorities—maybe we have not chosen the most pressing topic of concern. (For instance, in their interviews with Egyptian women about female circumcision, one woman asked, "Why do you think that is such a problem? That happened a long time ago and hurt for a short while. My husband's beatings are a much greater problem.") Lane and Rubenstein note further that we need to care about the other's feelings and pay attention to our choice of words. An approach needs to be constructed that is respectful of diversity, based on an awareness that our knowledge of different others is always contingent, tentative, and incomplete.

Drane,[61] a medical ethicist, believes that we need to find the right voice to speak about ethics, that when we are judging practices of another culture, like female circumcision, we need to use language that acknowledges the moral inadequacies of our own culture as well. He believes that the existing international dialogue in medical ethics provides a good opening for the consideration of a universal ethic. The experience of illness is a human commonality, and there are commonalities across cultures inherent in the relationship between the sick and those who help them. The professional commitment to help persons in distress is shaped by transcultural ethical standards, remarkably similar across history and cultures.

Some health professionals, of course, would disagree with him. Fan,[62] for instance, argues that ethical frameworks, at least in critical care medicine, must be local not global because one cannot share a content-rich bioethics with those committed to different moral premises and value rankings. Fan contrasts the Asian emphasis on the community with the Western value of individualism. Despite such arguments, however, steps have been taken to move from an international perspective in bioethics to a global one.

It was in 1984 that the first Health Policy, Ethics and Human Values Conference of WHO and CIOMS considered the possibility of an international perspective on bioethics. The need for dialogue regarding health policy making, ethics, and human values in different cultures was identified. A decade later, at a conference convened to review the progress on these issues, it was evident that a paradigm shift had occurred. An international perspective was no longer the goal; a "global agenda for bioethics" was developed, involving a search for a universal consensus on essential principles of bioethics, the application of bioethics concepts in human rights discourse, and a call for the World Bank and Regional Development banks to incorporate bioethical principles into project design and assessments. The need for intergovernmental organizations (eg, the World Medical Association, United Nations agencies) to play a substantial role in achieving this agenda was stressed.[63]

The conversation to derive a global health ethic should be a fruitful one, if it is grounded in a respect for all peoples as potential sources of wisdom. Tangwa,[64] for instance, points to the moral sensibilities of traditional Africa as something that Africans can offer a global ethical community. He notes that our contemporary world, while enjoying the benefits of Western science and technology, is allowing "the spirit of commerce and omnivorous discovery and experimentation"

to create greater inequalities between the prosperous and the poor.[64] He proffers as a better approach the traditional African egalitarian perspective, where moral consideration is indiscriminately due to all human beings, regardless of their personal characteristics, status, or social rank. Tangwa offers as a guiding image for resolving intercommunity disagreements and for reaching mutual understanding that of African elders sitting under a tree and discussing until they agree.

Tangwa would push Caplan's[55] concern for a renewed sense of brotherhood further. He notes that because the African worldview includes concepts of transformation (eg, reincarnation and transmutation), there is an awareness of the possibilities of brother/sisterhood with other beings. No hard and fast line separates human beings from other ontologic entities on the Earth. This raises an issue pertinent to any discussion of moral community: Should it extend beyond human life? Do we have an ethical obligation to live in a way that is mindful of other forms of life?

Living in harmony with nature and other life forms would seem to be an imperative in a global habitat. To date, however, we have failed to achieve a sustainable relationship with our environment. We are depleting earth resources, destroying other species, and leaving such large amounts of biologic and industrial waste products that they cannot be recycled expediently by natural processes.[65] The claims of nature need to be given voice in our ethical deliberations. JG Engel[66] maintained that we must make connections between our personal space and the needs of the community to recognize how our local space connects within the larger natural and cultural spaces. An understanding of our connectedness with the Earth and all its occupants might move us to a greater inclusiveness.

JR Engel describes how a Chicago regional planning project, Nature, Polis, and Ethics, is engaging citizens in the "most radical and elementary of social ethical questions: how ought we to govern ourselves within the conditions of life given to us on this planet and in this place?"[67] Such "ecological citizenship" moves us beyond the citizen as consumer, making choices on the basis of preferences and competitive advantage, to a concern for the common good, to a view of the good life as "humans mutually flourishing in a mutually flourishing world."[67] It seems necessary, as well, that we must recognize the effects of our actions on those who will come after us. Our descendants have no voice in what is happening at present, but the ramifications of the choices we are making will strongly affect them and the world in which they will live.

Hyakudai Sakamoto,[68] the founder of the Japanese Association of Bioethics, believes that for a global bioethics we need a revised humanism, one that is not so excessively human-centric. Coming from an Asian ethos influenced by Taoism, Buddhism, and Confucianism, he conceives of a "holistic harmony" as the foundation for worldwide ethics. This holistic harmony would mean that rather than the autonomous individual being the basic element of bioethics, a greater emphasis would be placed on nature, society, neighborhood, and mutual aid. He presumes the existence of feeling that is common to all people (eg, the feeling of pity) and proposes that such common feeling can be our ethical basis. Sakamoto admits that our initial goal in developing an ethic to serve in these global times realistically may need to be compromise more than harmonize.

Nevertheless, Sakamoto's metaphor of "harmony" seems a rich and useful one. It fits well with the idea of "improvisation," used by philosophers like Nussbaum[69] when stressing the need to be attentive to context in ethical situations. When persons such as jazz musicians or actors improvise, they must be more, not less, attentive to their group. They have to be committed to the other performers, to be acutely aware of and responsive to them. It is not that just anything goes; those who excel at improvisation have a deep understanding of the traditions that shape artistic form. Cultivating an attentiveness that supports harmony could be important to a universal ethic.

In describing the preconditions of moral performance, Vetlesen,[70] a Norwegian philosopher, says that there must be a receptivity, an attentiveness to action. Without it, we can fail to see ourselves addressed by situations that require a moral response. Until recently our efforts to promote ethical action in health care were primarily centered on the present and immediate issues affecting persons in our own particular communities. In this era of globalization, however, a significant shift is occurring. Our moral space is altering, and the constituents of our moral community are being redefined. We need to broaden our perspectives, to take the globe as our frame of reference as we answer the questions: How should we act? What is the right thing to do?

The Globe as Our Frame of Reference for Ethical Action

In nursing ethics, suggests Wurzbach,[71] moral metaphors have emerged over time that have strongly affected nursing practice. The military metaphor of the 1800s and the advocacy and academic metaphors of the 1960s are examples. She believes two new metaphors are arising today: the "individualist" and "community as caring" metaphors. She urges nurses to examine and reflect on the metaphors used to shape and guide practice. She warns that we must understand how they relate to the times in which we live.

Davis[72] points out that certain assumptions about values have been taken for granted in nursing. For example, she points to the strong influence of the United States and the United Kingdom evident in the stance that the self-reliant individual is the ideal. Now that influences are coming from other sources, she wonders what it will mean for the profession. "The question before us is: are there ethical notions of caring, ethical principles and virtues that could be endorsed as true for all nurses everywhere?"[72]

This article argues that the world has become a global village. If this is true, it seems necessary that nurses consider their changing roles and responsibilities within that village. Nurses must determine, for instance, whether they can actively imagine a world in which there is true opportunity for health for all.[73] One of the dangers of our times, however, is that we can become overwhelmed by the immense and rapid changes taking place, by the tremendous amounts of information available to us, and by the media-driven awareness of great human suffering. The temptation to moral minimalism can be strong.[6] We are at risk of developing an inhibiting "What can I do about it?" attitude. Nurses, however, are known for asking "What can I do about it?" in an active, rather than in a resigned, way. The mechanisms are in place for responding. The International Council of Nurses and Midwives and the WHO Collaborating Centers in Nursing and Midwifery are there to provide leadership as nurses come to address the new global health issues.

In *The Ethical Demand*, the philosopher Løgstrup[74] wrote that we all, inescapably, depend on one another. He said that we are mutually and, in an immediate sense, in one another's power. He was describing close-up ethical relationships, but we are recognizing how true this is not only close up, but also on a global scale. Now we have to act on that recognition.

REFERENCES

1. Skeat WW. *The Concise Dictionary of English Etymology.* Ware, Hertfordshire. UK: Wordsworth Editions; 1993.
2. McLuhan M, Powers B. *The Global Village: Transformation in World Life and Media in the 21st Century.* Oxford: Oxford University Press; 1989.
3. Albrow M. *The Global Age: State and Society beyond Modernity.* Stanford, CA: Stanford University Press; 1997.
4. Freidman T. *The Lexus and the Olive Tree: Understanding Globalization.* New York: Farrar, Straus & Giroux; 1999.
5. Jowitt K. *The New World Disorder: The Leninist Extinction.* Berkeley, CA: University of California Press; 1992.
6. Ignatieff M. *The Warrior's Honour: Ethnic War and the Modern Conscience.* Toronto: Penguin Books; 1998.
7. Beck U, Ritter M, trans. *Risk Society: Towards a New Modernity.* Newbury Park, CA: Sage; 1992.
8. Howson C, Fineberg H, Bloom B. The pursuit of global health: the relevance of engagement for developed countries. *Lancet.* 1998;351:586–590.
9. Midgley M. Transnational civil society. In: Dunne T, Wheeler N, eds. *Human Rights in Global Politics.* New York: Cambridge University Press; 1999.
10. Bauman Z. *Globalization: The Human Consequences.* New York: Columbia University Press; 1998.
11. Moore T, Stewart W. Nuclear missiles for sale by mail order. *Sunday Express,* July 23, 2000, 4.
12. Jonas H, Jonas H, Herr D, trans. *The imperative of Responsibility.* Chicago: University of Chicago Press; 1979.
13. Mahnaimi U, Colvin M. Israel planning "ethnic" bomb as Saddam caves in. *The Sunday Times, Scotland,* November 15, 1998, 1.
14. Delaney S. Scientists prepare to clone a human, *Washington Post,* March 10, 2001, A16.
15. Henderson M. Don't clone people, says man who made Dolly. *The Times,* March 29, 2001, 5L.
16. Specter M. Europeans revolt against test-tube-altered future. *The Globe and Mail,* July 21, 1998, A11.
17. Immen W. Consumers can't tell what's natural. *The Globe and Mail,* July 21, 1998, A11.
18. Dawson C. Vaccines growing on trees will take the sting out of immunizations—scientists. *The Edmonton Journal,* December 7, 1998, A1.
19. Young E. Genetically modified foods—the answer or the enemy. *The Ghanaian Times,* April 7, 2001, 11.
20. McMaster G. Confronting the drug dilemma: will the Third World get the drugs it needs? *University of Alberta Folio.* 2001;38(13). Available at http://www.ualberta.ca/FOLIO/0001/03.09/focus.html. Accessed August 2001.
21. McGeary J. Paying for AIDS cocktails: who should pick up the tab for the Third World? *Time,* February 12, 2001, 38.
22. Reutters, Amsterdam. Firms promise more cuts in AIDS drug prices. *The Ghanaian Times,* April 7, 2001, 4.
23. Cooper G. Embryos for sale at L300 on the Internet. *The Independent on Sunday,* November 22, 1998, 3.
24. The Associated Press release. United Daily News, Taipei, Taiwan, Sept. 11, 1998.
25. Gadamer HG, Gaiger J, Walker N, trans. *The Enigma of Health: The Art of Healing in a Scientific Age.* Stanford, CA: Stanford University Press; 1996.
26. Knoppers B. Human rights and genomics. In: Bhatia GS, O'Neill JS, Gall GL, Bendin PD, eds. *Peace, Justice and Freedom: Human Rights Challenges for the New Millennium.* Edmonton, AB: University of Alberta Press; 2000.
27. United Nations Educational, Scientific and Cultural Organization. *UNESCO Adopts Universal Declaration on the Human Genome and Human Rights.* November 11, 1997. Available at http://www.unesco.org/opi/29gencon. Accessed August 2001.
28. Beaglehole R, Bonita R. Public health at the crossroads: which way forward? *Lancet.* 1998;351:590–592.
29. World Health Organization. *The Jakarta Declaration on Leading Health Promotion into the 21st Century* (1997). Available at http://www.who.int/dsa/cat95/zjak.htm. Accessed August 2001.
30. Mahler H. The challenge of global health: how can we do better? *Health Hum Rights.* 1997;2(3):71–75.
31. Wilkinson R, Marmot M, eds. *Social Determinants of Health: The Solid Facts.* Geneva: World Health Organization, Europe; 1998.
32. United Nations Development Program, Human Development Report Office. *Human Development Report 1996.* Cary, NC: Oxford University Press.
33. Awuonda M. Helping the least developed. *West Africa.* March 26-April 1, 2001:27–29.
34. Kapstein E. A global third way: social justice and the world economy. *World Policy J.* 1999:XV(4):23–35.
35. Lindholm T. The emergence and development of human rights: an interpretation with a view to crosscultural and interreligious dialogue. Presented at the Diyarbakir Interna-

tional Conference on Human Rights; September 26–28, 1997; Diyarbakir, Turkey.

36. Nussbaum M, Sen A. *The Quality of Life*. Oxford: Clarendon Press; 1993.

37. Nussbaum M. Introduction. In: Nussbaum M, Glover J, eds. *Women, Culture and Development: A Study of Capabilities*. Oxford: Clarendon Press; 1995:1–15.

38. Tsikata D, Kerr J, eds. *Demanding Dignity: Women Confronting Economic Reforms in Africa*. Accra, Ghana: North-South Institute and Third World Reform-Africa; 2001.

39. Caldwell J. Health transition: the cultural, social and behavioural determinants of health in the Third World. *Soc Sci Med*. 1993;36(2):125–135.

40. World Health Organization. *Ottawa Charter for Health Promotion*. Ottawa, Canada: Canadian Public Health Association; 1986.

41. *Towards a Common Understanding: Clarifying the Core Concepts of Population Health: A Discussion Paper*. Ottawa, Canada: Health Canada; 1996.

42. Benetar S. The biotechnology era: a story of two lives. In: Bhatia GS, O'Neill JS, Gall GL, Bendin PD, eds. *Peace, Justice and Freedom: Human Rights Challenges for the New Millennium*. Edmonton, AB: University of Alberta Press; 2000:245–257.

43. *Universal Declaration of Human Rights*. Adopted and proclaimed by General Assembly resolution 217 A (III), December 10, 1948. New York: United Nations; 1948.

44. Bruntland GH. Fifty years of synergy between health and rights. *Health Hum Rights*. 1998;3(2):21–25.

45. Mann JM, Goskin L, Gruskin S, Brennan T, Lazzarini Z, Fineberg H. Health and human rights. In: Mann JM, Gruskin S, Grodin MA, Annas C, eds. *Human and Human Rights: A Reader*. New York: Routledge; 1999:7–20.

46. Gostin L, Mann J. Toward the development of a human rights impact assessment for the formulation and evaluation of public health policies. *Health Hum Rights*. 1994;1(1):59–80.

47. Peek L. US turns back on climate treaty. *The Times*. March 29, 2001, 20.

48. Reutter L. Socioeconomic determinants of health. In: Stewart M, ed. *Community Nursing: Promoting Canadians' Health*. Toronto, Canada: WB Saunders; 2000.

49. Labonte R. Health promotion and empowerment: reflections on professional practice. *Health Educ Q* 1994;21(2):253–268.

50. Routledge P. The third space as critical engagement. *Antiopode Radical J Geography*. 1996;28(4):399–419.

51. *The Ethics of Clinical Research in Developing Countries*. London: Nuffield Council on Bioethics; 1999.

52. Epp J. *Achieving Health for All: A Framework for Health Promotion*. Ottawa, ON: Health and Welfare Canada; 1986.

53. Death stalks a continent. *Time*, February 12, 2001, 28–37.

54. Benner P. The compassionate stranger: exploring caring practices and the ethics of care. Meeting the other in suffering and vulnerability: relational ethics in the Judeo-Christian tradition. Presented at the Kompendium of Sykepleiekonferanse PA Nordkalottens Tak. Tromsø, Norway; May 22–25, 1997.

55. Caplan A. *Am I My Brother's Keeper? The Ethical Frontiers of Biomedicine*. Indianapolis: Indiana University Press; 1997:ix, xi.

56. Oliner S, Oliner P. *The Altruistic Personality: Rescuers of Jews in Nazi Europe*. New York: The Free Press; 1988:144.

57. Washburn W. Cultural relativism, human rights, and the AAA. *Am Anthropol*. 1987;89:939–943.

58. Kaphagawani DN. Peace and violence in contemporary Africa: a possibility of intercultural dialogue? *J Humanities*. 2000;14:1–8.

59. Nussbaum M. Human capabilities, female human beings. In: Nussbaum M, Glover J, eds. *Women, Culture and Development: A Study of Capabilities*. Oxford: Clarendon Press; 1995:61–104.

60. Lane S, Rubinstein R. Judging the other: responding to female genital surgeries. *Hastings Center Rep*. 1996;26(3):31–40.

61. Drane J. Medicine and the possibility of a universal ethics (1999). Available at http://www.uchile.cl/bioetica/doc/med.htm. Accessed August 2001.

62. Fan R. Critical care ethics in Asia: local or global? *J Med Philos*. 1998;23(6):549–562.

63. Bryant J, Bankowski Z, eds. *Poverty, Vulnerability, the Value of Human Life, and the Emergence of Bioethics: Highlights and Papers of the Council for International Organizations of Medical Sciences (CIOMS) Conference*. Geneva: CIOMS; 1994.

64. Tangwa G. The traditional African perception of a person: some implications for bioethics. *Hastings Center Rep*. 2000;30(5):39–43.

65. Heltne P. Basic concepts of ecology and evolutionary biology. *Hastings Center Rep*. November-December 1998;(suppl): S12-S22.

66. Engel JG. Who are democratic ecological citizens? *Hastings Center Rep*. November-December 1998;(suppl):S23-S30.

67. Engel JR. The faith of democratic ecological citizenship. *Hastings Center Rep*. November-December 1998;(suppl):S31-S41.

68. Sakamoto H. A new possibility of global bioethics as an intercultural social tuning technology. Presented at Health Ethics: A Global Context, preconference to the 11th Annual Canadian Bioethics Conference; October 27, 1999; Edmonton, Canada.

69. Nussbaum M. *Love's Knowledge: Essays on Philosophy and Literature*. Oxford: Oxford University Press; 1990.

70. Vetlesen J. *Closeness: An Ethics*. Oslo, Norway: Scandinavian Press; 1997.

71. Wurzbach ME. The moral metaphors of nursing. *J Adv Nurs*. 1999;30(1):94–99.

72. Davis A. Global influence of American nursing; some ethical issues. *Nurs Ethics*. 1999;6(2):118–125.

73. Austin W. Using the human rights paradigm in health ethics: the problems and the possibilities. *Nurs Ethics*. 2001;8(3):181–193.

74. Løgstrup K, Jensen T, trans. *The Ethical Demand*. Philadelphia: Fortress Press; 1971.

The Author Comments

Nursing Ethics in an Era of Globalization

Although I had previously considered and presented ideas about nursing ethics and globalization, it was during my time as a Visiting Professor at the Department of Nursing at the University of Ghana that I wrote this article. In Ghana, I made the shift to a more global perspective on nursing ethics. I treasure that opportunity. My hope is that I have, in this work, opened some of the questions that nurses will need to address if they are to thoughtfully and effectively enact their changing role and responsibilities in our global village.

—WENDY AUSTIN

PHILOSOPHIES AND KNOWLEDGE DEVELOPMENT

CHAPTER 42

Nursing's Syntax Revisited: A Critique of Philosophies Said to Influence Nursing Theories*

Susan R. Gortner

Lodged within the syntax of a discipline are the value systems and research constraints that influence theory development and research strategies. Humanism and postmodern philosophy have challenged natural science philosophical influences on nursing's syntax. This paper examines the construction of nursing's syntax from empiricist, hermeneuticist, feminist, and critical social theory views. In this critique, two requirements are placed on the world views: (1) they must accommodate theoretical (realist) terms important to nursing; and (2) they should provide explanatory power for these terms within nursing's disciplinary substance. Arguments are continued for a "within-the discipline" structure, a substantive and syntactical structure for the discipline of nursing that recognizes the centrality of biobehavioral processes in the practice of nursing [Gortner, IMAGE: J. Nurs. Scholarship 22, 101-105 (1990)].

Introduction

Over a decade ago Donaldson and Crowley (1978) presented a landmark paper before the Western Society for Nursing Research, on the structural and syntactical features of nursing as a discipline, following characterizations developed by Schwab (1964). They identified the "substantive structure" as those conceptualizations, borrowed or invented, which are consonant with the perspective of the discipline; in contrast, the "syntax" of the discipline refers to "the research methodologies and criteria used to justify the acceptance of the statements as true

*Based on an invited paper presented at the First Symposium on Knowledge Development sponsored by the College of Nursing, University of Rhode Island, Newport Beach, U.S.A., 7 September 1990 and revised during a sabbatical as professeure invitée, faculté sciences infirmières, Universite de Montréal, Canada, Spring 1991.

About the Author

After graduating from Stanford University in 1953 with an AB degree in social sciences, SUSAN REICHERT GORTNER enrolled in the generic master's program at Frances Payne Bolton School of Nursing, Case Western Reserve University, graduating with honors in 1957. She completed a PhD in higher education from the University of California, Berkeley, in 1964, which coincided with the births of her children. She relocated with her scientist husband to Maryland and joined the Division of Nursing as a health scientist administrator, first to evaluate the 1964 Nurse Training Act and later to serve as Branch Chief for Research and Research Training. She was the first Associate Dean for Research (Nursing) at the University of California, San Francisco (UCSF). Dr. Gortner's many honors and recognitions include Frances Payne Bolton School of Nursing Distinguished Alumna, UCSF Helen Nahm Research Lecturer, Fulbright Association Lecturer/Research Scholar in Norway (Oslo University), and, most recently, the American Academy of Nursing "Living Legend" award in 2001. Internationally known for her views on nursing science and research, she developed a collaborative program of research on cardiac surgery recovery, examining patient and family treatment choices and outcomes and recovery processes. Dr. Gortner was honored for this work by the National Center for Nursing Research (now NINR) and the American Heart Association. She lives full-time in the High Sierras in California, enjoys summer and winter sports with her Border collies, and recently joined the Orvis School of Nursing as Endowed Chair (.50) to help faculty development in research.

within the discipline" (p. 119). Lodged within the syntax are the value systems and research constraints that influence theory generation and research designs; these "function to ensure that enquiry will result in conclusions and statements that are appropriate, valid, and reliable for the purpose of the discipline" (p. 119). Theories are both descriptive and prescriptive in this scheme, as shown in Figure 42-1, and intercept the substance and the syntax in Donaldson and Crowley's representation.

Both the substance and syntax, as the structural elements of the discipline, can reflect the nursing perspective of humanism and concern with the whole person. Yet this perspective can be problematic for the development of the discipline, since holism stands in direct opposition to objectivism and its associated reductionism. Accordingly social philosophy has become increasingly popular as a conceptual base for contemporary nursing. Natural science philosophy, including the philosophy of biology, appears now to have little conceptual value for nursing so that the associated view of humans as living organisms or entities is being sup-

planted by the view of humans as social beings. Hermeneutics has been proposed as an alternative syntax for the discipline, along with feminism and/or critical social theory and other non-naturalistic world views (Allen, 1985; Moccia, 1988; Benner and Wrubel, 1989; Holden, 1990; Holmes, 1990). What will these modifications of syntax accomplish for nursing as an emerging disciplinary field? How will the questions of substance be formulated and pursued? This is an issue first identified by Donaldson and Crowley in the conclusion of their 1978 paper and subsequently emphasized by Meleis (1987) nearly a decade later. Should particular phenomenological social philosophies continue their ascendancy in nursing, there will be ontological as well as epistemological consequences. The belief systems or ontologies may disallow reality outside of the human, the existence of biobehavioral patterns and regularities, and even theories. The belief systems or ontologies will determine the nature of explanations about phenomena, and whether explanations can become generalizations or not (Collin, 1992).

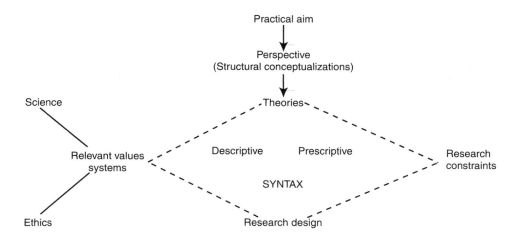

Figure 42-1 *Structure of a professional discipline.*

The purpose of this paper is to re-examine construction of the syntax (the value systems and research constraints), from empiricist, hermeneutic, feminist and critical social theory views. In this examination two requirements will be placed on the world views, in keeping with the author's scientific orientation. The requirements are that world views should accommodate theoretical (realist) terms important to nursing, and they should provide explanatory power for these terms within nursing's disciplinary substance.[1] Scientific realism maintains that theoretical terms and abstractions arising from scientific work exist, refer to the real world, and may or may not be true (Boyd, 1984). Explanatory power is the capacity of a set of propositions not only to account for a given event but to generalize to other events of the same set. Explanations therefore need to be nomothetic (that is law-like or general) as well as idiosyncratic (specific to the case, the particular, the singular). Explanations must cover the phenomena ["save the phenomena" in the van Fraasen (1980) terminology] and also predict what might happen the next time the same set of circumstances occurs (a traditional feature of scientific explanations). In the critique offered in this paper, arguments will continued for a "within-the-discipline" structure, a substantive and syntactical structure for the discipline of nursing that recognizes the centrality of biobehavioral processes in the practice of nursing (Gortner, 1990).

Origins of the Critique

Identification of supposed positivistic influences on nursing's syntax (i.e. theory and research) appears to have arisen from the Suppe and Jacox (1985) critique of nursing theories, in which the requirement of operationalization is said to be positivistic. Jacox subsequently has acknowledged that her earlier writings on theory development (Jacox, 1974) were unduly influenced by positivism. Interestingly, neither Whall (1989) or Meleis (1991) could find direct evidence of positivistic influ-

---

[1]Hesook Kim comments on these requirements, noting that scientific realism and explanatory power "represent major value systems of sciences that have contributed to the empiricist view of scientific knowledge." She suggests that hermeneutics, feminist (relativist) and critical social theory propose a different syntax. Donna Wells agrees, noting that the expectation of scientific realism for nursing's syntax construction gives "immediate primacy to a world view of empiricism." My contention is that these requirements, or some variation thereof, should be imposed on those views proposing a different syntax, to illustrate consequences and to aid in the choice of syntax. I would agree with Wells some conjoint view would be an improvement, as against a primordial view (one asserting primacy).

ence on nursing practice (Whall) or theory (Meleis), although Whall (personal communication, 1991) has observed that the "truth criteria" (i.e. are the relationships empirically verifiable) proposed for evaluation of nursing theories had positivistic overtones. Other critiques of natural science and positivistic science orientations have come from critical social theorists in nursing (Thompson, 1985, 1987; Allen, 1985; Moccia, 1988), from proponents of phenomenological and interpretive views (Benner, 1985; Benner & Wrubel, 1989; Leonard, 1989) and from some nursing philosophers who advocate caring as the leitmotif of nursing (Gadow, 1980; Eriksson, 1990; Newman et al., 1991).

These criticisms contain a central theme that positivism is antithetical to nursing's disciplinary orientation, an orientation or perspective that is framed by humanistic concepts, values and practices. Because of these humanistic intentions, it is argued that the research needs to be humanistic. The position that philosophical viewpoints necessarily should guide and direct research strategy may be termed the "purist" position. The "nonpurist" position has argued for theoretical and methodological pluralism, and toward a consensus regarding nursing philosophy of science (Gortner, 1990; Nagle and Mitchell, 1991). Still another position, "the radical separationist thesis," has been offered by Suppe at a knowledge development symposium (Suppe, 1990). This position argues that a discipline's theory and research are distinct and not necessarily congruent in philosophy (humanistic) and strategy (empiricist or phenomenological). Epistemology provides "no evidential role" for knowledge claims; rather philosophy can play a role in credentialing knowledge claims, a process of legitimatizing the claim into the shared body of information the discipline accepts and uses.[2] This position would allow humanism to be the dominant nursing perspective while allowing scientists to engage other themes and inquiry forms at various levels of analysis (Suppe, 1990).[3]

The stakes are high, for the arguments strike at the very belief systems of nursing scholarship and how we credential, accept as legitimate, the discoveries arising from scholarly work. How will we decide which is the more important question: "How is it that we know?", "What do we know?" or "What does it mean to be a person?" (patient or nurse). The first two questions have been the heart of Ph.D. training in the discipline. The third is raised by those advocating moral, social and political foundations for nursing's epistemology. How we respond will determine whether our conceptualizations can be microanalytic (e.g. cellular, biological) as well as microanalytic (e.g. social or cultural), whether the syntax can be objective and logical as well as interpretive and reflective, and whether we can model the human system/state at various levels (e.g. cell, organ, system) or rest with meanings and motives within the context of culture and society.[4]

Positivism/Empiricism

Suppe and Jacox's (1985) essay on philosophic influences on nursing theory development appears to be the major source for contentions that nursing theory has been influenced by positivism. Whether this contention of influence is accurate, despite assertions in our literature that it is, would depend on evidence that we don't have and preferably would have to be garnered from the theorists themselves. At the conference where this paper was originally presented, both Hesook Suzie Kim and Callista Roy were present; neither acknowledged the supposed influence of positivism on their own writings. Kim believes (personal communication, 1991) that the logical positivist influence on early theoretical works in nursing was selective and circumspective rather than dogmatic. Indeed, the reference by theoreticians to

---

[2]In her review of this paper, Kim notes that credentialing knowledge claims is a function of syntax, again supporting the importance of syntactical arguments for the discipline.

[3]Ann Whall's response to the "radical separationist thesis" is that such separation would make for a "very disparate and conflicting knowledge base"; perhaps this is what nursing has at present, but "is it a valid and worthy goal?". Probably not, but it does reflect current reality. Could the theories be reframed in the light of the evidence, I ask?

[4]Wells comments that more than meaning and motives would result: patterns of health and illness might be revealed through such examination, aiding explanation as well as understanding.

propositions and terms that are capable of empirical demonstration and testability might better reflect a (scientific) realist position rather than a logical positivistic or antirealist position. This skepticism about supposed positivistic influences prompted Whall to examine American nursing practice guides for the period 1950–1970; she failed to find evidence of positivistic influence and commented that it was strange, indeed, to have purported influence in one sector (theory) and not in the other (practice) (Whall, 1989).

In portrayals of philosophical positions, it is important to bear in mind that old distinctions no longer suffice. Much of the critique of positivism has been rendered against the form known as logical positivism, and the Vienna Circle. That form of positivism is no longer extant, and to continue to reference it (e.g. Sarnecky, 1990) is to ignore its demise in the late '60s (Glymour, 1980; Hacking, 1981; Schumacher & Gortner, 1992). Even in Benner and Wrubel's recent portrayal, positivism is equated with empiricism and illustrated through a mechanistic, reductionist principle: "the complex can be best understood in terms of its basic atomic components, components that bear no intrinsic relation to one another" (Benner and Wrubel, 1989, p. 32). This statement about contemporary empiricist views regarding the process of science continues fallacious equivocations of empiricism with reductionism, atomism, and quantification. There is no historical basis for the association of positivism with quantification; statistical theory and practices arose not from philosophy but from agricultural science.

Rather there is a postpostivistic view, a contemporary empiricist view (Schumacher & Gortner, 1992; Gortner & Schultz, 1988; Norbeck, 1986) that continues belief in observables, in careful scientific strategies that bear results that can be corroborated if not confirmed. This modern view has arisen in part through the historicist criticism of Kuhn (1970), Lakatos (1970), Laudan (1977) and others, including the positivists themselves. Contemporary empiricism recognizes the fallacies of the principle of verification, the impossibility of separating fact from theory and thus of making scientific endeavors antirealist (as the logical positivists attempted), acknowledges the theory-ladeness of observation and ex-

perience, and does not differentiate the context of discovery from justification in scientific work. Modern empiricists, along with clinical scientists, are concerned with complex phenomenon, some of which can be reduced and partitioned for study and some of which cannot. What guides a research program is a significant problem area, as for example pain or recovery or caregiving strain or postpartal depression, for which explanation and understanding are sought. Extant theory is used generally, hence the hypothetico deductive terminology. Yet generative theory is not ruled out; in fact Roy's experience with brain damaged adults during her Robert Wood Johnson Clinical Nurse Scholar's program is credited with the revisions and adjustments made subsequently in her theoretical position. Her work reflects clearly the thinking of an empiricist scholar (Roy, 1989).

In the following features are reflected the strengths of empiricist scholarship: (1) specification of factors assumed to be key to understanding and explanation of the phenomenon under study and (2) the expectation for theory testing and theory generation. Inherent is the belief that the event under study can be modelled or "objectified" (Schumacher & Gortner, 1992). The relevant syntax for nursing would consist of (a) generalized knowledge based on explanation of kind-phenomena; (b) human phenomena objectively identifiable and observable; and (c) predictions as well as explanation (Kim, personal communication, 1991; Schumacher & Gortner, 1992).

Because of this expectation, contemporary empiricism has the capacity for explanation that is so necessary for clinical practice. The observables (mood state, vital signs, laboratory and radiographic findings) must be linked with the unobservables, those normal and abnormal physiological and psychological processes to suggest causal factors and thus treatment. The efficacy of treatment is judged in terms of outcomes. Clinical practice has become more scientific and technologically dependent because of the need for identifying increasingly complex patient states (presumptive and competing diagnoses), which require prolonged periods of observation and assessment because of their complexity, and for which multiple therapies are needed. Acute care practitioners continually confront these complexities. Their scientific and clinical judgments are analytical, logical and empirical as often as they are intuitive and interpretive.[5,6] The latter forms of reasoning inform and extend the former, but generally lack specificity and logic. They answer the what of the phenomenon, not the why which is the impetus for therapeutic action. They also provide the equivalent of hypothetical counterarguments or counterfactuals, to support or weaken the clinical or scientific explanation.

Empiricism then is criticized for the very features that have made it the mainstay of scientific work. It is particularly relevant for the biological and behavioral sciences, for explicating fundamental human processes of biological and behavioral origin. It has appeal for subspecialties in acute and critical care, in which the human state is objectified and monitored painstakingly. It forces upon the investigator precision, caution and skepticism about outcomes; it seeks associations between theory and fact, acknowledging the importance of *a priori* propositions and hypothesized causal processes.

In the author's view, empiricism has been given short shrift in nursing, because of continued fallacious identification with logical positivism, because of lack of familiarity with primary sources on the perspective, and because of the critiques rendered by hermeneuticists, phenomenologists, and critical social theorists. Our historical reliance on the social sciences for our scientific base contributes to the anti-empiricist or anti-naturalist argument.[7] Also contributing to the critique of positivism is our inclination to adopt a philosopher of the month (Kuhn was our first white knight, followed by Laudan, Habermas, Toulmin and Foucault). We might take seriously Suppe's recent admonition not to take philosophy as dogma (Suppe, 1990).[8]

Hermeneutics

Hermeneutics has a century old tradition in continental philosophy (Palmer, 1969), and together with humanism is gaining appreciable interest in North American circles, especially in departments of philosophy, education, and social science (e.g. Phillips, 1987; Rosenberg, 1988). The reasons for this development are several, not the least of which is belief that the human world is one distinctly different from the natural world. Literary and artistic works are uniquely human creations, societies and cultures are human creations and so, goes the reasoning, are human responses to health and illness. Dilthey was one of the foremost proponents of a distinct human science philosophy in the last century; his "Geisteswissenschaften" was an attempt to set in place an epistemology for the human sciences that would complement that of natural science "Naturwissenshaften" (Dilthey, 1988):

> "The goals of the human sciences—to lay hold of the singular and the individual in historico-social reality; to recognize uniformities operative in shaping the singular; to establish goals and rules for its continued development—can be attained only by the devices of reason: analysis and abstraction" (Dilthey, p. 27).

This perspective on historical consciousness and the value of humanistic and historical knowledge in understanding human existence was an important contribution to understanding and explanation. Dilthey's hermeneutics reflect an accommodation of the "scientific" and the "human"; his anti-naturalism appears less fundamental and dogmatic than that of Heidegger

---

[5]Kim comments that this argument "suggests immediate linkages between 'idiosyncratic' features of practice and nomothetic/theoretical knowledge of science."

[6]Whall argues that nursing models need to incorporate physiological patterns as well as organismic relationships; valuing of one over the other will produce variations in outcomes and explanations that are insufficient or incomplete (Fitzpatrick & Whall, 1989, p. 11).

[7]Wells takes issue with this statement, noting that the social sciences have long believed that only empiricist methods will lead to progress in their disciplines. That the critical social theorist arguments were as much against scientism as against positivism is an important observation. I castigate contemporary empiricism and its proponents for the continuing equation of "good science" with "good method." This narrow view of science and scientific quality constrains novel designs and methods and accepts warrantable evidence more readily from programs of biomedical science than those of clinical or social science.

---

[8]Was Suppe "right" or "reasonable," asks Wells. When do we turn to philosophy and under what conditions?

(1962), who took an ontological rather than an epistemological turn with his conception of "Dasein" (Palmer, 1969). It is the power of the ontological sentiment of "being as being" (Palmer, 1969) that has brought hermeneutics close to the philosophical orientations of phenomenology, existentialism, and even critical theory. Indeed, the language and semantics requires disciplehood, making intersubjectivity difficult except among disciples (a phenomenon called "communicative entropy" by Suppe, 1990). Further, some proponents of Heidegerrian philosophy have operationalized features as method, contributing to the development of new scholars as well as to programs of scholarship of their own. There are several tenets of contemporary hermeneutics that have influenced nursing theorists and scholars: the appreciation of the human state or essence as supreme; the interactive circle ("hermeneutic circle") between patient and nurse or subject and scientist; shared meaning and embedded meaning, and self-reflection and understanding ("Verstehen") as the basis of knowing.[9] There is a common requirement of social discourse, generating a text or historical record for analysis.

Nursing theories increasingly address biology, behavior, and culture, frequently in interface with one another. They depict associations among factors and may suggest explanatory variables for human health and illness. Some require partitioning, objectification, and specification of relationships, hypothetical and real. The entire area of ecological knowledge known epidemiologically as "host factors" (or "risk factors") cannot be accommodated in a hermeneutic or phenomenology perspective. Human ecology requires identification of an antecedent state in the host/human, interrupting the process of lived experience which is continuous, has no antecedent or consequent, and is the "unit of analysis." Ideologically, hermeneutics captures the ethic of caring identified with nursing; it serves history, sociology, and art well; in this respect, it can frame the artform of nursing in rich and meaningful dimensions. It can frame the nature of human suffering, human health, human recovery in terminology that can enrich human understanding and thus discourse between sufferer, loved ones and clinicians. Because it will not objectify the human state or model it, it cannot supplant empiricism in explanatory power, only in understanding. Syntax based on this view would value contextual knowledge and understanding from the agent's perspective (Collin, 1992).

Had Dilthey pre-empted Heidegger in the nursing literature, might we have seen more accommodation of the empirical/historical in our writings? Our arguments around philosophies appropriate for the natural or human sciences appear to be classically American (Gortner, 1990). Colleagues elsewhere in northern Europe employ the Diltheyan "Geisteswissenschaften" in their scholarship and are not troubled by an apparent incongruity of philosophy and method as are we. They would appear to illustrate the Suppean "radical separationist thesis."

Feminism and Critical Social Theory

Rational philosophies employing feminist perspectives and critical social theory increasingly challenge traditional epistemology in a number of fields, including the social sciences (Marshall, 1988) and nursing (Allen, 1985; Thompson, 1987; Holter, 1988; Moccia, 1988; Campbell & Bunting, 1991). While these views have quite distinct origins and hold a variety of current positions, they have in common an emphasis on the subjective, on the social construction of reality, on socio-political and economic influences on science, and on the prevalence of racism and sexism in scientific as well as social activities. In recognition of these oppressive mechanisms, both views have an emancipatory purpose with that of critical social theory emphasizing the collective, the aggregate rather than the personal and individual. Here the commonalities cease and distinctions become important.

Critical social theory arose in Germany, specifically in Frankfurt, as a philosophical reaction to early

---

[9]This requirement and that of the hermeneutic circle, joining investigator and subject, eliminates virtually all of basic biology as a potential scientific base for nursing; does it disenfranchise basic nurse scientists from engaging in theory development and criticism within nursing?

20th century positivism and natural science and to traditional Marxism (Habermas, 1971; Marshall, 1988; Holter, 1988). Assumptions of critical social theory have been stated by Holter (1988), Stevens (1989) and Campbell and Bunting (1991) for the nursing audience. These hold that all research and theory are socio-political constructions, that human societies are inherently oppressive, and that all world interpretations (mythical, religious, scientific, practical and political) are open to criticism (Stevens, 1989). Perhaps the most powerful feature of contemporary critical theory is in the capacity and mandate for the critique; this emphasis on rationality is contrasted with the emphasis on relations, feelings and emotions among some feminist thinkers. While most contemporary scientists would acknowledge the need to consider the political and social consequences of their inquiry, there is not agreement that these features must be part of regular scientific activity (even though it is acknowledged that all theories reflect underlying ideologies and "truth" claims as an anonymous reviewer of this paper has pointed out). Opinions vary on the extent to which scientists should be obligated to consider the socio-political frameworks of their studies. In this respect critical scholars are "up front" in stating clearly for the reader the inherent assumptions governing a given investigation. Critical theorists and critically inclined scientists take seriously the charge for action; for them inquiry is incomplete without the consequential and liberating act. In this key feature critical social theory can become the basis for political and social action; for nursing situations involving group processes and societal organization, the dialectic as rationality and method is appropriate and creative. As rationality, critical theory provides a multidimensional lens for scholarship; as method it requires that oppositional and/or under-represented views on a given problem area are specifically represented. Syntax would acknowledge knowledge as action based.

The number of studies employing critical social theory as perspective is growing in nursing and related fields. As the findings are published and subject to scrutiny (to the process of legitimization and credentialing), the quality of the investigations will be judged. It is important that the style of presentation and argument be such as to encourage the intended discourse and debate rather than overwhelm and alienate intended audiences. In nursing's literature, critical rationality has taken a more moderate form of expression than was the case several years ago. Yet the requirement for social and liberating action remains and is one of the features this author finds troubling, especially for novice scholars. Why? Because if one knows ahead of time that one is going to undertake social action, then one does not need to carry out the justifying research. One can act as social and autonomous agent without the benefit of science.

Another feature that is troubling is the lack of modeling, and theory respecification, given the stated dissatisfaction with classical social and economic theories. Critical social theory has social, political and economic relations as the units of analysis. This feature has made its empirical application limited to date in our field. So the expectations of realism and explanatory power have yet to be demonstrated. Perhaps a new theory of rationality could be forged, incorporating some of the assumptions of postempiricist philosophy.

The feminist critique of society and science has many of the features of critical social theory, but places its emphasis on the world of women in a male dominated society (patriarchy). It shares with hermeneutics the belief in lived experience and history as the basis of knowing, generating and using language for documentation and analyses. As such it also has a requirement for social discourse and reflexivity among competent persons, presented in the context of the social situation with attendent embedded meanings. Feminist literature in nursing is seen in the writings of MacPherson (1983), Chinn and Wheeler (1985), Duffy (1985), Bunting and Campbell (1990), and Campbell and Bunting (1991). Feminist scholarship appears to be enlarging in nursing theory and research, representing liberal, cultural and radical views, which need to be differentiated for uninformed audiences. Central to the radical view is the belief that oppression (due to the patriarchy) is fundamental and pervasive; here the similarity to critical social theory is clear. Yet one perspective is based in social philosophy, and the other is moving to philosophical statements from sociopolitical arguments. Until recently, critical social theory and feminist theory were not examined for their similarities in social statements, assumptions and methodologies. Several thoughtful comparisons are now available from authors such as Marshall (1988) and Campbell and Bunting (1991). Both perspectives have too heavy a reliance on social relations and actions to serve nursing exclusively. On the other hand, feminism is attractive and meaningful for nursing as a predominantly female profession. Analyses such as that provided by McCormick (1989) and Lips (1989) can provide insights into how nursing science can contribute to improved understanding of human behavior in health and illness without forfeiting science values and strategies. Differences among men and women in moral and scientific reasoning have been demonstrated (Gilligan, 1982) as have gender differences in recovery from illness or treatment (e.g., cardiac surgery) (Rankin, 1990). Would a theory of gender be a major contribution, as Marshall (1988) suggests? Perhaps if it includes the "rapport de force," the social context in which gender is examined (Perreault, 1991). Whether feminist and critical social theory will become part of nursing syntax will depend less on the splendor of the rhetoric and more on the quality of the research and the extent to which the studies have interdisciplinary appeal.

Recapitulation

This critique has set the dual notions of scientific realism and explanatory power as requirements for nursing's developing syntax. Admittedly, these notions reflect empiricist traditions, although they need not be so represented in the position taken by this author. No single world view should have primacy in our syntax; rather the consequences of particular world views for substantive theory development in nursing science need to be considered. The anti-naturalistic positions

found within hermeneutics, critical social theory and some feminist views impose limitations on human science development even more consequential than those of empiricism and empirical inquiry.[10] Common to the hermeneutic position is the foundational place of human agency, an intensionality that has no reality outside the context of the lived experience. Central to the feminist and critical theory arguments is the foundational place of domination (in gender, social class, work place) and emancipation. These features of humanity, gender, class and society are appropriate to contemporary social science and to nursing, in so far as it is a social science. But nursing is not exclusively a social science. It has a biological science component, which it will continue to incorporate in its disciplinary structure until such time as it decides to be an exclusively social activity. Nursing will not be served well by substituting social determinism for biological determinism, any more than feminists will be so served (Marshall, 1988). We are biological as well as social beings; our cell structures and biochemistry exhibit regularities over and over; our social actions barring catastrophes tend to be more regular than otherwise. What is normative for the individual is just that, and should represent "baseline" for contrast against which to judge severity of illness or recovery.

Nursing theories must incorporate the relevant domains, including biology as well as individual and social action and specify the hypothesized links with reality that will encourage theory testing and expansion. Only one of the competing world views, hermeneutics, specifically disallows modeling of the human. In this respect, hermeneutics is an antirealist in its position as was logical positivism earlier in this century. Just as logical positivism expired by virtue of its own constraints, so too may hermeneutics if it disallows realism and explanations be-

---

[10]Antinaturalist is being used here in its original philosophical sense of being distinct from natural science (thus making inappropriate the methodology of natural science for study of the person). Hermeneutics and critical theory are decidedly antinaturalistic given this definition; radical feminism is as well. Hermeneutics also is antirealist, in that the world view does not allow belief in theoretic entities (noumena) external to the lived world.

yond the subjective. As Collin has argued recently (1992), an interpetive (hermeneutic) nursing science does not allow theoreticity or the building of theoretical constructs outside of the person and lived experience. A "normative" science structure would, and would use what Collin calls a "third-person" stance to explain "particular quirks in the patient's self-conceptions. Such theories would be causal theories, and we would want them to describe the mechanisms behind distorted self-conception in a way which is both conceptually simple and of general application" (Collin, 1992, p. 23). In essence the case is being made for nomothetic as well as idiographic understandings and explanations. Further, nursing is defined not as idiographic activity but as "individualizing activity" (p. 18), for which theorizing and specifically scientific theorizing is appropriate. "Generalized knowledge will be indispensable in the process of understanding the individual case" (p. 18). For disciplinary fields must build theories about the stuff and substance that intrigues them: for nursing it is the human state during illness and in health, the ecology of human health across the life span. We have acknowledged our need for prescriptive theories, in addition to descriptive ones (Gortner, 1984). Our developing syntax must hold that need intact.

Acknowledgments.   The author is indebted to Hesook Suzie Kim, Professor of Nursing at the University of Rhode Island, Ann Whall, Professor of Nursing at the University of Michigan, Donna Wells, Assistant Professor of Nursing at the University of Toronto and an anonymous reviewer for their careful readings of earlier versions of this paper. Philosopher of science Frederick Suppe's paper immediately preceded the presentation of the original paper; his observations about 'invisible colleges,' 'credentialling' of knowledge claims, and the 'radical separationist thesis' were important additions to the author's thinking. Colleague and professor of philosophy at the University of California, Riverside, Alex Rosenberg, reviewed the substantive critiques of the world views and reassured the author that her criticisms were valid as presented. Finally, the continued interest of colleagues Karen Schumacher, Inger Margrethe Holter and Afaf Meleis in the author's writings on philosophy of science is gratefully acknowledged. They have been compatriots in the quest for nursing's scientific philosophy and have provided immeasurable assistance.

REFERENCES

Allen, D. (1985). Nursing research and social control: alternative modes of science that emphasize understanding and emancipation. *IMAGE: J. Nurs. Scholarship 17*, 58–64.

Benner, P. (1985). Quality of life: a phenomenological perspective on explanation, prediction and understanding in nursing science. *Adv. Nurs. Sci. 8*, 1–16.

Benner, P. and Wrubel, J. (1989). *The primacy of caring: stress and coping in health and illness.* Addison-Wesley, Menlo Park, CA.

Boyd, R. N. (1984). The current status of scientific realism. In *Scientific Realism* (Leplin, J., Ed.), pp. 41–82. University of California Press, Berkeley, CA.

Bunting, S. and Campbell, J. J. (1990). Feminism and nursing: historical perspectives. *Adv. Nurs. Sci. 12*, 11–24.

Campbell, J. C. and Bunting, S. (1991). Voices and paradigms. Perspectives on critical and feminist theory in nursing. *Adv. Nurs. Sci. 13*, 1–15.

Chinn, P. L. and Wheeler, C. E. (1985). Feminism and nursing. *Nurs. Outlook 33*, 74–77.

Collin, F. (1992). Nursing science as an interpretive discipline: problems and challenges. *Vard I Norden 12*, 14–23.

Dilthey, W. (1988). *Introduction to the Human Sciences. An attempt to lay a foundation for the study of society and history* (Betanzos, R. J., Translator). Wayne State University Press, Detroit, MI.

Donaldson, S. and Crowley, D. (1978). The discipline of nursing. *Nurs. Outlook 26*, 113–120.

Duffy, M. (1985). A critique of research: a feminist perspective. *Health Care for Women Int. 6*, 341–352.

Eriksson, K. (1990). Systematic and contextual caring science. A study of the basic motive of caring and contest. Nursing science in a Nordic perspective. *Scand. J. Caring Sci. 4*, 3–5.

Fitzpatrick, J. A. and Whall, A. (1989). *Conceptual models of nursing: Analysis and application,* 2nd Ed. Robert J. Brady, Co. Bowie, MD.

Fraasen, B. C. van (1980). *The scientific image.* Clarendon Press, Oxford.

Gadow, S. (1980). Existential advocacy. Philosophical foundations of nursing. In *Nursing: Images and Ideals* (Stuart, E. and Gadow, S., Eds). Springer Publishing, New York, NY.

Gilligan, C. (1982). *In a Different Voice.* Harvard University Press, Cambridge, MA.

Glymour, C. (1980). Logical empiricist theories of confirmation. In *Theory and evidence,* pp. 10–62. Princeton University Press, Princeton, NJ.

Gortner, S. R. (1984). Knowledge in a practice discipline: philosophy and pragmatics. In *Nursing Research and Policy Formation: The Case of Prospective Payment.* Papers of the 1983 Scientific Session of the American Academy of Nursing (pp. 5–17). American Academy of Nursing, Kansas City, MO.

Gortner, S. R. (1990). Nursing values and philosophy: toward a science philosophy. *IMAGE: J. Nurs. Scholarship 22,* 101–105.

Gortner, S. R. and Schultz, P. R. (1988). Approaches to nursing science methods. *IMAGE: J. Nurs. Scholarship 20,* 22–24.

Habermas, J. T. (1971). *Knowledge and Human Interests* (Shapiro, J., Translator). Beacon Press, Boston, MA.

Hacking, I. (1981). *Scientific Revolutions.* Oxford University Press, Oxford.

Hagell, E. I. (1989). Nursing knowledge: women's knowledge. A sociological perspective. *J. Adv. Nurs. 14,* 226–233.

Heidegger, M. (1962). *Being and Time* (Macquarrie J. and Robinson, E., Translators). Harper & Row, New York, NY.

Holden, R. J. (1990). Models, muddles, and medicine. *Int. J. Nurs. Stud. 27,* 223–234.

Holmes, C. A. (1990). Alternatives to natural science foundations for nursing. *Int. J. Nurs. Stud. 27,* 187–198.

Holter, I. M. (1988). Critical theory: a foundation for the development of nursing theories. *Schol. Inq. Nurs. Prac. 2,* 223–232.

Jacox, A. (1974). Theory construction in nursing: an overview. *Nurs. Res. 23,* 4–13.

Kuhn, T. (1970). Introduction II, the route to normal science; I, The nature of normal science. In *Structure of Scientific Revolutions* (Kuhn, T., Ed.), pp. 1–34. University of Chicago Press, Chicago, IL.

Lakatos, I. (1970). Falsification and the methodology of scientific research programmes. In *Criticism and the Growth of Knowledge* (Lakatos, I. and Musgrave, A., Eds), pp. 91–196. Cambridge University Press, Cambridge.

Laudan, L. (1977). *Progress and its Problems.* University of California Press, Berkeley, CA.

Leonard, V. W. (1989). A Heideggerian phenomenologic perspective on the concept of person. *Adv. Nurs. Sci. 11,* 40–55.

Lips, H. (1987). Toward a new science of human being and behavior. In *The Effects of Feminist Approaches on Research Methodologies* (Tomm, W., Ed.), pp. 51–69. Wilfrid Laurier Press, Waterloo, Ontario.

MacPherson, K. I. (1983). Feminist methods: A new paradigm for nursing. *Adv. Nurs. Sci. 5,* 17–25.

Marshall, B. L. (1988). Feminist theory and critical theory. *Can. Rev. Sociol. Anthropol. 25,* 208–230.

McCormick, T. (1989). Feminism and the new crisis in methodology. In *The Effects of Feminist Approaches on Research Methodologies* (Tomm, W., Ed.), pp. 13–31. Wilfrid Laurier Press, Waterloo, Ontario.

Meleis, A. I. (1987). Revisions in knowledge development: a passion for substance. Schol. Inq. Nurs. Prac. I, 5–19.

Meleis, A. I. (1991). *Theoretical Nursing,* 2nd Edn. Lippincott, Philadelphia.

Moccia, P. (1988). A critique of compromise: beyond the methods debate. *Adv. Nurs. Sci. 10,* 1–9.

Nagle, L. M. and Mitchell, G. J. (1991). Theoretic diversity: evolving paradigmatic issues in research and practice. *Adv. Nurs. Sci. 14,* 17–25.

Newman, M. A., Sime, A. M. and Corcoran-Perry, S. A. (1991). The focus of the discipline of nursing. *Adv. Nurs. Sci. 14,* 1–6.

Norbeck, J. (1986). In defense of empiricism. *IMAGE: J. Nurs. Schol. 19,* 28–30.

Palmer, R. E. (1969). *Hermeneutics. Interpretation Theory in Schleiermacher, Dilthey, Heidegger, and Gadamer.* Northwestern Press, Evanston, IL.

Perreault, M. (1990). Les rapports sociaux de sexe comme fondement d'analyse. Commentaire critique du texte de Gladys Simons "Les femmes-cadres dans l'univers bureaucratique." Sous presse dans le cadre du colloque international: "L'Individu dans l'organization: les dimensions oubliees." Montreal Université.

Phillips, D. (1987). The new dynamics of the sciences. In *Philosophy, Science and Social Inquiry,* pp. 20–36. Pergamon Press, New York, NY.

Rankin, S. H. (1990). Differences in recovery from cardiac surgery: a profile of male and female patients. *Heart and Lung 1*(5), 481–485.

Roy, Sr. C. (1989). Nursing care in theory and practice: early interventions in brain injury. In *Recovery from Brain Injury* (Harris, R., Burns, R. and Rees, R., Eds). Institute for the Study of Learning Difficulties, Adelaide.

Sarnecky, M. T. (1990). Historiography: a legitimate research methodology for nursing. *Adv. Nurs. Sci. 12,* 1–10.

Schumacher, K. L. and Gortner, S. R. (1992). (Mis)conceptions and reconceptions about traditional science. *Adv. Nurs. Sci. 14,* 1–11.

Schwab, J. (1964). Structure of the disciplines: meanings and significance. In *The Structures of Knowledge and the Curriculum* (Ford, G. W. and Pugno, L., Eds). Rand McNally, Chicago, IL.

Stevens, P. E. (1989). A critical social reconceptualization of environment in nursing: implications for methodology. *Adv. Nurs. Sci. 11,* 56–68.

Suppe, F. and Jacox, A. (1985). Philosophy of science and the development of nursing theory. In *Annual Review of Nursing Research* (Werley, H. and Fitzpatrick, J., Eds), Vol. 3, pp. 241–267. Springer Publishing Company, New York, NY.

Suppe, F. (1990). Knowledge development in the context of shifting world views: the philosophy—theory linkage. Paper presented at the first symposium on knowledge development in nursing. Newport Rhode Island, September 1990.

Thompson, J. L. (1985). Practical discourse on nursing: going beyond empiricism and historicism. *Adv. Nurs. Sci. 7,* 59–71.

Thompson, J. L. (1987). Critical scholarship: the critique of domination in nursing. *Adv. Nurs. Sci. 11,* 27–38.

Whall, A. (1989). The influence of logical positivism on nursing practice. *IMAGE: J. Nurs. Scholarship 21,* 243–245.

Whall, A. (1991). Personal communication, 17 April 1991.

The Author Comments

Nursing's Syntax Revisited

This article originally was an invited paper at the first Knowledge Development Symposium at the University of Rhode Island in September 1990. It was further refined during a sabbatical at the University of Montreal in 1991 and is difficult reading. I had been teaching the philosophy of nursing science to first-year PhD nursing students at UCSF and had incorporated postmodern views and arguments along with modern ones. I was concerned that several of the postmodern positions failed to exhibit explanatory power (defined as the capacity of a set of propositions not only to account for a given event but also to generalize to other events in the same set). That theoretic terms and abstractions arising from scientific work may exist and may be true is the position of scientific realism and one that I consider important for the development and credibility of nursing science. Both explanatory power and scientific realism should be accommodated in the theories and worldviews that guide our inquiry. Alternatively, we can develop a "within-the-discipline" philosophic lens that recognizes multiple knowledge domains (biologic, as well as sociologic and humanistic).

—SUSAN REICHERT GORTNER

CHAPTER 43

Postmodernism and Knowledge Development in Nursing

Jean Watson

Postmodernism as a concept and periodizing point between centuries has been defined as both the beginning and the end of modernity. This article explores some of the dimensions of this moment and movement between centuries and the implications of the postmodern condition on the nursing profession. Amidst the health care reform angst of deconstructing and reconstructing, challenges and opportunities await nursing's evolution into its own postmodern paradigm. Manifestations of such a postmodern paradigm are already reflected in the epistemological shifts of nursing science and knowledge development. Challenges posed for nursing science by this disorientingly free-floating era are brought to light—away from the reaction worldview, past the reciprocal and into the transformative-simultaneous, whereby nursing can emerge within its own unique postmodern discipline.

Keywords: Epistemology, Knowledge Development, Nursing Paradigm, Ontology, Postmodernism

Postmodern—a response across disciplines to the contemporary crisis of profound uncertainty brought about by crash of modern hope of rationality and technology to solve human dilemmas and quest for a description of "Truth and Reality." Lather, 1991, p. 20)

Whether reading Derrida (1976), Foucault (1972, 1973), Saussure (1974), Sarup (1988), Smith (1982), Toulmin (1990), Lacan (Benvenuto & Kennedy, 1986), or Lather (1991); whether pondering quantum physics, holograms, literature, music, or art; whether reflecting upon medical or nursing science; whether at a confer-

About the Author

JEAN WATSON is Distinguished Professor of Nursing and holds the Murchinson-Scolville Chair in Caring Science at the University of Colorado Health Sciences Center (HSC). She is founder of the original Center for Human Caring and previously served as Dean of the University of Colorado HSC School of Nursing. She is a Past President of the National League for Nursing. Born in West Virginia, July 21, 1940, Dr. Watson earned undergraduate and graduate degrees in nursing and psychiatric-mental health nursing and holds her PhD in educational psychology and counseling. Dr. Watson is known for her theoretical work on the art and science of human caring. Her latest books and articles address empirical measurements of caring and new postmodern philosophies of caring and healing that bridge paradigms and point toward transformative models for the 21st century. Dr. Watson is the recipient of many awards and honors, including an international Kellogg Fellowship in Australia, a Fulbright Research Award in Sweden, five honorary doctoral degrees, the National League for Nursing's Martha E. Rogers Award, New York University's Distinguished Nurse Scholar Award, and the Fetzer Institute's Norman Cousin's Award. Her hobbies include international travel, skiing, hiking, biking, and writing.

ence in Finland or attending an academic seminar in Sweden, Copenhagen or Colorado; whether in a gallery or coffee bar, there is a prevalent worldwide discourse on postmodernism. From one century to another, there is a struggling to make new meaning, new sense of this modern world which William Butler Yeats captured in 1921, the sense we now share that "things fall apart; the center cannot hold" (Toulmin, 1990, p. 158).

Almost every field of human activity today is engaged in the issues related to postmodern thought, even if it is not labeled as such. Just exactly what is postmodernism is unknown and ambiguous at best. As with any *ism* there is a hesitation to engage in it at that level. However, prominent thinkers suggest postmodern thought is defined by both the beginning and end of modernity (Toulmin, 1990). Indeed, postmodernism has been dubbed the end of the Western mind with its dominance of one reality, primarily the Western worldview, leaving a multiplicity of realities (Tarnas, 1993).

The modern Western mind that stands in contrast to the postmodern has come to convey positivist reasoning with its neutrality of human values, its concern with control and dominance of one worldview for predicting and sustaining a given reality whereby knowledge = science = reality. Such a modern reality has come to value

facts over meaning, has come to value science over church, and physical over nonphysical/metaphysical. Lather (1991) notes that it is considered a periodizing concept and a descriptor for a cultural, aesthetic, philosophical (and the author would add scientific) movement.

One can see the modern-postmodern scientific shift reflected through worldview characteristics referred to in the nursing literature as organismic and mechanistic (Fawcett, 1993). Differing philosophic claims manifest in what Parse (1987) has labeled simultaneity and totality paradigms, informing approaches toward humans and toward health and in what Newman (1992) has identified as the three prevailing paradigms for nursing knowledge development; the particulate-deterministic, the interactive-integrative and the unitary-transformative. These philosophical worldview critiques in nursing, which Fawcett (1993) has named a plethora of paradigms, are reflective of the broader cultural, philosophical transdisciplinary shifts occurring worldwide among the public and academicians alike.

More succinctly, postmodernism/poststructuralism has become "the code name for the crisis of confidence in Western conceptual systems . . . creating a conjunction that shifts our sense of who we are and what is possible" (Lather, 1991, p. 159). Specifically, "the essence of the postmodern argument is that the dualisms which continue to dominate Western thought are inadequate for understanding a world of multiple causes and effects interacting in complex and non-linear ways, all of which are rooted in a limitless array of historical and cultural specificities" (Lather, 1991, p. 21).

The postmodern rise has been most evident in France and throughout Europe during this century, from the *angst* of the existential philosophical movements, to the descriptive, even transcendental phenomenological attempts to grasp the human experience, and beyond, into hermeneutics, critical hermeneutics, interpretative hermeneutics, to feminism, language and semiotics, to deconstruction, to constructivist thinking and onward, toward the disownment of theory, method and dominating systems. The result has been such a decentering of rationality in the predominant reality and worldview that there is a dramatic shift in the understanding of knowledge and science toward an uprising "against all the 'experts' who proposed to speak for or on behalf of others" (Lather, 1991, p. 23). We see a search for ontological and epistemological authenticity (Guba & Lincoln, 1989) whereby "postmodernism as an intellectual movement, challenges the ideas of a single correct approach to knowledge development, of a single truth, and of a single meaning of reality. . . . rejecting the ideal that there is one true story about reality" (Uris, 1993, p. 95). Such an ontological and epistemological shift invites and works with context, connections, relations, multiplicity, ambiguity, openness, indeterminacy, patterning, paradox, process, transcendence and mysteries of the human experience of being-in-the-world (Watson, 1992).

Another aspect of the postmodern in contrast to the modern has been most clearly articulated in the field of architecture (Klotz, 1988; Lather, 1991; Toulmin, 1990). Indeed, postmodernism first gained widespread attention through architecture. Toulmin (1990) pointed out that the American architect Venturi argued in the '70s that the age of modern is past and must yield to a new postmodern style. For example, modern architecture is noted to be anonymous, timeless, and indistinguishable—boring, featureless, sterile, and stark—disconnected from its landscape and previous historical referents. Medical facilities in particular during this modern era of the 20th century became distinguishable from hotels or comfortable places to be by adopting the look of "progressive modernity with a clean, efficient, and functional appearance that symbolized the time" (Kingsley, 1988, p. 83). The postmodern style reintroduced elements of beauty, local color, decoration, historical reference, and even fantasy. Such shifts are also now reflected in redesign projects in hospitals and in neighborhoods, whereby sterility, sameness, and functionality are being replaced by emergence of beauty, variety, connection—the use of diverse models of aesthetics toward an integration of the local landscape, color, culture, and even the use of historical archetypal designs, intentionally reconnecting human experiences to human history and myth, across time and space. Postmodern architecture attempts to make places where the soul can live, not just build warehouses in which bodies may dwell (Day, 1990).

While neither "modern" nor "postmodern" has any precise definition, there is general convergence from all parties to the debate that "the modern world committed us to thinking about nature, the human condition, and institutions in a new and 'scientific way' through the use of more 'rational and precise methods' to deal with the problems of human life and society" (Toulmin, 1990, p. 9). Thus, modernity has become a worldview, which some trace back to the French Revolution, to Kant, and even to Descartes' logic and rationality, which, according to Toulmin (1990) was even extended to politics and organization of nation states.

This modern era of course extended directly into the modern medical revolution, which became one of the pinnacles of the world for the 20th century and clearly influenced nursing's modern maturity. Now both fields are grappling with the end of modernity and how to transition from modern, with its assumption of rationality and functionality *in all things,* to the postmodern wherein the modern center no longer holds—things are falling apart.

Shadow Side of Postmodernism: Deconstruction

The falling apart represents what might be considered the down side, or shadow side, of postmodernism. It is commonly associated with what is called deconstruction. The deconstruction of reality, whether through analysis of language, knowledge, or power structures, emerged ironically from the despair of the human condition brought about through modern scientific and technological advances; it was further sparked through the implosion of knowledge, information transfer, and new insights and quests for new meaning of the human condition. All of these forces transformed the human landscape and generated new questions about humanity, nature, and survival. While enlightening insights can be obtained through deconstruction, without critique it can also lead to a void and moral confusion.

Historically, it has been pointed out that the information age and the technologies of electronic communication, which explode the space-time limits of messages and profoundly shape human experience through experiences of multidirectionality and simultaneity, constitute a different kind of human subject and what it means to be human. There is the despatializing of work; there is a language of signifiers that float in relation to referents (Poster, 1987-1988); there is a relativity of time and space which is revealed both in experience and in physics. All have become substitutes for certain forms of social relations, undermining the Cartesian ontology of subject and object (Lather, 1991, p. 21). In this postmodern domain there exist "linguistically transformed representations" (Lather, 1991, p. 21) whereby the unreal is constituted as real, where a virtual reality can recreate a surreal reality.

The formal concept of "deconstruction" (also framed as post-structuralism) gained attention as an avant-garde intellectual movement through the work of Derrida (1976) and Foucault (1972, 1973) in France in the late '60s. The close reading of text for meaning and for power and knowledge relationships became an attempt to discover another picture of reality; to analyze in terms of what is in the text as well as what is not said,

or on the margin; to analyze and deconstruct for how knowledge and language function as a form of power and disseminate the effects of power (Sarup, 1988, p. 55). Thus to deconstruct a text is:

> to locate the promising marginal text, to disclose the undecidable moment, to pry it loose with the positive level of the signifier, to reverse the resident hierarchy, only to displace; to dismantle in order to reconstitute what is always already inscribed. (Sarup, 1988, p. 56)

Such efforts toward deconstruction carry over into society and science generally wherein is finally seen that things fall apart and the center can no longer hold, acknowledging that there is *no known solution;* there is no one way of knowing, being, and experiencing reality; recognizing the rationalist model does not fit; people are not here to adapt, to focus on problems to be fixed, but rather to focus on solutions with open possibilities, for what might be. While aspects of deconstruction are liberating, revealing, and giving birth to a new reality, there is the other side. What can also be experienced socially, from such an unraveling of reality, is social and scientific confusion, human and environmental violence, and even moral anarchy, where it is possible to ponder that even humanity cannot hold.

> In summary, the other side of the postmodern era's openness and indeterminacy is thus the lack of any firm ground for a worldview. Both inner and outer realities have become unfathomably ramified, multidimensional, malleable, and unbounded—bringing a spur to courage and . . . unending relativism and existential finitude. (Tarnas, 1993, p. 398)

As Tarnas points out, with the ascendance of the postmodern mind, the human quest for meaning in the cosmos has devolved upon a hermeneutic enterprise that is disorientingly free-floating: the postmodern exists in a universe whose significance is at once utterly open and without warrantable foundation. Perhaps it is at this point that nursing's transformative paradigm of caring (healing) in the human health experience (Newman, Sime, & Corcoran-Perry, 1991), with its moral foundation and imperative of human caring with respect to human health experience, comes into such powerful light (Fry, 1993; Noddings, 1984; Watson, 1990). It is here, during this latter part of the 20th century, that perhaps the evolution of nursing's modern worldview is shifting from what Fawcett (1993) labeled a *reaction* worldview into the *reciprocal*. As such, the next turn in nursing's development holds great potential for nursing's postmodern paradigm to collapse toward the *transformative-simultaneous*. (See Fawcett, 1993.)

Into the Light of Postmodernism: Reconstruction

Thus, the other side of postmodernism, moving from the reaction worldview, through the reciprocal, and toward the simultaneous, brings with it an aim toward emancipation from oppression, from strict dualism, from domination of rationality, technological controls, and knowledge discourses which have been thrust upon humanity since the rise of modernity. The reconstruction of reality is now being called for, acknowledging that another reality is emerging, in that there is a search for meaning that calls forth personal experience as a truth of its own; that allows for an emergence of beauty, wholeness, and connectedness to replace the emptiness of the initial modern residual associated with the downside of the postmodern condition. The positive side of postmodernism is to acknowledge that this is a historic moment in human evolutionary history as well as nursing's; to realize that the ground of postmodernism and the condition which rises from it is to participate in an explosion of shifting change, complexity, and chaos. What is thus required is nothing less than a radical transformative process of constructing-reconstructing ourselves and our worlds. This reconstruction project for humanity is the light side that counters the down, despairing side of human deconstruction.

So, while we can now acknowledge that the center cannot hold, can we create, recreate, cocreate a new center and a new form of human experience and knowledge which will lead humanity toward emancipation and higher evolution, especially with respect to the art and science of nursing and its caring-healing practices and diverse ways of knowing and being within a wide universe of the human health experience? Or will we submit to further chaos and decline, deconstruction, if not destruction, of humanity and the planet Earth as we know it?

Postmodern Implications for Nursing Knowledge

Is it possible for [nursing science] to be different, that is to forget itself and to become something else—or must it remain a partner in domination and hegemony? —SAID, 1989, P. 225

The postmodern turn in the history of nursing is hallmarked by the fact that the knowledge that has been systematically excluded from the human consciousness now has to be restored and reconnected in order to reconnect with the human condition (Smith, 1982). Some of that knowledge is knowledge of what it means to be human that goes beyond the physicalist, material orientation and fixation of the modern era. Part of that knowledge is an awakening of nursing's moral consciousness and compassion that moves in concentric circles and chains (Noddings, 1984), from self care, to caring for others, to environment, to nature, to caring for and being a part of an evolving universe that people are cocreating.

Nursing, like all other disciplines, must now yield to a postmodern approach, even though it is perhaps yet to be fully redefined. During such redefining during the paradigm shift, even Kuhn (1970) believes that each field of inquiry is called to develop its proper methods, adapted to its special problems and phenomena.

Such postmodern directions are already evident in nursing science knowledge and contemporary nursing theories, even though they may not be labeled as postmodern. (See Newman, 1986, 1992; Newman et al., 1991; Parse, 1981, 1992; Rogers, 1970, 1989; Sarter, 1988; Watson, 1988, 1992). Sarter's (1988) critique of four contemporary nursing theories (Rogers' science of unitary human beings, Newman's health as expanding consciousness, Parse's theory of human becoming, and Watson's theory of transpersonal human caring) revealed shared themes related to what might be considered a redefining of nursing and nursing knowledge from the modern, to the postmodern. This shift in extant nursing science and knowledge matrix is reflected in such shared concepts as evolution of consciousness, self-transcendence, open system, harmony, relativity of space-time, patterning, and holism (Sarter, 1988). Such thinking stands in sharp contrast to previous themes in nursing science associated with concepts such as steady state maintenance, adaptation, linear interactions between humans and the environment, problem-based practice, stress-coping, bio-psycho-social need hierarchy, nursing problem diagnosis, and so on.

The art and science of nursing with its concern with caring-healing and health as a field of study, research, and practice within its own paradigm is realizing that in this postmodern time, science, knowledge, and even images of nursing, health, environment, person become one among many truth games. Thus truth becomes viewed at least as rhetorical as it is procedural (paraphrased from Lather, 1991). The postmodern truth for nursing reconnects with the truth of unfoldment, an expansion and fusing of horizons of meaning, an attending to the authenticity, ethos, and ethic of caring relations, context, continuity, connections, aesthetics, interpretation, and construction. Returning nursing to some of its finest art and artistry from the era of Nightingale is yet to be actualized. This would include acknowledging plasticity and constant change; recognizing all knowledge is constructed as a human endeavor; returning to the context rather than the abstract voice of theory, authority; celebrating ambiguity and pluralism for its openness and possibilities; questioning of all truth statements and assumptions; noting that nothing is fixed, but evolving and fallible—endlessly self-revising and self-reflecting.

The implications for knowledge development in nursing are already reflected in the epistemological shifting from:

- strict rationalist—toward ambiguity, poetic, aesthetic, imaginary;
- analytic, descriptive—toward critical, interpretative hermeneutics, co-constructed meaning;
- phenomena per se—toward lived experience, endlessly deconstructing-reconstructing;
- ontic (fixed) categories, entities—toward the ontologically authentic;
- structure—toward process, patterning, transformation;
- numbers, factual data—toward text, meaning, extracting embedded theory laden in the fact;
- profane—sacred (Watson, 1993).

In summary, as nursing locates itself within the postmodern condition of complexity, with its shadow and light side, and as nursing seeks a dwelling place which is open-ended, ambiguous, dynamically constructed, incessantly questioned, endlessly self-revising, never set, but floating and moving with the river of life:

- Will nurses extract from the margin, uncover, and reconstruct nursing's most ancient and contemporary extant caring-healing-health knowledge and practices?
- Will nurses construct and co-construct ancient and new knowledge of the human health-illness, caring-healing experiences, and thereby move knowledge with its artistry of practice to the center, further clarifying nursing for a new era?
- Will nurses be part of helping nursing to mature and grow up both ontologically and epistemologically, within its own transformative praxis paradigm?

Or will nurses remain as constituted and sustain themselves as highly trained technicians serving a newly "redesigned" medical care system, which has already moved from the modern to the postmodern, with respect to "mindbodyspirit—whole person" medicine as the emerging model for health care reform?

The postmodern challenge is our challenge: the issue is whether we will take advantage of the fact of change, chaos, and ambiguity, deconstruction, and so on, and participate in reconstructing, cocreating a novel and moral direction for knowledge and practice, leading us forward, toward an ever-evolving humanity of possibilities or, will "we go on acting as though nothing ha[s] happened?" (Toulmin, 1990, p. 208).

REFERENCES

Benvenuto, B., & Kennedy, R. (1986). *The works of Jacques Lacan.* London: Free Association Books.

Day, C. (1990). *Places of the soul: Architecture and environmental design as a healing art.* Northamptonshire, England: The Aquarian Press.

Derrida, J. (1976). *On grammatology.* Baltimore: Johns Hopkins University Press.

Fawcett, J. (1993). From a plethora of paradigms to parsimony in worldviews. *Nursing Science Quarterly, 6,* 56–58.

Foucault, M. (1972). *The archaeology of knowledge and the discourse on language* (A. M. S. Smith, Trans.). New York: Pantheon Books.

Foucault, M. (1973). *The birth of the clinic.* (A. M. S. Smith, Trans.). London: Tavistock.

Fry, S. T. (1993). The ethic of care: Nursing's excellence for a troubled world. In D. Gaut (Ed.), *A global agenda for caring* (pp. 175–181). New York: National League for Nursing.

Guba, E., & Lincoln, Y. (1989) *Fourth generation evaluation.* Newbury Park, CA: Sage.

Kingsley, K. (1988). The architecture of nursing. In A. H. Jones (Ed.), *Images of nursing: Perspectives from history, art, and literature.* Philadelphia: University of Pennsylvania Press.

Klotz, H. (1988). *The history of postmodern architecture.* Cambridge: M.I.T. Press.

Kuhn, T. (1970). *The structure of scientific revolutions.* Chicago: University of Chicago Press.

Lather, P. (1991). *Getting smart: Feminist research and pedagogy with/in the postmodern.* New York: Routledge.

Newman, M. A. (1986). *Health as expanding consciousness.* St. Louis: Mosby.

Newman, M. A. (1992). Prevailing paradigms in nursing. *Nursing Outlook, 40*(1), 10–13.

Newman, M. A., Sime, A. M., & Corcoran-Perry, S. A. (1991). The focus of the discipline of nursing. *Advances in Nursing Science 14*(1), 1–6.

Noddings, N. (1984). *Caring: A feminine approach to ethics and moral development.* Berkeley: University of California Press.

Parse, R. R. (1981). *Man-living-health: A theory of nursing.* New York: Wiley.

Parse, R. R. (1987). Nursing science: Major paradigms, theories, and critiques. Philadelphia: Saunders.

Parse, R. R. (1992). Human becoming: Parse's theory of nursing. *Nursing Science Quarterly, 5,* 35–42.

Poster, M. (1987–1988). Foucault, the present and history. *Cultural Critique, 8,* 105–121.

Rogers, M. E. (1970). *An introduction to the theoretical basis of nursing.* Philadelphia: Davis.

Rogers, M. E. (1989). Nursing: A science of unitary human beings. In J. Riehl-Sisca (Ed.), *Conceptual models for nursing practice* (3rd ed.) (pp. 181–188). Englewood Cliffs, NJ: Appleton and Lange.

Said, E. (1989). Representing the colonized: Anthropology's interlocutors. *Critical Inquiry 15,* 205–225.

Sarter, B. (1988). Philosophical sources of nursing theory. *Nursing Science Quarterly, 1,* 52–59.

Sarup, M. (1988). *Post-structuralism and postmodernism.* New York: Harvester Wheatsheaf.

Saussure, F. de, (1974). *Course in general linguistics.* London: Fontana/Collins.

Smith, H. (1982). *Beyond the post-modern mind.* Wheaton, IL: Theosophical Publishing House.

Tamas, R. (1993). *The passion of the western mind.* New York: Ballantine Books.

Toulmin, S. (1990). *Cosmopolis: The agenda of modernity.* New York: Free Press.

Uris, P. (1993). *Postmodern feminist emancipatory research: A critical analysis of nurses' moral experience of caring in a patriarchal society.* Unpublished doctoral dissertation, University of Colorado, Denver.

Watson, J. (1988). New dimensions of human caring theory. *Nursing Science Quarterly, 1,* 175–181.

Watson, J. (1990). The moral failure of the patriarchy. *Nursing Outlook, 36*(2), 62–66.

Watson, J. (1992). *Postmodern nursing and beyond.* Paper presented at the American Academy of Nursing Annual Meeting, Kansas City.

Watson, J. (1994). Poeticizing as truth through language. In P. Chinn & J. Watson (Eds.), *Art and aesthetics in nursing* (pp. 3–17). New York: National League for Nursing.

The Author Comments

Postmodernism and Knowledge Development in Nursing

This article was written after a Fulbright research and study in Sweden as part of a sabbatical. During that time, I was exposed to more European thinking within the postmodern discourse and philosophic traditions. I was seeing the connection between the rise of postmodern thinking and its consistency with nursing science's quest and critique of conventional thinking. This article, and the book that followed, *Postmodern Nursing and Beyond* (1999), offered an evolving model for nursing's future, consistent with futuristic directions in the evolution of human consciousness.

—JEAN WATSON

Paradigms Lost, Paradigms Regained: Defending Nursing Against a Single Reading of Postmodernism

Chris Stevenson
Ian Beech

Within nursing, postmodernism has been seen as both a freeing influence and a philosophy of rejection and relativism. Within this paper we consider readings of postmodernism that have been presented and offer a re-reading that retains the idea of 'the good' and is neither relativist nor rejectionist. Local knowledge is to be judged by the relevant community and theoretical knowledge becomes nursing knowledge through re-flexivity and improvization in practice. A story is good if it allows people to go on with their lives.

Keywords: postmodernism, deconstruction, philosophy in nursing, truth, validity.

Introduction and Foreword

In considering nursing texts (by which we mean text in its broader sense of a set of signals, whether written, spoken or enacted, that may be read) as part of our academic lives, we have become aware that postmodernism creates philosophical angst and moral panic. Postmodernism has been described as ' . . . a time of paradigms lost' (Reed, 1995, p. 71). There have been attempts from those positioning themselves outwith the postmodern turn to defend nursing from the postmodern hoax (Kermode & Brown, 1996). The three essential themes often ascribed to post-modernism, and the perceived threats, are:

- acceptance of multiple realities with loss of generalizable knowledge as local knowledge of nursing is fore-grounded, so that an anarchistic 'anything goes' attitude prevails (Holdsworth, 1997);
- relativism (Porter, 1996): creating an ethically free zone within which guidelines are not possible and

About the Authors

CHRIS STEVENSON was born on June 27, 1953. Dr. Stevenson earned an RMN, a BA (Hons), an MSc (Dist), and a PhD. The focus of Dr. Stevenson's scholarship is on describing the nature of nursing, the nature of nursing research and scholarship, and the nature of nurse education/training, from within the postmodern turn. Dr. Stevenson has a keen interest in social constructionism related to the practice of family therapy, especially with people with eating distress, a further research interest. He has worked closely with Professor Phil Barker in developing and evaluating the Tidal Model of psychiatric nursing, which has a developing profile nationally and internationally. Dr. Stevenson has an extensive publication profile, which includes many papers that challenge received nursing wisdom. Throughout life, Dr. Stevenson developed interests in reading, running, writing, quilting, and films.

IAN BEECH was born on September 30, 1960, and has earned an RMN, an RGN, and a BA (Hons). Mr. Beech is a PGCE Senior Lecturer in Mental Health Nursing in the University of Glamorgan, Wales, United Kingdom. His primary interests within nursing are working with people in depression using a logotherapeutic approach, spiritual aspects of people's lives and suffering, and the relationship between nurses and people receiving nursing care. Mr. Beech has conducted research into some of these areas using phenomenology and contributed widely within the UK to the debate on research methodology in mental health nursing. He is also facilitating the introduction of the Tidal Model within three separate clinical areas locally. Throughout his life, Mr. Beech developed interests in Buddhism, reading, playing folk music on Tenor Banjo and Octave Mandola, and walking the dogs.

health professionals are able, for example, to ignore the reality of abuse (Minuchin, 1991);

- a philosophy of rejection and destruction. For example, postmodernism signals the 'last post' for psychiatric nursing, leaving uncertainty and fragmentation (Clarke, 1996).

While respecting the issues that learned colleagues have raised, we think that some criticisms of postmodernism within nursing have been based on a single reading which, ironically (for postmodernists at least), purports to capture its *essence* as anarchistic, relativist and amoral, and destructive.

We think that this particular reading has its foundations in the ideology of positivist science. Shotter (1993) notes that when conversations become formalized into a particular discourse, ideological processes are likely to benefit some groups over others. Thus, when there is an orthodox, legitimated approach to knowing about the world, other approaches become subjugated. For example, elsewhere we have narrated our experiences of ethical and research awarding committees' lack of an understanding of qualitative research proposals because they do not value the kind of knowledge that would be generated (Stevenson & Beech, 1998). When one position becomes dominant, interesting questions arise in relation to epistemological hegemony (Birch, 1995). Do traditional ideas about truth become a normative imperative for all researchers? *Who* are the authentic voices in knowledge production? What benefits do they gain? How do nontraditionalist researchers establish their authority? Lather (1991) points out that traditional ways of knowing and being known necessarily involve a political dimension which includes some self serving bias. Cooper & Stevenson (1998) note that scientific knowledge in our society is seen as legitimate and disciplines adopting scientific methods are seen as respectable. In relation to psychology, they argue that this leads to a 'tidying away' of discrepant forms of knowledge, by overlaying them with science. For example, lay and folk psychological beliefs have been denigrated. We consider the critiques of postmodernism outlined above to be attempts to traditionalize nursing and as such are '...a self-descriptive, externalizing of the ideology of the day' (Rorty, 1982, 1-2). We suggest also that postmodernists are not insensitive to the 'real' world and its dilemmas. In the interest of balance, we revisit these 'dilemmas' and offer alternative, postmodern readings. However, we do not want to simply present another authorized version (grand narrative) of the nature of knowledge, from the academy. To do so would be to present a different marginalizing discourse. According to Lyotard (1984), what counts as knowledge is less important than an analysis of how the decision is made about what is classed as real, of who has the authority. For what is classed as not real becomes *second* class. Research falling within the postmodern turn points up the contradiction and presuppositions implicit to the production of any authorized version of the world, including its own (Heslop, 1997). Our aim is to keep the debate about postmodernism in nursing fluid. First, however, we set out what we mean by postmodernism in the context of this paper.

'What Are We Calling Postmodernity? I'm Not Up To Date.'

(Foucault in Schrag, 1992, p. 16)
Postmodernism has been seen as the modern turning upon itself to re-read its texts, reassessing their value in relation to current context.

> Postmodernism does not completely break with modernism . . . postmodernism 'begins' when the present ceases to be informed by the past. (Clarke, 1996, p. 257)

Bauman (1990) argues that postmodernity is not a successor regime to modernity rather modernity undergoing self-examination and resolving to change on the strength of that examination. Problematizing modernity

from within modernity is what Habermas (1981) described as the uncompleted project of modernism. For example, whilst Popper accepted the Humean objection to scientific inductivism, he used it as the foundation for a new logic of modernist science, i.e. falsificationism. For Habermas, the errors of modernity can be corrected by the use of reflective reasoning.

In common with Rolfe (2000), we reject the idea of postmodernism as modernism reflecting upon itself. We think that postmodernism entails a rejection of the values of modernism and this makes it more than the uncovering of contradictions within modernist science. We do not attempt to be definitive about postmodernism, because to do so would be contrary to the spirit of the postmodern turn. We prefer to give our *personal* description of postmodernism, drawing on the work of Stevenson & Reed (1996). Postmodernism is a rejection of the modern, post-Enlightenment concern with the rational and scientific. It is a movement away from grand theories or narratives that try to explain the world towards local and specific knowledge. Although there is much variation in postmodernism, there is sharing of nonfoundationalist ideas. For example, truth is seen as problematic and not necessarily progressively accessible through scientific exploration or logical reasoning. Complexity and ambiguity are celebrated and inconsistencies, paradoxes and contradictions are not of concern, because knowledge is inseparable from the specific context in which it comes into existence. We concur with Wittgenstein (1953) in his work *Philosophical Investigations* that language cannot be separated from a physical reality that it represents. In common with Wittgenstein, we see language as forming the world in which we live. What we know about our world lies in the relationship between the knower and the other. People co-create stories that are treated as negotiated or 'soft' realities which allow them to 'go on with' their lives. For example, this paper is itself a story that allows us to go on with our lives as academic researchers, in a context where there is disagreement about the value of different theoretical (or antitheoretical) inquiry positions. We think that our version of postmodernism can address the reading of postmodernism as antirealist, relativist, rejectionist and destructive, which we examine in the following sections.

One Truth or Multiple Realities?

There are many existing critiques of positivism (e.g. Chalmers, 1999). In a sense, positivism can be seen as a straw person, easy to criticize in its attachment to objectivity, representationalism, etc. when applied in the social sciences. However Rolfe (2000) suggests that some philosophers of science, e.g. Feyerabend and Kuhn, have taken a postpositivist position in criticizing the *methods* of positivist science whilst retaining a commitment to the *ideals* of science. If modernism and postmodernism are incommensurable, as argued above, then there is no way of formulating a description of modernist scientific knowledge within the postmodern *or* of criticizing the postmodern from within the modern. Lyotard (1989) described this impasse as *le différend*. Put simply, there are no rules equally applicable to each position that would allow a comparison between the positions. In such circumstances, decisions about what is 'good' or 'true' are based more on values as Rorty (1982) has argued. Yet, the reading of postmodernism outlined above ignores *le différend*. There are less traditional approaches that try to bridge the discrepant positions of modernism and postmodernism, engaging with the ideas of both. Critical realism, as developed by Bhaskar (1989a), entails the position that there is a real world 'out there.' Although Bhaskar rejects the idea that his view is positivist or empiricist, we would see him as occupying a postpositivist position, since he argues that the reality cannot be theorized about in an entirely objective way because of the limitations of human perception and cognition. Additionally, theoretical objectivity is impossible because of the collaborative process by which people make sense of their world. In this, Bhaskar accepts the social construction of knowledge. But critical realism was developed as an antidote to the perceived relativism inherent in some more 'anarchistic' approaches to 'knowledge' production (Bhaskar, 1989b). It entails an acceptance of an ontological reality, and so a scientific methodology in that there are rational grounds for preferring one belief to another. Truth is that which most closely *approximates* to the ontological reality.

Whilst Bhaskar massages concerns about what can be known, we believe that our world is not simply mediated by discourse, as in critical realism, but created through it. As Rorty (1982) describes it:

> So the real issue is not between people who think one view is as good as another is and people who do not. It is between those who think our culture, or purpose, or intuitions cannot be supported except conversationally, and people who still hope for some other support. (pp. 166–167)

Derrida (1978) challenged the taken for granted view that language is capable of expressing views without changing them. All language is metaphorical, referring to something that is not. By this we mean that language does not represent the world in a straightforward way. As an example we take the metaphorical language of AIDS/HIV:

> The papers are full of new drugs and new theories. The T-cell, it appears, far from being decimated by an HIV awakened from the languor of a 10-year slumber by some internal alarm clock, instead fights tooth and nucleus in a war of attrition against the invading virus, and then, after years of bloody battle, collapses in exhaustion as an army of replicants conquers the corpuscles. (Moore, 1996, pp. 74–75)

The inevitability of metaphor makes multiple meanings possible because, as de Saussure (1983) tells us, there is always a gap between the signifier (the word or act) and the signified (the concept to which the signifier refers). The signifier and the signified together make the sign that points to the object that is the reference. But because of the *inevitable* gap, gauging 'fit' against an external reality, as in positivism and postpositivism, is no longer a way of evaluating beliefs or interpretations. The power of language is demonstrated by an analysis of what happens when communication breaks down. We have given a clinical example elsewhere of a situation where a person encounters a professional and tells the story of being controlled by extraterrestrial forces (Stevenson & Beech, 1998). The professional has a choice. In following the language game (Wittgenstein, 1953) implicit in professional training, delusional or hallucinatory content is not discussed for fear of reinforcing the presentation of illness. In this circumstance, the person and professional usually enter into stalemate broken by the administration of medication. In entering into a discussion about the meaning of being controlled rather than a disagreement about the nature of reality the possibility for the co-creation of a new story emerges between the person and the professional with new possibilities for progress.

We accept that some readers may be unconvinced by our schizophrenia example given the debates ongoing within the scientific community on schizophrenia, in particular, the search for a marker gene for schizophrenia, the *disease*. Therefore, we offer an alternative example of diabetes mellitus, within which we use the work of Barthes (1977). Barthes rejected the idea of

> . . . the voice of a single person, the *author* 'confiding' in us. The aim of literary criticism was therefore no longer an attempt to arrive at the 'true' meaning of the text as intended by the author. (Rolfe, 2000, p. 38)

The death of the author allows the birth of the reader in the sense that responsibility for making sense of the text lies with the person making a personal interpretation. From our position, there are many different readings of, for example, diabetes mellitus. We do not dispute the body's failure to produce insulin in the way that might be expected. This need not dictate the nurse's approach to the person diagnosed as diabetic. Mitchell (1995) illustrates the approach of a nurse guided by a fairly traditional, scientific knowledge of diabetes to someone who planned to wean herself off insulin. In Mitchell's example, the nurse contacted the physician about the pending noncompliance and arranged a teaching session on the importance of insulin for the woman. After this inter-

vention had been carried out the woman found herself in conflict with the nurse and doctor and, in spite of being educated about the importance of insulin continued to plan to stop taking the drug. A nurse adopting the postmodern approach (advocated by Parse, 1995) entered discussion with the woman. Instead of finding that the woman was ignorant of scientific knowledge about insulin and its importance to her physiology, the nurse found that the woman, while being knowledgeable, did not value that particular story. Neither was the woman suicidal. She had made plans both to cut sugar from her diet and to keep detailed checks on her blood sugar levels. It emerged that the woman's father had died as a result of insulin and she now carried a conviction that insulin might kill her. The ongoing relationship between the nurse and the woman, rather than being based on an 'I'm right, you're wrong' monologue, enabled a set of future possibilities to develop. Superficially, the example is consistent with a realist analysis. The woman had a personal theory, or imperfect interpretation of the world, that guided her intention to stop taking insulin. However, a critical realist analysis invites a pathologizing discourse concerning the woman's case. Specifically, it allows a view that the woman's 'faulty' interpretation needs fixing. Some postmodernists acknowledge that there is a family resemblance (Wittgenstein, 1953) between nursing situations. In discussing diagnostic frameworks, Cronen & Lang (1994) note that there are similarities between people who are labelled as, for example, schizophrenic. However, and critically for these authors, the differences between these people are as great as the sameness and local nursing knowledge is needed. With this perspective there is less attachment to fixing pathology and more room to treat the individual albeit against a background of assumed similarity.

An emphasis on language is problematic for those outwith the postmodern turn. If there is no longer representationalism, then how can one version be better or worse than any other—anything goes with the tyranny of choice. We turn to this issue in our discussion of relativism and pragmatism.

Relativism and Pragmatism

A question arising from the single reading of postmodernism is 'What constitutes "good" postmodern nursing?' We turn to the work of William James (1907, p. 166) to help address this issue. In describing what pragmatism means, James set out a new way of dealing with conflict between ideas. He describes a heated debate about the following metaphysical problem:

> The *corpus* of the debate was a squirrel—a live squirrel supposed to be clinging to a tree trunk; while over against the tree's opposite side a human being was imagined to stand. This human witness tries to get sight of the squirrel by moving rapidly around the tree, but no matter how fast he goes, the squirrel moves as fast in the same direction, and always keeps the tree between himself and the man, so that never a glimpse of him is caught. The resultant metaphysical problem now is this: *Does the man go round the squirrel or not?* He goes round the tree, sure enough, and the squirrel is on the tree; but does he go round the squirrel?

Each side in the debate was definite that it was right. But James thought the best way to resolve the debate was to define what was *practically* meant by 'going round' the squirrel:

> If you mean passing from the north of him to the east, then to the south, then to the west, and then to the north again, obviously the man does go round him, for he occupies these successive positions. But if on the contrary you mean being first in front of him, then on the right of him, then behind him, then on his left, and finally in front again, it is quite as obvious that the man fails to go round him, for by making compensatory movements, he keeps his belly turned towards the man all the time, and his back turned away . . . . . .
> You are both right and both wrong according as you conceive the verb 'to go round' in one practical fashion or the other.

This is James' example of the pragmatic method derived from the work of Peirce 20 years before. It settles disputes which otherwise might be unresolvable. It works by tracing the practical, concrete consequences of respective positions. If no practical difference can be traced, then any dispute is idle. But beyond settling disputes, James' pragmatism has a theory of truth. Truth is ' . . . *one species of good,* and not, as is usually supposed, a category distinct from good . . . '. James justified this position by asking the rhetorical question, ' . . . if there were *no* good for life in true ideas, or if the knowledge of them was positively disadvantageous and false ideas the only useful ones, then the current notion that truth is divine or precious, and its pursuit a duty, could never have grown up or become a dogma.' Put simply, James conflated 'true' and 'good.' We look also to collapse true, good and useful. For example, Birch (1995) points out that there have been cases when people have survived after their parachutes failed to open. However, this is one discourse that is *better* marginalized. Death is not good for life and so postmodern skydivers pull their rip cords. We do not deny that aeroplanes fly, that rain makes you wet, that antibiotics can cure bacterial infections. But we consider also that the majority of our lives are lived in language about the 'real world.' That is why we are interested in how accounts of aeroplanes flying, rain wetting and antibiotics curing are generated and how these accounts allow us, indeed require us, to function in the social world.

Cronen & Lang (1994) consider that it is the *practice* of communication and conversation that allows people to live their lives. For example, a person diagnosed as schizophrenic and the psychiatric nurse engage in conversations about experiences and do not operate to change any physical (biological) reality of schizophrenia. Both the patient and the psychiatric nurse act into a set of future possibilities as in response to a set of past actualities (Shotter, 1986). Through this process, the dyad creates who they are and their social world. Such knowledge is local in that it arises from being in the situation. It is good/true in so far as it allows the pair to go on with their lives individually and together. It is not comparable to some gold standard of knowledge of schizophrenia, nor to knowledge of how to deal with schizophrenics as a whole. To ask whether such local knowledge is valid becomes a nonquestion. Stevenson & Reed (1996) suggest that validity can be re-authored as a story that fits for the people concerned. A good story is one that renders life meaningful not one that is factually true, one which is sufficient to allow people to get on with living (Parry & Doan, 1994). As the Irish saying goes 'Why let the facts get in the way of a good story!'.

Uncertainty and Fragmentation or Reflection and Responsibility?

A well-rehearsed criticism of postmodernism is that it deconstructs without ever giving an indication of what should stand in the place of the deconstructed phenomenon. With deconstruction, the moral fibre of society is at risk as uncertainty and fragmentation is taken as synonymous with anarchy and every person for her/himself. Rolfe (2000) notes that this position involves a confusion of deconstruction and destruction. Birch (1995) acknowledges the tendency to confuse deconstruction and destructive criticism. He notes, in analysing the power relationship between therapist and client, that:

> The task of liberation is to release the client from the yoke of the therapist, and the means of liberation is . . . the therapist. (p. 224)

But this deconstruction is not equivalent to destruction. It merely highlights that there is an area of ambiguity where we do not yet have the language to name the unnameable. For example, we cannot contemplate the therapist-less client. In Wittgenstein's (1953) terms a picture holds us captive and we cannot step outside of it as it lies in our language. For Wittgenstein the task of philosophy is to help us fight against the bewitchment of our intelligence by existing language conventions. How might this be accomplished? Rorty (1982) has suggested that we might evaluate our final vocabularies by means of critical irony. He suggests that we become sceptical about our own stories through listening to the alternatives offered by others in conversation or through reading; that we abandon evangelical intentions of converting others to our version through rejecting the idea that our own final vocabulary is closer to the truth than anyone else's. Rorty's ideas fit with the practice of reflecting team process. Andersen (1987) recommends that, as part of reflecting ideas back to families, the professionals involved make explicit the values and experiences that may be influencing their analysis. What does this mean for postmodern nursing practice?

Peplau (1988) noted that practice is the context in which scientific knowledge is transformed into nursing knowledge. For us, all knowledge is open to this application. The postmodern nurse, tooled with deconstruction, uses existing theory to inform practice without over applying theory in a ritualized fashion. S/he takes *responsibility* for reading and re-reading the evidence, rather than merely accepting it as received wisdom from the author. S/he is in a prime position to recognize how her particular area is similar to *and differs from* other areas and to practice accordingly. In this respect, we want to draw an analogy between the (postmodern) nurse and the jazz musician who improvises on a theme, originally set out by Schön (1987). A musical performance at time 1 could represent truth (in traditional terms) as described in the musical score. However, there are several reasons why this would be a limited and limiting activity. There is a general acceptance that the improvising musician will not want to replicate the improvisation but will improvise creatively and not recreatively at time 2. Other jazz musicians will improvise individually around the same theme. There is no expectation that the improvisation is representative or reflective of some underlying reality of 'good' music. Rather, the improvisation stands to be judged in its own right by each individual who hears it, on each occasion it is played. Neither will that judgement involve questions about why the improvisation is good. It is simply enough that it *is* good, within the particular social, political, economic context in which it is performed. The people best placed to judge the performance are the stake holding community (Atkinson & Heath, 1987). As Kuhn (1970) puts it in relation to science:

> There is no standard higher than the assent of the relevant [scientific] community. (p. 94)

If we apply improvisation to nursing practice, it is naïve to imagine that knowledge in nursing is of the type that can easily be generalized from one situation to another. Relativism seems inevitable. Few nurses would claim that the reality of working in an area one day was identical to that of the next/previous day, but they have to make responses and have them judged in a local framework of evaluation and hope that the response will be acceptable and accepted. Reed (1995) argues that good research is useful research in terms of certain patient important dimensions, e.g. informing about healing environments, inner human potential and the developmental/contextual nature of health. A similar set of dimensions might describe *useful* nursing practice.

Reflexivity, based upon critical, ironic reflection, can be the source of ethics. Nurses who reflect on their own contribution to the production of knowledge are placing their values and ideologies centre stage. In such circumstances, nurses can be held socially accountable for the distinctions that they make (Krippendorf, 1991).

Summary of the Postmodern Response to the Three Themes

In returning to the three themes that we identified at the start of this paper, we consider that postmodernism has been presented as: lacking in generalizability and giving primacy to local knowledge; relativist in its permissive-

ness for anything to be allowed; a philosophy of deconstruction that breaks down truth without replacing it with anything.

In response to the first theme of lacking generalizability we have shown that nursing ideas and nursing research are good if the stories they tell allow nurses and people in care to get on with their lives. If the story is useful it is used, if not it is rejected. While there is no overall generalizability there are family resemblances between stories that have resonance for practitioners.

The second theme alleges that postmodernism is relative and allows anything to go, including abuse. However abuse would be neither good nor useful to nurses and people in living their lives and would not be judged as such by nurses within the postmodern turn.

The third theme considers postmodernism to be destructive in its deconstruction of ideas. We have indicated that deconstruction should not be conflated with destruction and that the reflexive practitioner can improvise around the theme of existing theory while still deconstructing that theory.

So as a means of summarizing the paper's arguments, we want to offer our responses to the question, 'What is "good" postmodern nursing?'. Watson (1995) envisages nursing using the free-floating era of postmodernism as a means of nursing moving away from a reactionary worldview. Lister (1991) values postmodernism as an antidote to the unthinking application of models of nursing. Stevenson & Reed (1996) note that practitioners influenced by postmodern ideas may give the person in psychiatric distress more space to tell her/his story, because the professional is less attached to a single version of the truth of mental illness. If what counts as good nursing is less rule bound than is usually thought, nurses can take responsibility for their own practice based upon reflection in and on action.

REFERENCES

Andersen T. (1987). The reflecting: dialogue and metadialogue in clinical work. *Family Process, 26*, 415–428.

Atkinson B. & Heath A. (1987). Beyond objectivism and relativism: implications for family therapy research. *Journal of Strategic and Systemic Therapies, 6,* 8–17.

Barthes R. (1977). *Image Music Text.* Fontana, London.

Bauman Z. (1990). *Modernity and Ambivalence.* Polity, Cambridge.

Bhaskar R. (1989a). *Reclaiming Reality.* Verso, London.

Bhaskar R. (1989b). *The Possibility of Naturalism: a Philosophical Critique of the Contemporary Human Sciences.* Harvester Wheatsheaf, Hemel Hempstead.

Birch J. (1995). Chasing the rainbow's end and why it matters: a coda to Pocock, Frosh and Larner. *Journal of Family Therapy, 2,* 219–228.

Chalmers A. (1999). *What Is This Thing Called Science?,* 3rd edn. Open University Press, Buckingham.

Clarke L. (1996). The last post? Defending nursing against the postmodernist maze. *Journal of Psychiatric and Mental Health Nursing, 4,* 257–265.

Cooper N. & Stevenson C. (1998). New 'science' and psychology. *Psychologist,* 11, 484–485.

Cronen V. & Lang P. (1994). Language and action: Wittgenstein and Dewey in the practice of therapy and consultation. *Human Systems, 5,* 5–43.

Derrida J. (1978). *L'Écriture and Différance.* (tr. A. Bass). University of Chicago Press, Chicago.

Foucault M. cited by Schrag C. O. (1992). *The Resources of Rationality.* Indiana University Press, Bloomington, MD.

Habermas J. (1981). Modernity—an incomplete project. *New German Critique,* 22, 3–15.

Heslop L. (1997). The (im) possibilities of poststructuralist and critical social inquiry. *Nursing Inquiry, 4,* 48–56.

Holdsworth N. (1997). Postmodernity and psychiatric nursing: a commentary. *Journal of Psychiatric and Mental Health Nursing, 4,* 309–312.

James W. (1907). *What Pragmatism Means.* http://www.marxists.org/reference/subject/philosophy/index.htm (accessed 27/02/01).

Kermode S. & Brown C. (1996). The postmodern hoax and its effects on nursing. *International Journal of Nursing Studies,* 33, 375–384.

Krippendorf K. (1991). What should guide reality construction? In: *Research and Reflexivity* (ed. F. Steier). Sage, London.

Kuhn T. (1970). *The Structure of Scientific Revolutions.* University of Chicago Press, Chicago.

Lather P. (1991). *Getting Smart. Feminist Research and Pedagogy with/in the Postmodern.* Routledge, London.

Lister P. (1991). Approaching models of nursing from a postmodern perspective. *Journal of Advanced Nursing, 16,* 206–212.

Lyotard J.-F. (1984). *The Post-Modern Condition: a Report on Knowledge.* Manchester University Press, Manchester.

Lyotard J.-F. (1989). *The Differend: Phrases in Dispute* (tr. G. Van Den Abbeele). University of Minnesota Press, Minneapolis.

Minuchin S. (1991). The seductions of constructivism. *Family Therapy Networker,* September/October, 47–50.

Mitchell G. (1995). The view of freedom within the human becoming theory. In: *Illuminations: the Human Becoming Theory in Practice and Research* (ed. R. Parse). National League for Nursing, New York.

Moore O. (1996). *PWA: Looking AIDS in the Face.* Picador, London.

Parry A. & Doan R. (1994). *Story Re-Visions: Narrative Therapy in the Postmodern World.* Guilford Press, New York.

Parse R. (ed.) (1995). *Illuminations: the Human Becoming Theory in Practice and Research.* National League for Nursing, New York.

Peplau H. (1988). *Interpersonal Relations in Nursing.* MacMillan, Basingstoke.

Porter S. (1996). Real bodies, real needs: a critique of the application of Foucault's philosophy to nursing. *Social Sciences in Health, 2,* 218–227.

Reed P. (1995). A treatise on nursing knowledge development for the 21st century: beyond postmodernism. *Advances in Nursing Science, 17,* 70–84.

Rolfe G. (2000). *Research, Truth and Authority: Postmodern Perspectives on Nursing.* MacMillan, Basingstoke.

Rorty R. (1982). *Consequences of Pragmatism.* University of Minnesota Press, Minneapolis.

de Saussure F. (1983). *Course in General Linguistics.* Duckworth, London.

Schön D. (1987). *Educating the Reflexive Practitioner.* Jossey-Bass, San Francisco.

Shotter J. (1986). Speaking practically: Whorf, the formative function of communication and knowing of a third kind. In: *Contextualism and Understanding in Behavioural Science: Implications for Research and Theory* (eds L. Rosnow & M. Georgoudi). Praeger, New York.

Shotter J. (1993). *Conversational Realities.* Sage, London.

Stevenson C. & Beech I. (1998). Playing the power game for qualitative researchers: the possibility of a postmodern approach. *Journal of Advanced Nursing, 27,* 790–797.

Stevenson C. & Reed A. (1996). Editorial. *Journal of Psychiatric and Mental Health Nursing, 4,* 215–216.

Watson J. (1995). Postmodernism and knowledge development in nursing. *Nursing Science Quarterly, 8,* 60–64.

Wittgenstein L. (1953). *Philosophical Investigations* (tr. G.E.M. Anscombe). Blackwell, Oxford.

The Authors Comment

Paradigms Lost, Paradigms Regained: Defending Nursing Against a Single Reading of Postmodernism

Entering the 21st century, we were concerned with the growth in rhetoric in the United Kingdom about evidence-based nursing practice. It occurred to us that a narrow definition of evidence was being used, based largely in positivist or postpositivist ideas. In parallel, we noticed that there was a robust critique of postmodern ideas in nursing. However, to our (collective) mind, the critique was based in a reading of postmodernism through a traditional scientific lens. We wanted to argue that postmodernist nursing is not condemned to anarchistic relativism and retains a pragmatic notion of what is "good," that postmodernist nursing defines knowledge as transformable by nurses in everyday practice according to "peculiar" situation, and is what will enable them to sensitively help patients meet their needs.

—CHRIS STEVENSON
—IAN BEECH

Conversation Across Paradigms: Unitary-Transformative and Critical Feminist Perspectives

W. Richard Cowling III
Peggy L. Chinn

The purpose of this article is to convey a conversation that occurred over a period of months between a unitary-transformative scholar and a critical feminist scholar. The intention of our conversation was to uncover, through dialogue and engagement, ways in which these two paradigms might help us understand the forces and conditions which impede and may liberate full expression of health and well-being. Areas of essential tensions addressed were the relationships of action and theory, sense and soul, stories and numbers, and aesthetics and empirics. Critical conversational points were notions of liberation, consciousness and social conditions, unpredictability and acausality, and potentials for reconciliation that would serve nursing and society. We concluded that although there are significant differences that exist between the two paradigms, there are areas in which we might begin to speak with one voice for the betterment of nursing and health care.

At the National Forum on Doctoral Education in Nursing in 1992, representatives of four major paradigmatic perspectives in nursing shared the stage. The paradigms presented were the particulate-deterministic, interactive-integrative, unitary-transformative (Newman, Sime, & Corcoran-Perry, 1991) and feminist/critical theory. The focus of that conference was to articulate the impli-cations of these paradigms for the development of doctoral education in nursing. It was rare to have these four views discussed in one setting and, as representatives of two of these paradigms, we both found the experience illuminated the distinctions nursing knowledge and serving as context for the preparation of nursing scientists. It was the format of that particular conference that

Scholarly Inquiry for Nursing Practice: An International Journal, *2001, 15(4), 347–365.*

About the Authors

WILLIAM RICHARD COWLING, III, was born at Clark Air Force Base, Manila, Philippines, on December 10, 1948, where his mother and father were stationed after World War II. He received a diploma in nursing (1969) and then a BS from the University of Virginia (1972), an MS in psychiatric mental health nursing from Virginia Commonwealth University (1979), and a PhD in Nursing from New York University (1983). His hobbies and interests include gardening, feeding birds, reading, and watching movies that are unique in their presentation of life, and some of his other interests focus on his partner, daughter, 2 granddaughters, and animal companions Nina and V-tab. He is employed as a faculty member and teaches nursing concepts, theory development, and holistic and unitary perspectives and approaches applied to mental health issues and concerns. The focus of his scholarship is on unitary praxis related to the phenomena of despair and the life patterns of women living with despair. Key contributions made to the discipline are creating scholarship that provokes new and deepened understandings of despair in women, developing methods of inquiry specific to unitary research and practice, participating in promoting healing possibilities within women in despair, and supporting the development of students and others in learning about and using the unitary perspective in their work.

PEGGY L. CHINN earned her undergraduate nursing degree from the University of Hawaii and master's and PhD degrees from the University of Utah. She has authored books and journal articles in nursing theory, feminism and nursing, the art of nursing, and nursing education. Her recent research has focused on developing a method for aesthetic knowing in nursing and defining the art of nursing as an art. Her book, coauthored with Maeona Kramer, reflects this work and will be published in the sixth edition in 2003 under the title *Nursing Knowledge Development*. The fifth edition of her book *Peace and Power: Building Communities for the Future* was released in summer 2000. This book is used worldwide by women's groups and peace activist groups as a basis for group process, consensus decision making, and conflict resolution. With Richard Cowling and Sue Hagedorn, she cofounded the Nurse Manifest Project (http://www.nursemanifest.com), which incorporates emancipatory research projects to explore worldwide what it is like to practice nursing today. She is certified as a massage therapist and integrates therapeutic massage concepts and practices into teaching and peace work. She nurtures peace and tranquility in daily living by playing the harp, practicing yoga, gardening, walking, drumming and chanting, and petting her four-legged companions Cozie, Lavinia, and Sampson.

allowed presenters to give participants an encapsulated view of each paradigm represented and to describe implications for doctoral education after which the audience was given an opportunity to respond and/or ask questions of the four panelists. There was little time, however, for an in-depth conversation across these paradigms.

This article details a conversation between a unitary-transformative theory scholar and a critical feminist theory scholar. The dialogue focuses on areas of essential tension and mutuality between the two paradigms with the intent of creating the possibility of emergent reconciliation, elaboration, clarification, illumination, and innovation. A basic assumption underlying the conversation is that both of these paradigmatic perspectives individually have features which clearly serve nursing science and practice. Yet emerging ideas could arise from a conversation across the perspectives. We assumed that these ideas would serve to inform each perspective so that each individual perspective might be transfigured in unknown ways. We also thought there would be the possibility of an innovation in thinking that could contribute to a revolution in perspectives. We engaged in ongoing dialogue about these paradigms over several months. The article is a report and demonstration of the critical aspects of that conversation.

Comparison of Unitary-Transformative and Critical Feminist Perspectives

The authors wish to acknowledge that there are various interpretations of the essential elements of a unitary-transformative paradigm and a critical feminist paradigm. It is difficult to capture a singular set of assumptions that guides all practice and inquiry associated with the unitary-transformative paradigm. Newman, Sime, and Corcoran-Perry (1991, p. 4), however, outlined the major tenets of the unitary-transformative paradigm as follows:

- A phenomenon is a field embedded in a larger field and both are self-organizing.
- The field is characterized by pattern and its interaction with the larger whole.
- Fields interpenetrate and there is diversity within a unified field.
- Systems move through stages of organization and disorganization to more complexity creating change that is unidirectional and unpredictable.
- "Knowledge is personal, involves pattern recognition, and is a function of both viewer and the phenomenon viewed" (p. 4) and its substance includes thoughts, feelings, choices, and purpose.
- The reality of the whole is known through the inner reality.
- Caring in the human health experience could be understood and studied through viewing it as a unitary-transformative process of mutuality and creative unfolding.

One exemplar of the unitary-transformative paradigm is the science of unitary human beings (Rogers, 1970, 1992). Although the science of unitary human beings is an example of the unitary-transformative paradigmatic perspective, there are a few variations in view. These are critical assumptions of the science of unitary human beings:

- Humans and their environments are unitary, irreducible, indivisible, pandimensional energy fields.
- Humans and their respective environments are whole and cannot be understood through reduction to particulars.
- Human fields are distinguished by a unique pattern that is perceived through its manifestations.
- Humans and their environments are integral and always in mutual process.
- Change is continuous, relative, and innovative with increasing diversity of field patterning.
- Humans have the capacity to participate knowingly in change.
- The pandimensional nature of unitary fields implies an infinite nature that cannot be explained through causality; however, explorations of associations and connections among phenomena are useful in understanding, describing, and explaining unitary human beings and their world.

It should be noted that Rogers did not emphasize self-organization in her later writings (1992) and she preferred the phrase "mutual process" to the term "interaction" in describing the relationship between fields. Further, although Rogers relied heavily on systems theory as a foundation for her views (Rogers, 1992), it may be argued (Cowling, 1990) that her views more closely reflect a cognitive mode described by Koplowitz (1984) as transcending post-formal operations and systems thinking.

Berman and associates (1998) describe the major assumptions of the critical paradigm as:

- The focus of the critical paradigm, comprised of a variety of distinct modes of inquiry, is sociopolitical or structural change.

- The goal of the critical paradigm is to generate knowledge which contributes to emancipation, empowerment, and change.
- "All knowledge is value-laden and shaped by historic, social, political, gender, and economic conditions" (p. 3).
- Ideology is responsible for creating a social structure "that serves to oppress particular groups by limiting the options available to them" (p. 3).
- Knowledge is not generated for its own sake but is a form of social or cultural criticism.
- "Oppressive social structures can be changed by exposing hidden power imbalances and by assisting individuals, groups, or communities to empower themselves to take action" (p. 3).
- Research is viewed as praxis, embracing research and action in combination.
- The creation of knowledge that has the potential for producing change through personal or group empowerment, alterations in social systems, or a combination of these, is the primary agenda of the critical paradigm.
- People are valued as experts in their own lives and have an important stake in how issues are resolved.
- Causal explanation and interpretive understanding are acknowledged and valued as legitimate forms of knowledge.
- Critical scholars "do not wish to control and predict, or to understand and describe, the world; they wish to change it" (p. 3) and thus knowledge generated must meet this challenge.

In addition, Campbell and Bunting (1991) outline characteristics of a feminist perspective as follows:

- "women's experiences are the major 'object' of investigation;"
- "the goal of inquiry is to see the world from the vantage point of a particular group of women;" and
- "it is critical and activist in its effort to improve the lot of women and all persons." (p. 6)

Feminist approaches typically reflect the following threads and patterns:

- Unity and relatedness: dichotomies, exclusive categories, and absolutes are rejected—personal is political, and there are no sharp distinctions between work values and personal values, theory and practice, and knowing and doing.
- Contextual orientation: personal human relationships are valued and thought is directed away from independent discrete units to perceived relationships between objects, ideas, and action. Feminist thought has been described by Wheeler and Chinn (1984) as "oriented to the power of the whole as opposed to the power of division" (Campbell & Bunting, 1991, p. 7).
- Emphasis on the subjective: "Women value the lived experience, including the feelings of themselves, and other women" (Campbell & Bunting, 1991, p. 7).

Intentions and Structure of Conversation

The conversation was guided by the desire of both participants to illuminate the similarities and differences of the unitary-transformative paradigm and the critical feminist paradigm and to reach grounds of reconciliation. We viewed this conversation as vitally important, in part because nursing theory in general has remained essentially a-political and in part because feminism has remained essentially marginalized and not seriously integrated into nursing knowledge. Both of these issues are problematic from a critical feminist perspective. From a unitary-transformative perspective, in the absence of serious consideration of these issues, the unitary-transformative perspective remains situated in the realm of the individual person, a view which only marginally addresses the larger whole of context and society.

The goal of our conversation was to uncover, through dialogue and engagement, ways in which these two paradigms might help us understand the forces and conditions which impede, and which may liberate, full expressions of health and well-being. We both agreed that unitary theory specific to wholeness, uniqueness, and infinite possibilities and critical theory specific to emancipation, liberation, and empowerment had made and were making significant contributions to nursing and health care. Our intention was not to diminish the singular importance of each paradigm, but to push our own boundaries of understanding through these conversational encounters. And through pushing our own boundaries of understanding as they are informed by each paradigm, we hoped to envision new potentialities within a critical and unitary informed construction of nursing science and practice.

While we had thought there were some general reasons for engaging in such a conversation, we also wanted to acknowledge our individual commitments to such an endeavor. We wanted to go beyond the general reasons that we thought this would be a good idea to specific reflections we had related to the relevance of a conversation across these two paradigms. We also wanted to lay out our intentions clearly as a way of launching the conversation. At times throughout the conversation, we revisited this issue.

The structure for our conversation was an open-ended discourse associated with points of agreement and disagreement associated with the two paradigms as well as ways in which each paradigm may help inform some of the essential tensions in nursing science and practice. These essential tensions were defined as action and theory, sense and soul, stories and numbers, and aesthetics and empirics (Cowling, 1999). We had the conversation via e-mail and in two face-to-face encounters. We wanted the conversation to emerge naturally from our concerns. A structure emerged that shaped the content of the conversation and is reflected in this report of it. The structure developed around several key areas of discourse that surfaced:

1. Essential tensions in nursing science and practice related to action and theory, sense and soul, stories and numbers, and aesthetics and empirics.
2. Notions of liberation within each paradigm.
3. Issues of consciousness and societal conditions.
4. Implications of a unitary view of unpredictability and acausality for addressing the critical feminist's concerns with oppression.
5. Potential points of reconciliation.

Each of these key areas will be addressed in the sections that follow. Each section begins with a brief overview of the essential ideas that emerged in our conversation, along with a brief commentary concerning the limits of the conversation. Then, the conversation is presented as much as possible in its natural form to convey the true nature of this dialogue and engagement. There has been some modest editing for clarity and some elaboration of content at the suggestion of reviewers.

Essential Tensions in Nursing Science and Practice Related to Action and Theory, Sense and Soul, Stories and Number, and Aesthetics and Empirics

In this part of the conversation, we begin to explore the ideas of gender and social action (politics) that are central to a critical feminist perspective and the idea of wholeness that is central to a unitary-transformative perspective. We acknowledge common allegiances, at least implicitly if not explicitly, in each perspective to wholeness and social action.

Richard.   In a recent publication I articulated a view of essential tension that confronts the unitary-transformative scholar (Cowling, 1999). These tensions center on action and theory, sense and soul, stories and numbers, and aesthetics and empirics. I advocated for a posture in unitary science that would transcend the dichotomies inherent in these areas of tension. How do you see these tensions as relevant, if at all, to the critical feminist perspective?

Peggy.   I like how you have characterized these issues as tensions, but as you have explained, they are often felt as irreconcilable dichotomies. Each of the tensions you identified, and the unitary-transformative science perspective that you discuss as avenues to address each tension, are consistent with critical feminist ideas. For example, you propose a shift to a question of whether a theory offers provocative possibilities for action in addressing the theory/action tension. Your proposal to attend to all realms of data to address the sense and soul tension is consistent with a feminist commitment to view the whole. For the stories and numbers tension you suggest that both are needed, and both make valuable contributions to the development of science, which is at the heart of Ann Oakley's recent article titled, "Science, Gender, and Women's Liberation: An Argument against Postmodernism" (Oakley, 1998). You raise important questions and possibilities concerning the aesthetic and empirics tension. My own work with aesthetics suggests that aesthetics is an integrating pattern of knowing, bringing together all forms of knowing. From a feminist perspective, art and science have not always been viewed as separate, and need not be (Chinn, 1994). I am reminded here of Harding's wonderful chapter in the Omery, Kasper, and Page book. *In Search of Nursing Science*, titled "The method question" (Harding, 1995). Harding addressed the question, "Is there a unique feminist method?" and concluded that it is not method per se that accounts for the significance of feminist scholarship, but rather the epistemologic perspective that creates significant, albeit sometimes subtle, shifts in method. I think that your discussion of the tensions addresses epistemologies underlying nursing science, and the epistemologic stance that you propose is consistent with critical feminist perspectives.

To get more specific, feminist perspectives focus on healing the mind/body split, which you are suggesting can begin to happen with a unitary-transformative nursing science. What you have said about healing the tensions is consistent with feminist thinking in this regard, and in fact contributes quite significantly to this feminist "agenda." The two areas that don't come through here so clearly, and that critical feminist perspectives would bring to the discussion, are first, a deliberately political stance, and second, a gendered perspective. Having said that, I also subscribe to a feminist ideal held by some of transcending gender as we now know it. But in our present context a gendered perspective is necessary as a political stance.

Finally, I would like to comment that I think that there is an embedded feminist politic in the unitary-transformative perspective. The term "unitary" certainly implies wholeness, and the term "transformative" actually implies a powerful politic, particularly if one sustains Martha's notion of the wholeness of the person/environment. What is still missing is some guidance that defines the nature of transformations that we are seeking, which could be an essential tension between critical feminist and unitary-transformative perspectives.

Richard. Yes, I think that the nature of transformations being sought is a tension between the paradigms. In my own work I have tried to avoid the possibility of imposing what I think is the expected, or "best," transformation on the client/participant. I have tried to center the work in a highly participative fashion with the focus on the wholeness and uniqueness of the person as the primary vantage point. Yet, there could be an inherent tendency to project "unitary" expectations onto the situation and person.

One thing that I think is worth clarifying here is that with the unitary perspective it is implied that individuals are already whole and not reaching for wholeness. One of the issues that I keep seeing is that people don't often experience themselves as whole and that one of the experiences that creates liberation/transformation for some is to realize the interconnectedness of a variety of issues/experiences. This realization is a key attribute of the process of appreciation which is the essence of my unitary approach. Another entangled issue here is that of acausality. In the unitary-transformative perspective, it is most troublesome when you are dealing with change, and the source of change.

The gender issue is thorny within the unitary-transformative perspective. It occurs to me that while gender issues are not raised in a general way, being male or female is an aspect of the wholeness of experience. Perhaps, one avenue would be to look at society as a field and the ways in which gender beliefs/perceptions are associated with the field pattern. I concur that gender cannot be dismissed, and somehow a viable paradigm must account for this. I like the idea of looking at transcending gender. There is a theoretical view espoused by Wilber (1998) that addresses the universe as transcending and yet encompassing hierarchies or holarchies. I am not sure that this view would accommodate the unitary-transformative perspective because it implies level of being, rather than a unified, irreducible whole. But surely in a unified, irreducible whole perspective, the experience associated with, or specific to, gender must be included.

Peggy.   Actually, given our current gendered world, each of the tensions you identified carries gendered "weight," which renders quite a significant power imbalance. This, of course, implies a political tension as well, which also may explain some of the reasons that these tensions persist. As I think about this, there are nuances that need to be explored, but generally, "Action," "Soul," "Stories," and "Aesthetics" have feminine associations, and as a result, are the "disadvantaged" aspect of each of the tensions. It is interesting that nursing's growing acceptance of, and recognition of these aspects of the tensions, has coincided with the feminist movement of the past couple of decades. So I am wondering if some more discussion around the political potential within each of the tensions might provide one direction for our dialogue.

Richard.   Yes, it was clearly my goal in attempting to articulate the tensions that need attention in an evolving unitary-transformative science that we would face the question of our values and the agenda inherent in our worldview. Butcher (1999) has done an extraordinary job at discovering and enunciating the values of Martha E. Rogers that influenced her theoretical thinking. He did this through a process of ethical analysis and drew a substantive portrait of the value orientation of Rogers. I think that these values could be a starting point for explicating a unitary-transformative agenda.

What would the unitary-transformative take be on politics and the need for health care changes? One possible stance toward political change might be Williamson's (1997) idea of "dissent without contempt." It addresses the issue of the mutuality of human beings and how we might best knowingly participate with one another to serve needed change, rather than advocate for an argumentative process seeing those with whom we disagree as our political adversaries. The dissent without contempt notion would acknowledge the

right to dissent without having contempt for others. According to Williamson, "the greatest contribution a liberal can make to a political renaissance is to surrender his or her contempt for a conservative viewpoint, just as the greatest contribution a conservative can make is to surrender his or her contempt for a liberal viewpoint" (p. 111). I would say that in nursing we could substitute the words liberal and conservative with our various theoretical viewpoints and paradigm perspectives.

The reasons given for releasing ourselves from a stance of contempt are offered by Williamson (1997):

1. It undercuts our personal power by diminishing our insight and realization of our connection to others which is a foundation of true communication;
2. It is described as a low-level emotion (maybe low-frequency energy) or just simply better use of our personal energy; and
3. It creates a situation in which we are likely to withhold love or respect from our opponent.

Interestingly, Williamson says that to stay with contempt is to be stuck in the Newtonian paradigm, "keeping ourselves separate from the thing we wish to change and being therefore unable to do so" (p. 112). That notion of "non-separateness" or mutuality is an essential assumption of the unitary-transformative paradigm. This is described as waging peace.

Peggy.   Before we leave this topic, I want to reflect on the political nature of values. My favorite definition of "politics" is: the ability to enact one's values in the world. It seems to me that what you are describing above is a powerful politic based on a specific value and also suggests a clear agenda, waging peace.

Notions of Liberation Within Each Paradigm

In this part of the conversation we begin to explore a concept that is central to critical feminist perspectives, that of liberation. While not explicit in a unitary-transformative paradigm, transformation implies a major kind of change that is in an (implied) positive direction. We do not fully explain the concept of liberation, but rather focus here on exposing troublesome issues that emerge when we consider the notions of oppression and liberation (taken from a critical feminist perspective) and the notion of wholeness (taken from a unitary-transformative perspective).

Richard.   My opinion is that liberation is the goal of the unitary-transformative thinker, to overcome the oppression of narrowed, particularistic thinking. I think we accomplish that through engagement with those we care about, in an intimacy that awakens us to the oppression that exists, with an individual, or with a society. Critical social theory has much to offer us in general about liberation. In particular, I find the ideals of Paulo Freire in Pedagogy of the Oppressed (Freire, 1983) to have meaning for me as a unitary thinker and as a healing seeker from the standpoint of mutuality and knowing participation in change and what occurs in the praxis of appreciation. "A revolutionary leadership must accordingly practice co-intentional education. Teachers and students (leadership and people), co-intent on reality, are both Subjects, not only in the task of unveiling that reality, and thereby coming to know it critically, but in the task of re-creating that knowledge. As they attain this knowledge of reality through common reflection and action, they discover themselves as its permanent re-creators. In this way, the presence of the oppressed in the struggle for their liberation will be what it should be: not pseudo-participation, but committed involvement" (p. 51). To know one's being as unitary is ripe with potential for transformation.

Peggy.   Indeed, Freire's work has been a major influence in critical feminist perspectives, and is central to my own feminist theory of group process. There is a substantive criticism of his perspective that comes from feminist challenges to the patriarchal split of mind/body, self/other, and similar dichotomies. Freire's early work clearly painted a dichotomous oppressor/oppressed picture grounded in a Hegelian dialectic. While this can be interpreted as a dialectic whole, with one part of the dialectic dependent upon the existence of the other (which is Freire's interpretation), this per-

spective "places" people in one role or the other and in an adversarial relation to one another. Freire was quite clear that the oppressor could not and would not work on behalf of liberation of the oppressed, which to me contradicts the idea of interrelated wholeness fundamental to a unitary-transformative perspective.

Richard.   Yes, I agree that would be problematic from a unitary-transformative perspective. I think the idea of interrelated wholeness or mutual process would be a challenging point to Freire's view. I haven't thought about a unitary-transformative view of oppression. One thing I am sure of is that the unitary-transformative view would not separate out the oppressor and oppressed from the entire context of the wholeness of their existence and their mutual relationship with their respective environments. I think this raises serious issues for me and other scholars in this camp to tackle. More specifically, what would a unitary-transformative agenda have to say about the phenomenon of oppression? I don't have the answer yet.

Butcher (2000) has recently addressed issues raised by critical theorists in the context of the science of unitary human beings. He advocated forcefully for unitary research and practice that addresses "the need for emancipation or liberation of human beings from oppressive social systems and the patriarchal, racist, and authoritarian environments that suppress human caring values" (p. 50). He concludes that Rogers clearly promoted nursing's responsibility to deal with societal issues that might impede human health potentials. Further, he called for the reformulation and reconceptualization of issues of power and oppression within a unitary context and suggested that Rogerian praxis may be one avenue for transformation of oppressive perceptions.

Issues of Consciousness and Societal Conditions

At this point in the conversation, we move to a more fundamental issue that underpins any discussion of how individuals respond to social conditions and constraints: that of awareness or consciousness of social patterns. From a critical feminist perspective, in order to act to change oppressive social conditions, one must first become fully aware of the social conditions that limit one's freedom, and in so doing, acquire a very specific political agenda of social change. From a unitary-transformative perspective, all patterns, social and individual, constitute the whole, and there is not an explicit directive or agenda from which to develop social and political action.

Peggy.   Let's turn to the thorny issue of consciousness and false consciousness, and what is "real." If humans are, in fact, whole and one with their environment, then it seems to me that an agenda for unitary-transformative perspectives would be to fully realize this, and you talked about this earlier. If humans have to reach to realize their wholeness, this implies that we have been thoroughly socialized to see our reality as parts. Likewise, if being of one gender or another is truly socialized (which is the dominant feminist view of gender), then thinking of oneself as masculine or feminine would be a "false consciousness," that is, constructed for us by the socialization of our cultures. Actually this is roughly the perspective that David Allen, Karen Allman, and Penny Powers (1991) took in their article "Feminist nursing research without gender." This is truly a tension for me, because I resonate with their argument but still agree with Ann Oakley (1998) that retaining gender as a focus of concern is a vital feminist agenda that cannot yet be abandoned. From a critical theory perspective, all consciousness that sustains and creates oppression or advantage for some at the expense of others, is false consciousness, and coming to awareness of the circumstances of oppression brings forth an emancipatory interest that stimulates action toward liberation. Does this not imply a specific political agenda?

Richard.   I think the issue of "false consciousness" is an intriguing one. In the unitary-transformative view (which, by the way, I think is open to extension, elaboration, and evolution), a central idea is that we are energy existing in patterns of wholeness. In reality,

Martha Rogers never dealt with consciousness. It is Margaret Newman (1997) who made the leap into health as expanding consciousness. I think consciousness/awareness is a significant avenue for one to understand the wholeness of pattern, and it is simultaneously a tool to grasp the awareness of mutuality with one's environment (includes all beings and entities). When you realize that consciously we are all connected, this is a shift, perhaps responsible for the realization that harming another harms ourselves. I sometimes think that this perspective renders the issue of causality irrelevant. If everything is mutual, it is automatic that change is mutual. In addition, unitary thinking suggests that separateness of events or entities is an illusion. So one separate thing is not acting on another separate thing; all is one acting together. I admit that it is somewhat strange to think in this way.

My own experience in practice is that when the concept of appreciating the wholeness of the underlying pattern is applied to human experience/condition/situation that there is an awareness of the interrelatedness of events that contribute to the particular situation. For instance, one of my clients related the story of her experience as a little girl in which she is told that a boy who harasses her on the playground "only likes her" and that when she gets shoved on the ground and her chin is hurt and she ends up in a clinic, the doctor uses mercurochrome to paint over the injury creating a big orange smile on her face to show her what a good thing it is that she got this from an admirer. This makes everyone laugh. So this is an experience that has energetic manifestations that contribute to how this woman relates to male partners and how she sees herself in power relationships as well as in a myriad of other ways. Discovering this led the woman to literally rewrite stories of her life with different endings as part of the pattern appreciation process.

I think all this fits together with emancipation through knowing or being aware of the wholeness/oneness of everything. This might be considered a form of new consciousness. In Rogerian science terms, I think awareness through knowing participation in change would be the theoretical take on this situation. The woman had a deep appreciation of the relevance of this and other similar incidents throughout her life as an aspect of the wholeness of her experience. This theme of not being acknowledged, much less valued, was manifest throughout her dreams, in the way she thought about the world, in the way she carried her body, in the sensations of her body, in the choices she made about clothes or what to eat, and on and on. I think she experienced revelations in knowing wholeness that led her to think and act in different ways.

Peggy.   Societal patterns or political patterns are actually one with our individual patterns, which I guess accounts for acquiring a consciousness that is not consistent with our own liberation. What about the idea of a collective consciousness? How would unitary-transformative perspectives account for what we are socialized to see and what might otherwise be?

Richard.   It is clear that Martha Rogers thought that the concept of energy fields could be applied to individuals as well as groups. As a matter of fact, Rogers (1992) wrote that a group energy field could be a family, a social group, a community, or any other combination. So it would be possible, and fully understandable, for this irreducible societal field to have a collective consciousness. Again, Rogers favored awareness rather than consciousness because of the potential for misunderstandings associated with how the term consciousness has been used in non-unitary ways in other disciplines. The notion of consciousness from a unitary-transformative perspective, however, has been articulated by Newman (1994) and I think that her work has deepened our understanding of the phenomenon of consciousness. I think that a unitary view of consciousness would encompass many ways of knowing and avenues of awareness consistent with the wholeness of all experience.

Returning to the question of a specific political agenda, I think the agenda would most certainly embrace the idea that we need to move beyond the fragmentation inherent in our current health care system toward practices/actions that are essentially participa-tive and focused on uniqueness and wholeness of human experience.

Implications of the Unitary View of Unpredictability and Acausality for Addressing the Critical Feminist Concerns of Oppression

From the perspective "outside" a unitary-transformative stance, the notion of acausality is quite perplexing. From within a unitary-transformative stance, the notion of acausality is challenging in that it is a vast leap from the typical assumptions of cause and effect on which scientific logic is based. Critical feminist perspectives firmly situate problems of injustice and oppression, or of unequal power relations in the world, as arising from systematic patterns of social and political dominance, patterns that benefit a few at the expense of many. In this part of the conversation, we explore various views and interpretations that can be brought to bear on the concepts of "causality" and "acausality." We are reaching here for a potential frame from which to reconcile, or expand, or shift, how we understand these unitary-transformative ideas in light of critical feminist concerns for social justice.

Richard.   The unitary-transformative paradigm embraces an ontological view of acausality and unpredictability as reflective of the nature of change. This is a logical extension of the notion of a pandimensional universe (Rogers, 1992), a domain without spatial and temporal attributes. Rogers described pandimensionality as a "way of perceiving reality" (p. 31) and pandimensional as providing "for an infinite domain without limit" (p. 31). Moss (1995) communicates the connection between a pandimensional (infinite) domain and acausality and unpredictability (revelation) more directly in his writing. Moss points out that "causality ceases the moment we become referent to infinity" (p. 66) and that having infinity as the referent point means that "the universe and human beings are revelation happening" (p. 66). From the view of infinity (pandimensionality), "there is no definite causal explanation for our suffering or for our joy. Certainly we suffer, but we are not merely victims. We are that which is transformed in the suffering. Nothing is frozen; everything is unfolding, evolving" (p. 67).

In translation, the focus of nursing science is on the possibilities for revelation that exist in a pandimensional universe that would guide knowledge development and inform practice in new ways. Thus, for example, in dealing with the experience of despair as a nursing phenomenon, I am interested in the wholeness of the experience of despair or in unitary science terms, the unitary pattern that underlies all manifestations of human-environmental mutual process. I decided in my own work that I needed to develop myself as an instrument to appreciate and acknowledge the wholeness of human experiences consistent with the pandimensionality of the universe. Despair is an aspect of the pattern that provides an avenue for understanding the wholeness of human experience. Despair is examined in the context of this wholeness. This means a clear re-orientation to the experiences that a person would bring to my awareness. So rather than seeking the causes for despair, my goal is to understand the pandimensional nature of despair. This means appreciating how an individual's despair transcends time and space; that is that it is connected to a perceived past, an experienced present, and an anticipated future all at once.

An inclusive stance about what counts as evidence is requisite in reaching for the wholeness of human experience. Attention to the mutuality of persons and the environment, including all living and non-living entities, is significant to apprehending the nature of experience. In other words, the focus is upon the abundance of experiential, perceptual, and expressive phenomena that form the tapestry of the person's life. Inherent in the unitary-transformative worldview, change arises out of mutual human-environment process rather than being caused by environment. Individuals are considered to have the potential for knowing participation in change. Knowing one's wholeness creates an orientation that can lead to transformation, taking awareness beyond perceived boundaries and constraints.

Peggy.   Definitely, acausality is a problem from a critical feminist perspective. I feel like this is another space where I have been so thoroughly "taught" to see cause, or to think in terms of cause, that I can hardly imagine acausality, even though there are glimpses. If human experience evolves unidirectionally and in a patterned way, it seems somewhat inconsistent with the idea of acausality, which to me implies chaos, and, from the little I understand of chaos theory, even that implies some order emerging, otherwise, how would we even recognize chaos?! Sometimes it has helped me to think of "influence" as distinct from cause, but only momentarily! For example, if we take as plausible that consciousness is constructed, it seems to me that there are many influences that "build" the construction, but also, every little thing that comes together to build the construction can also be seen as an interrelated web (pattern) and is systematically coming together to sustain the construction, and that seems very deliberate. Marilyn Frye (1983) speaks of this very eloquently in her book of essays, *The Politics of Reality*. She likens all the "littler" things that construct oppression as being like a bird cage; if you look at each wire one at a time, you cannot see why the bird cannot fly free. But when you look at the entire cage, and realize that the wires are all connected to form a web, then it is perfectly obvious why the bird cannot fly free. The cage is not exactly a "cause," but it certainly is the systematic constraint that keeps the bird contained, and in that way can be viewed as a cause, a reason. Anyway, talk to me more about this issue of causality.

Richard.   Yes, the description of the birdcage is a perfect one! I do not think that the unitary-transformative world view would deny the existence of attempts to constrain human expression. Rather, it would offer a way to see the integral nature of these attempts and one's experience. Perhaps the stance would be toward understanding how these constraints contribute to experiential, perceptual, and expressive phenomena that comprise the pattern of wholeness of that individual. Also, as I said earlier, Martha Rogers (1992) thought that you could apply this to groups by seeing them as unitary energy fields. So it would be interesting to think of women as a field of energy and look at the ways in which constraints contribute to the central experiential features of women's lives. I think, regardless of an individual or group focus, a unitary-transformative understanding of the integral nature of constraints and experience of women would lead to action toward removal of these constraints.

Peggy.   This is very helpful. One caution that many feminists bring to the table is the problem of essentializing women, that is assuming that all women share common traits or experiences and ignoring or overlooking each woman's unique experience and perspectives. Women of color, who often bring this concern to the discussion, find race and class to be powerful factors in their experience that White feminists too often overlook. So it seems that energy fields could be defined with more and more parameters until you actually come right back to the individual in all of his or her uniqueness. And then, you add the dimension of time, I am a different person than I was when I was born, but I still have essential energy patterns that characterize me as me.

Richard.   Going back to Moss (1995), he described the potentialities of the present (or what Rogers called the relative present) in pretty dramatic terms that would be consistent with a unitary-transformative "take" on change. "The present is always infinitely potential, always as fresh and ripe with inception as the very moment of the Big Bang or the birth of life from the archaic seas billions of years ago. The present is ever ready to surprise us with a movement and a possibility we can never really imagine and never fully control. This is precisely our dread, and the good news" (p. 67). This has been the only thing that I have found that made me really comfortable with acausality and unpredictability. At the same time, I am troubled by the idea that somehow this could be used to excuse behavior that I view as harmful: the experience of the little girl above.

It is difficult as a practitioner of unitary nursing to reconcile the idea of the unitary theoretical position of acausality with the experience that what I do in practice, using strategies based on unitary thinking, creates a context for change. The way in which I act is important: washing and bathing an old person who has soiled him- or herself through uncontrolled defecation is not a mere physical act (as I argued once at a gerontological conference with someone who said theory was unimportant to nursing home workers). It is a holistic expressive energetic act that conveys a totally different message and experience when one views it as such (theoretically) and acts in concert with this theory. In other words, thinking of it as more than a physical act means I will likely treat it as more than a physical act and the client will experience it beyond the physicality of it. I am working to describe these experiences in which the "how we are" and the "making a difference" are linked without being causal.

Peggy.   I am thinking that we don't have a good language for this thing we are trying to call "cause." Causality (in the context of talking about acausality) seems to be linked with the idea of a specific agent that has a linear effect. But what about the meaning of that by which something is accomplished (I practice the harp to be able to play it well), or that which provides a reason (I need food for dinner tonight so I go to the market), or something that influences a decision or moves to action (I realized that other women have been subjected to ridicule and that the ridicule is unjust and that I can change my experience). All of these instances are not really "causes." From most critical feminist perspectives, social conditions (including socialization, cultures, governments, structures, institutions) create conditions that render advantage for some and disadvantage for others. Individual choices are often limited, and actually, I am wondering here if we might talk a bit about choice and free will. It seems to me that "will" implies the ability to exert one's effort to at least influence something to happen. I think that unitary-transformative science can be interpreted along these lines. You have said that within this paradigm, everything is possible. From a critical feminist perspective, when people become aware of the constraints of social and political conditions that limit what is possible, then their emancipatory interest is awakened and they begin to see possibilities beyond the limitations. Is this a point that can be reconciled between the two perspectives?

Richard.   Yes, I think this could be a point of reconciliation. I like your reaching to move beyond the concept of "cause" to something more meaningful both from a unitary-transformative and a critical feminist perspective. I think this warrants further conceptual and theoretical development within unitary-transformative science. Again, I am troubled by the difficulties of making a case for the relevance of unitary-transformative practice related to our "acausality" stance. There is something that happens in the encounters I have with clients/participants that I would not label as causal, but as participative action that supports expanded possibilities for change. Your suggestion of attending to the free will and choice issue reminds me of the work of Elizabeth Barrett (Barrett, Caroseli, Smith, & Smith, 1997), whose conceptual, theoretical, and empirical work on what is known as the "power to participate knowingly in change" theory is very useful. The dimensions of this view of power include awareness, choices, freedom to act intentionally, and involvement in change. This actually integrates consciousness or awareness with choice, freedom, and participation or involvement in creating change.

Potential Points of Reconciliation

Peggy.   First, I am wondering, are we really looking to reconcile the two perspectives? I think I have been assuming that we are, in part because of your interest in bringing a critical perspective to your work. But, it could be that your own emerging theory will be required to sort some of this out!

I want to go back to your point about wanting to respond to unjust situations (like the little girl who is hurt on the playground) more specifically than is implied in a unitary-transformative perspective. Clearly, responding to such situations is a major concern from

a critical feminist perspective. But I think that there is room for some reconciliation here. First, the unitary-transformative perspective regarding appreciating the whole, and patterns within the whole, is very closely related to what actually happens in the feminist process that we call consciousness raising. This process does deliberately seek, and deliberately interpret insight from a political perspective, and from a perspective that implies action to right the injustice. All too often, however, consistent with my comments earlier about Freire's work, the stance becomes an adversarial one, even among those of us committed to a feminist world characterized by cooperation, caring, and nurturing. I think we tend to respond to our rage, however justifiable. Maybe some rage would light a unitary-transformative fire, but seriously, your recognition that some sort of response to the specific situation of injustice as well as the need for response on a more global level, is perhaps the spark! What I would like to propose is that we draw on Williamson's work, and my work with Peace and Power processes (Chinn, 1999), and the Rogerian perspective of pattern and wholeness, and perhaps construct a feminist unitary-transformative "stance" toward injustice. There are other models, feminist and otherwise, that I think offer a lot to think about here, for example, the premises of civil disobedience. As you mentioned earlier, the idea is not to prescribe what to do, but rather to articulate, and then live, an attitude, one that comes from seeing all of us as part of a political/cultural pattern that addresses the other not as other but as a kindred spirit that seeks to make peace, that is grounded in values of human health and wholeness, and so forth.

As far as causality and acausality are concerned, I know that there is a very complex philosophic challenge here that I am not prepared to address, but my sense is that the idea of "knowing participation in change" from a unitary-transformative perspective and consciousness raising and political action from a feminist perspective offer some ground from which to construct an alternative notion that could help to understand how change comes about and the ways in which humans shape, change, or participate in their life patterns.

In addition, I think that some of our conversation around gender also informs an emerging concept related to cause. I think the problem with the dominant modern causal model (modern used here as used in postmodernism) is that it oversimplifies reality, seeking a linear model that provides a single explanation for any phenomenon. Feminist scholars who bring gender to the table also bring many other aspects of the world to the table and consistently search for awareness of all of the context, background history, human capabilities, spiritual forces, any aspect of the whole that one can imagine, that all of these be taken as part of what creates any experience or phenomenon—or, in Rogerian terms, what creates a pattern. Certainly this is central to a unitary-transformative perspective, but from a critical feminist perspective the dimensions that have been constructed to create advantage for some and disadvantage for others are clearly named and deliberately examined as part of the whole. Somehow it makes sense to incorporate a way to "name" the interrelated patterns as a way of bringing a political awareness into our emerging critical feminist unitary-transformative perspective.

Richard. I think your suggestions are compelling and represent an actual innovation in thinking that could be a bridge between the two perspectives. The critical feminist perspective brings to the unitary-transformative perspective the possibility of a consciousness that would ground social action and serve to make a strong case for the relevance of unitary-transformative thinking for humankind. I am intrigued and challenged by your proposal to explore ways to integrate the work of Williamson and your work on Peace and Power with the Rogerian perspective of pattern and wholeness. At the risk of being somewhat overly dramatic, but consistent with my own sense of passion, we may be forging a manifesto aimed at a revolution or liberation in nursing that would support the betterment of all people. I am also excited by the possibilities that your new conceptualization of change might bring. The alliance of the ideals of the unitary-transformative "knowing participation in change" with feminist "consciousness raising and political action," would be an-

other area rich with possibilities. Think how nursing could benefit by sharing the energies and passions of these two forces in nursing!

Summary and Conclusion

As we reflect on having this conversation and reporting it, we are struck by several revelations. First, the conversation provided an opportunity to explore and challenge each other's assumptions about the paradigms. We both came away with a deeper understanding of the paradigms. Second, the unitary-transformative and critical feminist perspective share in common a strong inclination toward transcending the dichotomies described as essential tensions in nursing science and practice. Third, a unitary-transformative scholar may make a unique contribution to the conceptualization of oppression through the lens of wholeness and mutuality. Fourth, unitary-transformative and critical feminist perspectives share in common a possible social agenda that calls for a participative health care system with a focus on the wholeness of human experience. This would require an examination of the notion of consciousness and its relationship to societal and political patterns. And finally, the alliance of the unitary-transformative ideal of "knowing participation in change" and the critical feminists' ideal of "consciousness raising and political action" could create a new model of change that would address issues of causation and prediction that are troublesome in both views. Although there are significant differences that exist between the two paradigms, we concluded that there are areas in which we might begin to speak with one voice for the betterment of nursing and health care.

One Voice. We came to this conversation open to the possibilities that might come from exchange across paradigms. We were uncertain, given the differences, that reconciliation in any form could occur. We certainly have not achieved reconciliation, but we have raised important issues and have suggested some possibilities. These possibilities deserve a much more in-depth philosophic exploration. But we see this as an inauguration of a promising integration of ideas that might address nursing's stance relative to social injustice and respond to the calls of society for a deeper appreciation of and a more passionate support of human experience in health care.

REFERENCES

Allen, D., Allman, K. K. M., & Powers, P. (1991). Feminist nursing research without gender. *Advances in Nursing Science, 13*(3), 49–58.

Barrett, E. A. M., Caroseli, C., Smith, A. S., & Smith, D. W. (1997). Power as knowing participation in change: Theoretical, practice, and methodological issues, insights, and ideas. In M. Madrid (Ed.), *Patterns of Rogerian knowing* (pp. 31–46). New York: National League for Nursing.

Berman, H., Ford-Gilboe, M., & Campbell, J. C. (1998). Combining stories and numbers: A methodological approach for a critical science. *Advances in Nursing Science, 21*(1), 1–15.

Butcher, H. K. (2000). Critical theory and Rogerian science: Incommensurable or reconcilable. *Visions, 8*(1), 50–57.

Butcher, H. K. (1999). Rogerian ethics: An ethical inquiry into Rogers's life and science. *Nursing Science Quarterly, 12,* 111–116.

Campbell, J. C., & Bunting, S. (1991). Voices and paradigms: Perspectives on critical and feminist theory in nursing. *Advances in Nursing Science, 13*(3), 1–15.

Chinn, P. L. (1994). Developing a method for aesthetic knowing in nursing. In P. L. Chinn & J. Watson (Eds.), *Art & aesthetics in nursing* (pp. 19–40). New York: National League for Nursing.

Chinn, P. L. (1999). *Peace & power: Building communities for the future* (4th ed.). Boston: Jones & Bartlett.

Cowling, W. R. (1999). A unitary-transformative nursing science: Potentials for transcending dichotomies. *Nursing Science Quarterly, 12,* 132–137.

Cowling, W. R. (1990). A template for unitary pattern-based nursing practice. In E. A. M. Barrett (Ed.), *Visions of Rogers' science-based nursing* (pp. 45–65). New York: National League for Nursing.

Freire, P. (1983). *Pedagogy of the oppressed.* New York: Continuum.

Frye, M. (1983). *The politics of reality: Essays in feminist theory.* Freedom, CA: The Crossing Press.

Hagedorn, S. (1995). The politics of caring: The role of activism in primary care. *Advances In Nursing Science, 17*(4), 1–11.

Harding, S. (1995). The method question. In A. Omery, C. E. Kasper, & G. G. Page (Eds.), *In search of nursing science* (pp. 106–126). Thousand Oaks, CA: Sage.

Koplowitz, H. (1984). A projection beyond Piaget's post-formal operations stage: A general system stage and a unitary stage. In M. L. Commons, F. A. Richards, & C. Armon (Eds.), *Beyond formal operations* (pp. 272–295). New York: Praeger.

Moss, R. (1995). *The second miracle: Intimacy, spirituality, and conscious relationships.* Berkeley, CA: Celestial Arts.

Newman, M. A. (1997). Experiencing the whole. *Advances in Nursing Science, 20*(1), 34–39.

Newman, M. A. (1994). *Health as expanding consciousness* (2nd. ed.). New York: National League for Nursing Press.

Newman, M. A., Sime, A. M., & Corcoran-Perry, S. A. (1991). The focus of the discipline of nursing. *Advances in Nursing Science, 14*(1), 1–6.

Oakley, A. (1998). Science, gender and women's liberation: An argument against postmodernism. *Women's Studies International Forum, 21*(2), 133–146.

Rogers, M. E. (1970). *An introduction to the theoretical basis of nursing.* Philadelphia: F. A. Davis Co.

Rogers, M. E. (1992). Nursing science and the space age. *Nursing Science Quarterly, 5,* 27–33.

Wheeler, C. E., & Chinn, P. L. (1984). *Peace and power: A handbook of feminist process.* Buffalo, NY: Margaretdaughters.

Wilber, K. (1998). *The marriage of sense and soul: Integrating science and religion.* New York: Random House.

Williamson, M. (1997). *The healing of America.* New York: Simon & Schuster.

Offprints. Requests for offprints should be directed to W. Richard Cowling, III, RN, PhD, School of Nursing, Virginia Commonwealth University, 1220 East Broad Street, P.O. Box 980567, Richmond, VA 23298–0567.

The Authors Comment

Conversation Across Paradigms: Unitary-Transformative and Critical Feminist Perspectives

I was inspired to create a real-life conversation relative to these two paradigms because of the values, perspectives in each as relevant to nursing science and art in general and my work with women in particular. I turned to Peggy as an expert in critical feminist perspectives and as a person who valued engagement and dialogue to have a conversation that would provoke extended understandings of these two paradigms. Peggy writes: I was inspired to engage in this dialogue with Richard because Rogerian theory and the unitary transformative perspectives have always inspired me. My own work has focused on theory development, aesthetic patterns of knowing, and community activism grounded in critical feminist theory, all of which share common elements and some values, bringing a unique emphasis which enlarges one's view of what is possible. We believe that this work makes a contribution to theory development in nursing because it moves away from an isolationist stance concerning paradigms. This conversation is ongoing, and, we hope, inspires others to join this dialogue and to pursue other dialogues across paradigms.

—WILLIAM RICHARD COWLING III
—PEGGY L. CHINN

Caring Science and the Science of Unitary Human Beings: A Trans-Theoretical Discourse for Nursing Knowledge Development

Jean Watson
Marlaine C. Smith

Background. *Two dominant discourses in contemporary nursing theory and knowledge development have evolved over the past few decades, in part by unitary science views and caring theories. Rogers' science of unitary human beings (SUHB) represents the unitary directions in nursing. Caring theories and related caring science (CS) scholarship represent the other. These two contemporary initiatives have generated two parallel, often controversial, seemingly separate and unrelated, trees of knowledge for nursing science.*

Aim. *This paper explores the evolution of CS and its intersection with SUHB that have emerged in contemporary nursing literature. We present a case for integration, convergence, and creative synthesis of CS with SUHB. A trans-theoretical, trans-disciplinary context emerges, allowing nursing to sustain its caring ethic and ontology, within a unitary science.*

Methods. *The authors critique and review the seminal, critical issues that have separated contemporary knowledge developments in CS and SUHB. Foundational issues of CS, and Watson's theory of transpersonal caring science (TCS), as a specific exemplar, are analysed, alongside parallel themes in SUHB. By examining hidden ethical-ontological and paradigmatic commonalities, trans-theoretical themes and connections are explored and revealed between TCS and SUHB.*

Conclusions. *Through a creative synthesis of TCS and SUHB we explicate a distinct unitary view of human with a relational caring ontology and ethic that informs nursing as well as other sciences. The result: is a trans-theoretical, trans-disciplinary view for nursing knowledge development. Nursing's history has been to examine theoretical differences rather than commonalities. This trans-theoretical posi-*

Watson J. & Smith M. C. Copyright © 2002; Journal of Advanced Nursing *37(5), 452–461*

About the Authors

JEAN WATSON is Distinguished Professor of Nursing and holds the Murchinson-Scolville Chair in Caring Science at the University of Colorado Health Sciences Center (HSC). She is founder of the original Center for Human Caring and previously served as Dean of the University of Colorado HSC School of Nursing. She is a Past President of the National League for Nursing. Born in West Virginia, July 21, 1940, Dr. Watson earned undergraduate and graduate degrees in nursing and psychiatric-mental health nursing and holds her PhD in educational psychology and counseling. Dr. Watson is known for her theoretical work on the art and science of human caring. Her latest books and articles address empirical measurements of caring and new postmodern philosophies of caring and healing that bridge paradigms and point toward transformative models for the 21st century. Dr. Watson is the recipient of many awards and honors, including an international Kellogg Fellowship in Australia, a Fulbright Research Award in Sweden, five honorary doctoral degrees, the National League for Nursing's Martha E. Rogers Award, New York University's Distinguished Nurse Scholar Award, and the Fetzer Institute's Norman Cousin's Award. Her hobbies include international travel, skiing, hiking, biking, and writing.

MARLAINE C. SMITH is Associate Dean for Academic Affairs and Director of the Center for Integrative Caring Practice at the University of Colorado Health Sciences Center School of Nursing. Born in Pittsburgh, PA, Dr. Smith received her BSN from Duquesne University, her MNEd and MPH from the University of Pittsburgh Schools of Nursing and Public Health, and her PhD in Nursing from New York University. Dr. Smith's prominent areas of research and creative work are nursing philosophy, metatheory, unitary theoretical perspectives, and processes and outcomes of healing. Her current scholarly work has examined healing outcomes of touch therapies and unitary perspectives on caring and healing. In 1999, Dr. Smith received the National League for Nursing's Martha E. Rogers' Award for excellence in the advancement of nursing science. She enjoys walking in the Colorado sunshine, the arts, crocheting, and Italian cooking.

tion moves nursing toward theoretical integration and creative synthesis, vs. separation, away from the 'Balkanization' of different theories. This initiative still maintains the integrity of different theories, while facilitating and inviting a new discourse for nursing science. The result: Unitary Caring Science *that evokes both science and spirit.*

Keywords: Rogers' science of unitary human beings, caring science, Watson's transpersonal caring theory, unitary caring science, trans-theoretical, trans-disciplinary

. . . While from the bounded level of our mind
Short views we take, nor see the lengths behind;
But more advanced, behold with strange surprise
New distant scenes of endless science rise!

—ALEXANDER POPE

Introduction

The focus of this paper is the exploration of the evolution of caring science (CS) and its relationship with the science of unitary human beings (SUHB). These two contemporary initiatives have generated two parallel, often controversial, seemingly separate and unrelated, trees of nursing knowledge. We offer a trans-theoretical view of these two, often-differing perspectives by considering commonalities. This trans-theoretical view offers a new discourse for nursing science. These two directions have emerged during the past three to four decades as nursing has made great strides in its knowledge and theory building. Part of this evolution has encompassed specific caring theories, as well as developments in nursing models, nursing science, and a variety of nursing theories.

Several frequently cited nursing writers represent developments of specific caring theories (for example, see earlier works of Leininger 1978, 1990, Watson 1979, Ray 1981; Gaut 1983, Gadow 1985, Roach 1987, Boykin & Schoenhofer 1993, Swanson 1999, Eriksson 1997, Eriksson & Lindstrm 1999). However, while there are various and differing perspectives on caring theory, caring itself is noted to transcend any particular model or theory and increasingly is acknowledged as central to the professional discipline of nursing (Watson 1990, Newman *et al.* 1991, Smith 1999).

Likewise, Roger's SUHB has informed the work of a cadre of nursing scholars and new generations of nurses and doctoral students who adopt a unitary view of human that transcends any one nursing model or specific theory. The past tendency in nursing theory and scholarship has been to examine theoretical differences, which separate, rather than unite ideas, thus inhibiting creative evolution of ideas. We offer a critique and overview of CS and SUHB, which maintains the integrity of differences, while also explicating shared themes that mutually inform and transform both perspectives. A trans-theoretical, trans-disciplinary discourse in nursing knowledge development is generated.

Background of Caring Theory and Its Evolution in Nursing Knowledge Development

Three major categories of caring knowledge development that transcend individual theories were identified by Boykin and Schoenhofer (1993) as: the ontological,

that is, caring as a manifestation of being in the world; anthropological, that is the meaning of being a caring person; and ethical or the obligative nature of caring. A fairly recent critique of caring research was completed by Swanson (1999). She completed a meta-analysis of 130 publications of empirical caring studies. Sherwood (1997) did a similar review by conducting a meta-analysis of qualitative studies of caring in nursing research. Their work helped to emphasize ethical aspects of caring processes and outcomes of caring in nursing and their intersection with empirical findings in the literature. For example, both of these meta-analyses acknowledged caring knowledge and ways of being that affect both personal and professional practices, for better or for worse, for patients as well as for nurses.

These empirical findings and conceptual orientations toward caring offer some directions for substantive nursing knowledge development and locate ethical and empirical caring within the context of nursing science. Further, these views of caring knowledge development help to reveal caring as a philosophical-theoretical-epistemic undertaking, not just a nice way of being. Rather, caring is an ethical, ontological and epistemological project requiring on-going exploration and expansion. As Mayeroff (1971) reminded us, we need knowledge to care.

> We sometimes speak as if caring did not require knowledge, as if caring for someone, for example, were simply a matter of good intentions or warm regard. . . To care for someone, I must know many things. . . such knowledge is both general and specific (Mayeroff 1971, p. 13).

> . . . Caring . . . includes explicit and implicit knowledge, knowing that and knowing how, and direct and indirect knowledge . . . (Mayeroff 1971, p. 15).

Critique of Caring Knowledge

In spite of the ontological, epistemological and ethical views, and diverse categories of caring knowledge, and in spite of Mayeroff's philosophical charge about needing different forms of caring knowledge (e.g. general, specific, explicit, implicit, direct, indirect) a recent publication by Paley (2001) critiqued both the pursuit of caring knowledge, as well as the approaches toward development of caring knowledge in nursing. By using Foucault's archaeological view of knowledge as his lens, Paley (2001) suggests that nursing scholars' view of knowledge of caring is dated and faulty. It can be reduced to ' . . . knowledge of things said, a chain of association, constantly expanded, constantly repeated (p. 9).' His conclusion is that the effort to generate caring knowledge is for all intents and purposes unattainable: thus, caring is ' . . . an elusive concept, which is destined to remain elusive-permanently and irretrievably (p. 9).'

Paley (2001) categorized the major approaches used in the nursing literature to generate caring knowledge. For example, descriptions of caring, collection of things said about caring, knowledge of caring via association, attributes of caring and aggregation via accumulation. In his critique he laments the fact that (1) this approach does not yield knowledge, and (2) each effort leads to continued efforts to constantly retrieve caring from its elusiveness (via these varying faulty approaches), ' . . . only to return, again and again' . . . (p. 2) to (the elusive concept) and conclude again it is elusive and needs additional study.

Paley's tautological conclusion and critique of caring knowledge is related to an earlier review by Morse et al. (1990) where they classified diverse nursing authors' work on caring into five categories of caring: caring as human trait; caring as moral imperative; caring as affect; caring as interpersonal interaction; and caring as therapeutic intervention. Morse et al. (1990) concluded, as did Paley (2001) that caring is left without any clarity as a concept because of its diversity.

It is important to respect the fact that both Paley (2001) and Morse et al. (1990) offer some new, provocative perspectives of information related to how caring is treated in the nursing literature. Further, these thorough, analytic critiques of caring knowledge mirror back to the profession the diversity and complexity and, yes, even more so, the elusiveness, of caring. They cause nursing and caring scholars to pause and reconsider the nature of caring and knowledge.

While both these efforts to critique caring literature highlight the diversity, complexity, and scope of perspectives, both critiques ignore any examination or discussion as to the unique philosophical-ontological, or paradigmatic worldviews in which the different work, or approaches to the study of caring, were located. The most serious weakness of these meta-level critiques is that they are a-contextual, and a-paradigmatic with respect to the moral-ontological foundation of the work. Caring looks differently depending upon the ontological and ethical perspective in which the 'approaches' and 'categories' are located. Without specifying the ontology one indeed cannot understand caring within it.

Foucault (1972) acknowledged that while the 'group of elements formed in a regular manner by a discursive practice . . . can be called *knowledge*, . . . knowledge is also the space in which the subject may take up a position and speak of the objects with which he (sic) deals in discourse . . . knowledge is also the field of coordination and subordination of statements in which concepts appear, are defined, applied and transformed . . . lastly, knowledge is defined by the possibilities of use and appropriation offered by discourse . . . its articulation on other discourses or on other practices that are not sciences' (Foucault 1972, p. 182, 183).

Thus, caring knowledge and its diversity and complexity can be seen in another, deeper context than Paley (2001) identifies, that is consistent with Foucault's broader view of knowledge. The above critiques did not seek to identify the underlying ethical, obligative, or ontological perspectives of caring as a relational way of Being Human, that engages out humanity; this being one of the most prominent core views of caring in the literature (see Smith 1999 for more depth discussion of these issues). Rather, both major critiques of caring literature (Morse *et al.* 1990, Paley 2001) paradoxically seemed to engage in the very exercise they critique. That is, at the meta-level, they accumulate words and total lists, categories, and approaches to study of caring. These were derived from a detached analysis of text, without an engagement of the ideas of caring or context espoused by the authors. This view of detached information is related to Lithuanian-French philosopher Levinas (1906-1995), and his critique of some of the writings on Heidegger and Husserl when he noted: 'To comprehend the tool is not to look at it but to know how to handle it' (in Nortvedt 2000, p. 6).

Foucault (1971) himself noted that there are dimensions (of knowledge) that are not invested in scientific discourses alone, but in a 'system of . . . values . . . an analysis that would be carried out not in the direction of the episteme, but in that of what we might call the ethical' (p. 193). Fleming's (2001) recent critique of nursing knowledge called for the notion of *phronesis* as a guide for critiquing nursing knowledge. He pointed out that *phronesis* emphasizes deliberation (reflection) and moral action—reminding us that *phronesis* requires that the ' . . . context of the situation be considered very carefully . . . ' (p. 251) with respect to knowledge and action. Indeed in the recent work of Nortvedt (2000) he claims that 'knowledge, and in particular clinical knowledge, rests on a precondition . . . ' (p. 10)—the precondition, being ethical sensitivity and value-laden experience.

Without addressing moral-ethical context, and ontological foundations, what results are more bits of information with a hard conclusion that has the impression of an attempt to totalize the discourse, which shuts off the debate as well as further pursuit of caring knowledge. De-contextualized bits of information, whether obtained at the specific level of analysis, or at the meta-level, do not equal understanding. As Critchley emphasized in his work on Levinas, 'ethics (and caring) is not a spectator sport' (p. 29). Human caring contains judgements, moral values as well as knowledge *per se*. There are moral, ethical insights that underpin the diverse approaches and categories, which are not acknowledged by these recent critiques of caring literature.

Thus, what is missing in these important critiques of caring in nursing literature is the fact, that first and foremost, and most deeply, caring is first and foremost an ethic, laden with moral values. Caring is a value-laden human condition which, according to Nortvedt (2000) is a precondition for proper clinical knowledge. Drawing upon the philosophy of Levinas (1969) we suggest the human encounter of caring exists as an 'ethic of first philosophy' (Levinas 1969) where caring is understood (with all its categories, lists, attributes, collection of words, approaches, meta-analyses, etc.) as a value-laden relation of infinite responsibility to self and others.

We do agree with Paley (2001) and Morse et al. (1990) for different reasons, that is, that engaged, ethical, value-laden caring, truly is ineffable and ultimately unknowable; it is unknowable because it is an engaged moral relational human to human living experience that is alive in the moment, not an objective phenomenon, *per se*. With Levinas (1969) the infinity of other as an ethical event, is the opening *towards* knowledge, *towards* epistemology, but it is not knowledge (Nortvedt 2000, author's italics).

Because of the deep relational, obligative ethical nature of caring, much of the caring literature does not claim to provide us with new knowledge *qua knowledge*, in terms of themes or categories, or even fresh discoveries. Rather, knowledge of caring is much like what 'Wittgenstein called *reminders*, of what we already know (at some deep human experiential level) but continually pass over in our day-to-day living' (Critchley 2002, p. 10).

Levinas (1969) reminded us *ethics is otherwise than knowledge* (Critchley 2002, p. 15) and ethics is not reducible to epistemology. Indeed, knowledge of caring is, like most of the important ideas in the history of humankind that seek to define and sustain our humanity, ineffable, difficult to describe and incomprehensible. However, just because concepts such as caring, suffering, love, beauty, God and so on are 'elusive' we struggle to capture their essence because of their importance. We always fall short, and will continue to fall short. Nevertheless, we strive to know them through many different methods and approaches, we seek descriptions, qualities, attributes, etc. as well as how they are experienced.

Perhaps the most important conclusion with this debate is to acknowledge that caring cannot be reduced to comprehension and empirical knowledge alone, that we so earnestly seek. It is perhaps because of the very reality of what Levinas framed as the 'face-to-face relation.' Indeed, perhaps it is because of this very elusive, deep unknowable, relational obligatory human-to-human aspect of caring that calls nurses paradoxically to continually pursue it. As Paley (2001) puts it ' . . . only to return, again and again, to a concept no less ambiguous and confused, than before, the goal to all intents and purposes unattainable' (p. 2). The one-to-one human engagement, in an ethical caring moment will forever remain unknowable, and elusive, but forever sought after, just as beauty and truth.

Evolution of Caring Science

In spite of critiques of caring in nursing and even attempts to eliminate caring as an essential concept for nursing, we witness that over the past two to three decades the focus on caring and caring knowledge development in nursing has indeed not ceased, but has continued to even accelerate. For example, the International Association of Human Caring is now into its 24th year of supporting scholarly publications and presentations. The relatively new journal *The International Journal of Human Caring* is dedicated to disseminating scholarship related to human caring. *The Scandinavian Journal of Caring Science* has been in existence since the eighties. In 1995 the American Nurses Association revised its definition and policy statement of nursing, to include caring. Major national conferences and think tanks have acknowledged caring as core in nursing theory and knowledge development (Stevenson & Tripp-Reimer 1990 report of American Academy of Nursing and International Sigma Theta Tau 1989 Wingspread Conference).

In spite of, or because of, the still controversial unresolved discourse about caring knowledge and caring as meta-level concept for the discipline, caring has become more formalized through nursing theories and research, and has been enhanced by scholarship in other related fields of study, such as ecology, education, ethics, and theology (For more information see Mayeroff 1971, Gilligan 1982, van Hooft 1995, Noddings 1984, Watson 2002). With this, there is a growing recognition of Caring as a philosophical-ethical-epistemic field of study. As work has advanced in multiple spheres, a more formal CS framework is emerging for nursing and other related fields; thus caring scholarship has moved toward cross-disciplinary activities and intersections. For example, CS departments and academic structures for nursing have become more prominent. The field of CS has been long standing in Scandinavian countries, e.g. Finland, Sweden, and Norway.

From a knowledge development standpoint, caring theory and knowledge are located within nursing science as well as other disciplines. Thus, caring knowledge is increasingly trans-disciplinary, that is, transcending several disciplines. Caring knowledge and practices affect all health, education, and human service practitioners. Thus, CS is emerging as a distinct field of study within its own right.

Nursing's disciplinary focus on the relationship of caring to health and healing differentiates it from other disciplines that relate caring to the unique concerns of their domain. However, because of recent trans-disciplinary developments in caring scholarship, it is helpful to identify some major foundational assumptions that seem to inform CS and scholarship.

A working set of assumptions for CS, include the following:

- Developing knowledge of caring cannot be assumed; it is a philosophical-ethical-epistemic endeavour that requires on-going explication and development of theory, philosophy, and ethics, along with diverse methods of caring inquiry that inform caring-healing practices.
- Caring science is grounded in a relational ontology of unity within the universe (in contrast to a separatist ontology that guides conventional science models); this relational ontology of caring establishes the ethical-moral relational foundation for CS (and for nurs-

ing) and informs the epistemology, methodology, pedagogy and praxis of caring in nursing and related fields.

- Caring science embraces epistemological pluralism, seeking the underdeveloped intersection between arts and humanities and clinical sciences, that accommodates diverse ways of knowing, being-becoming, evolving; it encompasses ethical, intuitive, personal, empirical, aesthetic, and even spiritual/metaphysical ways of knowing and being.
- Caring science inquiry encompasses methodological pluralism whereby the method flows from the phenomenon of concern, not the other way around; the diverse forms of caring inquiry seek to unify ontological, philosophical, ethical, and theoretical views, while incorporating empirics and technology.

A Working Definition of Caring Science

Caring science is an evolving philosophical-ethical-epistemic field of study that is grounded in the discipline of nursing and informed by related fields. Caring is considered by many as one central feature within the meta-paradigm of nursing knowledge and practices. The development of CS is informed by an ethical moral stance with a relation of infinite responsibility to other human beings (Levinas 1969); this view encompasses a humanitarian, human science orientation to human caring processes, phenomena, and experiences. It is located within a worldview that is nondualistic, relational, and unified, wherein there is connectedness of all. This worldview is sometimes referred to as a unitary transformative consciousness paradigm (Newman *et al.* 1991, Watson 1999) nonlocal consciousness (Dossey 1991) and Era III medicine/nursing (Dossey 1991, 1993, Watson 1999).

Caring science thus intersects with the arts and humanities and related fields of study and practices, including for example, ecology, peace studies, philosophy-ethics, women/feminist studies, theology, education, and mind-body-spirit medicine and the growing field of complementary medicine, health and healing.

Reconciling Caring Dissonance: Within the SUHB and Nursing Meta-Paradigm

While CS, including caring theories in nursing, has been emerging over these past decades, Rogerian Science has escalated as pre-eminent, revolutionizing nursing as well as related disciplines. But there has been little integration of the common foundational elements of CS and the SUHB.

Indeed, as already highlighted through the critiques of Morse *et al.* (1990) and Paley (2001), the inclusion of caring as a central and defining concept within the discipline of nursing continues to be contentious (Smith 1999). Rogers had serious concerns about caring being named within nursing's meta-paradigm, or as part of the essence of nursing. She was concerned that it would not advance the discipline of nursing nor generate substantive knowledge for practice.

Rogers' worldview offered, and continues to offer a new vision and conceptual system for generating and addressing phenomena related to unitary life processes. Thus, Rogers viewed caring as an important stance to the practice of any human service field, but not as a substantive area of knowledge development for nursing (Smith 1999).

What is more significant within the area of theory and knowledge development, is the fact that CS and SUHB have coexisted, over these past few decades, almost as two separate trees of knowledge. Both areas were pursuing their individual interests without exploring the common philosophical-ontological foundation and scientific assumptions that they may share. These common foundations may strengthen the advancement of nursing knowledge for this new century. For example, both the Society of Rogerian Scholars and the International Association of Human Caring hold scientific sessions. The papers presented have overlapping themes and yet there is little to no connections or communication between the two scientific groups.

This dissonance between CS and the SUHB, including the ambivalence about caring and its location with the disciplinary matrix of nursing, is still a tense undercurrent in nursing knowledge development circles. However, there are some noted exceptions.

Newman *et al.* (1991) offered a significant contribution to the evolution of including caring within the disciplinary matrix, by acknowledging in their critique of the existing meta-paradigm, that caring and health are linked within the theoretical literature of nursing. They then posed a manifesto of sorts with their well-known statement that sought to integrate caring into the meta-paradigm: 'Nursing is the study of caring in the human health experience' (Newman *et al.* 1991, p. 3).

Further, they acknowledged the use of different paradigms for knowledge claims and explication of (caring) knowledge. The three well-known paradigms they named are (Newman *et al.* 1991):

- particulate-deterministic—isolated phenomena, reducible entities with definable measurable properties;
- interactive-integrative—extension of particulate-deterministic, plus context, experience and subjective data; and
- unitary-transformative—representing a significant paradigm shift, whereby phenomena are viewed as unitary and self-organizing, embedded in a larger self-organizing field, which is whole and unified.

Another major work that attempted to explore new relationships between caring knowledge and its paradigm location is Smith's seminal work in 1999. She tried to break the exclusivity of these two separate trees of knowledge development within nursing, i.e. CS and SUHB.

Smith (1999) 'critiqued the critique' of caring in nursing. In contrast to the previously mentioned Paley (2001) and Morse *et al.* (1990) critiques, Smith located consistent ontological perspectives from extant caring theory, within the SUHB. By working at the onto-logical-ethical level she was able to clarify how caring resides within the SUHB; she explicated points of congruence between existing literature on caring and shared meanings in the SUHB. Smith identified five constitutive meanings of caring from a wide range of caring theories. Each of these meanings was conceptually lo-

cated within the SUHB system: (1) caring is a way of manifesting intentions; (2) caring is a way of appreciating pattern; (3) caring is a way of attuning to dynamic flow; (4) caring is a way of experiencing the infinite; (5) caring is a way of inviting creative emergence.

Smith (1999), recently Watson and Smith (2000), and earlier work of Newman *et al.* (1991) attempted to extend the discourse about caring at the meta-paradigm level. These works reflect the commonalities of a caring ontology that apply to a range of caring theories. Further, both locate particular scholarship on caring and the SUHB within the unitary-transformative framework, i.e. 'patterning, dynamic flow, manifesting intentions, and experiencing the infinite'; these features go beyond conventional particulate or interactive models for explaining phenomena, reflecting a world view that resides within the unitary-transformative paradigm.

This next section seeks to extend these intersecting connections between CS and SUHB, within the unitary-transformative paradigm. An overview of Rogers' SUHB will be followed by a summary of one specific theory of caring: Watson's transpersonal caring theory. The transpersonal caring theory will be used as an exemplar for the CS model to reflect the intersections with Rogers' SUHB.

By expanding the discourse on nursing knowledge development, a new evolution for nursing, caring knowledge and trans-theoretical theory development unfolds. Further, by exploring the convergence of ideas within the two systems, there is advancement of knowledge that transcends nursing, and contributes to a trans-disciplinary future for nursing in the wider arena of human health science.

Overview of Rogerian SUHB

Parallel with, and prior to, the evolution of caring theories in nursing, and the emergence of CS as a field of study, was the renowned work of Rogers (1970). Her views of nursing science and the concept of the SUHB (Rogers 1970, 1992, 1994) were posed as the disciplinary focus for nursing.

A review of basic principles of the SUHB is offered as a contextual backdrop for examining how the two specific systems can converge and extend each other for new possibilities. Rogerian science, from its inception, was located within the now emerging unitary consciousness worldview, labelled by Newman *et al.* (1991) as unitary-transformative: that is, phenomena are viewed as a unitary, self-organizing field, embedded in larger self-organizing field, recognized by pattern interaction within the whole.

Tenets of Rogerian SUHB and the unitary-transformative paradigm (Barret 1990, Rogers 1992) are shown in Table 46-1. Rogers' work initiated a new paradigm for nursing science. For example, her theoretical basis for nursing makes explicit the connectedness of all, a unitary, irreducible mutual human-environmental

Table 46–1
Tenets of Rogerian Science of Unitary Human Beings

Energy field	The fundamental unit of the living and the nonliving. Field is a unifying concept. Energy signifies the dynamic nature of the field; a field is in continuous motion and is infinite
Environment (environmental field)	An irreducible, indivisible, pandimensional energy field identified by pattern and integral with the human field
Pandimensionality	A nonlinear domain without spatial or temporal attributes
Pattern	The distinguishing characteristic of an energy field perceived as a single wave
Principle of resonancy	Continuous change from lower to higher frequency wave patterns in human and environmental fields
Principle of integrality	Continuous mutual human-environmental field processes
Unitary human beings (human field)	An irreducible, indivisible, pandimensional energy field identified by pattern and manifesting characteristics specific to the whole and which cannot be predicted from knowledge of the parts

field process. Further, her introduction of energy field as the fundamental unit of the living and nonliving, making 'energy field' an explicit unifying concept was revolutionary in its time.

The evolution within science itself, correspond with the ontology worldview articulated by Rogers's (1970). This revolutionary ontology propagates changes in epistemology, methodology, and practice that are consonant with it. To further explore the specific ontological connections between SUHB and CS it is helpful to highlight the internal features of CS vise a vise a specific caring theory.

Caring Science and SUHB: Transpersonal Caring Theory as Exemplar

Watson's theory of transpersonal caring (Watson 1979, 1985, 1988, 1995, 1999) is one extant caring theory, among others, that has emerged as a guide to practice and education for nursing and related fields. In addition transpersonal caring serves as a disciplinary framework to guide knowledge development related to both nursing and the emerging trans-disciplinary field of CS. Transpersonal caring theory is located within a CS framework. The next section provides an overview of some of the basic ingredients of transpersonal caring theory. For heuristic purposes it will be referred to as transpersonal caring science (TCS) to demonstrate parallel and intersecting connections with SUHB.

Central tenets of TCS are:

- The transpersonal caring field resides within a unitary field of consciousness and energy that transcends time, space, and physicality (unity of mind-body-spirit nature universe).
- A transpersonal caring relationship, connotes a spirit to spirit unitary connection within a caring moment, honouring embodied spirit of both nurse and patient, within the unitary field of consciousness.
- A transpersonal caring moment, transcends the ego level of both nurse and patient, creating a caring field with new possibilities for how to be in the moment

['. . . the process goes beyond itself, and becomes part of the life history of each person, as well as part of the larger, deeper complex pattern of life' (Watson 1985, p. 59)].

- A nurse's authentic intentionality and consciousness of caring has a higher frequency of energy than non-caring consciousness, opening up connections to the universal field of consciousness and greater access to one's inner healer.
- Transpersonal caring is communicated via the nurse's energetic patterns of consciousness, intentionality, and authentic presence in a caring relationship.
- Caring-healing modalities are often noninvasive, non-intrusive, natural-human, energetic environmental field modalities.
- Transpersonal caring promotes self-knowledge, self-control, and self-healing patterns and possibilities.
- Advanced transpersonal caring modalities draw upon multiple ways of knowing and being; they encompass ethical, and relational caring along with those intentional consciousness modalities that are energetic in nature, e.g. form, colour, light, sound, touch, visual, olfactory, etc. that potentiate wholeness, healing, comfort, and well-being.

Transpersonal Caring Science and SUHB

Drawing upon the above assumptions from TCS, it is now possible to extend more explicitly Smith's (1999) previous integration of caring and SUHB. For example, the following unifying statements amplify the integration of TCS and SUHB:

- The intention of transpersonal caring expands in open, resonating, concentric circles from self to other to Planet Earth to universe. It includes caring consciousness, and participating knowingly in human-environment energy field patterning;
- The nurse's authentic presence, consciousness and intention in a caring moment manifests caring field patterning;
- The nurse's presence and caring consciousness potentiate change in the field, by cocreating human-environment patterning from lower frequencies to higher frequencies (i.e. caring consciousness carries higher energy frequencies than noncaring consciousness);
- Transpersonal caring resides within a field of caring consciousness and energy that transcends time, space, physicality, and is one with the universal field of consciousness (spirit)—the infinite.

Table 46–2
Shared Notions of the Concepts in Both SUHB and TCS

Rogers SUHB	Watson's TCS
Pandimensionality	Transpersonal-transcends time, space, physicality, is grounded in the 'eternal now' of the caring moment
Infinity	Universal field of consciousness—connects with infinity
Resonancy	Consciousness is energy—caring consciousness manifests high frequency energy waves
Body—manifestation of energy field	Postmodern body = light, energy, consciousness (body resides in universal field of consciousness—see Watson 1999)
Integrality (mutual human-environment field process)	Mutuality of caring relationship within caring field.
SUHB: Healing modalities: noninvasive, meditative modalities, energy guided processes, therapeutic touch, healing environments: light, colour, harmony, intentional mutual patterning of human-environmental field; pattern manifestations appraisal and repatterning	TCS: Caring-healing modalities: Ethical relational, and energetic through caring consciousness, intentionality, presence, authenticity; noninvasive, nonintrusive, natural-environmental healing modalities; those modalities that help to connect with universal field to access inner healer; intentional conscious use of form, colour, light, energy, sound, touch, visual, consciousness, etc.

Through this process, we find shared notions of the concepts in both the SUHB and TCS in Table 46-2.

> To see a World in a Grain of Sand
> And a Heaven in a Wild Flower,
> Hold infinity in the palm of your hand
> and Eternity in an hour.   —WILLIAM BLAKE

SUHB and TCS: Trans-Theoretical Integration and Extensions of Shared Commonalities

In considering transpersonal caring as an exemplar of CS that intersects with some foundational aspects of SUHB, we find harmony in diversity that can advance the trans-theoretical discourse in theory and knowledge development in nursing science. In exploring relationships between the parallel nursing theoretic structures, we find philosophical and theoretical convergence. Some of the more specific commonalities between SUHB and TCS are as follows:

- both TCS and SUHB reside within a unitary-transformative paradigm, honouring the universal oneness and connectedness of all.
- both TCS and SUHB share unitary perspectives related to mutuality of human (caring) processes, whereby a caring moment potentiates the emergence of a new human-environmental energy field pattern.
- both TCS and SUHB are comingled and extended, by integrating principles of energy and resonancy (from SUHB), with caring consciousness (from TCS). For example, we extend the SUHB by asserting from TCS that the *caring consciousness of the nurse is a higher human-environmental field wave pattern than that of noncaring or ordinary consciousness. We extend TCS by integrating principles of resonancy into caring consciousness and caring field. Further, we make significant connections between SUHB and TCS

by attending to the human-environmental field pattern cocreated with the one-caring and the one-cared for.
- by relating transpersonal (caring) consciousness from TCS with pandimensionality from SUHB, we better understand that caring consciousness transcends time, space, and physicality and is open and continuous with the evolving unitary consciousness of the universe.
- by acknowledging caring as the ethical and moral foundation from TCS and relating that to SUHB we make explicit the imperative of an ontological-philosophical view for nursing, committed to knowledgeable, compassionate human service.
- drawing from both SUHB and TCS we make explicit an expanded view of what it means to be human, thereby acknowledging the unitary, transpersonal, evolving nature of humankind, both immanent and transcendent and continuous with the evolving universe.
- when energy field of SUHB and its continuous, infinite motion is integrated with TCS we see the connection with the mystery, the infinite, the universal field of cosmic consciousness energy, of living and nonliving.
- by integrating consciousness and energy from the two systems we evolve a unitary caring science that affirms a deep relational ethic and spirit, which transcend all duality, thus invoking the infinite, which in turn invites the sacred to return to our profession and our practices.

When nursing evolves to a point whereby it can embrace a model of knowledge development that includes both science and spirit, and incorporates both caring and unitary perspectives, we enter into a new level of deep knowing about the nature of reality. This turn makes explicit an expanding unitary, energetic worldview with a relational human caring ontology. As we evolve as a profession and discipline to this new level we are invited to consider new ways of knowing, being-becoming, and doing as *unitary caring human beings in continuous relation with an evolving universe.*

It is here in this new turn that caring and nursing knowledge development is transformed from frag-

---

*Note: Rogers did not incorporate consciousness into her system; the relationship between consciousness and energy is emerging within transpersonal caring theory as well as mind-body science.

mented bits of information into a unified framework for deep wisdom; here is where we more fully can experience and accommodate the empirical with the invisible; the subtle essence of the whole universe within each caring moment. It is here in these deeper dimensions that we are invited to explore the mystical with the empirical, the transcendent with the immanent, the embodied spirit of energy and consciousness and how they potentiate and mediate health and healing for self and others. If nursing continues to mature toward this deep nondualistic knowing, we shift from material particulate medicine/nursing to nonphysical phenomena and healing processes that requires new visioning, deep knowing, imagination, and creative trans-theoretical emergence for an open universe of possibilities.

Policy and Practice Implications

The policy and practice implications of this discourse results in further movement toward trans-theoretical and trans-disciplinary approaches and alliances in both scholarship and practice. By examining consistent ideas across theories, that are located within the same paradigmatic perspective, nursing moves away from fixed categories that set the debate and 'Balkanize' theoretical developments. By pursuing unities rather than theoretical differences nursing avoids locking theories into isolated 'silos' where there can be little dynamic flow. The movement toward transtheoretical integration and creative synthesis still maintains the integrity of each theory, while enabling nurses to join together on policy and practice issues that are important to multiple groups (e.g. International Association of Human Caring; Society of Rogerian Scholars; International Holistic Nursing Groups and Organizations; International Reflective Practice Conference Groups, etc.). Further, such efforts can unite nurses from different specialties, and even subspecialty groups to participate in trans-theoretical discourse and study by generating research/scholarship teams that cut across conventional units and systems. New theory-guided practice models may emerge that

integrate and synthesize unitary caring from two theoretical approaches that are internally consistent, thereby facilitating implementation and evaluation of advanced practice professional nursing *qua nursing* models.

Moreover, and most importantly, the trans-theoretical directions of CS and SUHB are congruent with the deep relational ethical caring covenant that nursing has held with its public across time around the world. By pursuing trans-theoretical unitary caring scholarship and practice, nursing is helping to sustain and live out its highest commitment to humankind and society.

Conclusions

Creative synthesis of TCS and SUHB can facilitate new directions for trans-theoretical knowledge development. The integration and extension of two previously disparate trees of nursing knowledge development, invite ethical-ontological and epistemological scholarship for further inquiry. By integrating nursing's unique TCS ontology with SUHB we point toward a new trans-theoretical discourse for nursing knowledge that is both discipline-specific, and trans-disciplinary in nature. In doing so, nursing's unique knowledge of transpersonal caring for unitary human beings can inform and extend other health and human service fields. Further, trans-theoretical scholarship can generate advanced theory-guided practice models that creatively unite ideas, rather than locking theories into fixed boxes, inhibiting their application and evolution.

Finally, as the search for trans-theoretical meaning continues, a *Unitary Caring Science* emerges. Together TCS and SUHB knowledge can advance contributions to human kind. Ultimately, while never fully comprehending the 'elusive' infinity of relational human caring, these continuing pursuits help to sustain nursing's relational caring ethic of infinite responsibility to other and humanity itself. One of Martha's hopes for the open-ended nature of all of science was that knowledge would continue to evolve to benefit the care of people in an ever-changing world (Rogers 1992).

REFERENCES

Bartret E. A. M. (ed.) (1990) *Visions of Rogers Science Based Nursing*. National League for Nursing, New York.

Boykin A. & Schoenhofer S. (1993) *Nursing as Caring*. NLN, New York.

Critchley S. (2002) Introduction. In *The Cambridge Companion to Levinas* (Critchley S. & Bernasconi R., eds), Cambridge University Press, Cambridge, in press.

Dossey L. (1991) *Meaning and Medicine*. Bantam, New York.

Dossey L. (1993) *Healing Words*. Harper, San Francisco, CA.

Eriksson K. (1997) Caring, spirituality and suffering. In *Caring from the Heart: The Convergence of Caring and Spirituality* (Roach S. ed.), Paulist Press, New York, pp. 68–84.

Eriksson K. & Lindstrm U. (1999) A theory of science for caring science. *Hoitotiede* **11**, 358–364.

Fleming D. (2001) Using *Phronesis* instead of 'research-based practice' as the guiding light for nursing practice. *Nursing Philosophy* **2**, 251–258.

Foucault M. (1972) *The Archeology of Knowledge* (translated by A. M. Sheridan Smith). Pantheon Books, New York.

Gadow S. (1993) Covenant without cure: letting go and holding on in chronic illness. In: *The Ethics of Care and the Ethics of Cure: Synthesis in Chronicity* (Watson J. & Ray M. A. eds), National League for Nursing, New York, pp. 5–14.

Gaut D. A. (1983) Development of a theoretically adequate description of caring. *Western Journal of Nursing Research* **5**, 313–324.

Gilligan C. (1982) *In a Different Voice*. Harvard University, Cambridge.

van Hooft S. (1995) *Caring. An Essay in the Philosophy of Ethics*. University Press of Colorado, Boulder, CO.

Leininger M. (1978) *Tran-Cultural Nursing*. John Wiley and Sons, New York.

Leininger M. (1990) Historical and epistemologic dimensions of care and caring with future directions. In *Knowledge about Care and Caring: State of the Art and Future Developments* (Stevenson J. S. & Tripp-Reimer R., eds). American Academy of Nursing, Kansas City, MO, pp. 19–31.

Levinas E. (1969) *Totality and Infinity*. Translated by A. Lingis. Duquesne University, Pittsburgh, PA.

Mayeroff M. (1971) *On Caring*. Harper & Row, New York.

Morse J. M., Solberg S. M., Neander W. L., Bottorff J. L. & Johnson J. L. (1990) Concepts of caring and caring as concept. *ANS* **13**, 1–14.

Newman M. A., Sime A. M. & Corcoran-Perrry S. A. (1991) The focus of the discipline of nursing. *ANS* **14**, 1–6.

Noddings N. (1984) *Caring*. University of California Press, Berkeley, CA.

Nortvedt P. (2000) Clinical sensitivity: the inseparability of ethical perceptiveness and clinical knowledge. *Scholarly Inquiry for Nursing Practice* **14**, 1–19.

Paley J. (2001) An archeology of caring knowledge. *Journal of Advanced Nursing* **36**, 188–198.

Ray M. A. (1981) A philosophical analysis of caring within nursing. In *Caring: An Essential Human Need* (Leininger M. M. ed.), Slack, Inc., Thorofare, NJ, pp. 25–36.

Roach S. (1987) *The Human Act of Caring*. The Canadian Hospital Association, Ottawa, Canada.

Rogers M. E. (1970) *An Introduction to the Theoretical Basis of Nursing*. F. A. Davis, Philadelphia, PA.

Rogers M. E. (1992) Nursing science and the space age. *Nursing Science Quarterly* **5**, 27–34.

Rogers M. E. (1994) The science of unitary human beings: current perspectives. *Nursing Science Quarterly* **2**, 33–35.

Sherwood G. D. (1997) Metasynthesis of qualitative analysis of caring. *ANS* **3**, 32–42.

Smith M. (1999) Caring and science of UHB. *ANS* **21**, 14–28.

Stevenson J. S. & Tripp-Reimer T. (eds) (1990) Knowledge about care and caring. In *Proceedings of a Wingspread Conference*, 1–3 February 1989. American Academy of Nursing, Kansas City, MO.

Swanson K. (1999) What is known about caring in nursing science? In *Handbook of Clinical Nursing Research* (Hinshaw A. S., Fleetham S. & Shaver J. eds), Sage, Thousand Oaks, CA, pp. 31–60.

Watson J. (1979) *Nursing: The Philosophy and Science of Caring*. Little Brown, Boston, MA. (1085) Reprinted. Colorado Associated University Press, Boulder, CO.

Watson J. (1985) *Human Science and Human Care*. Appleton-Century, Norwalk, CT. Reprinted (1988) NLN, New York. Reprinted (1999) Jones & Bartlett, Boston, MA.

Watson J. (1988) New dimensions of human caring theory. *Nursing Science Quarterly* **1**, 175–181.

Watson J. (1990) Caring knowledge and informed moral passion. *Advances in Nursing Science* **13**, 15–24.

Watson J. (1995) Nursing's caring-healing paradigm as exemplar for alternative medicine. *Alternative Therapies* **1**, 64–69.

Watson J. (1999) *Postmodern Nursing and Beyond*. Churchill-Livingstone/Harcourt Brace, Edinburgh, Scotland/New York.

Watson J. (2002) Caring and nursing science: contemporary discourse. In *Assessing and Measuring Caring in Nursing and Health* (Watson, J.), Springer, New York, pp. 11–19.

Watson J. & Smith M. (2000) Revisioning caring science and the science of unitary human beings. *Paper Presented at Boston Knowledge Development Conference*, Boston, MA.

The Authors Comment

Caring Science and the Science of Unitary Human Beings: A Trans-Theoretical Discourse for Nursing Knowledge Development

We were inspired to write this article for several reasons. First, the editor invited us to respond to an article by John Paley critiquing the caring literature. Second, we recognized and appreciated the convergent ontologic themes between Rogers' Science of Unitary Human Beings and Watson's evolutionary work on caring science. Finally, we wanted to advance the possibilities of transtheoretic work in nursing. For some time, nursing has focused on the differences among our paradigms and theories. It may be time to examine some common ideas across theories to strengthen the coherence of our disciplinary voice in health and healing care.

—Jean Watson
—Marlaine C. Smith

Nursing Theory and Practice

This unit addresses links between theory, knowledge development, and nursing practice. Theory is linked to practice through middle range theory, nursing aesthetics, pragmatism, and praxis. The theoretical ideas of two noted theorists of nursing's past, Rosemary Ellis and Hildegard Peplau, are presented in reference to their progressive notion about the dynamic link between practice and theory long before it was fashionable in nursing. Contemporary thought in other articles reveals that nursing is beginning to embrace their vision; practice is no longer the passive recipient of theory. Rather, practice and theory form a reciprocal process in the development of knowledge. Philosophies presented that support this thinking include moderate realism, neopragmatism and praxis.

The Practitioner as Theorist

Rosemary Ellis

When Gulliver traveled to Laputa, land in the clouds, he found rapt theorists wandering about construct-ing useless ideas. And, generally, that is what we think of theorists. This author, though, says that theo-rists in nursing are not the ivory-tower thinkers; they are the nurses who work directly with patients. With every patient, she explains, we select an approach, then use, modify, and expand it—whether or not we are conscious of doing so. Because theories in a field have a powerful, long-term influence on the di-rection that field will take, the author pleads that we struggle to make already-existing, implicit nursing theories—such as TLC, for example—clear and explicit, so that nursing will develop in the direction of more skilled bedside care.

Nursing has been called an applied science. It is, in the sense that it is the application of knowledge from the basic sciences. But nursing care, or nursing practice, is something more. It is not the simple transfer of basic science knowledge. The nurse does not practice chem-istry, anthropology, or sociology. She must sort out, se-lect, adapt, and infer from her basic science knowledge.

She uses some of the knowledge, orientations, processes of study, or models from these sciences as a guide to understanding patients, their pathology, and therapeutic practices.

This selection, adaptation, and sometimes interpo-lation from the basic sciences must be done by the prac-titioner. The physiologist or anthropologist cannot pre-

About the Author

ROSEMARY ELLIS was born in Berkeley, CA. She received an AB degree in economics and a BSN from the University of California, Berkeley-San Francisco, followed by an MA in nursing education and a PhD in human development from the University of Chicago. At the time of her death in the fall of 1986, she was a Professor of Nursing, a position she held at Case Western Reserve University since 1964. Dr. Ellis authored more than 30 articles, book chapters, and other scholarly works, including four in the *Japanese Journal of Nursing Research*. She emphasized the importance of pursuing questions about the substantive structure and description of nursing. Her metatheoretical writings have had a significant influence on nursing. The 1993 article "Rosemary Ellis' views on the substantive structure of nursing" by Donna Algase and Ann Whall, published in *Image: Journal of Nursing Scholarship, 25*(1), 69–72, addresses this significant contribution to nursing, drawing from both her published and unpublished works.

dict what specific knowledge or what concepts the nurse will need. The nurse must identify these, because what is needed depends on the specific purpose intended. The nurse, for nursing, uses some framework for her selection and adaptation. In this action she is a theorist. That is, some theory—often not made explicit—directs her selection of the knowledge or concepts to apply.

By "theory," I mean a coherent hypothesis, or set of hypotheses, or a concept, forming a general framework for undertaking something. Theory means a conceptual structure built for a purpose. For nursing, that purpose is practice.

But the practitioner cannot just select from a rack of ready-to-wear theories, because the knowledges and theories as we find them in the basic sciences are insufficient for practice. Instead, nursing practice requires that she structure converging, and sometimes conflicting, facts from the many fields which produce knowledge about human beings.

The nurse works within the framework of the inseparability and interdependence of one person's human life, so she attempts to relate aspects not yet clearly related in the separate sciences.

That is, we strive to act holistically, though our knowledge does not come for use from any holistic science of humans.

In this, the practitioner differs from the scientist. The scientist, due to reasons of control, feasibility, and measurement in study (due, as well, to the sheer impossibility of mastering all sciences, or even specialties within one science) isolates aspects for study. While the scientist may recognize the interrelationships of, for instance, physiologic and psychologic factors in man, he far less commonly studies these as a whole.

The practitioner of nursing, in contrast, may not have a complete science to nurse the whole man, but nurse the whole man is what she is striving to do. And, she sees the problems that result when one aspect or another is left out.

The practitioner of nursing thus finds herself working from a framework somewhat different from that within which knowledge is typically generated in the sciences. In this translation, the practitioner, of necessity, begins to restructure theory. She—often, at least—must apply the theory or concept in a way its originator may not have foreseen. She cannot simply take concepts from the sciences and directly apply them and hope to have the key to the biologic and psychosocial factors bound together in a patient, because this very interdependence is often a factor in response to and recovery from illness.

Generalities Don't Suffice

Further, because we attempt to nurse the individual, general theories cannot suffice. General theories of human behavior describe the typical or the norm, not the exception or the individual. Or, sometimes, they describe the extremes and not the middle range.

For example, it is a useful notion that self-preservation, both in a physical and psychologic sense, is a major element in human behavior that accounts for or explains much observed behavior. Yet it is not uncommon to see patients who do not act rationally for self-preservation. They appear to have some stronger motive for action. We also see heroic acts of self-sacrifice which are not easily explained by general theories of self-preservation.

As one moves from general theories about human behavior to those relevant to all of the helping professions, and then to those relevant to patient behavior, there is need for an increasing number of conditional statements. What applies is shaped by the context, roles, and, for patients, the physical status that presents. This is yet another reason why the professional is a theorist: she is the person who must identify the conditional factors; she has to make the conditional statements.

Related to this is the fact that the professional can encounter conflicting theories, with each supported by some evidence. If she is to take some action she must choose a theory, either consciously or not, for her action is not independent of history; it stems from some framework.

For example, the concept or theory that guides the common practice of encouraging patients to talk about their problems often is not made explicit. Verbalization is generally conceived to be a good thing. But does this concept support the practice in all circumstances for all patients, or explain clearly the exceptions? Theoretically, indiscriminate practice would seem to involve some risk. Do the reasons behind this concept identify the risks and the benefits? The practitioner who follows a practice based on theory must appraise and criticize the theory if she follows it in nursing patients. She must weight the risks and benefits in a manner not required of the scholar who theorizes about a phenomenon in the specific or in general, but who does not treat the individual.

The scholar is often concerned with describing and predicting phenomena. He seeks objectivity, so he reduces, to the extent possible, the influence he may have on the variance due to the experimenter. He seeks to eliminate the human, personal element of the investigator.

This is the converse of a practice discipline. As Conant (1967) has highlighted, a practice discipline seeks not only to describe or predict phenomena, but to introduce change. Practice is goal-directed, not to the accumulation of knowledge, but to the prescription and implementation of activity to change natural outcomes to desired outcomes.

Therefore, the clinical testing of a theory is essential if it is used as a guide to practice. It is the professional practitioner who is able to criticize the theory in use, and determine its value for directing actions to achieve defined outcomes. In this she is not only a *user* of theory, but she may be a *modifier* as well. She is also a *chooser* of theory.

Consider a practice of encouraging a patient to verbalize about his operation. Talking about one's operation occurs frequently enough to have become a folk expectation and to have provoked joking. The frequency and persistence of the behavior suggests that there is some potency behind it. One could speculate, too, that there is possibly a folk norm for the time at which such talking is acceptable, excusable, and tolerated by friends and family. There may also be social norms for what content is acceptable. If such norms exist, and the patient exceeds these norms, he runs the risk of being cut off verbally or avoided by others. One hears complaints to suggest this happens.

Can this be avoided through nursing? From one theory it can be argued that if the nurse encourages a patient to talk about his operation, some of the need to continue talking about it can be extinguished, and the risk for the patient of annoying family and friends can be reduced.

But, from another theory, one could argue that if the nurse, an important figure for the patient postoperatively, encourages the patient to talk, conveys the expectation that he will talk—and thus, in effect, rewards, the behavior—she may prolong or reinforce it, causing the patient to risk violating folk norms.

It is not the originators of alternative theories who can solve a possible dilemma for the nurse. It is the nurse as practitioner and user of theory who must resolve the dilemma—in action, in critique of action, and in further theorizing.

A universal practice of encouraging patients to talk about their feelings may be questioned from another orientation. A medical patient recently talked with one of my faculty colleagues about the graduate student who was caring for him. He could not understand what the student wanted of him. This student, in her clinical course work, had time to talk with patients, and had visited with the patient after she had completed the typical morning care activities of bathing and bed making. Her conversations were patient-focused but were not probing. She did not have any specific goal in mind except to interact with the patient and to get to know him.

This patient, however, told the instructor that he was an orphan, who had learned early that people do not do things for nothing. He interpreted the student's talking with him as evidence that she wanted something from him. This man viewed even conversation as something you get or give only in exchange for something or because you want something. For him, the nurse's attempt to learn more about him by talking with him was seen as a sexual advance. He could not imagine any interaction that did not have an exploitative motive. He was, therefore, made acutely uncomfortable by a very casual attempt by a nurse to encourage him to verbalize. Her motives were significantly misperceived, to the detriment of the patient (though one could argue that perhaps we learned more about the patient because of his discomfort).

There may also be instances where attempting to get a patient to talk about his feelings is contraindicated because it may dissipate the feeling. There may be instances where it is important for someone to experience and to recognize feelings *as feelings*. Talking about them may diminish them, objectify them, and so lose them as feelings. Joy is certainly one emotion that can be diminished by talking about it or attempting to explain it. I can recall an obstetrician father who was so profoundly moved by the birth of his own child that he burst into tears. The intensity of his own feeling totally surprised him, as well as his obstetrician colleagues. It seemed important for him to fully experience the intensity of his feeling and not diminish it until he had really felt it and absorbed it as his own feeling.

Lest I mislead, let me hasten to say that, in general, benefits seem to result from the practice of encouraging verbalization, but what are the exceptions? If benefits accrue, how are they explained? Practice could be more selective, and perhaps more effective, if we knew exactly what patient benefits to expect, and what dynamics would achieve them.

For example, benefits might be due to the patient's recognition, through talking, of the specific content of his feelings.

Benefits could also be due to the sense of companionship which can be achieved by talking with another, without regard for particular content. That is, would talking be effective without a listener? If not, what is supplied by a listener, even a nondirective listener, that is essential?

Is benefit derived from the recapitulation of an event which serves in some sense to produce mastery over, or integration of, the event, as in talking about one's operation? Or are benefits due to some reciprocal system where talking serves in place of some other potentially more detrimental form of discharge, such as acting out or somatization? Choose your theory. It is not likely to hold for all circumstances or cases, nor to support an invariate nursing practice of encouraging verbalization. Thus, the professional practitioner must become not simply a user of given theory, but a developer, tester, and expander of theory. This is not for the purpose of scholarship; it is an essential for intelligent practice.

The Need for Theory

It is essential because of the inadequacies in existing theories for the circumstances of nursing.

It is essential because of the need to synthesize, for practice, knowledge from diverse disciplines not yet fully related in theory.

It also is essential because the basic disciplines often are not pursuing the problems of importance to nurse and patient. For example, there is no extensive study, knowledge, or theory about appetite. As nurses we study nutrition, yet many of our observations and concerns with nutritional problems of patients are not solved by knowledge of nutrition. We need to know more about how to enable a patient to partake of the nutrients he needs, and about patterns of appetite in illness. For nursing, we need theories toward a science of appetite or of taste, and what happens to it in illness.

Conant (1967) gives an example of the complexities of a practice theory for back care: it must encompass maintenance of skin and underlying tissues, nutritional and fluid balance, and physical manipulation of the body. It is unlikely that the theory for back care will be developed from any other discipline than nursing. Existing theories guide the development of a field, because they guide what are seen as the interesting problems for study, the purposes for such study, and the ways in which problems are studied. Ways of defining problems, and of studying them, and what is considered worth pursuing are likely to differ from field to field. What may be significant problems for nursing may not fit with the theories, methods of study, or current focus of any other single field.

It is also unlikely that scientists in other disciplines will rush to collaborate with one another for study of a phenomenon because a nurse finds it important in nursing care. This is perhaps too pessimistic a view of collaboration in view of increasing evidence of interdisciplinary research. There remain, however, significant obstacles in orientation and method which impede cross-disciplinary research.

How Theory Is Built

Of course, we theorize without knowing we do it. A nursing student last fall was relating an experience she had while walking with a young child. The child had to smell every flower in a bush. The student told the child they would all smell alike, but he had to check out every blossom, just the same.

I commented that perhaps the child had made no generalization about flowers. He hadn't yet developed a notion that flowers that are shaped and colored alike, and grown on one bush, have a high probability of smelling alike. One could say the child was operating without any general concept of flower smell, and exploring each bloom was still an adventure.

Over time, the adventure may be lost and the child will conclude—or accept someone else's conclusion—that flowers that look alike, smell alike. And he'll spend time on other adventures.

Now it occurs to met that, not being a flower specialist, I have never really thought about similarities and differences in flower smells in any scientific way. As I think about it, I very much doubt that the visual cues I use to class flowers as the same—such as shape, color, type of petal, and so on—have very much to do with smell. I associate visual similarities with olfactory similarities—probably erroneously as to cause, but not erroneously from an empiric view. But it doesn't matter. I'm not the expert. I don't practice or teach others the practice of flower smelling. Only I suffer from my misconceptions. But if we all acted so confused about nursing matters, we'd be in trouble.

No skillful nurse could efficiently practice like the adventurous little child—testing every detail of every nursing action each time it appeared. Instead, she arrives at some generalizations and begins to accumulate some wisdom over time that allows her to group, to classify, to identify, to focus, and to select what she will spend time pursuing. She will reach at least my level of thinking about flowers and their perfumes—it may be erroneous, but it is at least a concept.

The professional practitioner quickly recognizes differences between patients, or their responses, and accounts for them. She may not do this deliberately or make her theory explicit but, nevertheless, she adjusts her approach, her expectations, and sometimes her activities, accordingly.

She also is theorizing when she *labels* patient behavior. Many nurses have learned to recognize and label behavior as rejection even when the cues the patient gives do not exactly duplicate any specific definition of rejection. We have in some sense extended this concept or the ideas about it.

Unfortunately, we often stop when we have categorized or labeled the behavior or speculated about its genesis, just as I stopped with color, shape, and odor because I had satisfied one level of understanding. But the skillful practitioner, contrary to me and my flowers, must test out her generalization, her framework. Further, she may have an obligation to change the behavior she has observed and labeled. But too often, when she does attempt to change it, she fails to make explicit the theory which guides her action, though she implicitly is operating from some framework toward some direction. Such framework is at least incipient theory. Recognition of patterns in patient behaviors is also incipient theory.

Everyday Theorizing

We are not sufficiently conscious of the extent to which we use theory in practice, nor of the extent to which we adapt theory in practice. We also rarely recognize when we create or develop theory in practice, yet it does happen.

It is not uncommon for a nurse to sense correctly that a certain patient is not going to be able to follow some prescribed regimen, or for the nurse to predict, correctly, a patient's negative reaction to some element of therapy. Sometimes these perceptions run counter to those of the physician or others. What has happened is that the nurse has related some element of behavior to acceptance of therapy or response to it, that the other persons have not included in their framework, for some reason. And, of course, the converse can be found. Such examples illustrate the differences in the theories that are used pervasively. When the nurse's perception and prediction differ from others, she has developed a different theoretical stance.

The failure to make theory explicit is sometimes from lack of awareness of how one structures something. We do not stop to think, or possibly are not really conscious of our framework. Much of our structuring may be preconscious. Certainly, some failure to make

theory explicit is because the practitioner (of necessity, and rightly so) is interested in the goal of nursing care, and not the analysis of the perceptions and processes used to achieve it. Our focus is on action, not on the analysis of it. But if we really have a commitment to the future beyond the personal accumulation of wisdom from patient to patient, and if we wish to communicate this wisdom we must try to analyze our actions and formulate theories from them. We must have practitioners in nursing who are willing to be scholars as well and who have the interest, skill, and time to pursue the analyses and formulations and test them in practice.

A New Look at the Familiar

But there is another reason why theory may not be made explicit. It is because we may overlook the familiar, or perhaps we devalue it.

There is some danger of neglecting, or even rejecting, some of the traditional, familiar components in nursing as we grow in our emphasis on science and research. One such component might be what is termed TLC—"tender loving care." This something or this concept, which someone (it would be fascinating to know who) has tried to capture by a phrase, is nonscientific. We are not likely to do research on it. We do not have tools to measure it. Yet many nurses, as well as non-nurses, recognize it as an essential component in nursing for many patients.

Recently in teaching I used this vague concept, TLC, as a possible example of something that occurs in nursing for which we do not yet have a theory or perhaps, more precisely, that we have not theorized about, yet which we can sense. I felt the idea embarrassed several students. I think this regrettable, but I was not totally surprised. One of my friends has been collecting data from entering, middle, and graduating students from nine schools of nursing, baccalaureate and diploma, religious-affiliated and secular. These data included many, many examples of student dilemmas about expressing their feelings for patients. It would appear that a significant number of students enter with compassion for patients but quickly get the idea they must never convey feelings to patients. Rightly or wrongly, such an attitude will affect one's view of "tender loving care."

My own view is that tenderness and love are essential ingredients in nursing care. We need to theorize about these elements in nursing. Others have valued them as effective components in care, and occasionally TLC is actually prescribed—though I doubt the effectiveness of ordering it.

Whether or not you agree with this view about TLC, it is an example of a concept that exists, that is associated with nursing, that has been felt to be rather specific to nursing, but that we have not yet made explicit, nor yet fully conceptualized. We probably know, at least at a preconscious level, more about it than anybody else, for we can see it in so many diverse actions and situations. It does not seem unreasonable to suggest that theorizing about something as vague and yet as familiar as TLC might be valuable for understanding nursing.

At this stage in theory development I could entertain, even, the use of jargon—in the sense of a special professional language—to express some of the ideas in nursing. For instance, I would endorse the use of this term TLC for the purposes of taking about it until we can more precisely or more elegantly describe what we are talking about.

At this time in theory development it will be profitable to borrow or adapt concepts and theories from whatever source we can, if they will help us to understand and produce nursing. They must, however, be tested for their usefulness in guiding nursing practice in the arena of practice.

Intuitive exploration, speculation, trial and error, introspection, subjective impression—all can be used toward development of theory.

What is needed are attempts to make theory explicit, with tests of theories for nursing *in the practice* of nursing, and with further development or theories emerging *from the practice* of nursing.

REFERENCE

Conant, L. H. (1967). Closing the practice-theory gap. *Nursing Outlook, 15,* 37–39.

The Author Comments

The Practitioner as Theorist

I wrote this article to demystify the then-prevalent ideas that theory should be "grand theory" or that what was needed was some "theory" to justify nursing. As was evident from the literature and conferences at national meetings, there was great confusion concerning uses of theory and why nurses as practitioners needed theory. With their emphasis on theory and research, nurse scientists often rejected or at least ignored the importance of phenomena of nursing practice.

—ROSEMARY ELLIS
1969

CHAPTER 48

Theorizing the Knowledge That Nurses Use in the Conduct of Their Work

Joan Liaschenko

Anastasia Fisher

The authors propose a classification of knowledge that they call case, patient, and person and that reflects the content of the knowledge necessary to the conduct of nursing work. This classification represents an attempt to theorize from their respective empirical research data. Case knowledge is general knowledge of pathophysiology, disease processes, pharmacology, and other therapeutic protocols. Patient knowledge is that knowledge that defines the individual within the health care system, the knowledge expressed in the individual's response to therapeutics, and the knowledge that enables nurses to move the recipient of care through the health care system and along the illness trajectory. Person knowledge is knowledge of the individual as a subject with a personal biography who occupies a certain social space and who acts with his or her own desires and intentions for reasons that make sense to him or her. Two types of social knowledge serve as relational knowledge, or a bridge that links case knowledge to patient knowledge and patient knowledge to person knowledge. Each type of knowledge is accessed differently and the extent to which each is attained and used is determined by the circumstances of the patient's illness and his or her location in the health care system. The authors make a case for why this classification might be useful to the discipline.

From Scholarly Inquiry for Nursing Practice: An International Journal, *13(1), 29(1), 29-41. Copyright©1999, Springer Publishing Co., Inc., New York. Used by permission.*

About the Authors

Joan Liaschenko joined the Center for Bioethics and the School of Nursing at the University of Minnesota as an Associate Professor in January 2001, coming from the University of Wisconsin-Milwaukee. In addition, she is an adjunct Associate Professor at the University of Calgary and the University of Toronto Schools of Nursing. She is also an Associate to the International Centre for Nursing Ethics at the University of Surrey, England. Dr. Liaschenko's research focuses on the moral dimensions of nursing work. Her PhD and postdoctoral research were conducted at the University of California, San Francisco, where she studied the ethical concerns encountered in the work of home care nurses and psychiatric nurses. Currently, she has National Institute of Nursing Research funding to study the ethical issues that arise in the work of nurses running clinical trials. Another project is looking at the correlation of the American Nursing Association and political action committee money and voting records of incumbents related to their support of health-related legislation. She has published widely, presents at numerous international conferences, and has been a visiting scholar at the Joint Centre for Bioethics at the University of Toronto and the School of Nursing, Flinders University, Adelaide, Australia. She is the coeditor of *Nursing Philosophy*.

Anastasia Fisher was born in Los Angeles, CA, where she completed her undergraduate and master's degrees in nursing. After several years as a practicing psychiatric nurse, she entered the doctoral program in nursing at the University of California, San Francisco. In her doctoral studies, she examined nursing practice with persons who are dangerous and mentally ill. She later completed a 3-year federally funded postdoctoral fellowship in addiction research at the University of Washington, Seattle. Recently, she and her colleagues at the University of Minnesota received National Institutes of Health funding to support their study, "Nurses: Research Integrity in Clinical Trials". Dr. Fisher is Principal Investigator at the Public Health Institute, Berkeley, CA, and Director of Clinical Education, Programs, Quality Outcomes and Research for Mental Health Services, Alta Bates Medical Center, Berkeley, CA.

In general, our intellectual project is concerned with theorizing the interaction between knowledge and the actions that constitute nursing work. We begin by naming some knowledges relevant to nursing practice; specifically, in this paper, we propose a designation of the content of knowledge used by nurses in direct patient care. We suggest that those actions constituting the work of direct care require three different types of knowledge that we call case, patient, and person. In our view these labels are representations of types of knowledge and do not refer to the actual recipient of care usually called the patient, client, or consumer. These names refer to knowledge that nurses use in meeting a variety of therapeutic goals for individuals or the recipients of care. We see these designations as useful for two reasons. First, this language came from empirical research designed to understand particular dimensions of nursing practice. In thinking about how knowledge and nursing action are organized and mutually interactive in specific temporal and spatial contexts of nursing work, these names came as an "aha" phenomenon allowing us to talk more easily about the complexity of the interactions between knowledge and action. Second, because the words, "case, patient, and person" knowledge provided us with insights, we believe they may likewise be useful to practicing nurses in articulating the work of nursing, a task that has typically fallen to the academics among us. One form this task has taken is debates about the theoretical, practical, objective, and subjective aspects of knowledge in nursing. But these debates are not helpful to those doing the work of nursing. We argue that in the absence of a way of talking about knowledge that makes sense to and is used by practicing nurses to articulate their work, the knowledge used in nursing and its connection to work remains invisible and undervalued (Wolf, 1989). Likewise, this absence also limits the ability of the discipline to articulate its practices to other disciplines, the public at large, third-party payers, and even to nurses themselves. We strongly believe that practicing nurses must be able to articulate their work in a language that they recognize as their own, thereby contributing to the development of nursing philosophy. We also believe that nursing will be developed and strengthened to the degree that practicing nurses can theoretically articulate their work.

Some will argue, however, that in addition to the more philosophical and technical debates on the nature of knowledge, the discipline already has a variety of conceptual means for articulating practice, including various nursing theories, nursing diagnoses and outcome measures, and the nursing process. Yet, in spite of the rich evolution of knowledge development within nursing over the years, it is evident to anyone who observes clinical practice that nurses rarely use the language of nursing theory, the language of nursing diagnosis, or the language of nursing process unless mandated to do so by accrediting bodies or institutional practice policies. Instead, working nurses talk about what they need to do using the language of nursing, which we view as an integration of everyday language and the language of science. The work of nursing, however, cannot be solely articulated in either of these languages. While the totality of knowledge used in the work of nursing cannot be fully described as scientific, neither can it be fully accounted for in everyday language. The proposed designation—case, patient, and person—offers the potential to theorize the interaction between knowledge and nursing actions in a way that connects the knowledge and work to the social reality in which nursing is situated.

Concern with the articulation of nursing work is not new, as nursing has been attempting to define itself since the beginning of organized, modern nursing (Nightingale, 1860/1969). We do not intend to convey the idea that there is one final articulation of nursing work that, when achieved, will assure nursing's place in health care once and for all. On the contrary, we believe that nursing is a historically situated social practice whose definition will change in accordance with social circumstances. Precisely because of this, however, we believe that articulation is important.

While the nature of knowledge in nursing has been debated since the beginning of the modern era of nursing (Johnson & Ratner, 1997), the contemporary dialogue was initiated with Carper's (1978) seminal paper identifying four patterns of knowing in nursing (Benner, 1984; Jacobs-Kramer & Chinn, 1988; Meerabeau, 1992; Wolfer, 1993). This work was particularly significant for its recognition of the need for multiple patterns of knowing in nursing, thus moving beyond the strictly scientific as sufficient knowledge for the practice of nursing. The study of practice is now commonplace and, indeed, it could be said that a tradition of such study has been founded. This literature has argued for the significance of the knowledge inherent in clinical practice (Benner, 1984; Benner & Wrubel, 1989; Jenks, 1993) and explored various aspects of the knowledge of practice including: personal knowledge (Gadow, 1990; Moch, 1990); intuition (Agan, 1987; Benner & Tanner, 1987; Rew, 1988, 1989); aesthetic knowledge or the "art of nursing" (Johnson, 1994); ethical or moral knowledge (Liaschenko, 1995a; Sarvimaki, 1995); and, knowing the patient (Jenks, 1993; Jenny & Logan, 1992; Liaschenko, 1997a; Radwin, 1995; Tanner, Benner, Chesla, & Gordon, 1993). This literature demonstrates the informal, practical knowledge that is not fully articulated but is nonetheless essential to nurses' ability to make judgments, act wisely, and get work done. This literature is significant for moving beyond the biomedical knowledge necessary to the conduct of nursing work. We are suggesting, however, that it does not go far enough, because it takes only limited account of the influence of the temporal and spatial organizational context on knowledge and action.

The Work of Nursing and the Origins of Our Language

The connection between knowledge and work is a critical one. Our concept of work is taken from Strauss,

Fagerhaugh, Suczek, and Weiner (1985/1997), where work is understood as involving "a sequence of expected tasks, sometimes routinized but sometimes subject to unexpected contingencies" (p. 9). In the context of health care, work is the organized sequence of activities aimed at managing illness trajectories. Yet, work is too often conceived of only as an endpoint or outcome measure rather than as a process (Wadel, 1979). Our claim is that the proposed designations provide a conceptual organization that is useful because it links the actions of nursing to the knowledge used in the conduct of those actions, thus legitimating them as work. It has the potential to be theoretically more complete and yet parsimonious, because it recognizes and describes the processes constituting nursing work and not merely the outcomes. Most important, it does so in a language that is used by nurses and is understandable to others.

While it is indisputable that nursing requires scientific, biomedical knowledge, the discipline's nearly exclusive focus on this form of knowledge leaves unrecognized other kinds of knowledge necessary to patient care. In an earlier paper, Liaschenko (1998) argued that nurses know much more than a certain portion of scientific knowledge. In addition to the knowledge of anatomy, physiology, pathophysiology, and so forth, nurses know how to get things done; they know how to move patients through a health care system, how to connect patients with resources. This knowledge is not scientific knowledge, but is knowledge absolutely essential to patient care that is organized, continuous, safe, and humane. Of course, nurses are familiar with this type of action; it is commonly referred to as the coordination of care and involves the transmission and coordination of information. Coordination of care is rarely articulated as work and rarely counts in institutional structures as work (Jacques, 1993). The cultural assumption is that the critical work is the scientific work, all other kinds being of secondary importance, of the kind that "just sort of happens." It is further assumed that there is no knowledge involved in arrangements that "just happen."

Jacques (1993), an organizational theorist who studied nurses, noted the critical importance of this work to the functioning of health care institutions, call-

ing attention to the fact that this work is completely external to the reward structures of institutions. Fletcher (1994), another organizational theorist, studied female engineers and found that while they do the interpersonal work essential to the successful completion of projects, this work "gets disappeared" by institutional structures that refuse to recognize these relational practices as work. In her research on the particular household labor of feeding families, DeVault documented that although a major portion of that work consisted of "thought work," it was viewed as so natural that the women themselves failed to see it as work. One consequence of the lack of a commonly accepted, useful articulation of nursing work is that the nurses themselves, like others who do gendered labor, fail to recognize what they do as work (DeVault, 1991). This invisibility is not total, however, as some nurses have shown themselves to be astute observers of what work they are being paid to do and what work they are not being paid to do (Liaschenko, 1997b).

The studies by Jacques (1993) and Fletcher (1994) were studies of practices specifically concerned with the concept of work, including the knowledge necessary for the work. Likewise, our approach is decidedly empirical in that it was generated from research (Fisher, Fonteyn, & Liaschenko, 1994; Liaschenko, 1993). Our designation of knowledge arose from discussions about the empirical studies of nursing practice that we conducted. Fisher and her colleague, Marsha Fonteyn, did ethnographic fieldwork in a psychiatric emergency service, and in cardiovascular and neurosurgical intensive care units, while Liaschenko conducted a narrative study of home care and psychiatric nurses using unstructured interviews. The design, method, and analyses used in these studies are described elsewhere (Fisher & Fonteyn, 1995; Liaschenko, 1993). Although the aims of the respective research were different, with Fisher and Fonteyn studying clinical reasoning and Liaschenko examining moral dimensions of nursing practice, "knowing the patient" was a central feature for the nurses in both studies. We came to see through our discussions, however, that knowing the patient was used by nurses to refer to different types of knowing that they used in the conduct of their work. We labeled these knowledges case, patient, and person (Fisher, Fonteyn, & Liaschenko, 1994; Liaschenko, 1997a). While "knowing the patient" has received increasing attention in the literature, our work shows that "the patient" is understood in ways that reflect the kind of knowledge needed to do the work of nursing in the confines of contemporary health care structures.

Case Knowledge

Case knowledge, which we consider biomedical knowledge, is the generalized knowledge of anatomy, physiology, pathophysiology, disease processes, and therapeutics (see Figure 48-1). It is concerned with the causation of disease and its treatment. It is gained through the principles of science and the scientific method and is generalizable because it is based on statistical probabilities. Elsewhere, Liaschenko (1997a) has claimed that case knowledge is "disembodied" knowledge in that no particular physical body, nor indeed any body, is required to have case knowledge. One could know, for example, all the facts about cardiac disease without seeing that disease as embodied in a particular individual. One could start with the anatomy and physiology of the heart, follow this with the pathophysiology of various disease entities, and proceed through the therapeutics. Biological norms are implicit in the anatomy and physiology, while pathophysiology reveals the disease processes. The effectiveness of therapeutics is based on the percentage of the population that responds favorably to a given therapeutic. This knowledge is the standard against which the particularities of an individual recipient of care are evaluated. This case, or biomedical, knowledge is the primary knowledge of the contemporary health care system in that it legitimizes the practice of medicine which, in turn, controls this knowledge. It also legitimizes that aspect of nursing work that is concerned with monitoring disease processes and therapeutic responses.

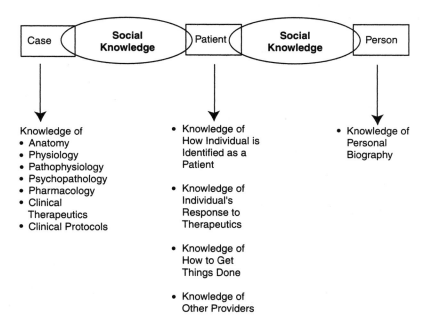

Figure 48-1. *Knowledge That Nurses Use Within the Social-Temporal-Spatial Context of Their Work.*

In their research conducted in cardiovascular and neurosurgical intensive care units and a psychiatric emergency service, Fisher and Fonteyn (1995) identified case knowledge as the basic knowledge nurses need to meet the primary goal of stabilizing, maintaining, and moving critically ill patients to another level of care. In these settings, aspects of knowing the case included nurses' knowledge of the disease processes, physiology, clinical protocols, indicators and range of expected patient outcome (i.e., the usual clinical therapeutics and anticipated complications). All of this knowledge is biomedical and it is the most straightforward and, in many ways, the easiest knowledge to work with. In this aspect of nursing work, the work is essentially biomedical in that disease is understood as a deviation from a biological norm. We suggest that for nurses, case knowledge serves as a code or cue that sets up expectations about actions that will be necessary.

Social Knowledge Linking Case and Patient Knowledge

As mentioned, case knowledge is highly general and it is not until the nurse encounters the actual body of the recipient of care that a shift is made from the exclusive use of case knowledge to patient knowledge, which includes case knowledge. This transition requires knowledge other than biomedical knowledge; specifically, it requires knowledge of the social actors involved in the work. For example, in Fisher and Fonteyn's research (1995) knowledge of which surgeon performed the procedure included information relevant to the specific recipient of care, such as the surgeon's previous experience with this type of surgery, his or her usual technique, and typical postsurgical protocols. Knowledge of the surgeon tells nurses how much leeway they have in their decisions and actions toward meeting the goal of stability. The particularities of the surgeon, such as his or her competence, incision and drain preferences, what medications were likely to be ordered, and approaches to pain management, shape nurses' definitions of the situation and the actions they will take in response. Knowledge of the surgeon allows nurses to formulate expectations of what had been done in surgery and therefore to anticipate the condition of the patient on arrival at the ICU (intensive care unit). Likewise, nurses could anticipate what actions they could and could not take during the initial recovery process without calling for additional orders. This anticipated knowledge provided a map which served to guide their actions. In other words, knowledge of the surgeon allowed nurses to organize their actions in a very specific way in response to the particularities of the situation at hand. In this way, knowledge of the surgeon is a link between case and patient knowledge.

Because nursing work involves the organization of care for multiple individuals across time and space, knowledge of other social actors such as other nurses, nursing assistants, respiratory therapists, social workers and so forth is critical. Such knowledge involves knowing the skill and working patterns of these providers, so that nurses are able to match the required care or service with the appropriate provider.

Patient Knowledge

In our view, patient knowledge is the largest, most complex domain and is absolutely critical to the work of nursing. While case knowledge is limited to biomedical knowledge, the content of patient knowledge includes knowledge of how an individual becomes identified as a patient, knowledge of the individual's response to treatment, knowledge of how to get things done for the individual within and between institutions, and knowledge of the many others who are involved in providing services across time and space (see Figure 1). The health care system consists of a network of relationships that (a) use a certain kind of language, (b) define and label disease according to a set of rules, and (c) are characterized by recognizable practices (Young, 1993). The recipient of care upon interaction with the system acquires an identity that enables him or her to move through the system. This "patient" identity includes, among other things, an identification number, a diagnosis, a physician, a location point within the system, (for example, unit 4A), and a location exit. In addition to this, a certain amount of information or demographics about the recipient of care (for example, address, socioeconomic status [SES], and marital status) is recorded to facilitate the work of the health care system. This information endows the individual with a particularity that becomes concrete in the body, and knowledge of this identity of the particular body is knowledge of the patient. Viewed in this way, patient knowledge is not only knowledge of the patient, it creates the patient.

Part of the complexity of patient knowledge is due to the fact that its content is no longer limited to generalized case knowledge and the expectancies for action which it generates. Rather, it consists of the nurse's interaction with a particular body, the responses of which will be compared to generalized case knowledge. At the point of this interaction, the nurse monitors how a particular individual is responding to a therapeutic regimen using the established norms of biomedical knowledge. This monitoring of the recipient of care is what is commonly referred to in the literature as "knowing the patient" (Jenny & Logan, 1992; Liaschenko, 1997a). Monitoring the patient in this way is the most visible work that nurses do. Society recognizes this work as needed and desired and grants authority to nurses to do it.

Patient knowledge, however, is far more comprehensive than knowing how the recipient of care is responding to therapeutic interventions. Part of nursing work is the work of negotiating a patient through the system, which requires knowledge of the interactions between social actors and institutional practices. This is complex, social knowledge that includes knowledge of people's commitments, priorities, competencies, styles of working, vulnerabilities, emotions that accompany human interaction, and the appropriate languages to use with these multiple others. This knowledge requires attention to the multiple audiences to whom nurses must speak to get things done. It consists of how the institution works, as well as knowledge of the key people involved in various decision-making capacities affecting the individual's care and is analogous to the way ICU nurses know the surgeons. In order for nurses to accomplish this work, they must know the formal rules of conduct such as who can talk to whom and under what

conditions, what can be said, and what are the risks and consequences of undertaking certain courses of action.

Although the recipient of care is situated in a particular time and space, the goal of the health care system is to move the individual from one level of care, usually more intense, to a less intensive level. Yet the resources of the health care system can be temporally discontinuous and are often geographically dispersed. The work of actually moving someone through the system, marshaling appropriate resources and attempting to stave off what seems to be the inherent fragmentation of care (Liaschenko, 1997b), is part of nursing work and requires a great deal of practical knowledge which is gathered largely through role-modeling, experience, and trial and error.

When nurses "know the patient," they know the recipient of care through the realm of their work, a set of routines and practices that are also temporally and spatially structured by the institution and, in particular, specific work sites within the institution (Strauss et al., 1985/1997). ICUs, for example, are temporally and spatially organized differently from an OR (operating room), which is different from a pediatric unit. The particular constellation of a structure sets parameters on what can be known of and can be done to a patient in that unit. For example, in Fisher and Fonteyn's study, the units were designed to deal with highly specialized conditions necessitating craniotomies, open-heart procedures, and emergency psychiatric management. Individual recipients of care in these units were clinically unstable, on the units for short periods of time (sometimes for no longer than 24 hours), and were often unconscious, paralyzed, or mute for the duration of their stay. Thus, what nurses can know and do is both constituted and constrained by the institution's view of what the goals are for a particular disease.

This aspect of nursing work and the knowledge it takes to do it is akin to the work that Fletcher (1994) calls relational practices. This work and knowledge is not legitimated, not visible, not part of nurses' job descriptions, and not what gets acknowledged in evaluations. Nonetheless, it is essential both to the recipient of care and to meeting institutional goals.

Social Knowledge Linking Patient Knowledge to Person Knowledge

In our view, the nurse's ability to envision the everyday world of the recipient of care necessitates knowledge of the illness trajectory as extending beyond the boundaries of the health care system and into his or her world. This includes knowledge of (a) the social conditions in which a recipient of care lives, (b) the impact of a particular disease on the individual's ability to function and manage his/her disease in a variety of contexts, (c) the stigma attached to a given disease, and (d) the degree to which the individual takes up the dominant cultural discourse about his or her particular disease. These are not static entities, but dynamic interactions of social life. The fact that disease and illness will mean different things to different people is particularly important, because it encompasses acquired knowledge and marks the intersection between the work of nursing and an individual's own management of illness. It is the awareness that these factors impact individual lives that constitutes the knowledge that can potentially bridge patient and person knowledge. The link is constructed as the nurse begins to wonder what living with this disease or disability is like for the individual. To ask the question is to visualize that individual as someone more than a patient in a health care system or as something more than an object of biomedical science. This visualization, or imagination, if you will, forms a background, a repertoire of possible explanations that facilitate nurses' formulation of hypotheses regarding the individual's experience and action when this is necessary in the conduct of their work. Once these hypotheses are validated by relevant details of the individual's biography, the nurse can be said to have person knowledge. While we are aware that the choice of "hypotheses" might be cause for objection because of its association with certain philosophies of science, we, nonetheless, use it because it is not entirely inaccurate and it is also understood by working nurses.

Before continuing with person knowledge, it might be useful to compare this type of social knowledge with that previously noted linking case knowledge to patient knowledge. The noteworthy distinction is that the latter is a form of localized and unique knowledge that allows nurses to apply general case principles to an individual in a way that particularizes that individual in order to accomplish nursing work. In contrast, linking patient to person knowledge is generalized and abstract knowledge, but it nonetheless works to further particularize the individual. What makes these two kinds of knowledge the same is that they are both social; that is, they are both knowledge of human beings as social actors in social contexts. Moreover, this knowledge can be accessed only within localized interaction, or, to use Fletcher's (1994) words, "relational practices."

Person Knowledge

In contrast to case and patient knowledge, person knowledge is knowledge of the individual as a self with a personal biography (Brody, 1987; Bury, 1982) who occupies a certain social space and who acts on her or his own desires and intentions for reasons that make sense to him or her (see Figure 1). When we know a person, we know something about what it means for the individual to have a specific history, live a particular life, and engage with the world in which he or she is situated. In her paper, *Knowing the Patient?*, Liaschenko (1997a) suggested that knowledge of this engagement included knowledge of how individuals enact their agency within the spatial and temporal dimensions of their lives. Access to this knowledge is by direct interaction with the individual in order over time, either through multiple encounters or over some extended period, and it necessarily involves the subjectivity of the nurse. When the nurse has this knowledge and begins to wonder about the individual's experience along the illness trajectory, the nurse is imagining the position of the individual in order to understand it from his or her perspective, and is not merely applying theoretical knowledge.

As we saw from earlier examples, knowledge of the person is not always possible nor, we would add, desirable. On the other hand, while the nurse may have knowledge of the person, it may not impact in a significant way on the nurse's day-to-day work with that individual. Having said this, we might ask to what end this knowledge of the person, when available, is used in the conduct of nursing work? Liaschenko's research demonstrated that person knowledge was used when there was some conflict or potential conflict between courses of action desired by the individual and those desired by the providers or among the providers themselves. Knowing the person offered a perspective that served to keep the recipient of care central. Interestingly, the imagining of the position of the other seemed a reflexive practice in which nurses were also aware of the position they occupied in the social structure of health care and in their respective institutions. It served as a reminder that neither the nurse nor the recipient of care are separate from or beyond the network of relationships that form the health care system. The nurses in her study saw themselves as institutional representatives of the cultural and personal authority that stands behind scientific medicine and health care institutions (Liaschenko, 1995b, 1997b). In this capacity, they were aware of how easy it was for them to undermine or negate patient agency. Person knowledge is a potent reminder that the life being lived is the life of the recipient of care. Nurses use person knowledge to defend their arguments for an alternative management of disease trajectories and to justify their actions when those actions support an individual's agency, even though this can conflict with established biomedical or institutional courses of action.

Summary

We have theorized a content for the knowledge necessary for the conduct of nursing work that we designate case, patient, and person. This designation originated in discussions of our respective empirical research. Case knowledge is general knowledge of pathophysiology, disease processes, pharmacology, and other therapeutic protocols. Patient knowledge is the knowledge of how an individual becomes identified as a patient, knowledge of the individual's response to treatment, knowledge of how to get things done for the individual within and between institutions, and knowledge of the multiple others who are involved in providing services across time and space. Person knowledge is knowledge of the individual as a self with a personal biography who occupies a certain social space and acts according to his or her own desires and intentions for reasons that make sense to him or her. We suggest that knowledge of social actors and the nurse's work context serve to link case to patient knowledge and patient to person knowledge. Each of these knowledges are accessed in different ways and the extent to which they are attained and used by nurses is determined by the circumstances of the patient's illness and his or her location in the health care system.

Because these knowledges are linked to nursing work, we believe they will make sense to practicing nurses enabling them to think more theoretically about their work and, therefore, to articulate it. Theorizing nursing work has always been a challenge, because much of the work is not scientific; rather, it is concerned with how to get things done within extremely complex systems, work described by Fletcher as relational practices. It is our intention that case, patient, and person knowledge may offer a useful way to begin to theorize about the interaction of knowledge and action that constitutes nursing work, a task that requires the attention of the entire discipline, and not merely of the academics among us. For this reason, we believe the content of this paper has important implications for the what and how of nursing education, a topic for some other time.

REFERENCES

Agan, D. R. (1987). Intuitive knowing as a dimension of nursing. *Advances in Nursing Science, 10,* 63–70.

Benner, P. (1984). *From novice to expert: Excellence and power in clinical nursing practice.* Menlo Park: Addison-Wesley Publishing Company.

Benner, P., & Wrubel, J. (1989). *The primacy of caring.* Menlo Park, NJ: Addison-Wesley.

Benner, P., & Tanner, C. (1987). Clinical judgment: How expert nurses use intuition. *American Journal of Nursing, 87,* 23–31.

Brody, H. (1987). *Stories of sickness.* New Yaven: Yale University Press.

Bury, M. (1982). Chronic illness as biographic disruption. *Sociology of Health and Illness, 4,* 167–182.

Carper, B. (1978). Fundamental patterns of knowing in nursing. *Advances in Nursing Science, 1,* 13–23.

DeVault, M. (1991). *Feeding the family: The social organization of caring as gendered work.* Chicago: University of Chicago Press.

Fisher, A., & Fonteyn, M. (1995). An exploration of an innovative methodological approach for examining nurses' heuristic use in clinical practice. *Scholarly Inquiry for Nursing Practice, 9,* 263–276.

Fisher, A., Fonteyn, M., & Liaschenko, J. (1994, May). *Knowing: The case, the patient, the person.* Symposium presentation at the International Nursing Research Conference, Vancouver, BC.

Fletcher, J. (1994). *Toward a theory of relational practice in organizations: A feminist reconstruction of "real work."* Unpublished doctoral dissertation, School of Management, Boston University, Boston.

Gadow, S. (1990). Response to "Personal knowing: Evolving research and practice." *Scholarly Inquiry for Nursing Practice, 4,* 167–170.

Jacobs-Kramer, M. K., & Chinn, P. L. (1988). Perspectives on knowing: A model of nursing knowledge. *Scholarly Inquiry for Nursing Practice, 2,* 129–143.

Jacques, R. (1993). Untheorized dimensions of caring work: Caring as a structural practice and caring as a way of seeing. *Nursing Administration Quarterly, 17,* 1–10.

Jenks, J. M. (1993). The pattern of personal knowing in nurse clinical decision making. *Journal of Nursing Education, 32,* 399–405.

Jenny, J., & Logan, J. (1992). Knowing the patient: One aspect of clinical knowledge. *Image: Journal of Nursing Scholarship, 24,* 254–258.

Johnson, J. L. (1994). A dialectical examination of nursing art. *Advances in Nursing Science, 17,* 1–14.

Johnson, J. L., & Ratner, P. A. (1997). The nature of the knowledge used in nursing practice. In S. Thorne & V. Hayes (Eds.), *Nursing praxis: Knowledge and action* (pp. 3–22). Thousand Oaks, CA: Sage Publications.

Liaschenko, J. (1993). *Faithful to the good: Morality and philosophy in nursing practice.* Unpublished doctoral dissertation, University of California, San Francisco.

Liaschenko, J. (1995a). Ethics in the work of acting for others. *Advances in Nursing Science, 18*(2), 1–12.

Liaschenko, J. (1995b). Artificial personhood: Nursing ethics in a medical world. *Nursing Ethics, 2,* 185–196.

Liaschenko, J. (1997a). Knowing the patient? In S. Thorne & V. Hayes (Eds.), *Nursing praxis: Knowledge and action* (pp. 23–38). Thousand Oaks, CA: Sage.

Liaschenko, J. (1997b). Ethics and the geography of the nurse-patient relationship: Spatial vulnerabilities and gendered space. *Scholarly Inquiry for Nursing Practice, 11,* 45–59.

Liaschenko, J. (1998). The shift from the closed to the open body—ramifications for nursing testimony. In S. D. Edwards (Ed.), *Philosophical issues in nursing* (pp. 11–30). Basingstoke, UK: Macmillan.

Meerabeau, L. (1992). Tacit nursing knowledge: An untapped resource or a methodological headache? *Journal of Advanced Nursing, 12,* 108–112.

Meleis, A. (1987). ReVisions in knowledge development: A passion for substance. *Scholarly Inquiry for Nursing Practice, 1,* 5–19.

Moch, S. D. (1990). Personal knowing: Evolving research and practice. *Scholarly Inquiry for Nursing Practice, 4,* 155–165.

Nightingale, F. (1969). *Notes on nursing: What it is and what it is not.* New York: Dover Publications. (Original work published 1860)

Radwin, L. E. (1995). Knowing the patient: A process model for individualized interventions. *Nursing Research, 44,* 364–370.

Rew, L. E. (1988). Nurses' intuition. *Applied Nursing Research, 1,* 27–31.

Rew, L. E. (1989). Intuition: Nursing knowledge and the spiritual dimensions of persons. *Holistic Nursing Practice, 3*(3), 56–68.

Sarvimäki, A. (1995). Aspects of moral knowledge in nursing. *Scholarly Inquiry for Nursing Practice, 9,* 343–353.

Strauss, A., Fagerhaugh, Suczek, & Weiner (1997). *The social organization of medical work.* New Brunswick: Transaction Publishers. (Originally published by the University of Chicago Press, 1985)

Tanner, C. A., Benner, P., Chesla, C., & Gordon, D. R. (1993). The phenomenology of knowing the patient. *Image: Journal of Nursing Scholarship, 25,* 273–280.

Wadel, C. (1979). The hidden work of everyday life. In S. Wallman (Ed.), *The anthropology of work* (pp. 365–384). London: Academic Press.

Wolf, Z. R. (1989). Uncovering the hidden work of nursing. *Nursing and Health Care, 10,* 463–467.

Wolfer, J. (1993). Aspects of "reality" and ways of knowing in nursing: In search of an integrating paradigm. *Image: Journal of Nursing Scholarship, 25,* 141–146.

Young, A. (1993). A description of how ideology shapes knowledge of a mental disorder (posttraumatic stress disorder). In S. Lindenbaum & M. Lock (Eds.), *Knowledge, power, and practice: The anthropology of medicine and everyday life* (pp. 108–128). Berkeley, CA: University of California Press.

Acknowledgments.   The authors wish to acknowledge the contributions of Dr. Marsha Fonteyn to early conceptualizations of this work. In addition, we would like to thank Mr. John Paley and especially the editor, Dr. Sara Fry, for their very helpful comments in the preparation of this manuscript. During the preparation of this article Dr. Fisher received support from NIH-NIDA 5T32 DA07257–08.

The Authors Comment

Theorizing the Knowledge That Nurses Use in the Conduct of Their Work

Our interest has been the actual work of nursing practice. The thrust of our work has been to understand what nurses do for people and what happens to nurses in the complex environments in which they work. Theorizing is our attempt to understand practice, but it is not itself theory. Our goal is to continue theorizing the knowledge, action, and moral stances that constitute nursing work rather than to develop theory. However, should some of our colleagues find our work useful in theory development, we would be pleased—to us, it would mean that we have articulated some aspect of the world of nursing work that makes sense to others.

—Joan Liaschenko
—Anastasia Fisher

Transforming Practice Knowledge into Nursing Knowledge— A Revisionist Analysis of Peplau

Pamela G. Reed

Nursing practice typically has been viewed as applying knowledge. However, currently, there is increasing awareness that nursing practice is also a process of knowledge development. Still, research and practice are not always connected. Analysis of Peplau's works illuminates a scholarship of nursing practice that is relevant today. This paper focuses on a specific strategy and philosophic perspective, as derived from Peplau, for integrating nursing practice more fully into today's knowledge development. Emphasis is on the need for nursing practice-based theory, as well as nursing theory-based practice.

Keywords: theory development; knowledge development; H. E. Peplau; philosophy (nursing)

Peplau (1952) fostered a scholarly interest in nursing practice and the nurse-patient relationship that continues to grow today. Although nursing practice generally is not considered a research endeavor, it is in part a scientific and scholarly endeavor (Peplau, 1988). Over the past 40 years, Peplau has described nursing practice as a caring and systematic process that produces knowledge for the benefit of patients and the nursing discipline. Unfortunately, a "depth of disconnectedness" between current research activities, theory, and practice threatens nursing scholarship (Maeve, 1994; Schmitt, 1994, p. 319).

Analysis of Peplau's ideas can further illuminate the scholarship of nursing practice and the role of nursing practice in contemporary approaches to knowledge development. Of particular interest are Peplau's ideas about nursing practice in reference to the current philosophic context for developing nursing knowledge.

About the Author

PAMELA G. REED was born in Detroit, MI, in June 1952 and grew up in an environment enriched by the sociopolitical and musical events of Motown. She is a three-time graduate of Wayne State University in Detroit, receiving a BSN in 1974, an MSN in 1976 (with a double major in child-adolescent psychiatric mental health nursing and teaching), and her PhD, with a major in nursing (focus on lifespan development and aging, nursing theory) in 1982. She worked as a psychiatric-mental health clinical nurse specialist and was an Instructor in Nursing at Oakland University, Rochester, MI, from 1976 to 1979. From 1983 to the present, she has been on the faculty at the University of Arizona College of Nursing in Tucson, including 7 years serving as Associate Dean for Academic Affairs. With her doctoral work, she pioneered nursing research into spirituality and its role in well-being. Dr. Reed has developed a theory of self-transcendence and two widely used research instruments, the *Spiritual Perspective Scale* and the *Self-Transcendence Scale*. Her publications reflect her three main passions and contributions to nursing: the conceptual and empirical bases of the significance of spirituality in health experiences, a lifespan developmental perspective of well-being in aging and end of life, and the philosophic dimensions of the development of the discipline. Dr. Reed also enjoys classical music, hiking in the Grand Canyon, swimming, and raising her two daughters, Regina and Rebecca, with her husband, Gary.

From a revisionist perspective of Peplau's ideas, practitioners are more than "working scientists," as Peplau (1988) described; practitioners not only "use the knowledge that 'producing scientists' publish" (p. 12), but they, along with patients, create many of the contexts that initiate the formation of nursing knowledge.

Postmodernism and Nursing Knowledge

Revisiting Peplau's ideas about knowledge development is instructive in postmodern 1996. In postmodernism, there is an emphasis on pragmatics and the unadorned events of everyday life as sources of knowledge (Doherty, Graham, & Malek, 1992; Waugh, 1992): Truths, ideals, and overarching conceptual schemes, called "metanarratives," that explain reality as stable, holistic, and universal are criticized and cast aside. These metanarratives, once revered in various disciplines, are being traded for other truths that espouse the instability of meaning, the value-ladeness of perception, and the power of language.

Postmodernism is evident in nursing. Some nurses question the value of nursing theory (King, 1994; Koziol-McLain & Maeve, 1993), particularly "high theory," as found, for example, in the familiar nursing conceptual models or grand theories critiqued in Fawcett (1995a; 1995b) and Fitzpatrick and Whall (1989). These theories are viewed as too remote or too stagnant for application. Instead some are turning to the culture of nursing practice for knowledge development (Kim, 1994; Maeve, 1994).

Peplau's theory may be one of those nursing theories that seems to lack relevance to today's nursing practice. However, existing nursing theories and conceptual models provide insight into the links between practice, research, and theory. Specifically, a closer look at Peplau's theory demonstrates an approach to knowledge development through the scholarship of practice; nursing knowledge is developed *in* practice as well as *for* practice. In this postmodern era, knowledge development is no longer only a concern of theoretical nursing; it is a concern in practice. Knowledge development increasingly is recognized not merely as a product to apply in practice, but as an activity in the everyday life of the practicing nurse.

Once viewed more narrowly as a psychodynamic theory, Peplau's (1952) "interpersonal process" has broader implications and can bridge nursing's modernist past with current postmodern influences on knowledge development. In modern times, the focus was on identifying universal and unique theoretical concepts that distinguished nursing from other disciplines and provided a scientific base for nursing practice. Peplau's theoretical ideas—such as the interpersonal process between patient and nurse, the developmental capacity of patients, and the centrality of anxiety in health and illness—contributed to a unifying base of knowledge. Peplau's theory also has kept pace with postmodern influences that have reinforced nurses' awareness of the knowledge-laden context of practice, at the level of the patient. Thus, Peplau has provided nursing with a model of scholarship in which knowledge development is nourished by both the practical and the theoretical. It is a scholarship that embraces the unique characteristics of individual patient situations: it employs theoretical insights and generalized meanings that have proven useful to nursing over time.

A Strategy for Linking Knowledge Development and Practice

Peplau's interpersonal process is a strategy for knowledge development that incorporates a modernist emphasis on theory as a source of truth with a postmodern emphasis on the significance of everyday contexts. Although Peplau (1952) made use of the contemporary wisdom of her day, it is equally evident from her 1952 work onward that she applied knowledge in a way that is congruent with recent philosophic trends. Peplau synthesized ideas from the "high theories" of, for example, Harry Stack Sullivan, Abraham Maslow, and Erich Fromm. Yet her approach to inquiry for nursing let the patient and the "voice of nursing" (Johnson, 1993) be heard above the theory. In doing this, Peplau introduced

an approach to knowledge development that was anchored in nursing practice, and in the science and art of the nurse-patient interaction. Development and testing of explanations through the interpersonal process between patient and nurse was done for therapeutic purposes. But, by revisiting Peplau's theory, it can be seen that this interpersonal process is also a strategy for generating nursing knowledge, which can then be examined further and refined through research. Steps 1, 2, and 3 describe the strategy of transforming practice knowledge into nursing knowledge.

Step 1:
Observation of Fundamental Units

Knowledge development, according to Peplau, began with observations made in the context of practice. For Peplau, this context was primarily the nurse-patient relationship. Observation preceded conceptual interpretations. Peplau (1952) outlined various methods of observation that yielded knowledge, including spectator observation, role-playing, and random observation. However, Peplau (1952, 1992a) emphasized participant-observation, in which a nurse uses' self as both the instrument and object of observation while participating in the interpersonal process with a patient. According to Peplau (1952), a nurse enters a situation with theoretical understanding, personal bias, and previously acquired nursing knowledge. Patients enter with their knowledge and with the powers and capabilities of a developing human being. Patients possess the principle data for inquiry in the form of underdeveloped or unused competencies, subconscious meanings, and personal knowledge. Nurses possess knowledge of methods to help patients make use of their competencies and to regain well-being.

Peplau (1992c) explained that, while on a philosophic level human beings are not reducible, elements about human beings can be studied and measured to develop nursing knowledge at the theoretic level (p. 88). Relevant units of observation are those that are meaningful and useful to patients, measurable, and definable, and that can be replicated and compared with other data (Peplau, 1952, p. 270). Fundamental units of inquiry within Peplau's theory (1952, 1988) are "processes" and "patterns" and the problems that can emerge from them.

Processes refer to behaviors that develop over time in observable phases (Peplau, 1987, 1992a). Examples include what Peplau called language-thought processes—referring, for example, to development of less ego-centric verbal expressions and thinking. Other examples are personality development, learning processes, and perceiving. Peplau (1992a) also included nursing therapeutic processes, such as the four-phased interpersonal relationship, as that which "cooperates with and assists" other processes to move the patient toward health (p. 125).

Patterns are comprised of separate thoughts, feelings, or actions that share the same theme or aim (Peplau, 1987, 1992a). Peplau (1994), also citing Sullivan (1953), defines pattern as "the envelope of insignificant particular differences" (p. 104). Examples can be observed in a person's behaviors of withdrawal or guilt. Patterns also may be shared by two or more people; these are then referred to as "pattern-integrations." Pattern-integrations may be mutual (when both parties exhibit the same set of behaviors), complementary, or antagonistic.

Thus, building knowledge entails observation of human processes that follow a developmental progression, and observation of human patterns. Patterns consist of connected though seemingly isolated events that occur within the patient or between patient and others.

Problems in processes and patterns arise when anxiety is excessive and cannot be transformed into energy needed for development (Peplau, 1988). Instead, anxiety is manifested in symptoms called "relief behaviors" (Peplau, 1952; 1987). Relief behaviors point to the source of the problem while providing, for some, a sense of well-being. For example, delusions and hallucinations indicate problems in the language-thought process while protecting a patient from destructive levels of anxiety. Frustration, loneliness, and helpfulness are natural human experiences that can become chronic problematic patterns (Peplau, 1952). As fundamental units of concern in nursing, then, patterns and processes can be observed, studied, understood, and influenced by pa-

tients and nurses (Peplau, 1992a). Ultimately, "nurse's work" is in assisting patients to develop knowledge about destructive patterns and processes, and about the means for enacting more healthy behaviors.

Step 2:
Peeling Out Theoretical Explanations

Once initial observations are made by a nurse in an interpersonal relationship, theoretical concepts are then "peeled out and drawn into the interpersonal process to explain observed phenomena (Peplau, 1973; 1988). Peeling out refers to abstracting concepts from clinical knowledge and from existing scientific theories and conceptual frameworks; these concepts represent the phenomena observed in practice. Earlier, Peplau (1958) discussed this as part of a nursing process of "interpreting observations." This process includes such investigative activities as creative invention, decoding, subdividing data, categorizing data, identifying layers of meaning at different levels of abstraction, and applying a conceptual framework to explain phenomena.

Through peeling out, hypotheses are drawn from the nurse's observations (Peplau, 1952, p. 269). Tentative explanations are formulated that are then validated with the patient and tested for their meaningfulness and usefulness in the context of the nurse-patient relationship. Peplau's approach to developing theoretical explanations reflects a broader focus for understanding phenomena than was typical within positivist philosophy (Suppe & Jacox, 1985). Her theorizing was not limited by a strict adherence to formulating operational definitions or deducing testable statements from existing "high theories." Rather, Peplau's regard for universal patterns in psychosocial development, learning, and other human experiences was tempered by her emphasis on the clinically-based reality created during encounters with patients (Reed, in press).

Step 3:
Transforming Energy and Transforming Knowledge

For Peplau (1973; 1988) application of theoretic knowledge through interactions with patients serves as a critical step in transforming practice knowledge into nursing knowledge. The term, application, hardly captures this transformation, because it requires the aesthetic perspective, intellectual competencies, and clinical judgment (Peplau, 1988, p. 13).

The truthfulness of knowledge, according to Peplau (1952; 1988), was not based upon how well the knowledge corresponded to a preexisting theory but how effective it was in helping patients enhance their self-understanding and developmental progress. Developmental progress occurs when symptom-bound energy is transformed into growth-promoting patterns and processes—and the patient's dormant powers and capacities become competencies. Knowledge that facilitates this transformation of the patient's energy acquires the status of nursing knowledge (Peplau, 1988). Nursing knowledge is developed in the context of practice through synthesis of (a) existing scientific theories, clinical observation, and judgment of nurses, and (b) knowledge and active participation of the patients. Thus, Peplau's interpersonal process provides a context for both the transformation of anxiety into productive energy and the transformation of practice into nursing knowledge.

Cycle of Inquiry

Peplau did not elaborate on the strategies used by researchers outside practice. However, her writing suggests they were equally as important as the inquiry that occurred in nursing practice (e.g., Peplau, 1952; 1988; 1992b; 1992c). A cycle of inquiry compatible with Peplau's theory is one in which the nursing knowledge that is generated through nursing practice is further refined through research. The resulting knowledge, then, becomes part of a practicing nurse's repertoire of nursing knowledge, which undergoes transformation and validation in subsequent nurse-patient encounters, as the cycle of inquiry begins again.

During the early modern era of nursing, nursing researchers not infrequently tested knowledge borrowed from other disciplines and practitioners used this knowledge. Peplau's cycle of inquiry is proposed here as one approach to producing nursing knowledge rather than borrowing knowledge. It is "nursing" knowledge by virtue of its link to nursing processes and nursing practice. It was unlikely, given the positivist views in the 1950s and 1960s, that nursing researchers would have embraced Peplau's practice-oriented strategy of nursing knowledge development. However, philosophic thought in the 1990s legitimates theories from practice for building theory—as Peplau, Ellis, and others did decades ago.

Philosophic Perspectives on Linking Knowledge Development and Practice

Although Peplau developed her theory of interpersonal relations when logical positivism was endorsed by nursing researchers (Whall, 1989), Peplau's ideas about nursing knowledge extended well beyond positivist philosophy. Positivists, in their quest for emancipating truth, separated values and truth, scientific process and product, knowledge development and application, theory and practice, science and art (Hempel, 1966). Peplau, however, espoused what today may be labeled a "postpositivist" philosophy of science. In this view (Cook, 1985; Phillips, 1990; Popper, 1968), science is not separated from other intellectual endeavors, and theory is fallible and value-laden. There is a belief in a natural world order but this reality is not fully knowable by patient or nurse. Although we use systematic methods to build knowledge, the processes and products of inquiry are interrelated and interpersonally constructed, and must be open to critical reflection and validation through consensus.

Peplau's (1952; 1988) participatory approach to inquiry and intervention denoted a shift away from positivist "epistemology" or philosophy of knowledge. The positivist regard for objective and value-free observations contrasted with Peplau's epistemology, in which knowledge was believed to be embedded in a social, temporal, and situational context (Peplau, 1975). Before nursing had incorporated postpositivist philosophy in its science, Peplau had embraced it in her practice.

Readings of Peplau's 1952 work without benefit of the broader context of her other writings have led some to conclude that Peplau's approach to nursing was positivistic and mechanistic (e.g., Meleis, 1991; Sellers, 1991). However, over the past four decades, Peplau has clarified her philosophy of nursing as an intellectual, interpersonal process of inquiry that integrates science and art. And this philosophy, as evident in her practice theory, extends beyond the descriptive and interpretive purposes of science to embrace a critical approach to inquiry as well.

Nursing Knowledge as Emancipatory Knowledge

Peplau's goal was not only to describe and understand the world, but also, to change the world. The interpersonal relationship was the avenue for this to occur. Critical science is concerned not only with the intellectual production of ideas but with practical efforts to transform interpersonal situations (Habermas, 1973; Popkewitz, 1984). Critical science is not unlike a professional discipline, particularly nursing. Emphasis is not on the instrumental use of knowledge for control and manipulation, but on its emancipatory use to liberate a person through enhanced self-knowledge. Congruent with this, Peplau (1952) defined nursing as a "maturing force and educative instrument" (p. 8) for the best interest of patients. Patients may have acquired knowledge of processes and patterns of thinking and acting that constrain their developmental progress and diminish well-being. Insights gained through the critical application of language in nurse-patient relationships often render these views inapplicable and, in this sense, change the world for the patient. The nurse's world changes as well, through self-assessment and personal growth in the relationship (Peplau, 1992a). Mutual learning and self-understanding are considered common outcomes for both patient and nurse (Beeber, Anderson, & Sills, 1990; Forchuk, 1994; Peplau, 1952).

Peplau (1952) proposed a nurse-patient relationship to "facilitate forward movement . . . in ways that displace feelings of helplessness and powerlessness with feelings of creativeness, spontaneity, and productivity" (Peplau, 1952, p. 32). It is a relationship "in which neither nurse nor patient feels helpless" (p. 33). Thus, both process and product of knowledge development are liberating. Patients are encouraged to formulate their own explanations and to "express and amplify their powers" (Peplau, 1952; 1969). Nurses do not presume to have authority over patients (Peplau, 1962; 1992a). Peplau (1952) was cognizant of the imbalances in power in nurse-patient relationships. She embedded strategies to check the nurse's potential misuse of power as well as enhance the patient's sense of power over the course of the investigative process of the relationship (p. 135).

Knowledge generated through the interpersonal relationship, then, reflects a critical theory approach to inquiry. Knowledge is tested for its emancipatory effectiveness throughout Peplau's (1952) four phases of the interpersonal relationship, which outline criteria of emancipatory knowledge for patients. For example, the orientation phase focuses on knowledge that fosters a feeling of acceptance and hope in oneself; the identification phase focuses on enhancing a sense of identity with others and a recognition of inherent capabilities in self and others; the exploitation phase encourages a patient to enact one's powers and make full use of available resources; and the resolution phase fosters a willingness to participate in the ongoing developmental change process. The emancipatory nature of nursing knowledge is evident when participants in the interpersonal process achieve an understanding that is "therapeutic and effects a cognitive, affective, and practical transformation" (Bernstein, 1976, p. 199; 1983).

Tender-Hearted and Tough-Minded

Peplau (1952, 1988) revealed another of her philosophic views in her discussion of "tough-mindedness" and "tender-heartedness." She used these terms to explain a two-parted approach to knowledge development that is incongruent with positivism. Being tender-hearted is being open, accepting, attending to personal knowledge, and sensitive. Being tough-minded is to emphasize critical thinking and reflection, rationality, and verification.

As part of the tough-minded approach, Peplau (1988) cited the importance of objectivity and emotional detachment, but not in the positivist sense that inquiry and values must be independent. Rather, Peplau's use of these terms is more consistent with a hermeneutic understanding of the distance that exists between two people interacting (Allen & Jensen, 1990; Reeder, 1988). Peplau (1952) acknowledged that "in the struggle toward developing a common understanding" (p. 290), not all experiences can be shared or understood. The "text" of the interpersonal relationship must be interpreted with the awareness of inherent differences between two people's social, historical, and personal contexts.

Peplau's (1988) tough-minded stance also incorporates existing theories about regularities and shared experiences. Peplau did not eschew the grand narratives of modern science; theories, for example, from Sullivan on personality development and Maslow on needs gratification were valued for informing nurses about potentially relevant "commonalities in human patterns" (Peplau, 1952). Peplau's (1988) tender-hearted approach was used to translate this existing theoretical information into a more individualized and contextually-based understanding of the "unique and highly personal variations in patterns and problems" of a patient (p. 14).

In this postmodern time, there is an intensified appreciation for the truths found in the everyday contexts of nursing. William James' (1908) original distinction between tender-mindedness and tough-mindedness is becoming blurred (Denzin & Lincoln, 1994). Today, nursing scholarship means embracing the philosophic view that each dimension informs the other in knowledge development. Knowledge gained through tender-heartedness is not subordinated by or reduced to knowledge gained through the more traditional tough-minded approach. Peplau helps nurses see that both are legitimate elements in transforming practice knowledge into nursing knowledge.

Practice in Scholarship

Contemporary nursing epistemology reflects a perspective of knowledge development that Peplau (1952) began over 40 years ago with *Interpersonal Relations in Nursing*. It is increasingly being recognized that practice knowledge as well as other patterns of knowing (e.g., Carper, 1978; Cowling, 1993; Munhall, 1993) are integral to nursing scholarship.

The logical positivist view held by mid-twentieth century nursing scientists may have obscured some of Peplau's contributions to knowledge development. And postmodernist skepticism of nursing models and theories may further relegate the potential insights from these sources to "nursing's intellectual underground" (Rawnsley, 1994). This would be a waste. Nurses in the 21st century should more fully "exploit" nursing metanarratives of past and present.

Peplau's philosophy of nursing and strategy for developing nursing knowledge provide an original basis for new methods that connect theory, research, and practice. These methods employ the interpersonal relationship as a mode and context for building knowledge; examples are found in Newman's (1990) research as praxis, Boyd's (1993) research practice methods, Kim's (1994) nursing practice theories, and Titchen and Binnie's (1994) action research. The patient's search for truth, as Peplau (1990) envisioned it, is a metaphor for nursing's development of knowledge; both require an interpersonal context, systematic processes, and a combination of science and sensitivity.

Nursing practice is more than a context for applying a tested and refined theory: Practice is a context for initiating and testing theory (Peplau, 1988). In her theory of interpersonal relations, Peplau (1952) operationalized a concept of practitioner that was later described by Ellis (1969) as "not simply a user of given theory, but a developer, tester, and expander of theory"

(p. 1438). As such, a practitioner is a participant in a cycle of inquiry that develops nursing knowledge and has a responsibility to make practice knowledge "explicit" (Ellis, 1969). Peplau (1992b) states that she reawakened nursing to the importance of science-based practice after Nightingale.

From this revisionist analysis, it can be seen that Peplau (1952) modeled a philosophy and designed a strategy for practice-based science. As long as what is practiced is nursing, practice will play an essential role in the scholarly transformation of knowledge into nursing knowledge. There is need not only for scholarship in practice, but also for practice in nursing scholarship.

REFERENCES

Allen, M. N., & Jensen, L. (1990). Hermeneutical inquiry: Meaning and scope. Western Journal of Nursing Research, 12, 241–253.

Beeber, L., Anderson, C. A., & Sills, G. M. (1990). Peplau's theory in practice. Nursing Science Quarterly, 3, 6–8.

Bernstein, R. J. (1976). The restructuring of social and political theory. New York: Harcourt Brace Jovanovich, 1976.

Bernstein, R. J. (1983). Beyond objectivism and relativism: Science, hermeneutics, and praxis. Philadelphia: University of Pennsylvania Press.

Boyd, C. O. (1993). Toward a nursing practice research method. Advances in Nursing Science, 16(2), 9–25.

Carper, B. (1978). Fundamental patterns of knowing in nursing. Advances in Nursing Science, 1(1), 13–23.

Cook, T. (1985). Postpositivist critical multiplism. In R. Shotland & M. Mark (Eds)., Social science and social policy (21–62). Beverly Hills, CA: Sage.

Cowling, W. R. (1993). Unitary knowing in nursing practice. Nursing Science Quarterly, 6, 201–207.

Denzin, N. K., & Lincoln, Y. S. (1994). The fifth moment. In N. K. Denzin, & Y. S. Lincoln (Eds.), Handbook of qualitative research (575–586). Thousand Oaks, CA: Sage.

Doherty, J., Graham, E., & Malek, M. (1992). Postmodernism and the socialsciences. New York: Macmillan.

Ellis, R. (1969). The practitioner as theorist. American Journal of Nursing, 69, 1434–1438.

Fawcett, J. (1995a). Analysis and evaluation of conceptual models of nursing (3rd ed.). Philadelphia: F. A. Davis.

Fawcett, J. (1995b). Analysis and evaluation of nursing theories. Philadelphia: F. A. Davis.

Fitzpatrick, J. J., & Whall, A. L. (1989). Conceptual models of nursing: Analysis and evaluation. Norwalk, CT: Appleton & Lange.

Forchuk, C. (1994). Peplau's theory-based practice and research. Nursing Science Quarterly, 7, 110–112.

Habermas, J. (1973). Theory and practice (J. Viertel, Trans.) Boston: Beacon Press.

Hempel, C. G. (1966). Philosophy of natural science. Englewood Cliffs, NJ: Prentice-Hall.

James, W. (1908). Pragmatism and the meaning of truth. Cambridge, MA: Harvard University Press.

Johnson, R. (1993). Nurse practitioner-patient discourse: Uncovering the voice of nursing in primary care practice. Scholarly Inquiry for Nursing Practice, 7, 143–158.

Kim, H. S. (1994). Practice theories in nursing and a science of nursing practice. Scholarly Inquiry for Nursing Practice, 8, 145–158.

King, M. (1994). Nursing theories outdated (letter to the editor). Journal of Psychosocial Nursing, 32, 6.

Koziol-McLain, J., & Maeve, M. K. (1993). Nursing theory in perspective. Nursing Outlook, 41, 9–82.

Maeve, M. K. (1994). The carrier bag theory of nursing practice. Advances in Nursing Science, 16 (4), 9–22.

Meleis, A. I. (1991). Theoretical nursing: Development and progress (2nd ed.). New York: J. B. Lippincott.

Munhall, P. L. (1993). "Unknowing": Toward another pattern of knowing in nursing. Nursing Outlook, 41, 125–128.

Newman, M. A. (1990). Newman's theory of health as praxis. Nursing Science Quarterly, 3, 37–41.

Peplau, H. E. (1952). Interpersonal relations in nursing. New York: Putnam.

Peplau, H. E. (1958). Interpretation of clinical observations. (Original paper presented at The University of Nebraska College of Medicine, Omaha, NE: In A. W. O'Toole & S. R. Welt (Eds.) (1989). Interpersonal theory in nursing practice: Selected works of Hildegard E. Peplau, 149–163.

Peplau, H. E. (1962). Interpersonal techniques: Crux of psychiatric nursing. American Journal of Nursing, 62, 50–54.

Peplau, H. E. (1969). Professional closeness. Nursing Forum, 8, 342–359.

Peplau, H. E. (1973). Letter to Geraldine Ellis. Cited in S. R. Welt & A. W. O'Toole (Eds.) (1989). Hildegard E. Peplau: Observations in brief. Archives of Psychiatric Nursing, 3, 254–264.

Peplau, H. E. (1975). Investigative Counseling. (Original paper presented at the University of Leuven, Belgium). In A. W. O'Toole & S. R. Welt (Eds.) (1989). Interpersonal theory in nursing practice: Selected works of Hildegard E. Peplau, 205–229. New York, NY: Springer.

Peplau, H. E. (1987). Interpersonal constructs for nursing practice. Nursing Education Today, 7(95), 201–208.

Peplau, H. E. (1988). The art and science of nursing: Similarities, differences, and relations. Nursing Science Quarterly, 1, 8–15.

Peplau, H. E. (1990). Interpersonal relations model: Principles and general applications. In W. Reynolds & D. Cormack (Eds.), Psychiatric and mental health nursing: Theory and practice (87–132). London: Chapman & Hall.

Peplau, H. E. (1992a). Interpersonal relations: A theoretical framework for application in nursing practice. Nursing Science Quarterly, 5, 13–18.

Peplau, H. E. (1992b). Notes on Nightingale. In J. Watson (Ed.), Florence Nightingale's Notes on Nursing: What it is and what it is not (Commemorative Edition) (48–57). Philadelphia: J. B. Lippincott.

Peplau, H. E. (1992c). Perspectives on nursing knowledge (interview by T. Takahashi). Nursing Science Quarterly, 5, 86–91.

Peplau, H. E. (1994). Quality of life: An interpersonal perspective. Nursing Science Quarterly, 7, 10–16.

Phillips, D. C. (1990). Postpositivistic science: Myths and realities. In E. G. Guba (Ed.), The paradigm dialog (31–45). Newbury Park, NJ: Sage.

Popkewitz, T. (1984). Paradigm and ideology in educational research: The social functions of the intellectual. London: Falmer.

Popper, K. R. (1968). The logic of scientific discovery (2nd ed.). New York: Harper & Row.

Rawnsley, M. M. (1994). Response to "The nurse-patient relationship reconsidered: An expanded research agenda." Scholarly Inquiry for Nursing Practice, 8, 185–190.

Reed, P. G. (in press). Peplau's nursing practice theory of interpersonal relations. In J. J. Fitzpatrick & A. L. Whall (Eds)., Conceptual Models of nursing: Analysis and application (3rd ed.). Norwalk, CT: Appelton & Lange.

Reeder, F. (1988). Hermeneutics. In B. Sarter (Ed.), Paths to knowledge: Innovative research methods for nursing (193–238). New York: National League for Nursing.

Schmitt, M. (1994). The connectedness of nursing research: Revisiting an old issue (editorial). Research in Nursing & Health, 17, 319–320.

Sellers, S. C. (1991). A philosophical analysis of conceptual models of nursing. Unpublished doctoral dissertation, Iowa State University, Ames, IA.

Sullivan, H. S. (1953). The interpersonal theory of psychiatry. New York: Norton.

Suppe, F., & Jacox, A. K. (1985). Philosophy of science and the development of nursing theory. In H. H. Werley & J. J. Fitzpatrick (Eds.). Annual review of nursing research: Vol. 3 (241–267). New York: Springer.

Titchen, A., & Binnie, A. (1994). Action research: A strategy for theory generation and testing. International Journal of Nursing Studies, 31(1), 1–12.

Waugh, P. (1992). Postmodernism. New York: Edward Arnold.

Whall, A. L. (1989). The influence of logical positivism on nursing practice. Image: Journal of Nursing Scholarship, 21, 243–245.

The Author Comments

Transforming Practice Knowledge Into Nursing Knowledge—A Revisionist Analysis of Peplau

As a psychiatric mental health nurse clinician at the master's level, I was familiar with Peplau's ideas on interacting with patients in a psychiatric setting. Then, as a doctorally prepared nurse interested in the philosophic dimensions of the discipline, I revisited Peplau for her insights into the process of knowledge development. I believed that her statements reflected much more than simply the positivist views of her day and the belief in separation of knowledge development and application. A closer reading of Peplau offered a wealth of ideas on the scholarship of practice and its integral role in nursing knowledge development. I envision a future in nursing where all clinicians are educated to not only apply knowledge but also use their practice to build knowledge.

—Pamela G. Reed

Toward an Understanding of Art in Nursing

Jeanne J. LeVasseur

The art of nursing is a term on which there is little definitional agreement. Nursing includes both artistic and scientific traditions; at times, the balance between these two approaches is an uneasy one. An examination of aesthetics offers a perspective to ground practice in nursing art through John Dewey's philosophy of art as experience. Differences and similarities between science, art, and craft are examined. Nursing art is defined as helping patients create coherence in lives threatened by illness and change.

Key words: art, craft, nursing, philosophy, theory

The opposition between science and art has existed from the beginning of modern nursing. Nightingale championed the view of nursing as a moral art, while Fenwick argued for registration and insisted that nursing was an independent profession allied with science and technology.[1] Peplau[2] states clearly that art values subjectivity and involvement while science emphasizes objectivity and detachment. Nurses often have struggled to achieve a theoretical stance between art and science

that permits appropriate and skillful help. An attempt to claim both these paradigms has produced abundant discourse, diversity of opinion, and heightened awareness to alternatives, which is evident in the nursing literature.

This article proposes to demonstrate that nursing art is inseparable from nursing science and that its claim to be both an art and a science has never been wrong. To accomplish this, this article will examine

About the Author

JEANNE J. LEVASSEUR was born in Hartford, CT. She has alternated educational study in the arts with the study of nursing, receiving her first degree from Beloit College in Theater, followed by an MS in nursing from Pace University, an MFA in writing from Vermont College, and a PhD in nursing from the University of Connecticut. She is interested in theoretical problems that challenge and expand our conception of nursing. Her recent articles include work on professional authenticity among combat nurses in Vietnam, a methodologic problem of bracketing in phenomenology, and Nightingale's philosophic legacy. She has also published poetry in literary and nursing journals, including the anthologies *Between the Heartbeats: Poetry and Prose by Nurses* and *Uncharted Lines: Poems from the Journal of the American Medical Association.* She is currently the director of graduate nursing at Quinnipiac University in Hamden, CT.

some of the dominant theories in aesthetics and critique their applicability in nursing. This article will locate a theory of aesthetics that promises to be productive for nursing practice and then will contrast ideas on art and craft in order to assess the application of these concepts in nursing.

In what way can nursing be said to be an art? By invoking the term "art," nurses have referred to qualities of intuition, caring, embodied skill, and the evaluative idea of something well done.[2,3] Often, use of this term is a kind of rhetorical attempt to capture all that is ineffable in nursing. Katims[4] observed that the concept of nursing art is at once familiar and yet mysterious and ill defined. She suggests that the concept evokes such immediate understanding among nurses that this tends to curtail further attempts to define and deepen its meaning. In the nursing literature, authors have used the phrase "the art of nursing" to refer to those elusive things that cannot be accounted for by science and in this way, a schism has developed between the notions of artful and scientific nursing. Here is found the dilemma in nursing: reasoned application of scientific principles can be accused of indifference to the individual, variable patient and thus of indifference to nursing's ultimate concern. On the other hand, empathy and intuition can be accused of excessive subjectivity that is liable to arbitrary, unverifiable, and therefore untrustworthy conclusions.

Currently, the idea of nursing art is unformed theoretically. Nursing theorists have limited theoretical understanding or agreement on nursing art, but there is abundant agreement that it exists.[2,5-8] Johnson[3] examined the nursing literature on the art of nursing through the work of 41 authors, from Nightingale[9] to the present, and outlined patterns of agreement and disagreement. She calls her approach a dialectical one in that she attempted to present views in a nonpartisan manner and considered the various theoretical perspectives to be in dialogue with each other regardless of their position in history. Johnson's examination revealed five quite separate senses of nursing art. Her work makes apparent the lack of agreement on the art of nursing in the professional literature.

While it is essential to look for nursing art in practice, it is also necessary to use theoretical constructs to shape one's notion of art and use such theory to research and extend applications in practice. Kuhn[10] claimed that one of the tests of scientific theory is its ability to solve long-standing puzzles or anomalies. He also acknowledged that a theory that can address rigorously problems in the discipline also must be good on another count: it must be productive. A productive theory not only answers old questions but also poses new ones. Therefore, one of the tests one could put to a theory of aesthetics in nursing would be whether it illuminates something essential about nursing and opens a space for further productive inquiry.

If one is to employ the word "art" with accuracy, nursing art should be elucidated within the traditions of aesthetics. Discourse in the field of aesthetics frequently considers art in terms of a manifest object or event and also as the principles and methods governing any craft. In nursing, the discussion of nursing art has centered on the methods or processes of art rather than on the outcome. Every art has a particular craft tradition and mastery of these techniques and their application is a necessary precondition for art. The craft of nursing involves knowledge, skills, techniques, materials, and specific settings. But the tangible manifestation or result of nursing art has been ignored largely in the professional literature.

If nurses can clearly distinguish what is nursing art, they can deepen their understanding and improve both the practice and teaching of it. Johnson[3] has identified five conceptual meanings of art in the nursing literature but Chinn and Kramer[11] have suggested that at least two of these themes are not related strictly to aesthetic knowing. Recent work has examined the actual experience of the art of nursing among practicing nurses.[12-17] While these studies have advanced the discourse on nursing aesthetics, they have not forged a strong link to traditional aesthetic literature in an attempt to define the concept of nursing art before asking participants to reflect on their experience of it. To define nursing art, one may well profit by a working knowledge of existing aesthetic theories and how they could help solve problems within the discipline. It is hoped that such definitional focus will reveal a specific aspect of nursing art and allow both the process and outcome to become more visible.

Art as Representation of Reality

Philosophic inquiry in the field of aesthetics is far from agreement on the nature of art. In the first millennium, the mimetic theory or the theory of representation dominated western views on art. These views began with Plato,[18] who believed that art was an imitation removed from reality. For Plato, the forms represented the highest and most conceptually pure reality. Like Plato, Aristotle also regarded the arts as essentially mimetic. But unlike Plato, who believed that most art should be banned in the ideal republic because it inflamed the passions and subverted reason, Aristotle[19] believed good art elicited an ethical response precisely by prompting an emotional response to imagined events.

The central difficulty with the representational view is that not all artworks portray a version of reality or even claim to represent truth. Many artworks are concerned with unique patterns of sound, color, image, or form and do not refer to the world of meaningful human experience. But perhaps more importantly, people cannot philosophically agree on what reality is; for Plato, the ideal forms represent ultimate reality and are accessible only through the insight of reason. But the empiricists, Aristotle included, would protest that reality is located in the physical world and experienced through the senses.

Aside from the problem of which reality art should represent in nursing, the representational theory does not permit the kind of fluid, future-oriented world that nursing art needs to embrace. Representation holds that art renders structures that imitate reality. Thus, art, in this view, is not instrumental to claiming experience except in so far as artwork reveals reality. Given the phenomenological world of nursing, in which meaning is difficult if not impossible to specify in advance, this theory does not offer as much interpretative latitude that other theories do. Nor does it fit with the evolving, uncertain world of a patient's lived experience.

One of the chief problems in defining an art of nursing is making the artwork visible. It seems clear that the art of nursing will take many shapes, most of which will not include a visible artifact or object. Representation depends on a tangible artwork that can be viewed as distinct from reality. Only in this way does it refer to and depict reality. It is a theory that, by definition, relies on a certain distance or division between reality and art; thus, it does not permit a reality enmeshed in or continuous with art, which is the actuality in most nursing situations.

Formalism and Autonomy of Art

Early in the 19th century, the idea that art occupied an autonomous realm, sufficient unto itself, came into being. In *The Critique of Judgement*, Kant[20] argued that beauty is independent of utility, morality, and truth; this idea promoted the development of formalism. He developed the idea that aesthetic judgment should be free from external considerations; the artwork should not have to correspond to anything external to itself. If art is going to be free from external conditions, then art needs to have an internal subject that is sufficient to it. This leads naturally to the idea of form. Bell[21] argued that "significant form" is the defining attribute of art. By "significant," Bell does not seem to imply "meaningful," but more the notion of "sufficient." Bell does not deny that art can be representational, but he believes this kind of art appeals to "emotions of life." Objects that elicit these emotions are inferior art, according to Bell. He believes that representation in art is always irrelevant to a rapturous appreciation. When people are unable to fall into rapture, they use art as a means to the "the snug foothills of humanity."[22(p276)]

Formalism emphasizes the organic unity of art and the necessity of focusing on its formal properties rather than on its meaning or connection to the world. In short, it posits form as the distinctive element essential to art. In this view, an artwork is essentially an integrated and patterned structure that affects people by its overall organization rather than by its meaning. The famous aphorism "art for art's sake" captures this idea and became the rallying cry for aestheticism in France early in the 19th century.[23]

One of the difficulties with the theory of formalism is its inability to distinguish between an artwork and a theorem. Science, math, and logic all are worked predominantly through form and yet one's common language meaning of the word "art" distinguishes it from these other entities. Eisner[24] holds that all made things have form, whether in art, science, or practical life, and when well made, these forms have aesthetic properties. Eisner believes that the common function of the aesthetic is to modulate form so that it, in turn, informs one's experience. This certainly extends the significance of a formal arrangement of elements into the realm of experience, but it discredits the notion that form can be that elusive essence by which art can be defined and distinguished.

One of the most problematic notions of formalism for nursing is its lack of connection to the world of experience and human meaning. The distinction between aesthetic rapture and the emotions of life seem to make it a poor fit with a practice discipline very much concerned with ordinary human emotions. Tolstoy[15] held that the artist has moral responsibilities, but formalism eschews these obligations and holds that art occupies a separate and autonomous realm. The essential autonomy of art under this conception makes it a poor match for a field in which art and craft are yoked in a conjoint effort to alleviate suffering and promote human welfare. Nursing has a tradition of purposeful, moral activity. Benner, Tanner, and Chelsa use the term "ethical comportment"[25(p233)] to refer to the skilled know-how of nurses who relate to others in ways that are "respectful, responsive, and supportive of their concerns." As an aesthetic theory, formalism would deny the concept of ethical comportment in nursing. Given that the historical focus and current project of nursing is devoted to furthering the welfare of the patient, this theory presents too many contradictions to the spirit of nursing to be viable as the dominant aesthetic framework.

Art as Expression of Emotion

If representation and formalism are inadequate aesthetic theories for nursing art, could the theory of emotional expression possibly capture what is needed for nursing? Several theorists have put expression at the center of their aesthetic theory and certainly art does seem to engage and express emotion. Collingwood[26] argues for a conception of art as imaginative expression. In his analysis, the artist struggles to identify unrealized and shapeless feelings by articulating them through artwork. Collingwood also is careful to distinguish between expressing emotion and betraying or exhibiting emotion. Here he defines expression as "lucidity or intelligibility,"[26(p122)] which allows the audience to discover the emotion in the art for themselves. Through art, an artist comes to know both self and world because experiences are clarified by the artful expression of emotions. Collingwood believes that art is not a luxury and there is no division between intellectual and emotional elements; emotions are connected to ideas and the artist does not merely express the emotional residue of thought but fuses the two together.

As theory for nursing art, certain versions of expressionism have much to offer. The connection to a human world of emotions and the clarification of these emotions could be productive for nursing. However, one problem of expressionism is its focus on the emotions of the artist, for it is the meaning and significance of *these* emotions on which expressionism dwells. And although there are times when the nurse will want to clarify his or her understanding of patient care situations through artistic expression, this is not the essential purpose of nursing or nursing art. Rather, nursing is oriented to the concerns of the patient and it can be hoped that the art of nursing will respond to these concerns. If nursing art is to be a vital part of a practice discipline, then the art must serve the needs of practice.

Art As An Open Concept

The aesthetic theories of representation, formalism, and expressionism set for themselves the problem of defining an essential concept of art. An essential concept consists of a set of conditions that are necessary and jointly sufficient for something to be a work of art. But can art be defined this way? Weitz[27] has argued that one must reject the problem of the essential definition of art and instead recognize the open, loose textured nature of art. Weitz holds that art is a concept that defies definition in the traditional sense and that no essence can be distilled that would be true in all instances of it. He invokes a similar argument made by Wittgenstein[28] about games and argues that the same is true of art. There are no absolute common properties, Weitz comments, "only strands of similarities."[27(p31)] He asserts that if one forces an essential definition of art, then one

forecloses "on the very conditions of creativity in the arts"[27(p32)] and new arts and new unimagined expressions of art always will and should develop.

The problem with this idea for nursing is that art is already an open concept in nursing; witness the many meanings of the term in the professional literature.[3] Unfortunately, the concept is so open that it is difficult to see overlapping strands of meaning. This has the effect of making the art of nursing all but disappear into the many professional activities. While this theory offers a great deal of latitude, it does not sharpen or clarify the meaning of nursing art and it is not a theoretically productive way to examine art within a *specific* discipline. As a theory, its chief value is a broad, flexible perspective of art across multiple disciplines and its ability to accommodate the wide varieties of art found in many fields. Its open stance is congruent with an evolving art form such as that found in nursing, but it does not offer a sharp enough focus to illuminate the field and define the terrain.

The Institutional Theory of Art

The institutional theory sidesteps the problem of denoting a set of properties common to all art and yet also goes beyond the notion of art as an open concept. Dickie[29] defined a work of art as an artifact that has had conferred upon it the status of art by persons acting on behalf of certain social institutions. By "social institutions," he means the art world, which includes critics, exhibitors, producers, and even to some extent, the public. Art then is whatever the art world agrees it is, Danto[30] asserts that what constitutes art is a wider theoretical world of history, tradition, philosophy, and criticism. Artwork articulates with this world in a particular way that prevents the art from collapsing into mere artifact. Danto emphasizes the interpretive quality of art, particularly the way in which it converses with history; this permits a fluid art world that is subject to evolution and revision. Danto insists that some art could not have been called by that name 50 years ago, as the world was not ready for it. Thus, art depends on its context for its very definition. He likens the theories in art to those in science and postulates that when a whole new class of artworks arrives on the scene, people have to address their prior theories either by abandoning them for something better or by adding auxiliary hypotheses. He even goes so far as to say that the upheavals in the art world are similar to those in science, in which a well-established and powerful theory threatened by new ideas constitutes a crisis that may result in a scientific revolution.

One problem with the institutional theory of art is that it often does little to reveal the nature of art and instead concentrates on its evaluation by expert groups of critics in separate disciplines. While criticism is an excellent way of refining and extending definitional meaning, it is not always the most useful way of founding it. The institutional theory focuses less on the definition of art and more on its evaluation within specific artistic traditions. The institutional theory identifies a reality within the art world similar to Kuhn's[10] notion of scientific progress through revolutionary paradigm shifts. At present, though, nursing has no recognized art world so the institutional theory does not apply. However, efforts to define the art in nursing may in time create and make visible an art world for the discipline. If nursing art can be described for practitioners and the public, a widely based institutional theory of art might become possible. Certainly, nursing has a practical and theoretical world as well as a history and tradition, which could modulate the development of a nursing aesthetic.

Art as Experience

John Dewey, a 20th century American pragmatist, believes art is embedded in experience and should not be isolated into a realm of its own. Dewey remarks that "contempt for the body, fear of the senses and the opposition of flesh to spirit"[31(p20)] have conjoined to separate the higher things of experience from their vital roots. Dewey places at the center of his theory a project to recover for art its continuity with ordinary living and turns to everyday experience to examine the origins of art. He believes art is misunderstood apart from its place in human experience and proposes to restore a sense of connection between aesthetic experience and works of art.

Dewey has argued that aesthetic form is what unifies the otherwise disparate events of ordinary life into what he calls "lived experience."[31] Much of ordinary life passes unmemorably and half distracted, one's attention dispersed among various and competing claims. People start, stop, and shift their attention, events interrupt them, or they do not have the desire or passion to pursue the experience creatively. But when people have *an* experience, events become organized toward an end; the parts relate to each other in meaningful ways, each contributing to the whole. Dewey writes that in such experiences, all the parts flow together into what happens next. This is to say, in an experience, there are points of rest or pause, but the events are conjoined and become part of each other and what comes next. The experience forms a unity that can be named: *that* meal, *that* storm. The ending of an experience is thus a consummation, not a cessation.

One of the things that makes Dewey especially important to a discussion of nursing art is the way that he develops an idea of human experience as essentially related to aesthetic form. For Dewey, experience is not the passive reception of sense data, as it was for the empiricists, nor is it primarily mental insight, as it appears to be for many of the rationalists. Rather, for Dewey, experience is necessarily structured and therefore nameable, so that people speak of *that* experience. The clearest, most revealing model of experience for Dewey is found in the experience of art. Dewey does not think of art as a collection of visual or auditory objects removed from practical life. Rather, for Dewey, a work of art is primarily a mode of experience; conceived of as an object, it is a source, origin, or possibility of experience. But the key pragmatic idea is that the nature of art is to offer itself as an experience with all the dimensions of experience: temporal, spatial, and meaningful. The practical value of art, according to Dewey, becomes clear when one reflects that all human experience at its best—when most heightened, enlivened, and memorable—takes on aesthetic form in which means and ends are combined into a comprehensive unity. Aesthetic form for Dewey is not merely form, as it was for Bell, but is continuous with the practical structure of human experience at its most conscious.

While Dewey[31] believes that aesthetic experience is the origin of art, he agrees with Collingwood that art involves the expression of emotion. He also takes care to differentiate aesthetic expression from the thoughtless discharge of emotion that occurs in much ordinary life. A mere gesture of frustration or pleasure is not necessarily an aesthetic expression. Nonetheless, Dewey recognizes that aesthetic expression does not occur without the excitement and turmoil of emotion. Aesthetic expression results from the carrying forward and development of emotion rather than the discharge or dismissal of it. Dewey believes expression begins with turmoil and that it can become a productive ferment when something is at stake for the person. When people are staked in the situation, they are motivated to clarify and deepen their understanding. The successful result of this is *an* experience; a deeply felt, conclusive, and integrated whole. Its failure likewise would be a failure of experience and understanding.

Illness and Experience

Aesthetic experience matters in nursing because both patients and nurses are stakeholders in the situation. Experiences of illness have the potential to become lifted from ordinary life simply because so much is at stake. The details and nuances of relationships between patients and nurses are significant because they are part of this experience of illness and this is why the deeply engaged stance of caring matters. Without engagement, the nurse is no longer a stakeholder and nursing art is not possible. Engagement is a precondition of experience. Benner and Wrubel argue that caring creates a world and that "without care, the person would be without projects and concerns."[32(p1)] Their view implies that care is fundamental to meaning and that meaning comes to be on the basis of some prior structure of care. A person may be regarded as constituted by their involvement and commitments in the world and without such engagements, one remains, in the profoundest sense, a mere possibility of a person. Similarly, Dewey believes that art must be "loving;" that is, "it must care deeply for the subject matter upon which skill is exercised."[31(p48)] An engaged, emotional commitment is a precondition for nursing art and effective intervention.

Art invites action and Dewey believes that a "beholder must *create* his own experience;"[31(p54)] without this act of re-creation, an object is not perceived as a work of art. This means that emotion is not separate from comprehension. "Perception is an act of the going out of energy in order to receive, not a withholding of energy."[31(p53)] This anticipates Benner's[33] expert nurse who utilizes and learns from clinical exemplars. In Benner's account, expertise depends on an inquiring and engaged mind brought into contact with particular situations in which understanding can be refined, extended, and revised. This is why art seems rigorous and demanding of nursing's attention, because it calls forth those same qualities of attentive openness coupled with an outgoing of energy that helps nurses move toward conclusions.

Dewey[31] contrasts perception with recognition, which he believes is satisfied with a tag or label. For instance, it is common practice in medicine to structure the medical interview in such a way to limit information from the patient. Thus, the interviewer seeks answers only to preconceived and standard questions considered useful in constructing a differential diagnosis for the patient's chief presenting symptoms. Coles[34] recounts his insecurity as a psychiatric resident and his need to construct theoretical interpretations even as his patients were in the midst of telling him their problems. Being able to recognize these problems and convert them into medical language offered a great sense of control and purpose. This way of proceeding appears to promote an efficiency of time and attention by screening out unnecessary details not crucial to diagnosing biomedical disease. But it also produces inefficiency by imposing a dogmatic structure that sharply limits the emergence of new information about illness in the life of the patient.

A patient's negotiation of his or her illness can be a powerful experience that is dramatically different from the flow of ordinary, less reflective life. Sometimes it is only at moments of illness that patients stop to reflect, to take stock of their life, and so become newly awakened to life and to experience. Broyard, diagnosed with cancer, felt clarified and awakened by his illness: "Suddenly, there was in the air a rich sense of crisis, real crisis . . . Time was no longer innocuous, nothing was casual anymore . . . I now felt as concentrated as a diamond . . . ."[35(p32)] Broyard goes on to speculate that such concentration and alertness was likely only a phase, or as he says, "a rush of consciousness, a splash of perspective, a hot flash of ontological alertness."[35(p32)]

Perhaps one of the aims of nursing art is to help people shape the potentially powerful experience of illness into *an* experience, to come alive to the possibilities in it, and thus not miss it. Chinn, Maeve, and Bostick found that nursing art often was a deliberate attempt to "shift or shape the experience of the patient."[14(p88)] Whether aesthetic experience becomes art depends on one's ability to clarify and fully express experience. This, Dewey believes, takes time. He means here more than time to scribble the poem but also a "prolonged interaction"[31(p65)] between self and objective conditions, whereby both self and media are transformed. Thus, Dewey does not underwrite the idea of art as a passive object of contemplation, but instead articulates an aesthetic that permits nursing art as the product of caring engagement that can shape the experience of the patient and nurse alike.

Not Art Or Science

Dewey takes issue with dualism of many types and opposes the "division of everything into nature *and* experience, of experience into practice *and* theory, art *and* science, of art into useful *and* fine, menial *and* free."[36(p304)] He observes that modern thinkers celebrate science, rationality, and fine art in contrast to practical knowledge and he would remind us that the fine arts are also "affairs of practice."[36(p302)] In Dewey's conception, everything belongs to the practical world because that is what people are intent on changing. He would have people see that "science is an art, that art is

practice, and the only distinction worth drawing is not between practice and theory,"[36(p303)] but between meaningful practice and practice that is without enjoyment or intelligence. Dewey believes that aesthetics is the organizing principle and culmination of all vivid experience including scientific thought. Nurses may appreciate a special irony in his claim that science acts as a "handmaiden"[36(p304)] to art.

The art/science dichotomy that implicitly frames much theoretical writing in nursing historically has posed difficulties for achieving a clear, theoretical self awareness for the practice of nursing.[2,6,7,37,38] Many nurse theorists have remarked on the difficulty in defining the essence or focus of nursing today.[39,40-43] The divide between art and science in nursing undoubtedly has contributed to this problem of focus and definition in the discipline.

While Dewey does make distinctions between art and science, he is reluctant to draw sharp divisions and points out that Plato considered both to be forms of *techné*. Dewey wants one to understand that thinking in all its forms is predominately an art. Thinking is a series of progressions and conclusions in which meaning is clarified and concentrated so that it illuminates other ideas; in this way, it becomes aesthetically organized. Dewey believed that intellectual experience and aesthetic experience are similar. The two merely differ in their materials. The materials of the fine arts consist of qualities such as color and texture, while those of the intellect consist of signs or symbols that have no intrinsic quality of their own but stand for things that otherwise may be experienced.[31]

Dewey[31] notes that thinking in terms of "qualities," as artists do, is as demanding as thinking in terms of verbal or mathematical symbols. Knowledge, science, and art all go forward into the practical world and confer new qualities and potentials on things that did not belong to them previously. This opening into new awareness is how art can change people's lives. Not only are people changed by their appreciation of art but the making of art also involves a process of protest and self expression whereby they become engaged in remaking the world.

Eisner agrees that works of science are also works of art and he believes that art and science do not occupy distinctively separate spheres. "All scientific inquiry culminates in the creation of form: taxonomies, theories, frameworks, and conceptual systems. The scientist like the artist must transform the content of his or her imagination into some public, stable form, something that can be shared with others . . . "[24(p26)] Eisner believes that all things made by human beings have form. If form is by nature aesthetic, this demonstrates that the ideas within disciplines are human constructions, "shaped by craft, employing techniques, and mediated through some material."[24(p35)]

Others do not see an aesthetic framework as an essential organizing principle for thought. In discussing nursing, Rogers[6] states that science is an organized body of knowledge arrived at by research and analysis, while art is the creative application of this body of abstract knowledge. This relates art to practice, yet there is an incongruity in Roger's later comment that "the study of nursing is not the study of nurses and what they do any more than biology is the study of biologists and what they do."[6(p100)] This is a faulty comparison. Nursing is a practice discipline and part of practice is the interaction between the nurse and the patient. Nurses' interventions often are interpretive and deserve to be researched. Although Rogers relates art to practice, she excludes nursing art as something worthy of study when she discourages the study of nursing practice. It is crucial that nurses understand how they affect patients and how they can facilitate and promote transitions from one state of health to another. To comprehend this fully, nurses need to understand the art of nursing.

Art and Craft in Nursing

More than 100 years ago, Nightingale claimed that nursing was the finest art. She did this in her inimitable prose in which she only half claimed the idea, thereby securing it all the more.

"Nursing is an art; and if it is to be made an art, it requires as exclusive a devotion, as hard a preparation, as any painter's or sculptor's work. For what is the having to do with dead canvas or cold marble compared with having to do with the living body—the temple of God's spirit? It is one of the fine arts; I had almost said, the finest of the fine arts."[44(p504)]

The notion of "the fine arts" originated in the 18th century. Art such as painting and poetry, in which the aesthetic characteristics are more significant than the utilitarian ones, was dubbed "fine" and this created the impression that art had no function other than to be art.[23] One can presume that Nightingale, an educated woman writing nearly 100 years later, was not unaware of this use of terminology and that she did not use the term thoughtlessly in her writing. By obliquely claiming that nursing is the finest art, she at once celebrated the human medium in which nurses work and also, perhaps more subtly, claimed a utilitarian purpose to art.

In *Notes on Nursing,* Nightingale[9] has written a manifesto on the importance of purposeful nursing activities, in which she describes the need for close observation of the sick, proper nourishment, light, cleanliness, and air. Because it is inconceivable, in Nightingale's view, that nursing is without a purpose—given the demanding role of the nurse in observing patients and managing environments—she combines nursing art with the utilitarian function of craft and considers them inseparable. That she should do this is not surprising because Nightingale was educated classically, read Plato in Greek, and was influenced by Socratic thought in her vision for nursing;[45] the Platonic idea of *techné* does not separate art from craft but rather, includes notions of art, craft, and science.

In modern aesthetic theory, however, there is considerable controversy over whether there is a difference between art and craft. Collingwood[26] believes there is a principled difference between art and craft and argues for the necessity of making clear distinctions between them. Collingwood's[15] distinctions can be summarized by the following: craft results from skillful use of method or technique to produce a pre-specified product from some kind of raw material. Thus, the endpoint of a craft is visualized before the methods of achieving it are determined, so the way to proceed is planned from the beginning. Judging a work of craft is therefore less a matter of interpretation than a matter of fit between artifact and preconceived models of particular craft objects. According to Collingwood,[26] craft implies clearly understood goals and methods and this makes evaluation straightforward. The results of art, on the other hand, cannot be specified before creation; and means and ends are not always thought out separately. The artist does not always know what to make, or the most effective way to go about it; rather, ends and means evolve simultaneously. According to this definition, art is both more creative and difficult to evaluate.

By Collingwood's[26] definition, the craft of nursing might be exemplified by giving an injection well. By this definition, the art of nursing will need to involve something more because the end results for an injection and most technical procedures can be pre-specified. It is important that a nurse competently master such technical procedures. But is such competence what nurse theorists wish to call the art of nursing? In the discovery of art in nursing, one may need to consider a process that does not rely so much on a technique suited to pre-specified purposes, but develops goals simultaneously. Describing this process would seem to emphasize the creative aspects of art, the sense that it ventures into new terrain and cannot be judged by preconceived criteria.

Drawing distinctions between craft-like competence and artistic open-endedness raises the question of whether a project to separate art and craft in nursing is misdirected. For moral reasons, there is little tolerance for error in nursing and little freedom to experiment. Nurses have serious responsibilities and they are not free in their creative efforts in the way most traditional artists are. "Art for art's sake" is not a slogan that could ever be appropriate in nursing. Dewey[31] believes that the difference between art and craft is not simply that craft serves a utilitarian function, but rather that art also serves the purpose of spurring immediate and vital experience. Because of this, art serves aesthetic and not merely useful ends. Dewey draws some distinctions between art and craft but on the whole, he considers these unnecessary to the definition of a work of art.

One consequence of Dewey's view of art is that the distinction between art and craft becomes blurred; art and craft are now related on a continuum of experience. Craft is what art becomes when it is habitual or routine and no longer engages a heightened comprehension of the whole. Craft is not creative but is secondary to the creative moment of aesthetic awareness. Nonetheless, craft has the structure of art and remains a possibility for aesthetic experience when the practitioner gains insight into, or envisions new possibilities for, the craft.

Dewey deems the usefulness of an artifact immaterial to determining whether it is called craft or art. Rather, what he feels is critical is the "live creature's" experience of producing art and the way in which a work of art ignites experience in an observer.[31] This kind of aesthetic experience should cause a person to feel more alive and contribute to an expanded life. Without aesthetic experience, living may be put aside for the sake of production. In this, Dewey implies that by itself, craft tends to be repetitive, routine, and focused on production rather than experience. Art appears to be a way of cracking the purposeful activities of craft open to possibility and vivid aesthetic experience.

Chinn, Maeve, and Bostick[14] have defined nursing art as a spontaneous, in-the-moment act that requires deliberate rehearsal. In discussing nursing art, Breunig[46] tells the story of the Zen master who draws the bow and waits without purpose until the moment of highest tension. Her point is that every great artist is a great craftsperson who knows how to draw the bow perfectly. The practical task of learning to draw the bow usually is overshadowed by the goal of hitting the target, but the lesson of the story is that practice and craft are inseparable from the moment "it" moves through the craftsperson and the arrow is shot. This story indicates that while both art and craft have purpose, art occurs to the prepared mind as a moment unencumbered by its overriding purpose and open to possibility and experience. Benner, Tanner, and Chesla's[25] idea that expertise flows from experience is a crucial addition to this story. Their concept of nursing experience as a turning around, nuanced amendment of preconceived notions is a critical element in understanding how craft or practical know-how should not be separated from art—the ability to let the arrow fly at the right moment. Nursing situations are marked by an individual, never-the-same-again quality. Part of the art of nursing is knowing how to respond in these infinitely variable situations.

Chinn and Kramer[11] have commented that art draws a person into new realms and expands perceptual capacities. If the object of nursing art is to transform the lived experience of health and illness, as Chinn claims, this explains why art is potentially so important for nursing. Not only do nurses need art to expand their perspectives on caring for patients, but patients also need nursing art to help them perceive the possibilities in their situation. A nurse who is artistically creative may set new standards for how things can be done. Art can change the ethos of what is considered good practice and alter the conceptions of what nursing outcomes ought to be. This means that the "audience" for nursing art will be not only patients and family members, to whom nurses hope to show possibilities so that they may move forward and transform their futures, but also other nurses, from whom nurses learn and with whom they transform practice. By maintaining a fluid openness in nursing situations, it may be that nurses' own experiences and that of their patients is enlarged.

Dewey's[31] answer to the problem of differentiation between art and craft is congenial to the problems raised by separating them in nursing. His ideas do not mandate that art and craft be wholly separated and differentiated, nor do they restrict art to unplanned and open-ended activity as Collingwood would have it. Rather, he has chosen to focus on the way in which art ignites vital experience. By these lights, art in nursing would coalesce around problems where something is at stake; and in an effort to clarify these issues, the nurse creates an experience of progressive and vital movement toward a conclusion. What comes most easily to mind are those intense, dramatic moments of health illness transition when a nurse can, by virtue of his or her privileged and intimate relationship with the patient, help resolve, move, or restructure the experience. But also consider the everyday version of nursing art related by Lumby, who sees "this art every time I walk into an environment where a nurse is busy 'creating,' the day

for another person. They are busy using light, space, sound, words, movement and touch to deliver the message of care."[47(p1009)]

This depiction depends on an understanding of the environmental deprivation and disorientation commonly experienced by ill or hospitalized patients. It also brings up Nightingale's[9] early concerns with light, space, and air. Nightingale's message was that nurses need to manage the environment in order to create the conditions under which recovery from illness can occur. But more than that, Dewey's ideas show how nurses' attention to these basic needs creates an environment of care in which experience actually is constituted. Aesthetic experience and art are significant to Dewey[31] precisely because they do more than indicate experience; they constitute it. Not all experience will be aesthetically organized, but to the extent that nurses can aesthetically organize experience and "create the day" for their patients, nurses will have helped bring order, unity, and meaning to their lives.

One of the difficulties in defining this aspect of nursing art has been the invisibility of the art object. The *process* of art is visible enough in nursing. The tools, techniques, and craft-like approach can be described, but the outcome of the art is very difficult to specify. Nurse theorists are reluctant to identify the patient as the object of nursing art. It is contrary to their philosophical tradition to objectify patients in this way, nor would this identification be correct.

But how is art manifest in nursing? To answer this question, one needs to consider the disruption to the life world of the patient during illness. Cassell[48] wrote of the unpredictable suffering patients experience during illness because of the threat to various aspects of personhood. He makes the point that suffering is not only the physical experience of pain but also the grave threat that illness and its treatment pose to the many facets of a person. Specifically, he mentions the disturbance that illness provokes in a person's experience of body, relationships, social roles, activities, work, and sense of the future.

Nurses endeavor to nurse patients through an illness to a satisfactory outcome, whether this is regaining health and function or coping with disability or the ultimate transition of a peaceful death. To do this, nurses rely on the craft of nursing, which involves knowledge, skills, and specific techniques. The tangible manifestation of this work is a satisfactory outcome, however that is measured. Outcomes long have been associated with the resolution of pathobiological disease and physical dysfunction and this narrows the potential application of artful nursing. Nurses help patients navigate a variety of disruptive transitions and the art of nursing is manifest in helping patients regain coherence and meaning in lives threatened by illness and change.

In summary, the author has argued that many prevalent aesthetic theories are incompatible with the notion of art in nursing. In contrast, Dewey's theory of art as vital experience is a congenial one with which to examine and claim the practice of nursing art. Dewey does not insist on a fundamental distinction between art and craft, nor does he deny art the fulfillment of needs or purposeful activity. Because nursing activity is highly purposeful and connected to human experience, Dewey's philosophy of aesthetics is a better fit with a theory of nursing art than some of the others examined earlier in this article. In addition, distinctions between science, art, and craft have been examined and common ground has been established in the idea that all human constructions have aesthetic form. Moreover, art is linked to the practical world under Dewey's notion of experience, and thus, is as deeply teleological as science and craft have been assumed to be. The art of nursing is not an indulgent nicety, but instead, an essential activity grounded by practice and manifest in helping patients create coherence and meaning in lives threatened by transitions of many kinds.

REFERENCES

1. Rafferty AM. Art, science and social science in nursing: occupational origins and disciplinary identity. *Nurs Inquiry.* 1995;2:141–148.
2. Peplau H. The art and science of nursing: similarities, differences, and relations. *Nurs Sci Q.* 1988;1(1):8–15.
3. Johnson J. A dialectical examination of nursing art. *ANS,* 1994;17(1):1–14.
4. Katims I. Nursing as aesthetic experience and the notion of practice. *Sch Inquiry Nurs Prac.* 1993;7(4):269–278.
5. Carper BA. Fundamental patterns of knowing in nursing. *ANS.* 1978;1:13–23.
6. Rogers ME. Nursing science and art: a prospective. *Nurs Sci Q.* 1988;1(3):99–102.
7. Watson J. The lost art of nursing. *Nurs Forum.* 1981;20(3):244–249.
8. Weidenbach E. *Clinical Nursing: A Helping Art.* New York: Springer; 1964.
9. Nightingale F. *Notes on Nursing: What It Is and What It Is Not.* New York: Dover Publications; 1969.
10. Kuhn TS. *The Structure of Scientific Revolutions.* Chicago: The University of Chicago Press; 1970.
11. Chinn PL, Kramer MK. *Theory and Nursing: A Systematic Approach.* New York: Mosby, 1998.
12. Appleton C. The art of nursing: the experience of patients and nurses. *J Adv Nurs.* 1993;18:892–899.
13. Bournaki M. Germain C. Esthetic knowledge in family centered nursing care of hospitalized children. *ANS.* 1993;16(2):81–89.
14. Chinn PL. Maeve K, Bostick C. Aesthetic inquiry and the art of nursing. *Sch Inq Nurs Pract.* 1997;11(2):83–95.
15. Chinn PL, Watson J, eds. *Art and Aesthetics in Nursing.* New York: National League for Nursing; 1994.
16. Skillman-Hull LE. She walks in beauty: nurse-artists lived experience of the creative process and aesthetic human care. [Dissertation]. Denver, Co: Univ. of Colorado Health Sciences; 1994.
17. Sorrell, IM. Remembrance of things past through writing: esthetic patterns of knowing in nursing. *ANS.* 1994;17(1):60–70.
18. Plato. *The Republic* (Larson R, trans.). Arlington Heights, IL: Harlan Davidson, Inc.; 1979.
19. Aristotle. *Poetics* (Janko R, trans.). Indianapolis, IN: Hackett Publishing; 1987.
20. Kant I. *The Critique of Judgement* (Pluhar W, trans.). Indianapolis, IN: Hackett Publishing Co.; 1987.
21. Bell C. *Art.* London: Chatto & Windus; 1949.
22. Fisher JA. *Reflecting on Art.* Mountain View, CA: Mayfield Publishing Co.; 1993.
23. Cooper D, ed. *A Companion to Aesthetics.* Oxford, UK: Blackwell Publishers; 1992.
24. Eisner E. Aesthetic modes of knowing. In: Eisner E, ed. *Learning and Teaching the Ways of Knowing.* Chicago: University of Chicago Press; 1985.
25. Benner PA, Tanner CA, Chesla CA. *Expertise in Nursing Practice: Caring, Clinical Judgement, and Ethics.* New York: Springer Publishing Co.: 1996.
26. Collingwood RG. *The Principles of Art.* Oxford: The Clarendon Press; 1938.
27. Weitz M. The role of theory in aesthetics. *J Aesthetics Art Criticism.* 1956;15(1):27–35.
28. Wittgenstein L. *Philosophical Investigations* (Anscombe E, trans.). London: Oxford University Press; 1953.
29. Dickie G. *Art and the Aesthetic.* Ithaca, NY: Cornell University Press; 1974.

30. Danto A. The artworld. *J Philosophy*. 1964;61:571–584.
31. Dewey J. *Art as Experience*. New York: Perigee Books; 1934.
32. Benner P, Wrubel J. *The Primacy of Caring: Stress and Coping in Health and Illness*. Menlo Park, CA: Addison-Wesley Publishing Co.; 1989.
33. Benner P. *From Novice to Expert: Excellence and Power in Clinical Nursing Practice*. Menlo Park, CA: Addison-Wesley Publishing Co.; 1984.
34. Coles R. *The Call of Stories*. Boston: Houghton Mifflin Co.; 1989.
35. Broyard A. Intoxicated by my illness. *NY Times Mag*. 1989; Nov. 12:32.
36. Dewey J. Experience, nature and art. In: McDermott J. ed. *The Philosophy of John Dewey: The Structure of Experience*. New York: GM Putnam's Sons; 1973.
37. Gortner SR. Nursing values and science: toward a science philosophy. *Image*. 1990;22(2):101–105.
38. Newman MA. Prevailing paradigms in nursing. *Nurs Outlook*. 1992;40(1):10–13.
39. Fawcett J. From a plethora of paradigms to parsimony in worldviews. *Nurs Sci Q*. 1993;6(2):56–58.
40. King JM. Nursing theory 25 years later. *Nurs Sci Q*. 1991;4(3):94–95.
41. Meleis A. Facilitating transitions: redefinition of the nursing mission. *Nurs Outlook*. 1994;42(6):255–259.
42. Newman MA. Sime AM. Corcoran-Perry SA. The focus of the discipline of nursing. *ANS*. 1991;14(1):1–6.
43. Packard S, Polifroni C. The dilemma of nursing science: current quandaries and lack of direction. *Nurs Sci Q*. 1991;4(1):7–13.
44. Breslin ET. Aesthetic methods as a means of knowing for nursing. *Issues Ment Health Nurs*. 1996;17:503–505.
45. LeVasseur J. Plato, Nightingale and contemporary nursing. *Image*. 1998;30(3):281–285.
46. Breunig K. The art of painting meets the art of nursing. In: Chinn PL, Watson J. eds. *Art & Aesthetics in Nursing*. New York: National League for Nursing: 1994.
47. Rose P. Parker D. Nursing: an integration of art and science within the experience of the practitioner. *J Adv Nurs*. 1994;20:1004–1010.
48. Cassell EJ. *The Nature of Suffering*. New York: Oxford University Press; 1991.

The Author Comments

Toward an Understanding of Art in Nursing

I was interested in understanding more fully what might be meant by the often-used phrase "the art of nursing." Recently, the notion of "science" in nursing has captured our imagination, and we have embraced the rigor, replicability, and status of science as a worthy model for nursing. Yet, we also frequently regard nursing as a holistic, individualized, caring process—words that strongly imply a dash of art mixed with our science. To decide whether the words "the art of nursing" were philosophically justified, I read a good deal in the philosophy of art to determine whether there was a congenial theory that could illuminate the phenomena of art in a discipline such as nursing. This definitional work became the basis for my further research on the art of nursing, as it exists in the experience of practicing nurses.

—JEANNE J. LEVASSEUR

CHAPTER 51

The Art of Nursing

Paul Wainwright

It is a common assumption that nursing is an art. Art in this sense is sometimes taken to mean a fine art, and sometimes a skill or craft. This paper reviews some of the arguments for nursing as an art and concludes that nursing is not a fine art, but that it is an art in the more general sense of a craft or skill performed by people. It is further argued that, in most instances, to say that nursing is an art tells us little or nothing that is useful and the word 'art' is redundant in this context. © 1999 Elsevier Science Ltd. All rights reserved.

Keywords: Nursing art; Nursing aesthetics; Nursing philosophy; Nursing theory

Introduction

The assumption that nursing is an art, evident from the nursing literature of the last 20 years, has gone largely unchallenged and the majority of writers have concentrated on describing the implications of this belief for nursing knowledge and practice. However, recent contributions to the literature have for perhaps the first time seriously challenged the shibboleth of nursing art (e.g. Edwards, 1998; De Raeve, 1998; Van Hooft, 1998) and expressed doubts about the validity of claims about nursing art and aesthetics. The purpose of this paper is to develop the debate and to offer some further thoughts on the possibility of nursing as an art.

Copyright © 1999, Elsevier Science LTD. International Journal of Nursing Studies, 36, *379–385.*
With permission from Elsevier Science.

About the Author

PAUL WAINWRIGHT was born on the south coast of England in 1948. He trained as a general nurse in Southampton from 1971 to 1973 and subsequently earned his master's degree at Manchester and his PhD in Wales. He has worked extensively in clinical practice and health services management but now works as a Senior Lecturer in the Centre for Philosophy and Health Care, part of the School of Health Science at the University of Wales, Swansea, where he has been for 10 years. His hobbies include sailing, reading, listening to music, gardening, walking, and cycling. The focus of his scholarship is the concept of practice (particularly nursing practice, but the central ideas are transferable). He is interested in how a practice is defined, what it means to be a practitioner, what makes different kinds of practice different, what makes for good practice, how practice is evaluated, the ethics of practice, and any related issues. He hopes that his key contribution to the discipline will be philosophic (although he is also engaged in empirical research), particularly in the aesthetics of practice and, generally, in philosophy of nursing and medical humanities.

Is Nursing an Art?

Many people seem committed to the notion that nursing is an art. Nightingale's observation that nursing is both art and science is frequently cited, the argument received impetus from the work of Carper and Johnson has compiled a review of work by 41 authors in the field (Carper, 1978; Johnson, 1994). Chinn and Watson (1994) edited a collection of 18 articles on "Art & Aesthetics in Nursing" and anyone who has discussed the topic with groups of students will know that nursing's status as an art is taken for granted by many. Edwards (1998) however, from an examination of theories of art and in particular the work of Collingwood (1958), comes to the conclusion that nursing cannot be properly described as an art, a view supported Tschudin and Hunt, and Van Hooft (Tschudin and Hunt, 1998; Van Hooft, 1998).

Edwards' analysis relies on philosophical accounts of the fine arts (Edwards, 1998, p 395). He discusses Collingwood's distinction between the historical meaning of the term 'art' in Latin and Greek and its current usage. He points out that the Ancients applied the term to any skilled activity and thus included many activities in the category of arts that today we might call crafts. Edwards develops his argument from Collingwood's analysis of the distinctions between art and craft and comes to the conclusion that by Collingwood's terms

nursing cannot be seen as an art and that there are even problems with its characterisation as a craft.

Edwards' conclusion is perhaps not surprising, given the grounds on which he has chosen to base his argument. Tschudin and Hunt agree with Edwards' conclusion but they deny that when people refer to the art of nursing this means it "should be classified together with poetry and painting" but merely that "good nursing has a creative and discretionary edge that responds to a unique moment in a balanced way" (Tschudin and Hunt, 1998, p. 384). Van Hooft claims that when people talk about the art of nursing they do not mean 'Art' at all and the word could be replaced with 'skilled activity'. According to Van Hooft it is all a matter of the ambiguity of the English language and nursing has as much to do with "Art in the aesthetic sense" as do book keeping or tree pruning (Van Hooft, 1998, p. 545).

Nursing: 'Art' or 'art'?

Tschudin and Hunt and Van Hooft are perhaps not aware that many nurses do claim that nursing is a fine art, an Art Form rather than merely a technical skill, while many others appear to see it more as a skill or craft. Collingwood (1958) refers to the distinction between 'art proper' and 'the obsolete sense' in which the word refers to what he calls a craft. This other usage of the term may be obsolete for philosophical aesthetics, but as Kristeller points out the contemporary usage of the label 'Art' to signify the fine arts is relatively recent, originating in the 18th century (Kristeller, 1997). The term, he suggests, is often identified with the visual arts alone, but is quite commonly understood in a broader sense. It includes, above all, the five major arts of painting, sculpture, architecture, music and poetry, which Kristeller (1997, p. 91) refers to as "The irreducible nucleus of the modern system of the arts." Others are sometimes added, such as gardening, engraving, decorative arts, dance, theatre, opera, eloquence and prose literature. The notion that the five major arts are an area by themselves clearly separated by common characteristics from crafts, sciences and other human activities, suggests Kristeller, has been taken for granted from Kant to the present day.

It might seem unlikely that even the strongest advocate of nursing as an art would claim that nursing belongs with the fine arts in this strict sense. Paraphrasing Kristeller, to speak of "the six major arts of painting, sculpture, architecture, music, poetry and nursing" clearly lacks credibility. However, as Collingwood acknowledges and Kristeller points out, the relevant Greek and Latin terms do not specifically denote fine art in the modern sense, being applied to all kinds of human activities now called crafts or sciences. The Ancients understood by art something that can be taught and learned, unlike the modern view of art as something that cannot be taught. The Greeks contrasted art and nature, thinking of human activity in general and as opposed to the natural world; when Hippocrates contrasted art with life, according to Kristeller, he was thinking of medicine as the art in question.

There are dangers in applying concepts from antiquity to a contemporary debate. However there is much that we do take from Platonic and Aristotelian thought and it is clear that a more general use of the word art was common at least up to the middle of the 18th century. In 1746 Abbé Batteux said that it was the arts that "build towns, bring together widely dispersed people, make them polite, civilised, capable of living in society" (Batteux, 1997, pp. 102–103). In general, he says, an art is "a collection or assemblage of rules for doing well

what can be done well or badly, because what can only be done well or done badly has no need of art." He described three kinds of art: the mechanical arts; the fine arts; and the arts that are both useful and agreeable. The mechanical arts he said meet the basic needs of mankind: " . . . man could not remain long in inactivity. Feeling forced to seek solutions, he found some. When he found them, he perfected them, to make them of greater, surer, more complete use, whenever the need arose again" (Batteux, 1997, p 103).

Another 18th century writer, Jean le Rond D'Alembert, suggests that "In general the name Art may be given to any system of knowledge which can be reduced to positive and invariable rules independent of caprice or opinion. In this sense it would be permitted to say that several of our sciences are arts when they are viewed from their practical side" (D'Alembert, 1997, p. 107). He also suggests that the arts are related to our needs. More recently Valéry points out that the word art originally meant simply a way of doing. This usage evolved to mean "ways of doing that involve voluntary action or action initiated by the will" (Valéry, 1935, p. 25), which implied that there was more than one way of achieving something and that some form of preparation and training was involved. "Medicine is said to be an art, and we say the same of hunting, horsemanship, reasoning, or the conduct of life" (Valéry, 1935, p. 25).

Nursing Art: Contemporary Usage

To demonstrate that such use of the word 'art' was commonplace in the mid-1700s or even the 1930s is not sufficient to demonstrate its relevance today. However, everyday speech has many examples of such use. Words such as 'artificial,' 'artefact,' 'artifice' and 'artisan,' from the Latin, and 'technology', 'technique' and 'technical' from the Greek, are all in current use and all relate to the things that are the work of people rather than of nature, precisely the distinction made by the ancient Greeks. Such activities require training and the acquisition of knowledge and skills. We would not think it strange if someone wanted to explain to us the art of making a good soufflé or the art of growing fuchsias. There is thus a straightforward way in which nursing can be construed as an art, not in the technical sense of the fine arts but in the everyday sense understood by most people. Valéry sums up this account of art as "that quality of the *way of doing* (whatever its object may be) which is due to *dissimilarity in the modes of operation* and hence in the results—arising from the *dissimilarity of the agents*" (Valéry, 1935 p. 25–26).

One gets the sense that some authors seek to make a more significant claim than that nursing is just something done by people. However I would argue that even such a modest claim has value. To call nursing an art in this sense is to say that it requires a body of knowledge with rules and principles to inform its practice. It is something above mere routine or that which "can be done by hand alone" (D'Alembert, 1997, p. 107). Nursing meets some of "the basic needs of mankind," and is to be perfected to make it of "greater, surer, more complete use" (Batteux, 1997, p. 103). To contrast nursing art with nursing science as Nightingale did could become problematic since by this analysis science itself is an art. However the comparison becomes more meaningful when one remembers that scientific method, though carried out by people, seeks to eliminate the impact of the human presence from the process. The philosophers of science may decide to what extent this is possible, but the distinction reminds us that nursing practice is not only performed by people, but depends for its results upon the effect of the interactions between people, with all their unpredictability, spontaneity and particularity, that science attempts to exclude. Crucially, to paraphrase Valéry, there will be differences in the way nursing is performed, and hence different results of that nursing, that arise from the differences between different nurses.

Tolstoy's "What is Art?"

There is also a way in which the mundane use of the word 'art' to describe human activity overlaps with the more formal definition of fine art. Tolstoy defines art as "a human activity consisting in this, that one man consciously, by means of certain external signs, hands on to others feelings he has lived through, and that others are infected by these feelings and also experience them" (Tolstoy, 1994, p. 59). He says (Tolstoy, 1994, pp. 60–61):

> "We are accustomed to understand art to be only what we hear and see in theatres, concerts, and exhibitions, together with buildings, statues, poems, novels . . . but all this is but the smallest part of the art by which we communicate with each other in life. All human life is filled with works of art of every kind—from cradle song, jest, mimicry, the ornamentation of houses, dress, and utensils up to church services, buildings, monuments, and triumphal processions. It is all artistic activity. So that by art, in the limited sense of the word, we do not mean all human activity transmitting feelings, but only that part which we for some reason select from it and to which we attach special importance."

Tolstoy's account has clearly been influential in the nursing literature (e.g. Watson, 1988; Chinn and Watson, 1994). Compare for instance the passage from Chinn and Watson quoted by Edwards: "The art of nursing is the capacity of a human being to receive another human being's expression of feelings and to experience those feelings for oneself" (Chinn and Watson, 1994, p. xvi) with Tolstoy's "And it is upon this capacity of man to receive another man's expression of feelings and experience those feelings himself, that the activity of art is based" (Tolstoy, 1994, p. 57). In an earlier work Watson acknowledges the influence of Tolstoy's account (Watson, 1988). She begins a passage headed "The art of transpersonal caring" with a reference to Tolstoy and most of what follows is a very close paraphrase of Tolstoy, albeit with words such as 'person' or 'human being' substituted for 'man' and references to 'nursing' and 'caring' inserted where appropriate (Watson, 1988, pp. 67–68; Tolstoy, 1994, pp. 57–59). In particular she says "It is on this capacity of one human being to receive another human being's expression of feeling and to experience those feelings for oneself that the artistic activity of nursing and caring is based" (Watson, 1988, p. 67).

One can see why Tolstoy's account might be attractive to nurses trying to develop theories of art and aesthetics in nursing, although his approach has been shown to have limitations and Lyas (1997) gives an account of the problems. However quite apart from technical philosophical difficulties there are problems for those who wish to recruit Tolstoy to the cause of nursing art. For example, Edwards complains that it is questionable as to whether it is possible for one person to experience the feelings of another in the way they do themselves. He takes the phrase "to receive another human being's expression of feelings and to experience those feelings for oneself" (Chinn and Watson, 1994, p. xvi) to mean that the art of nursing is in the ability of the nurse to experience the feelings of the patient, an interpretation that given the context is quite reasonable. This would be in keeping with other claims in the literature regarding the importance of empathy, sensitivity and intuition in nurses, but Edwards doubts for example that one person can ever experience another's pain. However to base a suggestion that the nurse could experience the feelings of the patient on Tolstoy's definition of art is to misunderstand Tolstoy. In the relevant passage we find that Tolstoy is not claiming that anyone has the capacity to experience the feelings of another in the sense of knowing how the other person feels. What he says is that one person, the artist, can conjure up and express an emotion or a feeling, such as fear or anger, and express that feeling so powerfully that members of an audience also feel fear or anger, or at least recognise that that is the feeling being conveyed. When one person says "I am afraid" and another says "So am I" we know only that each is feeling what he or she imagines to be fear. We have no way of knowing that each is feeling the same as the other. What Tolstoy is saying is that artists have the ability to express an emotion in a way that others can recognise and share. This is not usually what is envisaged when nurses talk about their understanding of or empathy with the patient who is suffering. There are occasions when a nurse will express feelings or emotions, which she hopes that the patient may also experience, such as confidence, hope, courage, calmness and so on, but she does not do this in the way as would an artist in Tolstoy's sense of the word.

There are other difficulties with Tolstoy's position. Collingwood argues that one of the distinctive features of art proper is that it is essentially self centred, self-regarding. The artist is at the centre of matters and it is the expression of the emotions of the artist that are of primary importance. The imaginative work done by the artist is crucial and, where nursing is essentially other-regarding, art is self-regarding (Collingwood, 1958). This egocentric stance of the artist represents a difficulty for nurses committed to a patient-centred approach to care. However just such a self-regarding approach is reflected in Tolstoy's description of art. According to Tolstoy the activity of art requires that one evokes in oneself "a feeling one has once experienced, and having evoked it in oneself, then, . . . transmit that feeling that others may experience the same feeling." It requires that one "consciously, by means of certain external signs, hands on to others feelings he has lived through, and that other people are infected by these feelings and also experience them" (Tolstoy, p. 59). Those who are "infected by those feelings" Tolstoy refers to as the audience. Lyas summarises Tolstoy's account as having three components, which consist of: the artist's feelings, emotions or attitudes; the work in which the artist embeds these and which is passed on to the audience; and the audience that comes to share the artist's feelings, emotions or attitudes (Lyas, 1997, p. 61).

Lyas notes that there is nothing in Tolstoy that requires that the artist must actually feel what the work expresses. In Tolstoy's example of a boy telling a story about being frightened by a wolf, Tolstoy is clear that when he tells the story the boy imaginatively recreates the fear. It is not necessary that the boy had ever even seen a wolf—he could simply invent an encounter and then tell the story and this for Tolstoy would be art. Lyas suggests that all Tolstoy needs "is the pretty obvious claim that the artistic creator must have had a sufficient actual acquaintance with the emotions in order to have the materials out of which to build imaginative expressions of them" and he goes on to note that there can be emotions expressed in a work that could not be emotions had by the artist. Munch's painting 'Puberty' for example portrays the confusion experienced by a girl at the onset of puberty that Munch as a man could not experience (Lyas, 1997, pp. 62–63). Once again this would seem at least to limit the acceptability of Tolstoy's approach for nurses who stress the importance of honesty, sincerity and authenticity in nursing practice.

Art as a Way of Knowing in Nursing

Chinn and Kramer, drawing on Carper's original work, conflate the concepts of art and aesthetics in a way that makes them appear almost synonymous. They suggest that "Aesthetic knowing in nursing is the comprehension of meaning in a singular, particular, subjective expression that we call the art/act (sic)" (Chinn and Kramer, 1991, p. 10). They go on to talk of the possibility of "knowing what to do with the moment, instantly, without conscious deliberation" and say that "Perception of meaning in an immediate encounter is what creates an artful nursing action." The art of nursing involves engaging, which is "a direct involvement of the self within a situation" which does not depend on "mental structures or cognitive representations or explanations." The meaning of the moment "comes from deep within the subjective experience, is interpreted from the context of the individual's human experiences and becomes expressed through in-the-moment being in the situation." Finally they say that "aesthetics is not expressed in language but artistically in the moment of experience-action . . . nursing's art form tends to be the artful ways in which nurses interact with people and perform skilled tasks" (Chinn and Kramer, 1991, pp. 10–11).

There seem to be several problems with this as an account of an art form. From Tolstoy's point of view art involves the artist consciously evoking the emotion and then expressing it in a way that others can appreciate. Spontaneous acts appear specifically to be excluded from Tolstoy's conception of art. He says "If a man infects another or others directly, immediately, by his appearance, or by the sounds he gives vent to at the very time he experiences the feeling . . . that does not amount to art" (Tolstoy, 1994, p. 57). Chinn and Kramer clearly

see the nurse as the performer, but they emphasise the immediacy of the moment and the spontaneity of the nurse's response, while the expression of feelings and emotions comes from the patient. Carper herself says "Empathy—that is the capacity for participating in or vicariously experiencing another's feelings—is an important mode in the aesthetic pattern of knowing. One gains knowledge of another person's singular, particular, felt experience through empathic acquaintance" (Carper, 1978, p. 17). She quotes Wiedenbach as claiming that the art of nursing "is made visible through the action taken to provide whatever the patient requires to restore or extend his ability to cope with the demands of his situation." But for this to count as art, says Carper, "requires the active transformation of the immediate object—the patient's behaviour—into a direct, nonmediated perception of what is significant in it—that is, what need is actually being expressed by the behaviour" (Carper, 1978, p. 15). Such approaches would clearly seem to depend on sincerity and authenticity on the part of the nurse in her expressions of feeling.

To be fair to Carper, she does not refer to Tolstoy in her account, but justifies her use of the concept of art in nursing on arguments from Weitz. This approach involves the denial of any essential characteristic by which art may be defined and takes the position that art is too complex and variable to be reduced to a single definition (Carper, 1978, p. 16). Weitz's claim is that art is an open concept and however we view art at one moment there is nothing to say it will not evolve in the future in ways we may not imagine. Any attempt to confine definitions of art to some essentialist account simply restricts creativity. This may be true, but Weitz does not make clear exactly what he means when he says that art is an open concept, and the fact that new works of art and new types of art continue to appear does not mean there can be no defining features of art or that there are no limits or constraints on the application of the term. The fact that we acknowledge new art forms merely demonstrates that we recognise something in the new form that qualifies it as art. Thus Carper cannot use Weitz's open concept approach as an excuse for saying that nursing can be an art because anything can be art: she must give some justification to show that nursing shares sufficient family resemblances with other art forms to justify its inclusion in the family. The qualities of empathy and sensitivity may well form a vital part of nursing, but they might just as easily be explained by reference to social psychology and theories of human relationships as to theories of art.

Carper's reliance on the open-concept account of art suggests that she recognises that nursing is not typical of the fine arts. Descriptions of nursing do not fit the essentialist account of writers such as Tolstoy or Collingwood and so Carper needs Weitz if she is to argue that nursing is an art. However writers such as Chinn take as their starting point the foundations laid by Carper (e.g. Chinn and Kramer, 1991) but go on to use definitions that are clearly taken from Tolstoy (Chinn and Watson, 1994). Such philosophical accounts of nursing as an art are, therefore, contradictory: Carper has based her argument on a rejection of essentialist definitions and must therefore reject accounts such as Tolstoy's, so those who follow Carper must also reject essentialist accounts or at least attempt some justification of their use.

Claims that Nursing is a Fine Art

It might seem unlikely that anyone would claim that nursing is a fine art in the strict sense. Tolstoy is clear that there is a difference between formal art and everyday life and that "by art, in the limited sense of the word" we mean "only that part which we for some reason select from it and to which we attach special importance" (Tolstoy, 1994, p. 61). However Chinn and Kramer speak of nursing's "art form" and nursing as a "work of art" (Chinn and Kramer, 1991) and Watson refers to "the feelings that *the nurse as an artist* inculcates in others" (Watson, 1988, p. 68, my emphasis). Thus these authors and others wish to elevate nursing to something other than the general artistic activity that occurs throughout life. Chinn and Watson quote Stewart, who in 1929 wrote of "The real essence of nursing, as of any form of fine art . . . " (Stewart cited in Chinn and Watson, 1994, p. xiv). Many writers quote Nightingale's claim that "Nursing is an art, and if it is to be made an art it requires as exclusive a devotion, as hard a prepa-

ration, as any painter's or sculptor's work" (Nightingale 1859 quoted in Chinn and Watson, 1994, p. xv). Chinn and Watson claim that these words "place nursing, the oldest art, among the fine arts" (Chinn and Watson, 1994, p. xv). It is not clear how one would judge whether nursing was really the "oldest art," but although Nightingale compared the degree of devotion required to be a nurse with that required of artists and sculptors it does not follow that nursing is the same kind of activity. One might just as well say that a nurse requires as much devotion and preparation as an athlete, but this would not mean that nursing was a sport.

An extreme form of the nursing as fine art movement is illustrated by Parse. She says (Parse, 1992, p. 147)

> "To call nursing practice a performing art is to place it in the company of drama, music, and dance, among others. Within the practice of these arts, the artist cocreates something unique. The uniqueness arises from the knowledge base and cherished beliefs of the artist whose way of being present with an idea, person, object, or situation expresses the art form. All artists perform from a knowledge base which is the science of the art. Dance, for example, is the execution of knowledge related to choreographed movements, as well as cherished beliefs about the meaning the artist gives to the movement in the movement . . . So too, the nurse, an artist like the dancer, unfolds the meaning of the moment with a person or family consistent with personal knowledge and cherished beliefs . . . The performing art of nursing is the creative life of the science; it is a unique contribution to the health care of people".

There may be some value in the use of dance as a metaphor for nursing. Nurses move, sometimes with grace, rhythm and expression. These movements may involve one person or complex interplay between two or more. But the dance as a performing art involves just that—a self-regarding performance created for an audience. It may be frivolous and witty, or highly charged with emotion, or it may deal with profound issues of human existence, but it remains a performance in

which composer, choreographer and dancers collaborate to evoke emotions and feelings with which they are
familiar and which they hope to convey to a sympathetic
audience. To call nursing "a performing art" and to
compare the nurse to a dancer in any serious way
would seem to demean nursing. As Valéry argues, "The
most evident characteristic of a work of art may be
termed uselessness" (Valéry, 1935, p. 26), but it seems
unlikely that those who argue that nursing is a fine art
or a performing art would want to accept that nursing's
most evident characteristic was its uselessness.

A Way Forward?

Having argued that nursing is not a fine art or a performing art we are left with the question of how to go forward.
One of the problems with the ambiguity of the word 'art'
is the amount of confusion it can cause. Chinn and Watson (1994, p. 20) says "Art is not something that stands
opposed to science . . . indeed it is part of all human experience" and one thinks she may be using the word in
the general sense that Tolstoy means when he talks of
human life being "all artistic activity." However Chinn
continues (Chinn and Watson, 1994, p. 20)

> Art expresses what words usually fail to express. Art
> brings wholeness to human consciousness. Art is
> powerful, profound, moving, and deeply political.
> Art is both feared and revered because it moves
> consciousness into realms not imagined and reali-
> ties not predicted. Art is also feared, and sometimes
> revered, because it is associated, in the depths of
> the human consciousness, with women, with the
> ability to create, to generate, to bring forth life.

This is not the mundane use of art in the general
sense of everyday life. Now Chinn is talking about some
higher form, of fine art. It may be the case that nursing
can express what words fail to express (but so can
mathematical formulae), can bring wholeness to
human consciousness (but so might meditation or psychotherapy), and can be seen to be powerful, moving
and deeply political (as is some of the content of a
newspaper). It is certainly associated with women, with

the ability to create, to generate and to bring forth life.
But this does not make it fine art.

The human activities that we classify as arts in the
broad sense might be further subdivided into those that
require the effective use of interpersonal skills and the
communication of feelings between those involved, as
opposed to technical procedures for which such communication is unnecessary. One might speak of the art
of teaching, counselling, or nursing, as being qualitatively different from the arts of driving, cookery or
growing vegetables. As activities involving artistry both
categories might be thought superior to potato picking,
hod carrying or sweeping the floor. It may be good to
recognise the place of such activities in human life and
to understand the importance, in occupations such as
teaching or nursing, of the human element and all that
goes with it—sensitivity, creativity, interpersonal communication and so on. However we do not need continually to stress the fact that these are arts.

Much of what is written about the art of nursing
would be as meaningful if the word 'art' were to be replaced with 'nursing.' The problem with the use of 'art'
as a term to distinguish an activity from the natural
world or from unskilled activities is not so much that
this usage, as Collingwood claims, is obsolete, as that it
is frequently redundant. If nursing is an art it is the
whole of nursing; it is not informative to describe it as if
the art was only one aspect of nursing. It helps to remind ourselves from time to time that nursing is an art
and that this has implications for our understanding of
it as an activity, but most of the time we do not need to
make this explicit. The term 'art' in this context
amounts to meta-data, that is it is data that tells us
something about the nature of data, information about
information. Trees are made of wood, but we do not
continually draw attention to "the wooden trees."

Conclusions

In this paper I have argued that nursing is not a fine art.
It has many features that distinguish it from the fine arts
and the performing arts and claims to the contrary lack
credibility and demean nursing. Such claims are con-

fused, mistaken and based on misinterpretation of philosophical accounts of art and aesthetics. However I have argued that there is a sense in which nursing is an art and in which the common, sincere view held by many to that effect makes sense in a non technical context. This weaker, general sense of nursing art is drawn from the long-standing distinction between those things that are part of the natural world and those that are made or done by people, the art versus nature distinction that predates the eighteenth century conception of the fine arts. This claim, although less dramatic, is useful because it highlights the importance of the human element in nursing and helps to differentiate the interpersonal approach from scientific methods that by definition attempt to exclude the personal and interpersonal. It also helps to clarify the difference between practices such as nursing, other more technical activities and routine manual labour.

However I have also argued that, having recognised the nature of the art of nursing, we would do well not to make mention of this claim too often. In particular we do not need to raise the issue of nursing as an art when we are discussing matters that are internal to nursing. If not exactly tautological, the use of 'art' as in 'the art of nursing' or 'the art of nursing practice' is certainly redundant. If nursing is an art then by definition it is the whole of nursing that is an art, not some particular aspect of it and it is sufficient to refer to it as nursing.

REFERENCES

Batteux, A., 1997. The fine arts reduced to a single principle. In: Feagin, S., Maynard, P. (Eds.), Aesthetics. OUP, Oxford, pp. 102–104.

Carper, B., 1978. Fundamental patterns of knowing in nursing. *Advances in Nursing Science 1* (1), 13–23.

Chinn, P., Kramer, M., 1991. Theory and nursing: a systematic approach. Mosby, St Louis.

Chinn, P., Watson, J., 1994. Art and aesthetics in nursing. NLN, New York.

Collingwood, R. G., 1958. The principles of art. OUP, Oxford.

D'Alembert, J. I. R., 1997. The arts and the fine arts. In: Feagin, S., Maynard, P. (Eds.), Aesthetics. OUP, Oxford.

De Raeve, L., 1998. The art of nursing: an aesthetics? *Nursing Ethics 5* (5), 401–411.

Edwards, S., 1998. The art of nursing. *Nursing Ethics 5* (5), 393–400.

Johnson, J., 1994. A dialectical examination of nursing art. Advances in Nursing Science 17 (1), 1–14.

Kristeller, P. O., 1997. The modern system of the arts. In: Feagin, S., Maynard, P. (Eds.), Aesthetics. OUP, Oxford, pp. 90–102.

Lyas, C., 1997. Aesthetics. UCL, London.

Parse, R., 1992. Editorial: The performing art of nursing. *Nursing Science Quarterly 5* (4), 147.

Tolstoy, L., 1994. What is art? Bristol Classical Press, London.

Tschudin, V., Hunt, G., 1998. Editorial. *Nursing Ethics 5* (5), 383–384.

Valéry, P., 1935. The idea of art. In: Osborne, H. (Ed.), Aesthetics. OUP, Oxford.

Van Hooft, S., 1998. The art of nursing: aesthetics or praxis? A response to Steven Edwards, Louise de Raeve and Per Nortvedt. *Nursing Ethics 5* (6), 545–550.

Watson, J., 1988. Nursing: human science and human care, a theory of nursing. NLN, New York.

The Author Comments

The Art of Nursing

I was motivated to write on the aesthetics of nursing after conversations with colleagues in my centre and with students in our MSc program in nursing, with whom we had been discussing the questions of art and aesthetics and the work of Barbara Carper. I believed that there was considerable confusion about what aesthetics of practice might involve and of what use an account of such an aesthetic might be. I believe that aesthetic quality is a necessary condition of practice for it to be judged good practice, and I want to develop a much fuller theoretic account of that claim.

—PAUL WAINWRIGHT

PRACTICE, PRAGMATISM, AND PRAXIS

CHAPTER 52

Practical Nursing Judgment: A Moderate Realist Conception

June F. Kikuchi
Helen Simmons

Under the influence of idealist mainstream thinking that reality is mind-dependent, many nurses are dismissing the possibility of attaining objectively true judgments. A worrisome trend that has emerged from such thinking is to recommend that nursing practice decisions ultimately be based solely on subjective judgments. We present a conception of practical nursing judgment based on the common-sense philosophy of moderate realism, which has the potential to help offset the trend. It allows for nursing decision making in which nursing principles and rules are modified in light of the contingent circumstances of a nursing situation, resulting in decisions which have both a subjective and an objective aspect to them. This feature, plus the fact that the nursing principles are grounded in common natural needs, rights, and obligations, provides nurses with a basis for nursing care which is individualized, just, benevolent, and sensible, a means requisite to making our lives good.

Nowadays, under the influence of idealist mainstream thought that reality is mind-dependent, many nurses (e.g., Appleton & King, 1997; Barnum, 1994; Mitchell, 1994; Moccia, 1988; Munhall, 1982; Sandelowski, 1996) are dismissing the possibility of attaining bias-free or objective truths (i.e., judgments which are objectively true by virtue of their correspondence with reality as it exists independent of the mind). Objective truths are said to be unattainable because reality and measures of truth are a matter of whatever worldview one has chosen to adopt based on one's own values. Since values are held to be subjective (a matter of taste or preference and unarguable), as opposed to being objective in nature (a matter of truth and ar-

About the Authors

JUNE F. KIKUCHI was born on the west coast of Canada in 1939 and, being of Japanese ancestry, she spent some of her early years in an internment camp in the interior of British Columbia during World War II. She received her BScN degree in 1962 from the University of Toronto and her MN and PhD degrees in the nursing care of children in 1969 and 1979, respectively, from the University of Pittsburgh. Postdoctorally, she studied philosophy at the University of Toronto. She has held various nursing positions, including staff nurse, instructor, head nurse, clinical nurse specialist, clinical nurse researcher, and, most recently, professor. With Dr. Helen Simmons, she cofounded the Institute for Philosophical Nursing Research at the University of Alberta in 1988 and served as its director until 1997, when she retired early to engage leisurely in philosophic nursing inquiry, gardening, and volunteer work with hospitalized children. The aim of her scholarly work continues to be raising nurses' awareness of the need to think philosophically about their world.

HELEN SIMMONS was born in 1927 into a family of 15 children living on a homestead near Fort Saskatchewan, Alberta. By good fortune, some 25 years later, she enjoyed a liberal education, receiving a bachelor and master of art degrees (with majors in psychology and philosophy) from the University of British Columbia. She worked for several years in mental health settings in Alberta and Minnesota and then held teaching positions at the University of Oregon and Oregon State College while pursuing a PhD in educational psychology at the University of Oregon. Returning to Canada in 1971, she held a joint appointment with the Faculty of Nursing at the University of Alberta and the Mental Health Division of the Edmonton Board of Health, where she developed and taught the philosophy of public health nursing. In 1988, with Dr. June Kikuchi, she cofounded the Institute for Philosophical Nursing Research at the University of Alberta and, in 1999, was awarded an honorary life membership in the Alberta Association of Registered Nurses "in recognition of distinguished service and valuable assistance to the nursing profession." Her pursuits in work and leisure have always been focused on three cooperative arts: nursing, teaching, and farming. Since her retirement from professional life in 1992, she has continued to live on and operate a grain farm northeast of Edmonton.

guable) and, as Adler (1990) states, the worldview itself is a construction of individual imagination about what can be, not what is, any particular perspective based in a worldview (and any judgments emanating from it) is seen to be subjective. Thus, nurses speak of all knowledge as value-laden and being of "multiple realities," multiple conceptions of reality—all equally valid, acceptable, and unarguable. The "truth" of a judgment is determined solely on the basis of the individual's say-so.

Born of such idealist thinking is a worrisome trend recommending that nursing practice decisions (i.e., practical nursing decisions or judgments) ultimately be based *solely* on judgments emanating from an individual's or a group's perspective of a(n) situation, experience, or entity. In other words, since perspectives (and judgments emanating from them) are thought to be subjective in nature, nurses are being urged to ultimately base their decisions solely on subjective judgments. In this philosophical essay, we present the result of our philosophizing: to develop a conception of practical nursing judgment that has the potential to help offset the trend. We begin by setting down the fundamental philosophical underpinnings of our thinking. We then describe some bases for nursing decision making illustrative of the current trend of relying on subjective judgments. Next, we outline a conception of justice and present salient aspects of a conception of practical judgment upon which our conception of practical nursing judgment rests. Finally, we outline our conception and explain why it has the potential to help offset the trend.

Fundamental Philosophical Underpinnings

Our essay is based on the assumptions and tenets of moderate realism, a common-sense philosophy which attains its principles by reflecting on common-sense knowledge and reasoning therefrom in light of available evidence. Common-sense knowledge consists of those judgments we all form as a result of our common sense: our proclivity to develop opinions based on our common experience (e.g., everyone suffers good and bad fortune), experience gained simply from living day to day (e.g., the experience of physical pain). Judgments can also take other forms: (1) mere opinion, opinion expressing emotional predilection or personal prejudice (e.g., I prefer nurses in white rather than green uniforms), (2) probable truth, opinion with evidence and/or reason to support it beyond a reasonable doubt (e.g., all human beings need love); and (3) absolute truth, opinion which is beyond a shadow of a doubt (e.g., the whole is greater than any of its parts) (Adler, 1965b, 1981).

Moderate realism maintains that philosophy can attain probable truths about what exists and what happens in the world and about what we ought to do and seek in human life. Probable truths about the former are attained by comparing our descriptive judgments against reality as it exists independent of the individual mind and determining where the weight of the evidence and reason falls; probable truths about the latter are attained by comparing our prescriptive judgments against right desire as set down in the self-evident truth, "*we ought to want and seek that which is really good for us (i.e., that which by nature we need)*" [italics added] (Adler, 1981, pp. 79–80). This truth is self-evident in the sense that the opposite is unthinkable. According to moderate realism, what is really good for us are goods that meet our natural needs. Thus, we ought

to desire them to make our whole life good. By combining this *prescriptive* truth with *descriptive* truths about human needs, other *prescriptive* truths are attainable. Value judgments of this normative kind are judgments of truth and, consequently, are arguable. When we disagree about them, we can, and ought to, seek agreement in light of available evidence about human needs. Value judgments which are statements of preference are matters of taste. It would be unreasonable to argue about them or to anticipate agreement (Adler, 1965b, 1981, 1990).

Contrary to those idealist philosophies that adhere to the notion of world views, moderate realism takes the position that, although we view reality differently as a consequence of how we are *nurtured,* we can, nonetheless, attain an objective view of reality which is probably true by testing our various subjective views against reality which common sense tells us exists, and is the way it is regardless of how any one of us views it. Further, although the content of our individual minds varies across person, time, and place, the nature of our minds, like the nature of any other entity in reality, does not. We all possess the natural cognitive powers of conception, judgment, and reason (though not to the same degree) which allow us to compare our various views against reality and to base our judgments on available evidence and reasons (Adler, 1990). Having set down the philosophical underpinnings of our thinking, we now describe some proposed bases for nursing decision making illustrative of the current trend recommending that practical nursing decisions ultimately be based solely on subjective judgments.

Relying Solely on Subjective Judgments

The recommendation in question is apparent in the different bases for nursing decision making being proposed by various nurse scholars. There is the advisement by Fawcett (1995) that nurses analyze and evaluate nursing theories (all based on one or another worldview) according to specified criteria. Of those theories that meet the criteria, nurses are to adopt one that fits their own or their institution's preferred view of the world and of nursing, as the basis for making nursing decisions. Along this line of thinking, Cody (1993), Mitchell (1995), and Parse (1992) implicitly recommend that the human becoming theory be adopted. In that theory, the nurse is advised to talk with the patient in such a way that he or she does not let his or her opinions intrude and interfere with gaining an understanding of the patient's subjective perspective and judgments, which are to serve as the ultimate basis for nursing decisions.

On the other hand, Bishop and Scudder (1990) propose a different kind of dialogue. They suggest that, in accordance with their particular areas of "legitimate authority" (p. 135), health care professionals and patients disclose their subjective perspectives and judgments on the matter under discussion and decide together on "the treatment which best fulfills the moral sense of benevolent concern for each other" (p. 116). But they also specify that the decision must fit what the patient views as the good life and what he or she desires out of life. In so doing, regardless of the difference in dialogue, the ultimate basis of decision making that they propose appears to be the same as that of Cody (1993), Mitchell (1995), and Parse (1992): the patient's subjective perspective and judgments. Gadow (1995), however, puts a somewhat different spin on this whole matter.

Like Bishop and Scudder (1990), Gadow (1995) proposes that both the nurse and patient bring their particular subjective perspectives to bear on the nurse-patient dialogue. The nurse and patient are to discuss their particular perspectives ("narratives") with a view to developing a common perspective (narrative) acceptable to both parties, in light of which they can together decide on a course of action. The nurse's perspective and judgments and those of the patient are treated in an egalitarian fashion. Additionally, Gadow suggests that, in the sense in which the commonly developed narrative transcends the subjective narratives of the nurse and patient, it can be thought of as objective in nature. But, since it is developed by simply synthesiz-

ing the subjective narratives, one can only conclude that it actually is subjective in nature, still leaving the nurse with only a subjective basis for decision making.

As will become apparent later, we, like Bishop and Scudder (1990) and Gadow (1995), are of the mind that, in making practical nursing decisions, the perspective and judgments of both the nurse and the patient must be heard and considered. Our view differs profoundly from theirs (and from other purely subjective views), however, in that we hold that nurses must consider both perspectives in light of objectively true principles related to the pursuit of happiness by human beings and must ground their nursing decisions in those principles. We contend that unless they do, they cannot avoid acting unjustly. Our reasoning has its basis in the moderate realist conception of justice. What follows is an outline of salient, objectively true, principles which constitute that conception as described by Mortimer Adler.

Conception of Justice

Central to the moderate realist conception of justice are a number of fundamentally linked philosophical notions: natural needs, real goods, natural rights, and duties or moral obligations. How they are integrally connected will become apparent as we outline that conception in terms of its foundational base—the natural moral law, a law inherent in our common human nature (Adler, 1970).

Three obligations follow on the three precepts of the natural moral law. The first precept charges us to *seek* that which is good and to *avoid* that which is evil. In other words, we are to pursue those things that are really good for us because they meet our needs, our natural desires. The inclination of our needs is to seek fulfillment whether or not at any particular time we are aware of that inclination. Real goods are goods that fulfill our *needs*. In contrast to real goods are apparent goods, goods that meet our *wants*, our acquired desires. Our wanting them makes them appear to be good (Adler, 1981). An example of a real good is vigor; it helps satisfy our natural need for health. An example of an apparent good is a substance that someone who is addicted to it wants.

Since our natural needs are inherent in our common human nature, we all have the same natural needs and are all obligated by nature to seek the real goods that satisfy them. By meeting this obligation, we fulfill our primary obligation—to pursue happiness, to make good lives for ourselves. Happiness here does not refer to happiness in the psychological sense but to happiness in the ethical sense, a good life consisting of the possession of all the real goods (including apparent goods as long as their attainment does not interfere with that of the real goods) over the whole of one's life. By virtue of our primary obligation to pursue happiness, we all possess a basic natural right to pursue happiness. (A natural right is a right which is inherent in our human nature, as opposed to a legal right which society confers upon us.) Stemming from this basic right are other natural rights, which we all possess, to the things we need to discharge our obligation to make good lives for ourselves, for example, the right to life, to health care, and to political liberty (Adler, 1970, 1971, 1981).

Adler (1981) points out that the first precept of the natural moral law is not considered a principle of justice, because it concerns the conduct of an individual with regard to him or herself, whereas justice pertains to an individual's conduct with regard to others and to the community as a whole. It does, however, serve as the foundation for the principles of justice: the two remaining precepts of the natural moral law. According to the second precept, we are to *do* that which is good and avoid *doing* that which is evil. In other words, we are obligated to act justly in relation to others: (1) not violate their rights (natural or legal) and thus not interfere with their pursuit of the good life; and (2) treat them in a fair manner in transactions of goods or services, which entails "treating equals equally and unequals unequally in proportion to their inequality" (p. 176). In acting unjustly toward others by way of violating their rights (e.g., violating their natural right to health by assaulting them) or treating them unfairly (e.g., distributing nursing services according to irrelevant criteria such as race and religion), "the ultimate injury done the

unjustly treated individual lies in the effect it has upon his or her pursuit of happiness" (p. 189). A third form of injustice results from acting contrary to the third precept of the natural moral law.

The third precept charges us to act for the good of the community as a whole (i.e., the common good). In following this directive, we act justly and *indirectly* benefit others in their pursuit of happiness. Our contribution to the good of the community as a whole (a real good) benefits (flows back on) the individual members of the community. When, however, we act so as to *directly* help others as they pursue happiness, we act out of love or benevolence, not justice. We go beyond what justice requires; in addition to respecting their rights and giving them what is due them, we provide direct help. Finally, when we act contrary to the common good, we act unjustly and impede not only others' pursuit of happiness but our own as well (Adler, 1970, 1971, 1981).

The domain of justice has another sphere of interest besides that of the just conduct of the individual: the just conduct of the state in relation to its population. The just state is one that, by various means (e.g., laws and public institutions) meets its obligations: (1) to secure the natural rights of its members; and (2) to advance the community by maintaining and improving it and by assisting its members to secure those real goods which they are unable to acquire wholly on their own. When the state helps its members in this way, it is acting out of justice, not benevolence (Adler, 1970, 1981).

From the foregoing conception of justice, it is apparent that, as Adler (1981) asserts, in order to act justly, knowledge of what is really good for all human beings is necessary, because it is that knowledge that tells us what any human ought to seek and to avoid to make a good life, and what natural rights and moral obligations each of us has in that regard. Since this knowledge consists of objectively true principles, nurses who are denying the possibility of attaining such principles and recommending that nursing practice decisions ultimately be based solely on subjective judgments would be bereft of this knowledge. Consequently, they could not avoid acting unjustly no matter how well intentioned they are. It is beyond the scope of this paper to detail the supporting arguments.

What we require in nursing is a conception of practical nursing judgment which makes possible nursing care that is just and, at the same time, benevolent, sensible, and sensitive to patients' values and wishes. We present such a conception, after setting down salient aspects of a moderate realist conception of practical judgment upon which it is based.

Conception of Practical Judgment

Simply stated, a judgment is an assertion. It can be about any number of things: reality, values, knowledge, conduct, and so forth. When we assert that something is the case, is desirable, ought to be desired and sought, or ought to be sought in a particular way—or not, we are putting forward a truth claim. What then is a *practical* judgment and how is its truth value determined? All judgments that have to do with ends and means of human acts or work and therefore regulate human acts or work, are practical in nature (Adler, 1981; Maritain, 1953/1970). Practical judgments can be distinguished in terms of their particular foci of concern. Good human acts, acts in line with the good of humankind, are the focus of practical *moral* judgments. Good human work, work in line with the particular good to be effected, is the focus of practical *artistic* judgments (Maritain, 1953/1970).

Practical judgments, moral and artistic, can take a descriptive form ("is") or a prescriptive form ("ought"). Practical *descriptive* judgments state (1) what is desirable, and (2) what as a matter of fact is desired—or not. On the other hand, practical *prescriptive* judgments are injunctions that stipulate (1) what we ought to desire and seek, and (2) in what way the desirable ought to be sought—or not. The truth of practical *descriptive* judgments is determined in terms of their correspondence with reality as it exists independent of the individual mind; the truth of practical *prescriptive* judgments is determined in terms of their alignment with right desire (Adler, 1990). In the moral realm, right de-

sire is desiring (willing) aright, desiring that which is in line with the good of humankind; in the artistic realm, it is desiring that which is in line with the particular good to be effected (Maritain, 1930, 1953/1970).

The final distinction to be described pertains to the fact that the regulative function of practical judgments demands a process of practical reasoning which entails reasoning successively forward from one level of judgment to another: from (1) the universal level where judgments take the form of principles which apply universally, that is, the principles apply to all members of a class (e.g., all human beings) at any time and place, to (2) the general level where judgments take the form of rules which apply generally, that is, they apply to a specific subgroup of a class (e.g., a specific group of human beings) at a particular time and place, to (3) the particular level where judgments take the form of a decision which pertains to a specific member of a specific subgroup of a class (e.g., a specific member of a specific group of human beings) at a particular time and place. On each of these levels, reasoning proceeds practically and syllogistically. Although the content of the practical syllogism varies from level to level, the structure does not. On all three levels, the major premise is a *prescriptive* judgment regarding that which ought to be desired or sought, the minor premise is a *descriptive* judgment (a factual assertion) related to the subject matter of the major premise, and the conclusion is a further *prescriptive* judgment regarding that which ought to be desired or sought. This structure allows us to attain *prescriptive* judgments, the truth of which is dependent on their alignment with right desire and on the validity of the factual assertion contained in the minor premise (Adler, 1970, 1990).

Successive movement from one level to the next is accomplished as follows. The prescriptive conclusion (judgment in the form of a principle) established as true at the universal level serves as the major premise of the syllogism at the next level, the general level. The prescriptive conclusion (judgment in the form of a rule) established as true at the general level then serves as the major premise of the syllogism at the particular level. Further, as we move from the universal to the particular level, the descriptive judgment comprising the minor premise of the practical syllogism changes from conveying relevant (1) universal facts at the universal level, to (2) general facts at the general level, to (3) particular facts at the particular level (Adler, 1990).

Adler (1990) reminds us that as we descend from the level of the universal to the particular case with contingencies entering (via the minor premise), we can be less and less certain about the rightness of our judgments. Also, Simon (1991) states that at the point of making the ultimate decision, because contingencies render it impossible to make a *direct* logical connection to principles, so prudence or practical wisdom is required. Further, because there is no science of prudence in the form of principles or rules (Maritain, 1962), prudence must rely on other resources such as past experience, memory, imagination, and consultation in its deliberations (Maritain, 1962; Simon, 1991).

With the above conception of practical judgment serving as its base, an outline of our conception of practical *nursing* judgment follows.

Conception of Practical Nursing Judgment

Besides being grounded in the assumptions and tenets of moderate realism and in its conceptions of justice and practical judgment, our conception of practical nursing judgment also rests in the moderate realist conception of cooperative art and in our assumption that nursing is primarily an art—a cooperative art. According to Adler (1985), there are three kinds of cooperative arts: "farming, healing, and teaching" (p. 1). Unlike other arts which proceed by "*operat[ing] on* nature" (p. 1), cooperative arts are arts of doing which cooperate with the processes of nature to facilitate nature's development of desirable goods (e.g., fruit, health, and knowledge). The cause of the development is primarily nature and, secondarily, the cooperative artist, for example, the teacher in the acquisition of knowledge (Adler, 1965a, 1985).

As cooperative artists engaged in healing, nurses, guided by the natural moral law, cooperate with the processes of nature to facilitate nature's development of some aspect of health, health being the common end of the healing arts. Since health is a real good that meets a natural need, nursing's unique contribution to nature's development of health is a *health-related particular real good,* a means to health, which in turn is a constitutive means to happiness. In this regard, a concern and obligation of nursing as cooperative art is to do *good nursing work,* to work in line with nursing's unique end, its contribution to health. But, a higher concern and obligation is to commit *good nursing acts:* to do nursing's work in line with the good of humankind. This means that practical nursing judgments are, at once, moral and artistic in nature, analytically separable into nursing moral and nursing artistic judgments. Both nursing moral and artistic judgments consist of (1) descriptive assertions about the desirable and the desired, and (2) prescriptive assertions regarding the desirable. The desirable and the desired pertain to good nursing acts, in the case of nursing *moral* judgments to good nursing work, in the case of nursing *artistic* judgments. The truth of *descriptive* nursing judgments is determined by comparing them with reality as it exists independent of the individual mind; the truth of *prescriptive* nursing judgments, by comparing them with right desire—desiring that which is in line with (1) the particular real good that is nursing's end to attain, and (2) the good of humankind.

At the universal level of judgment, practical nursing judgments (descriptive or prescriptive, moral or artistic) take the form of nursing principles. They are completely objective and apply to all nurses at any time and place. This is because, at this level, practical nursing judgments are most intimately connected to natural human needs through nursing's unique contribution to health, a particular real good that helps to fulfill our natural need for health. At the general level, the judgments take the form of nursing rules applicable to a designated group of nurses practicing at a particular time and place. At the particular level, they take the form of a nursing decision that pertains to a specific nurse who is a member of a designated group of nurses practicing at a particular time and place. Underlying the three levels of judgment are the precepts of the natural moral law.

By reasoning successively forward from the universal level to the particular level, as described earlier, practical nursing judgments in the form of principle-based nursing rules and decisions are attained. Further, because facts of a contingent nature (including those about what is in fact desired) enter into the making of these rules and decisions, they are necessarily partly objective and partly subjective in nature. Their objective aspect has to do with their ground, nursing principles; their subjective aspect, with the contingent facts. The subjective aspect is greatest at the particular level, because one has entered here the realm of decision and of action and production, the realm of concrete existence complete with all its contingencies (Maritain, 1959). Also, since there are no principles or rules of prudence, nurses must rely on other resources to make a prudential nursing decision, resources which vary from nurse to nurse (e.g., the nurses's propensity to consult the patient about his or her perspective of the situation, wishes, and dreams; the patient's ability to communicate in a meaningful way; and the availability of consultants).

Making a prudential nursing decision entails getting to know the contingent circumstances, the patient, and one's self. Also, as Wallace (1983) states, "Nursing art represents the practical 'know-how' of a nurse who knows what to do in a particular situation, considering all of the attendant circumstances, so as to achieve the best possible result. It presupposes some knowledge of the rules or principles of nursing practice. . . . The better one possesses the art, the more prudence she or he will manifest in making nursing decisions, in knowing what rules to apply, what exceptions to make, and so on" (pp. 286–287). Adler (1970, 1981) would add that prudence also requires temperance, fortitude, and justice, all existentially inseparable moral virtues. Further, benevolence would complement justice. Having outlined our conception of practical nursing judgment and its bases, we proceed to explain why it has the potential to help offset the current trend recommending that practical nursing decisions ultimately be based solely on subjective judgments.

Practical Nursing Decisions: Sound, Sensitive, Sensible

In our estimation, our conception of practical nursing judgment has the potential to help offset the current trend in that it addresses those aspects of nursing decision making which make possible nursing care of a kind that nurses should and do strive to provide: individualized, just, benevolent, and sensible. We are cautiously optimistic that the potential alluded to can be brought to fruition if the ideas presented so far are given due attention and developed further. The reason for our thinking so is that the conception, for all practical purposes, is not only tenable, but allows a way of thinking about practical nursing judgments that gives traction to nursing action, which the kind of care nurses strive to provide demands. It identifies the kinds of practical nursing judgments such care requires, how those judgments are attained, and the philosophical justification for seeking them. In other words, the conception informs nurses about what is entailed in making sound, sensitive, and sensible nursing decisions upon which the provision of individualized, just, benevolent, and sensible nursing care essentially depends. The relationship between this kind of nursing care and nursing decisions becomes apparent when we consider what constitutes a sound, sensitive, and sensible nursing decision.

Nursing decisions are sound, sensitive, and sensible when they: (1) are based in practical nursing principles (descriptive and prescriptive, artistic and moral) that are true beyond a reasonable doubt and in nursing rules derived therefrom; (2) are made not only in light of nursing's unique contribution as cooperative art but also in light of what all human beings need in order to make their lives good (e.g., health, knowledge, benevolence, just treatment, and right to self-determination); (3) prudently take into account the relevant contingencies (including the patient's wishes and dreams) in applying nursing rules in the particular case; and (4) are based in and congruent with our common experience, common sense, and common-sense knowledge. Whether indeed nurses are able to, and do, make nursing decisions so characterized would depend upon factors under their control (e.g., the extent to which they are prudent and virtuous) and outside their control (e.g., the extent to which the society in which they live is just). A significant determining factor largely outside the control of the individual nurse would be the availability of nursing principles and rules. In this regard, our conception again will help nurses gain the traction they require to move forward.

Our conception provides a tenable framework for nurse scientists, nurse philosophers, and nurse artists to work together worldwide to develop a body of nursing knowledge consisting of a coherent set of objectively true, practical nursing principles (based on common natural human needs, the natural moral law, and natural rights) to serve as a transcultural basis for making just nursing rules and decisions. To arrive at just nursing rules, various groups of nurses could modify the nursing principles according to the unique circumstances under which they practice. Different sets of nursing rules would then exist and, being based in nursing principles, would be sound, as would the nursing decision that results from prudently modifying the rules, as needed, to accommodate the contingencies always operative in situations calling for a decision.

We believe that our conception has the potential to help offset the trend toward relying solely on subjective judgments because it addresses matters recognized to be central to nursing practice. First, common human needs, nursing principles, and particularizing nursing decisions to fit the patient, nurse, and nursing situation have long been recognized as fundamental aspects of nursing practice (Schlotfeldt, 1987, 1988). Second, there is evidence that nurse researchers (e.g., Polifroni & Packard, 1995; Schumacher, Stewart, & Archbold, 1998; Wolfer, 1993) are realizing that it is essential to pay heed to both the subjective and objective aspects of nursing practice. Third, despite the advocation in the nursing literature (e.g., Bartol & Richardson, 1998; Brunt, Lindsey, & Hopkinson, 1997; Princeton, 1993)

that nurses respect cultural notions of health and health practices, the fact that practices such as infanticide pose moral problems for nurses signals their awareness that such practices violate natural human rights and must be addressed. Fourth, there are other moral problems thought to be vital for the nursing profession to resolve. There is the conflict between individual good and common good identified by Fry as early as 1983 as one demanding resolution, but which to date remains unresolved. Another unresolved problem is finding a way to accommodate both duty and virtue in nursing ethics (Salsberry, 1992). Lastly, As Olsen (1993) states, the pitting of justice against caring evident in the nursing literature is problematic, and a synthesis of the concepts of caring and justice based in our common humanity is required.

Summary and Conclusion

In this essay, we examined the current trend recommending that nursing decisions ultimately be based solely on subjective judgments. We presented a conception of practical nursing judgment which holds the potential to help offset the trend. It makes possible individualized, just, benevolent, and sensible nursing care, a means requisite to making our lives good. If the trend is offset, the future of the nursing profession and all those it serves looks promising indeed.

Note. [1]June Kikuchi and Helen Simmons, both currently retired, were Director and Associate Director respectively of the Institute for Philosophical Nursing Research, Faculty of Nursing, University of Alberta, Edmonton, Alberta, Canada.

REFERENCES

Adler, M. J. (1965a). *Poetry and politics.* Pittsburgh, PA: Duquesne University Press.

Adler, M. J. (1965b). *The conditions of philosophy.* New York: Dell.

Adler, M. J. (1970). *The time of our lives. The ethics of common sense.* New York: Holt, Rinehart, & Winston.

Adler, M. J. (1971). *The common sense of politics.* New York: Holt, Rinehart & Winston.

Adler, M. J. (1981). *Six great ideas*. New York: Macmillan.

Adler, M. J. (1985). The arts of farming, healing, teaching. *Viewpoint, 3*. Chicago: Institute for Philosophical Research.

Adler, M. J. (1990). *Intellect. Mind over matter*. New York: Macmillan.

Appleton, J. V., & King, L. (1997). Constructivism: A naturalistic methodology for nursing inquiry. *Advances in Nursing Science, 20*(2), 13–22.

Barnum, B. S. (1994). *Nursing theory. Analysis, application, evaluation* (4th ed.). Philadelphia: Lippincott.

Bartol, G. M., & Richardson, L. (1998). Using literature to create cultural competence. *Image, 30*, 75–80.

Bishop, A. H., & Scudder, Jr., J. R. (1990). *The practical, moral, and personal sense of nursing*. New York: State University of New York Press.

Brunt, J. H., Lindsey, E., & Hopkinson, J. (1997). Health promotion in the Hutterite community and the ethnocentricity of empowerment. *Canadian Journal of Nursing Research, 29*, 17–28.

Cody, W. K. (1993). Norms and nursing science: A question of values. *Nursing Science Quarterly, 6*, 110–112.

Fawcett, J. (1995). *Analysis and evaluation of conceptual models of nursing* (3rd ed.). Philadelphia: Davis.

Fry, S. T. (1983). Dilemma in community health ethics. *Nursing Outlook, 31*, 176–179.

Gadow, S. (1995). Clinical epistemology: A dialectic of nursing assessment. *Canadian Journal of Nursing Research, 27*(2), 25–34.

Maritain, J. (1930). *An introduction to philosophy*. London: Sheed & Ward.

Maritain, J. (1959). *The degrees of knowledge* (G. B. Phelan, Trans.). New York: Charles Scribner's Sons.

Maritain, J. (1962). *Art and scholasticism and the frontiers of poetry* (J. W. Evans, Trans.). Notre Dame, IL: University of Notre Dame Press.

Maritain, J. (1970). Art as a virtue of the practical intellect. In M. Weitz (Ed.), *Problems in aesthetics* (pp. 76–92). London: Macmillan. (Reprinted from *Creative intuition in art and poetry*, chap. 2, by J. Maritain, 1953, New York: Pantheon)

Mitchell, G. J. (1994). Discipline-specific inquiry: The hermeneutics of theory-guided nursing research. *Nursing Outlook, 42*, 224–228.

Mitchell, G. J. (1995). Reflection: The key to breaking with tradition. *Nursing Science Quarterly, 8*, 57.

Moccia, P. (1988). A critique of compromise. Beyond the methods debate. *Advances in Nursing Science, 10*(4), 1–9.

Munhall, P. L. (1982). Nursing philosophy and nursing research: In apposition or opposition? *Nursing Research, 31*, 176–177, 181.

Olsen, D. P. (1993). Populations vulnerable to the ethics of caring. *Journal of Advanced Nursing, 18*, 1696–1700.

Parse, R. (1992). Human becoming: Parse's theory of nursing. *Nursing Science Quarterly, 5*, 35–42.

Polifroni, E. C., & Packard, S. A. (1995). Explanation in nursing science. *Canadian Journal of Nursing Research, 27*(2), 35–44.

Princeton, J. C. (1993). Promoting culturally competent nursing education. *Journal of Nursing Education, 32*, 195–197.

Salsberry, P. J. (1992). Caring, virtue theory, and a foundation for nursing ethics. *Scholarly Inquiry for Nursing Practice, 6*, 155–167.

Sandelowski, M. J. (1996). Truth/storytelling in nursing inquiry. In J. F. Kikuchi, H. Simmons, & D. Romyn (Eds.), *Truth in nursing inquiry* (pp. 111–124). Thousand Oaks, CA: Sage Publications.

Schlotfeldt, R. M. (1987). Defining nursing: A historic controversy. *Nursing Research, 36*, 64–67.

Schlotfeldt, R. M. (1988). Structuring nursing knowledge: A priority for creating nursing's future. *Nursing Science Quarterly, 1*, 35–38.

Schumacher, K. L., Stewart, B. J., & Archbold, P. G. (1998). Conceptualization and measurement of doing family caregiving well. *Image, 30*, 63–69.

Simon, Y. R. (1991). *Practical knowledge*. New York: Fordham University Press.

Wallace, W. A. (1983). *From a realist point of view*. Lanham, MD: University Press of America.

Wolfer, J. (1993). Aspects of "reality" and ways of knowing in nursing: In search of an integrating paradigm. *Image, 25*(2), 141–146.

The Authors Comment

Practical Nursing Judgment: A Moderate Realist Conception

When we were teaching graduate nursing philosophy courses, we were consistently told by the majority, if not all, of the students that as undergraduate students, they had been instructed to respect and not make any judgments about patients' beliefs, values, wishes, perspective, and so forth. However, they found they could not carry out this imperative in practice. Moreover, apparently, the judgments they were making were almost exclusively subjective. Their confusion about the place of judgment in nursing practice led to our desire to try to clarify that place and, subsequently, to our writing this article. Today, as understanding of the importance of prudent judgment in nursing practice is deepening, our article serves as a philosophic basis for further development of nursing theory in the 21st century regarding nursing artistic and moral judgment in nursing practice.

—June F. Kikuchi
—Helen Simmons

Bridging the Gulf Between Science and Action: The "New Fuzzies" of Neopragmatism

Catherine A. Warms

Carole A. Schroeder

Rather than a philosophy, pragmatism is a way of doing philosophy that has major implications for solving disputes involving nursing science, theory, and practice that may otherwise be interminable. Pragmatism weaves together theory and action so that one modifies the other continuously, but both maintain their mutual relevance. Pragmatism emphasizes pluralism and diversity, and depends on an ethical base for determination of what is reasonable. Recently repopularized by the philosopher Richard Rorty and others, pragmatic ideals seem inherent to nursing. We propose that a better understanding of the history and utility of pragmatism will enhance both clinically relevant nursing theory and theoretically relevant nursing practice.

Key words: knowledge development, neopragmatism, nursing, philosophy, practice, pragmatism, theory

Pragmatism may be the most misunderstood philosophical movement in the history of philosophy. Unlike most philosophy, pragmatism is not based on theoretical notions of truth or falsity, and it refuses to offer a method for discovering truth. Instead, pragmatism is a way of *doing* philosophy. On its most basic level, pragmatism is the theory that the meaning of a proposition or course of action lies in its observable consequences. Moreover, the sum of these consequences constitutes the meaning of the proposition or action. Pragmatism is a method for evaluating philosophical problems by tracing the practical consequences of each question. In the words of William James, "The question is not, "Is that true?" but *What difference* would it make if that is

About the Authors

CATHERINE ANN WARMS was born in Bremerton, WA, and attended the University of Washington for all her undergraduate and graduate nursing education. She received a BA in social welfare in 1971, a BSN in 1981, an MN in Family Nursing in 1986, and a PhD in nursing science in 2002. She has been a rehabilitation nurse for more than 20 years and has worked in multiple nursing roles, including inpatient nursing, outpatient nurse practitioner, and research study nurse. Currently, she is a postdoctoral scholar in biobehavioral nursing at the University of Washington School of Nursing, focusing on health promotion for people with disabilities and/or chronic conditions, with an emphasis on physical activity, its measurement, and its effect on health in populations with mobility impairments. Her hobbies include gardening, cooking, and reading.

CAROLE A. SCHROEDER was born in the San Francisco Bay Area and grew up in Reno, NV; received her doctorate at the University of Colorado Health Sciences Center; and did postdoctoral study at the University of Washington in health systems before taking a faculty position. She has been a single parent for most of her adult life, an experience that leaves her with a unique understanding of issues of gender, class, power, and privilege. The focus of her scholarship is to promote social justice and decrease inequalities in health and health care access. Her key contributions include her theoretical writings, work with vulnerable populations, and teaching approach using the Peace and Power philosophy and methods developed by Dr. Peggy Chinn.

true?"[1(p112)] For the pragmatist, belief in a truth cannot be separated from intent, performance, and consequences. Considering the immense ethical contradictions inherent in both the theory and practice of nursing, pragmatism may be a way of grounding our work in a new coherence.

The purpose of this article is twofold: (1) to discuss the history of pragmatism as a philosophical movement, and (2) to argue its relevance to the advancement of nursing knowledge and action in a postmodern world. Pragmatism is a way of "doing" philosophy that weaves together theory and action so that they intertwine, each modifying the other, continuously maintaining their mutual relevance.[2] In contrast to the criterion-based conception of reality, which creates a gulf between scientific objectivity and everyday human activity by its continual search for a defined "truth," the pragmatist conception of reality bridges that gap through inquiry that is a continual reweaving of different versions of the truth, one that incorporates new ideas and better explanations in the context of human encounters and activities. Pragmatism may be a means for nursing to abandon stale theoretical and scientific debates that have inhibited our progress toward philosophical and clinical relevance.

Definition: Confusion and Clarification

The words pragmatism and pragmatic have been co-opted into common usage with meanings that have lost their original richness. Today, pragmatic is commonly used to mean practical or utilitarian. This association of pragmatic with practical assumes knowledge must be limited to promote action. But, as conceived by the early pragmatists, action is creative, complex, knowledgeable, and expansive; it is directed toward new applications of knowledge that bridge the gap between the "actual good and possible better."[9(p43)] The tendency for the term to be used only in its most basic sense of "practical" has separated pragmatism from its history and transformed it into a term of disparagement. A person who is considered pragmatic may also be thought atheoretical, narrow minded, and dogmatic. In actuality, in the philosophical sense of the word, a pragmatic person is very open minded and willing to listen to as many ideas or versions of the "truth" as possible to better solve problems.

History of Pragmatism

Pragmatism began as a uniquely American philosophical movement that appeared near the end of the 19th century, peaked in popularity just before World War II, and then lay dormant for 25 years. In 1977, pragmatism reemerged in a postmodern cloak as neopragmatism, largely because of the efforts of philosophers Richard Rorty at the University of Virginia in Charlottesville, Hilary Putnam at Harvard University in Cambridge, Massachusetts, and Richard Bernstein at the New School for Social Research in New York. As a philosophical movement, pragmatism has been evolutionary in nature, changing with each philosopher who contributes to its tenets. In its earliest stages in the 19th century, pragmatism was popularized by the work of three major philosophers, Charles Sanders Peirce, William James, and John Dewey. We briefly discuss the contributions of each to the development of both pragmatic thought and the pragmatic method below.

Pragmatism was first named by William James (1842–1910) in a lecture given at Berkeley in 1898. In this lecture James presented what he called Peirce's principle of pragmatism, giving Charles Sanders Peirce (1839–1914) credit as originator of the philosophical movement. In 1877, Peirce and several other scientists and philosophers formed the Metaphysical Club in Cambridge, Massachusetts. During discussions with James and others, Peirce began to piece together a method "for making ideas clear."[3(p109)] The earliest versions of pragmatic thought emphasized respect for the views of others and the notion that conversations, not dogma or universal truth, are the basis for developing beliefs.

After James had named this way of "doing" philosophy pragmatism in the Berkeley lecture, Peirce outlined the pragmatic method. This method involved carefully defining conceptual terms and then imagining the practical, ethical, and theoretical consequences of affirming or denying a concept. Unlike previous thought that emphasized definition and preset evaluative criteria, the pragmatic method emphasized that inherent in those *consequences* was the whole of the concept.

Although Peirce has been credited as being the originator of pragmatism, William James popularized the movement. James emphasized that pragmatism was a way of doing philosophy, a method of "settling metaphysical disputes that otherwise might be interminable."[1(p94)] Graduate students in nursing may appreciate James' descriptions of such disputes:

Is the world one or many? Fated or free? Material or spiritual? Disputes over such notions are unending. The pragmatic method in such cases is to try to interpret each notion by tracing its respective practical consequences. *What difference would it practically make to anyone if this notion were true?*[1(p96)]

James claimed pragmatism to be "anti-intellectualist." He believed rationalism to be pretentious, for pragmatism has no dogmas or doctrines, only method. James also coined the term "cash-value," a term that relates to the worthwhileness of a theory, meaning theories are only worth what they can be used for. He stated, "Theories thus become instruments, not answers to enigmas, in which we can rest. Pragmatism unstiffens all our theories, limbers them up and sets each one at work."[4(p27)] He describes this "work ethic" as the standard for value:

Pragmatism is willing to take anything, to follow either logic or the senses and to count *the humblest and most personal experiences.* She will count mystical experiences if they have practical consequences.[1(p111)]

James also tackled the notion of truth, heretically claiming that truths are plastic and made, rather than discovered by using the rigorous methods of science. James' work predated our postmodern relinquishment of the notion of universal truth, handed down by higher authority.

The philosopher John Dewey (1859–1952) was the final member of the founding triumvirate of pragmatism. Dewey was a student of Peirce at Johns Hopkins

University in Baltimore and later taught at the University of Chicago and Columbia University in New York. For Dewey, the essential feature of the pragmatic way of knowing was "to maintain the continuity of knowing with an activity which purposely modifies the environment."[5(p216)] For Dewey, reason was the ability to apply prior experience to a new experience, and a reasonable person kept an open mind.

Although denied entry into academic halls because of gender, Jane Addams (1860–1935) was also extremely influential in pragmatic thought. An early social worker and women's suffrage advocate, Addams opened Hull House, a settlement house that was a community service center for the poor in Chicago. She envisioned Hull House as a place of possibility, one where people, working together, could produce meaningful change. She viewed action as integral to life:

> The settlement stands for application as opposed to research; for emotion as opposed to abstraction, for universal interest as opposed to specialization . . . it is an attempt to express the meaning of life in terms of life itself, in forms of activity.[6(p276)]

Addams' life work exemplified the tenets of pragmatism by her willingness to value humble experiences and disciplinary pluralism, and to examine the ethical and practical consequences of an act.

Richard Rorty, Richard Bernstein, and the Pragmatic Revival

By the 1930s, the popularity of pragmatism appeared to wane. Existentialism, structuralism, Marxism, and psychoanalysis also emerged in the 1930s, and all of these schools of thought competed with pragmatism for public attention. In actuality, pragmatism did not disappear at all, but became so ingrained in the American way of life that its tenets were inherent in all of the major schools of thought and philosophical approaches.

Richard Rorty, a professor of humanities at the University of Virginia, is credited with the recent revival of pragmatism as a way of doing philosophy in the United States. This reemergence of pragmatic thought is popularly referred to as neopragmatism.[7] With the publication of *Philosophy and the Mirror of Nature* in 1979, Rorty successfully adapted pragmatism to the postmodern environment of the late 20th century:

> The aim . . . is to undermine the reader's confidence in the *mind* as something about which one should have a philosophical view, in *knowledge* as something about which there ought to be a theory and that has foundations and in *philosophy* as it has been conceived since Kant.[7(pxxxii)]

Rorty used irony to carry on the anti-intellectualist tradition of William James, and developed his own particular version of pragmatism that is tolerant of alternative views and humanistic, "not in the sense of trying to bring about something already defined, an essential human nature, but in the sense of *creating* something better than what we have known before."[8(p78)]

In 1987, Rorty described 20th century pragmatism as "new fuzziness,"[9] and claimed that pragmatism blurs the distinctions between objective and subjective and fact and value. See Table 53-1 for Rorty's version of pragmatism.[9]

Perhaps the most radical aspect of Rorty's work is a set of moral values, rather than preordained criteria, used by the new fuzzies as the basis for judgment of logic. These values include:

- tolerance
- respect for the opinions of those around us
- willingness to listen
- reliance on persuasion rather than force
- emphasis on communication over agreement or truth.

Rorty promotes broad intellectual tolerance and, above all, leaves room for alternative narratives.

> Rorty qualifies as a legitimate heir to the pragmatic tradition by virtue of his implicit focus on a problematic deeply embedded in the American experience: the fact and consequences of *plurality* in its psychological, social, and political forms.[10(p66)]

Table 53-1
Rorty and the New Pragmatism

Tenet	Explanation
No theory of truth, instead, an ethnocentric view of truth ("work by our own lights," no better lights to work from).	Humans are responsible only to our selves. Each person will hold as "true" those beliefs we find good to believe.[9(p42)] Ethnocentric view is that there is nothing to be said about truth separate from our own descriptions of procedures of justification.
Distinctions between objective/subjective, rational/irrational, true/false unhelpful.	Beliefs can be agreed upon without being true or rational in the methodological sense. The best way to find out what to believe is to listen to as many suggestions and arguments as possible, contrast our beliefs to proposed alternatives and choose that which offers the best solution or answer for that time, place, and situation—not that which is most true.
Redefine inquiry	Inquiry is a matter of "continually reweaving a web of beliefs"[9(p44)]—trying out new beliefs as they are suggested and incorporating or discarding them as we see fit. The goal of inquiry is the attainment of an appropriate mixture of un forced agreement with tolerant disagreement in a community which encourages "free and open encounters."[9(p44)]
Pragmatism has an *ethical* base, not an epistemological or metaphysical base.	Pragmatism depends on moral values or virtues for determination of what is reasonable: "tolerance, respect for the opinions of those around us, willingness to listen and reliance on persuasion rather than force."[9(p40)]
Disciplinary diversity is the goal.	All disciplines participate in cooperative human inquiry and all are equally objective if there is unforced agreement. "Fierce competition" between disciplines is vital.[9(p45)]
Redefine progress.	Progress cannot be judged by forward direction but by the fact of richer human activity, the opportunity for humans to do more interesting things and to be more interesting people.

The emphases on plurality and tolerance figure prominently in the works of another neopragmatist, Richard Bernstein. Professor of Philosophy at the New School for Social Research, Bernstein declines to identify a pragmatic essence or a set of propositions shared by all pragmatists, because " . . . there can be no escape from plurality—a plurality of traditions, perspectives, philosophic orientations."[11(p389)] Like Rorty, Bernstein suggests that disciplinary boundaries dissolve so that richer conversations can take place across them. He calls us to

> nurture the type of community and solidarity where there is an engaged fallibilistic pluralism—one that

is based upon mutual respect, where we are willing to risk our own prejudgments, are open to listening and learning from other and we respond to others with responsiveness and responsibility.[11(p400)]

Narrative, or dialogue, is the method espoused by Bernstein for encounters between individuals and disciplines. He characterizes a community as "a group of individuals locked in an argument,"[12(p66)] and suggests that a vital pragmatism is "the ongoing process of being locked in argument."[12(p66)] The variety of voices constituting the narratives is the primary basis for vitality. Rather than truth, the reason for inquiry is the *application* and *usefulness* of beliefs held by a discipline.

The history of pragmatism is found in the writings of its founders. Peirce emphasized respect for all viewpoints and conversation as the pathway to developing beliefs. For James, pragmatism was not a philosophy in and of itself, but a way of settling disputes. James believed theories to be instruments, valued only for their utility. James also initiated the important emphasis on pluralism. Dewey added an educator's perspective with his approach to learning as doing, a way of applying experience to life. The neo-pragmatists Rorty and Bernstein revived the notion of narrative, tolerance for all viewpoints, and truth as what we *choose* to believe. They added an emphasis on communication and free and open encounters as methods to achieve interdisciplinary cooperation in human inquiry. Both philosophers remind us that pragmatism relies on an ethical base of moral values, rather than specific criteria to evaluate the worth of knowledge.

> We should relish the thought that the sciences as well as the arts will *always* provide a spectacle of fierce competition between alternative theories, movements, and schools. The end of human activity is not rest, but rather richer and better human activity. We should think of human progress as making it possible for human beings to do more interesting things and be more interesting people, not as heading toward a place which has somehow been prepared for us in the past.[9(p45)]

Pragmatism and Nursing

> the usefulness of theory . . . is ultimately answerable to those whose lives are supposed to be bettered by it.[13(p263)]

The tenets of pragmatism are not new to nursing. Nursing has always attended to the cash value or the worthwhileness of nursing theories to achieve desired results in clinical nursing. Clearly, nurses are interested in doing what works. Donaldson (1995) posits that nurse scholars and scientists who intend to build the discipline of nursing "keep in mind that the centrality

and value of this knowledge will be determined by the nurse pragmatist."[14(p6)] For Donaldson, a nurse pragmatist is willing to use any existing theory or knowledge relevant to the situation, "spanning distinct philosophies, paradigms, and disciplines."[14(p6)] For nursing science to be relevant, it must have utility, usually for the achievement of mutually determined clinical outcomes. For Donaldson, a nurse pragmatist is a nurse in practice, "one who is caring for patients and requires a useful knowledge base from which to make applications to "do" nursing."[14(p10)] Donaldson's discussion of the nurse pragmatist emerges from the early pragmatists' assertions of theories as instruments, learning by doing, and the notion of valuing interdisciplinary knowledge.

Although pragmatism seems embedded in the ideals and reality of nursing practice, it also has great utility for furthering the longstanding debates regarding nursing theory and research. In the following sections, we offer four noteworthy examples from the nursing literature that seem to use pragmatic ideals to solve problems in nursing science.

In a 1992 article, Schumacher and Gortner[15] discuss recent shifts in philosophy that replace the tenets of traditional, positivistic science with so-called scientific realism. Shumacher and Gortner move away from the old view that universal laws apply to all situations regardless of circumstance, to a view of science and research that takes into account the context of the phenomena under discussion. Discussing causality, they assert that the notion of causation in "human science is complex, multifaceted, and possibly multidirectional."[15(p7)] At the same time, they defend the traditional notion of causality, stating it is required to make science clinically relevant and because clinicians need to know "the likely consequences of certain events under given conditions."[15(p7)] This approach is pragmatic, illustrating a pluralistic approach that solves problems using ideas from both traditional positivistic science and scientific realism. Schumacher and Gortner weave their ideas into a conception of nursing science that they believe is relevant and useful for nursing. Our task in nursing becomes one of encouraging free and open encounters while listening to as many conversations as possible to discern the utility of Schumacher and Gortner's ideas for nursing.

Utility is also foremost in the 1995 treatise from Ford-Gilboe et al on the pragmatics of science in nursing.[16] The authors discuss the postpositivist, interpretive, and critical paradigms and the use of qualitative and quantitative methods. They conclude that combining strategies across paradigms enhances the value of a study. Ford-Gilboe et al, like Schumacher and Gortner, seem to believe that "good" nursing science is pragmatic. They expand their argument for a pragmatic nursing science by advocating the critical paradigm as an appropriate perspective for advancing nursing knowledge.[17] Under the umbrella of the critical paradigm, the authors propose methods for the purpose of accomplishing a "critical agenda"[17(p13)] to create knowledge that will be persuasive for the purpose of producing change. They emphasize respect for the opposing opinions and reliance on persuasion rather than force, both moral values inherent in pragmatism.

Missing from pragmatist writings is a comprehensive analysis of the inescapable power dynamics inherent in the process of communication. Henderson opens the conversation in nursing with a presentation of participatory action research as a research method that may reduce power hierarchies between researcher and researched.[18] She describes consciousness raising as a method that precedes other forms of data collection, for it is the format in which research takes place: "By engaging in critical and liberating dialogues, individuals uncover the hidden distortions within themselves that help to maintain an oppressive society."[18(p63)]

Critical and liberating dialogues, similar to Rorty's notion of free and open encounters, are both based in ethical notions of unshackled communication and tolerance for diversity. The ideals of feminism and critical theory could advance pragmatic tolerance by addressing power imbalances that create rifts between the researcher and the researched. The tolerant pragmatist would not object to this agenda as long as she can evaluate its value in the given situation.

Boyd also presents a structure for nursing research that is congruent with pragmatist ideals.[19] Boyd uses multiple approaches to research and emphasizes the utility of each approach for specific types of situations depending on context. Her ideas are pragmatic in their respect for pluralism and notions of theories as instruments. Boyd portrays nursing encounters as opportunities for communication and for constructing theories that will be useful in future encounters. For Boyd, nursing becomes a mutual search for both meaning and action, by "adding a research agenda to one's nursing work merely provides for the communication of what is learned so that other nurses, other patients may profit from it."[19(p20)]

Boyd's approach to nursing science is an example of a willingness to use the "humblest and most personal experiences"[1(p111)] to create a knowledge that is tolerant, inclusive, and contextual in nature.

Nursing at the Crossroads

In a discussion of shifting paradigms in the fields of bioethics and health law, Wolf[20] describes these fields as standing at a crossroads between

> the well trod road of conversations among experts, governed by top-down theory . . . abstract pronouncements, inattentive to differences . . . (and) a new more complex path, wide enough to accommodate multiple proposals and critiques as to method, willful attention to feminist, race-attentive and other contributions . . . teeming with people.[20(p415)]

Nursing stands at that same crossroads. The struggle for nursing science to find itself, to be able to name a tradition or paradigm into which nursing knowledge belongs, has proven interminable and impractical. As nursing science evolves into the millennium, an enhanced willingness to use knowledge from other disciplines and share that knowledge with all disciplines seems to be emerging in nursing.[21] As professional nursing matures, we welcome the fact that our old fascination with long-standing debates regarding appropriate methodologies and methods of inquiry in nursing seems to be waning. Pragmatism is an approach that holds promise for developing innovative and useful nursing knowledge in the future, and we would do well to heed Peirce's words: "The willful adherence to a belief and the arbitrary forcing of it upon others, must both be given up and a new method of settling opinions must be adopted."[3(p10)]

Writing on pragmatism and feminism, Seigfried[13] discusses the interrelationship of theory and practice in words that seem particularly relevant for nursing.

> emancipatory theory arises out of practice as much as it reflects back on it. It is a tool for directing practice, not a privileged insight into reality. As a tool it is instrumental to an outcome desired, rather than a hegemonic imposition of a predelineated order. Therefore, theories should be capable of revision as outcomes surpass or undercut expectations . . . The usefulness of theory, therefore is ultimately answerable to those who lives are supposed to be bettered by it.[13(p263)]

Nurse-philosopher Dr. Sally Gadow (unpublished poem, 1995) says words similar to those of Seigfried in a more poetic form:

Musings on Theory

Theory speaks as if a theorist's words are more
        true, more important,
than the words a particular patient and nurse will
        say with each other
in their experience together.

Ambiguity is the possibility for a different
        meaning: ambiguity is freedom.
Can theory have a different meaning?
Can theory emancipate instead of coerce, open
        instead of closing the door to meanings?
        Can there be a critical theory?

I think so—if a theory is just another story,
        one meaning among many,
        without authority,
        always surpassed by the stories each
                nurse and patient compose in their
                situation together.*

_____
*Courtesy of Dr. Sally Gadow © 1995.

Pragmatism is proposed as one way of assisting nursing to emerge from the old constraints of modernism, and begin to act on what is known, rather than act upon what has been told. No longer concerned only with the truth or falsity of a proposition or situation, nurses can begin to ask the pragmatists' question, "*What difference* would it make if this were true?" Pragmatism is a way of doing philosophy that weaves together theory and action, each continuously modifying the other and maintaining their mutual relevance.[2] Considering the immense ethical contradictions inherent in the theory and practice of nursing, pragmatism may be a means for nursing to move toward a higher level of philosophical and clinical relevance.

REFERENCES

1. James W. Pragmatism's conception of truth. In: Menand L, ed. *Pragmatism: A Reader.* New York: Vintage Books: 1997:94–131. (Original work by James written in 1907).
2. Mahowald MB. So many ways to think. An overview of approaches to ethical issues in geriatrics. *Clin Geriatr Med.* 1994;10(3):403–418.
3. Peirce C. The fixation of belief. In: Houser N, Kloesel C, eds. *The Essential Peirce: Selected Philosophical Writings, Vol. 1 (1867–1893).* Bloomington: Indiana University Press; 1992:109–123. (Original work by Peirce written in 1877).
4. James W. Pragmatism. In: Burckhardt F, ed. *The Works of William James: Pragmatism.* Cambridge, MA: Harvard University Press; 1975:20–30. (Original work by James published 1904).
5. Dewey J. Theories of knowledge. In: Menand L, ed. *Pragmatism: A Reader.* New York: Vintage Books; 1997: 205–218. (Original work by Dewey written in 1916).
6. Addams J. A function of the social settlement. In Menand L, ed. *Pragmatism: A Reader.* New York: Vintage Books; 1997:273–286. (Original work by Addams written in 1899).
7. Menand L, ed. An introduction to pragmatism. In: *Pragmatism: A Reader.* New York: Vintage Books: 1997:i–xxxiv.
8. Kolenda K. *Rorty's Humanistic Pragmatism.* Tampa: University of South Florida Press; 1990.
9. Rorty R. Science as solidarity. In: Nelson J, Megil A. McCloskey D. eds. *The Rhetoric of the Human Sciences: Language and Argument in Scholarship and Public Affairs.* Madison: University of Wisconsin Press. 1987:38–52.
10. Hall DL. *Richard Rorty: Prophet and Poet of the New Pragmatism.* Albany, NY: State University of New York Press; 1994.
11. Bernstein RJ. Pragmatism, pluralism and the healing of wounds. In: Menand L. ed. *Pragmatism: A Reader.* New York: Vintage Books; 1997:382–401. (Original work by Bernstein written in 1988).

12. Bernstein, RJ. American pragmatism: The conflict of narratives. In: Saatkamp J. ed. *Rorty and Pragmatism*. Nashville. TN: Vanderbilt University Press; 1995:54–68.
13. Seigfried C. *Pragmatism and Feminism*. Chicago: University of Chicago Press: 1996.
14. Donaldson SK. Nursing science for nursing practice. In: Omery A, Kasper C, Page G, eds. *In Search of Nursing Science*. Thousand Oaks. CA: Sage Publications; 1995:3–12.
15. Schumacher K, Gortner S. (Mis)conceptions and reconceptions about traditional science. *Adv Nurs Sci*. 1992;14(4): 1–11.
16. Ford-Gilboe M, Campbell J, Berman H. Stories and numbers: coexistence without compromise. *Adv Nurs Sci*. 1995; 18(1):14–26.
17. Berman H, Ford-Gilboe M, Campbell J. Combining stories and numbers: A methodologic approach for a critical nursing science. *Adv Nurs Sci*. 1998;21(1):1–15.
18. Henderson D. Consciousness raising in participatory research: Method and methodology for emancipatory nursing inquiry. *Adv Nurs Sci*. 1995;17(3):58–69.
19. Boyd C. Toward a nursing practice research method. *Adv Nurs Sci*. 1993;16(2):9–25.
20. Wolf S. Shifting paradigms in bioethics and health law: The rise of a new pragmatism. *Am J Law Med*. 1994;20(4): 395–414.
21. Moody L. The quest for nursing science. In: Woody LE. ed. *Advancing Nursing Science through Research*. Newbury Park, CA: Sage Publications; 1990:15–46.

The Authors Comment

Bridging the Gulf Between Science and Action: The "New Fuzzies" of Neopragmatism

This article began as a class project for a course on the philosophy of nursing science taught by Carole Schroeder, my first attempt to write a scholarly paper after more than 20 years of practice as a nurse clinician. My need to find a way to bridge my own gulf between my past nursing practice and my hope for a relevant nursing science was clearly addressed by Rorty's writings and the philosophic tenets of neopragmatism that Dr. Schroeder presented in class. Together, we built upon the original class project by merging the ethical basis for pragmatism with the notion of emancipatory theory emerging from and reflecting back on nursing practice. This article presents an approach for development of nursing knowledge in the 21st century that argues for disciplinary postmodernity, diversity, free and open conversations, and tolerance of ambiguity. We hope that by adopting a neopragmatic approach to philosophy, nursing science will evolve beyond truth seeking and instead will find a way to interweave theory and action by developing knowledge that is ultimately "answerable to those whose lives are supposed to be bettered by it."

—Catherine Ann Warms
—Carole A. Schroeder

CHAPTER 54

Nursing as Normative Praxis

Colin Holmes
Philip Warelow

The purpose of this paper is twofold. First, it introduces a variety of concepts of 'praxis,' and argues in support of those which reflect the normative dimension of the critical social perspective. This begins with the Aristotelian concept, and moves through a variety of sources, including Hannah Arendt and Paulo Freire, but focuses primarily, and uniquely in the nursing literature, upon the work of the Yugoslavian 'praxis Marxists'. Second, specific ways of conceiving nursing as praxis are outlined, including political, aesthetic and ethical forms which have immediate import for nurses. The paper concludes with brief suggestions as to how these ways of conceiving praxis may be used by nurses to develop a more intimate and productive understanding of their own practices.

Key words: critical theory, ethics, Marxism, nursing, praxis.

A number of authors have suggested that nursing can usefully be conceived as constituting a form of praxis (Holmes, 1992; Bent, 1993; Holmes, 1993; Rolfe, 1993; Lutz, et al. 1997; Thorne and Hayes, 1997; Warelow, 1997; Penney and Warelow, 1999). In this paper we explore the value of conceiving nursing as a form of praxis, undertaking some groundwork about what this may entail, and in particular trying to elucidate the part played by praxis in relation to nursing ethics. Many types of ethical viewpoint are 'normative'; that is, they are predicated on a particular view as to how a person should lead their life. In the case of praxis, the norma-

Holmes C and Warelow P. Nursing Inquiry 2000; 7: 175–181
Reproduced with permission from Blackwell Science.

About the Authors

COLIN ADRIAN HOLMES was born in Southampton, England, trained as a psychiatric nurse in 1972, and subsequently specialized in working in secure environments. He moved to Australia in 1989, and, in 1997, Dr. Holmes was appointed Foundation Clinical Professor of Nursing (Mental Health) at the University of Western Sydney. He is currently Professor of Nursing at James Cook University, Townsville, Queensland, and an Honorary Visiting Professor at the University of Central Lancashire, England. In addition to nursing and teaching qualifications, he holds an honors degree in psychology and philosophy, a research master's degree in history, and a PhD in nursing ethics. His research interests center on the care of mentally ill offenders, the history of psychiatry, and ethical and philosophic issues in health care. Dr. Holmes is married, with two adult children, and his hobbies include philately, the music of the 1920s and 1930s, and collecting materials relevant to the history of psychiatry.

PHILIP JOHN WARELOW was born in Kingston upon Hull, Yorkshire, England, but has lived for many years in Geelong, Victoria, Australia, where he works as a Lecturer in nursing, teaching undergraduate and postgraduate courses at Deakin University. He holds qualifications in psychiatric and general nursing and is currently undertaking a PhD through James Cook University, Townsville. His main area of scholarly interest is caring and how it may be conceptualized as nursing comes to grips with emerging intellectual, sociopolitical, and cultural challenges. Dr. Warelow cherishes lighthearted times with his family and friends, enjoys sports and fishing, and generally promoting the Australian value of giving people "a fair go."

tive element is the claim that human beings should become 'beings of praxis'. For this perspective, praxis can be seen as a standard of excellence, an ideal ethical goal for which to strive; it is also what Marxists would describe as an attempt to make an irrational world more rational, or a way of making useable sense of one's practice world.

Normative ethics is founded upon questions concerning how a person ought to live, what a person may or may not do, and especially how to define what constitutes a 'good life'. During the twentieth century, as a concomitant to the development of linguistic methods of philosophical analysis, this question gave way to a concern for the meaning and nature of ethical statements. Since the mid-1970s, however, normative ethics has gradually re-emerged as an important topic of political and ethical debate, focusing on problems arising from new technology and increasing public awareness of social injustices. More particularly, recent popular critiques of a whole range of social policies and practices

by peace campaigners, advertising watchdogs, civil rights movements, governmental inquiries and so on has meant that the meta-ethics of philosophical analysis has become largely an irrelevance for all but the professional philosopher. The question 'what ought we to do?' has once again become one of the central questions of political and moral philosophy. It is not, however, simply a restatement of the classical debate: unlike previous generations, we are today faced with options that have the power to transform the world in all its aspects; and, at personal, social and global levels, the question of the good life is resurrected in a new and awesome way. Not surprisingly, the normative basis of personal and political decision-making is therefore under intensive scrutiny.

The guidance afforded to policy-makers by the broad objectives of traditional political ideologies has been outstripped by the variety of choices with which they are faced, and we discern a widespread acknowledgement that neither conservatism, liberalism, nor utopianism constitute an amalgam of politico-ethical principles adequate to the demands of modern political decision-making. Decisions as to the extent and nature of social, technological, political, and ecological change generate an increasing need for a normative social philosophy, which goes beyond traditional political ideologies. The need for a normative basis to political action has thus intensified considerably since Marx made the first attempts to construct a truly theoretico-practical political philosophy in the mid-nineteenth century, his political stance being based on a desire to eschew abstract theorisation in favour of applied philosophy, in accord with his famous observation that philosophers had hitherto only tried to describe the world, whereas the point was to change it.

There are three strands to the response of Marxists to these developments: critique of the present, a vision of the future, and a means by which theory and practice may unite in the realisation of that vision. First, it insists that before we consider the future, we must ask what exactly we find unsatisfactory about present conditions. This has led to Marxist critiques of just about every aspect of modern life, aiming to expose the pervasiveness of oppressive social processes, and to relate these to the material conditions of life. Second, Marxism offers a vision of a better form of society, in which inequalities and injustices are transcended by an egalitarian socialism within which each individual may find personal fulfilment. Third, it avoids the charge of utopianism or philosophical abstraction by making political practice inherent in its theory, and this is the notion of 'praxis.'

How might this notion of 'praxis' be useful as a means of conceiving the work of nurses? We may reasonably say that praxis is theory and practice in an intimate relationship, and this sounds promising as a way of describing nursing. The exact nature of that relationship is surprisingly elusive, however, and a number of interpretations are offered in the nursing literature (Warelow, 1997; Penney and Warelow, 1999). Nursing has not generally been sensitive to the distinctions on which these alternatives are based, however; nor to the social-political theories from which they have emerged (Holmes, 1992). Working through these shades of

meaning will, we believe, lead us to a notion that may be of the utmost importance to our understanding of our practice as nurses. Carr and Kemmis (1986) promoted a concept of praxis as informed action, which, by reflection on its character and consequences, reflexively changes the knowledge base that informs it. We suggest here that the more humanistic elements that many nurses advocate in their daily practice such as those of 'caring,' 'doing good,' and being guided by unwritten moral rules, are all nursing dispositions that contribute to praxis. They all encourage nurses to act truly and justly, incorporate the ideal of doing the right thing by others, notably patients, and are an essential element of being a theoretico-practical person or a 'being of praxis.' In this paper, praxis entails thought and action, or theory and practice, operating in a dialectical and complementary relationship.

On the Relationship between Theory and Practice

Aristotelian Praxis

Views as to the relationship between theory and practice have a long history, centring on the unifying concept of praxis. In vernacular Greek, praxis was the action of free men in contrast to that of slaves. Indeed, Aristotle conceived praxis as constituting the moral and political life of the free man, made possible through a kind of disciplined knowing (practical knowledge or prudential judgement) called phronesis. It excluded the manual activities of slaves, and the domestic activities of women, which were considered basic activities of daily living. Aristotle also distinguished it from poesis, the production of artefacts, using techne or craftsman's skills. For Aristotle, praxis was citizenship itself, and the outcome was irrelevant: the good is in the exercise of praxis itself. Good actions (eupraxia) are those performed in accordance with phronesis, or good judgement, and praxis comes a strong second to theoria as the ultimate good. Theoria (theoretical knowing) is the supreme good because it transcends humanity through the pursuit of those things, which are unchanging and divine, whereas praxis is concerned with the moral and political organisation of the state/polis. We could say, then, that the contrast is between abstract knowledge (knowing) and concrete applications (doing).

Hannah Arendt

This Aristotelian notion of praxis was revived and developed by Hannah Arendt (1958) in *The human condition,* where she distinguishes between the contemplative life and the active life, and describes three varieties of the latter: labour, work and action (i.e., praxis). Labour produces the necessities of life; work produces artefacts, which transcend bodily requirements; and praxis seeks to solve the problem of meaninglessness generated by the instrumentality of labour and work by engaging in activities that are good in themselves. Praxis for Arendt is thus a means of confirming the humanity and uniqueness of the actor in relation to others. According to Crocker (1983), one of our distinctively modern dilemmas is that the pre-eminence of action in the Greek polis has been replaced by the superiority of labouring in a society of jobholders and consumers, and the opportunity to engage in true praxis has suffered accordingly.

Marx's Notion of Praxis

In *The German ideology* Marx refers to material praxis and social praxis, and some theorists have identified these with his notion of the labour process described in *Das Kapital.* Such labour is both biological, because it is the means to physical sustenance, and instrumental, in that it results in a product. It may be either unalienated, or (as at present) alienated. Although the Frankfurtian critical theorists, such as Marcuse and Habermas, make an advance on this notion of praxis as productive labour and as practical activity, they posit a relatively value-neutral concept, which refers to a 'normal' human mode of being. From their perspective, praxis is not the interaction with, or fashioning, an ordinary object but the generation of 'object domains'. This operates on the basis of two quasi-transcendental, 'knowledge-constitutive' cognitive interests: the technical and the practical, which result in two different types

of science, the empirical-analytic and the hermeneutic, respectively. Technical interests are associated with purposive-rational action of which there are two forms—instrumental action and strategic action. Instrumental action occurs when a person employs rules in order to achieve some desired, predicted state of affairs or goals. Strategic action involves a rational choice on the basis of information and values. The aim is not to control reality but to make a rational decision. Practical interests require a different form of praxis; this time aimed at securing personal identity and shared understandings. This is what Habermas (1972) calls 'communicative action,' and in a modern technocratic society it has tended to disappear under the weight of technical interests evidenced in the pervasive influence of positivism in the humanities and social sciences.

Praxis as Transformative Reflective Action: Freire

Freire's (1972, 1973) conception of praxis draws from the work of Lukács on the task of explaining to the people their own action, from Mao Tse Tung on antidialogical action, and from the humanistic Marxism of the Yugoslavian philosopher, Petrovic. For Freire, praxis is characterised by certain fundamental types of relation between persons, their actions, and the world, and Grundy (1987) describes it as the act of reflectively constructing or reconstructing the social world. Authentic praxis must involve both action and reflection, and a dialectical relationship between subjectivity and objectivity which is achieved through what Freire calls 'conscientisation,' or learning to perceive social, political, and economic contradictions, and the taking of action against the oppressive elements of reality as outlined by Ramos (Freire, 1972, p. 15), thereby changing the status quo.

Praxis is generally described by Freire as neither action nor reflection, but rather their synergistic combination in the human mind and body. Indeed, Freire (1973, p. 111) has gone so far as to say that men (sic) 'are praxis.' He is not entirely consistent concerning the epistemological status of his notion of praxis, however, and also says, for example, that 'men's activity consists of both action and reflection: it is praxis' (Freire, 1972, 96). Nevertheless, he is clear that praxis is a combination of reflection and action and that this combination may take the form of dialogue. Dialogue in which action is sacrificed is simply empty verbalism, he suggests, and dialogue in which reflection is sacrificed is blind activism; true dialogue only occurs when action and reflection are in combination. For Freire, therefore, to utter a true word is to engage in both action and reflection, i.e., praxis, and therefore to transform the world. Freire insists that there can be no dialogue without humility, love of life, or faith in one's fellow human beings. Dialogue is the motor force of social change, i.e., of revolutionary action, and such revolutionary praxis must stand opposed to the praxis of the dominant elites, for they are by nature antithetical.

Yugoslavian 'Praxis Marxism'

The humanistic Marxists in the former Yugoslavia, the 'Praxis Marxists,' most notably Markovic (1974a, 1974b) and Stojanovic (1981), tried to establish a normative concept of praxis in which their theory of the good life is combined with the epistemological and transformative concept described by Freire. They insist that the good life is achievable through human beings becoming 'beings of *praxis*.' The norm of praxis represents on one hand a standard for individual excellence, and on the other an axiological principle for social critique of present formations and possible futures. The principle that the optimal society is a praxis society, reflects this dual focus on the individual and the community, arguing that a praxis society promotes lived praxis rather than alienation, and creates structures and institutions which maximally exemplify communitarian principles, such as freedom, equality and justice.

The Marxist doctrine of the unity of theory and practice, which is basic to the concept of praxis, is understood by these writers in three ways, each embodying the notion that theory is the passive reflection of economic practice. First, for good or ill, theory directly influences human action. Second, social theory seeks to influence social behaviour: thus, Habermas, for example, has the practical intention that his theory play an emancipatory role enabling the surpassing of existing social formations, while for Markovic and Stojanovic, the whole point of theory is to make an irrational world more rational. Third, the theorist's task is a dialectical one, not only deriving philosophical principles from life, but also raising life to the level of philosophical principles. In order to be what Crocker (1983, p. 29) calls a 'theoretico-practical being,' the theorist must practice his/her theory, and this is what we take to exemplify the meaning of the term 'praxis.'

For Markovic and Stojanovic, praxis is an ideal human activity because it realises in action one's best latent and actual dispositions, among which Markovic counts intentionality, self-determination, creativity, sociality, and rationality. It involves the realisation of some human potentials at the expense of others, and thus requires a valuing of some human qualities above others. It is 'ideal human activity . . . in which [wo]man realises the optimal potentialities of his[her] being, and which is therefore an end in itself' (Markovic, 1974a, p. 64). Markovic suggests that this ideal may be realised in a whole range of activities which Aristotle or Arendt would have excluded, such as domestic, intellectual and artistic activity, and therefore the concept does not elevate one particular aspect of life over others. It does exclude 'alienating activity' and value-neutral work, which are depicted as antipraxis. Markovic and Stojanovic both regard 'alienation' as occurring when others have control over one's work and creations, and as characteristically involving activities that are aimless, routine, and irrational, that lead to estrangement from others, and detract from the realisation of one's own optimal potentialities (Crocker, 1983, pp. 57–58). Value-neutral activity is equivalent to Marx's concept of labour as the means of survival: whilst it need not be alienating, it can never be praxis because it is purely instrumental. When one's work is also enjoyed for its intrinsic qualities, then it is regarded as praxis, but then it ceases to be defined by its qualities as work and is defined by its qualities as leisure or some other type of praxis. In other words, work can include praxis, but is never itself praxis. Markovic himself seems to regard work as morally neutral, in contrast to praxis, which is a moral ideal. It should be noted that, although it is normative and aspires to certain 'ideals,' praxis Marxism purports not to be utopian idealism, because it offers a way of determining a future which is not fanciful, but founded on a rational and feelingful evaluation of the concrete situations which face individuals, the communities and society as a whole.

Although praxis is not an ontological concept for Markovic, as it is for Habermas (1972), he regards persons as 'beings of praxis' even when they are not acting but are merely characterised by a dominance of optimal dispositions. Hence, he conceives the good life to comprise good character as well as good action, dialectically related. Crocker argues further that ' . . . good action is the realisation of optimal dispositions, and optimal dispositions are tendencies or capacities to act in certain ways in certain situations (Crocker, 1983, p. 59).

The Components of Praxis

Markovic (1974a) suggested six dispositions that are necessary and sufficient for actions to constitute praxis.

(1) *Intentionality:* For Markovic, intentions are both causal and goal-directed or purposive, although for Stojanovic (1981), intentions are never causes of actions. Apart from this difference they are agreed that conscious intention is a precondition of praxis.

(2) *Freedom:* Freedom is conceived as self-determination, and both theorists argue for free choice in human affairs. This relates to their view of critical social science as considering possible alternative futures and the options open in their pursuit. Markovic attempts to reconcile strict determinism with freedom of the will, in order to substantiate a comprehensive account of political and social liberty. Marx himself had been unable to resolve the contradictions created in his theory by the problem of free will, either in respect of socio-historical processes and revolutionary action, or in respect of ethical theory and the concept of the person, but Marxist revolution only makes sense if people can influence the course of history.

(3) *Creativity:* For Markovic, creative activity is novel and has definite aesthetic qualities, involving innovation and beauty: innovation allows the individual to transcend the immediate circumstances and develop new potentialities. Thus, praxis involves the creation of new needs and new potentialities. Beauty is regarded as a value in itself, and constitutes the norm by which the aesthetic value of novelty may be judged.

(4) *Sociality:* Markovic argues that 'all the features by which he [man] is constituted are social products: language, forms of thought, habits and tastes, education, values, and norms of behaviour' (Markovic, 1974a, p. 74). Thus,

[T]o perform an act of praxis is not only to act intentionally, freely, and creatively but also to realize one's disposition for sociality . . . establishing, maintaining, and developing human relationships marked by coordinated effort, open communication, and reciprocal nurturing of individual self-realization (Crocker, 1983, p. 78).

Crocker discusses sociality in the Markovician concept of praxis, using theatrical performance as an illustration. The conscious intentional acts of individuals are coordinated by a common goal, employing a common means, and the performance is a collective expression of these commonalities. Without co-ordination the performance would comprise the chaotic renditions of individuals; with coordination, however, the performance not only facilitates pursuit of common goals in effective ways but also develops a life of its own such that no one alone can significantly alter it. For Markovic (1974b, p. 120), this loss of control in social processes is the result of the statistical effects on the individuals of large classes of chance events. It arises because their purposive, free actions are not purposively and freely co-ordinated in social action. A prerequisite for this to happen is some degree of mutual understanding through effective communication. Praxis thus requires *verstehen,* or mutual understanding, which is achieved through communicating in what Habermas (1972) calls the 'ideal speech situation'. *Verstehen* aims at deepening and extending our understanding of social life and why it is perceived and experienced as it is.

(5) *Rationality:* Praxis also realises the generic disposition of rationality. Theory and practice are unified in rational activity. Reminiscent of Habermas' knowledge of constitutive interests, Markovic (1974a) identifies three forms of rationality: scientific, technical and ethical. Scientific rationality identifies what is and what might be; technical rationality identifies the most effective means for achieving a certain goal, whilst ethical rationality concerns the best ends, as well as the best means.

(6) *Self-realisation:* There are two elements to this: self-realisation and the self-realisation of others. Praxis is self-realising because it is 'activity in which one actualizes the full wealth of his best potential capacities' (Markovic, 1974a, p. 65). Note that it is not all one's potentials that are to be developed, but rather the best: distinctive capacities must be worth realising and must not conflict with any of the criteria for praxis that Markovic identifies.

The social element of praxis also requires that individuals participate in the nurturance of the self-realisation of others. This is not an injunction to self-sacrifice however, but a call to balance self-interest with humane interest in the well being of others. Postponement of the pursuit of one's own goals, and subjugation of personal interests in favour of those of others, are expected only in the short term. Again, Markovic (1974a) sees 'self' and 'other' considerations as mutually compatible, leading ultimately to each person's self-realisation. He argues convincingly that morality involves a conscious, free choice from alternatives, and that this choice transcends the immediate selfish needs of actual existence: it expresses long-range needs and dispositions of our potential being. As Crocker (1983) argues, praxis is an activity with a threefold social dimension including co-ordinated action, undistorted communication, and a reciprocal nurturing of self-realisation.

Both Markovic (1974a) and Stojanovic (1981) interpret Marx as combining social science and moral criticism in a genuinely critical social theory. In contrast to the pluralism of Stojanovic, however, although never given explicit definition, Markovic sees praxis as representing a single ethical standard in Marx's work, positing a morality founded on the interests, inclinations and potentialities of real people. It is a teleological morality, which serves people, and which people serve, rather than a deontological morality imposed through categorical imperatives derived from abstract reasoning.

Nursing as Praxis

Although it would be easy to miss this from examining the use nurses have made of it, praxis is a profoundly political notion. It acts as a bridge between the idea, familiar to nurses, that the personal is the political, and conversely that the political is not about oneself but about the whole of the global community. Praxis is about a person's relationship with themselves, and whether they are authentic, striving for the transformation of their existence both by reflecting upon and revising the practices, beliefs and attitudes upon which that existence is founded. Such a person asks, 'Am I "true to myself"?' and questions whether the relationship in which they stand to their own feelings, beliefs and practices (*vis-à-vis* others) optimises their synergistic action toward self-realisation. Praxis is also about one's relationship with the wider community; whether one strives for the optimal contribution that one can make to the common good as well as one's own. Such a person asks, 'Am I true to others as well as to myself?' and questions whether the relationship in which they stand to their own feelings, beliefs and practices optimises their synergistic action toward the self-realisation and development of other people.

Nurses are engaged in a theoretico-practical process, which has the potential to be developmental and self-realising in a profound and critical way: it is also part of the healthcare system which is itself political in both senses described above. Dealing with the personal-political first: a normative philosophy of praxis, of the kind described by the Yugoslavian Marxists and to some extent by Freire, would have nurses undertake a twofold dialectical critique, aimed at maximising the quality of their healthcare practices. In order to meet the normative standards of praxis, nurses must first critically reflect upon their practice in order to elaborate the implicit and often complex theories and attitudes, by which it is established, developed and sustained. It takes a considerable amount of effort, integrity, self-discipline and courage to work out anything which comes close to a comprehensive picture since, quite apart from the psychological difficulties involved, clearly, nursing's technical, aesthetic, ethical, communicative and other caring elements are linguistically differentiated, diverse and difficult to pin down. Second, nurses would need to critically reflect upon their feelings and beliefs about these linguistically differentiated elements, revising them in the light of the associated discourses, and bring this reflection to bear upon their nursing practices. Were they not to refer to the associated discourses, their reflections would be purely solipsistic, without regard for the experience and wisdom of others, thereby depriving nurses individually and collectively of a means for the realisation of their potential and subsequent improvements in nursing practice.

As we noted previously, praxis may take the form of dialogue, and by uttering true words and engaging in genuinely theoretico-practical actions—that is, by becoming beings of praxis—we transform the world of nursing, for ourselves, other nurses and patients, now and in the future, because we inevitably challenge dominant elites and demonstrate effective liberating alternatives. To paraphrase Freire, from a normative perspective, 'nurses are praxis,' actualising the full wealth of their best potential capacities, encompassing their distinctive talents and skills and engaging an emancipatory position in which they challenge received ways of thinking, feeling and practising. An approach to nursing based on the notion of praxis could thus take its cue from Freire's work.

One way in which nursing can be seen as constituting a form of praxis has been intimated by Holmes (1992), who introduces the notion of nursing as 'aesthetic praxis,' in which the performance of the task of nursing is viewed as an art form, combining practice skills, knowledge and values. The focus is on nursing as a skilled 'performance' along the lines described in Goffman's (1961) theory of 'dramaturgy,' but embodying the principles of a critical theory concept of praxis, as described above. Holmes refers to this performance as 'aesthetic praxis' and suggests that it represents 'a powerful form of self-expression, which has the potential to become liberating for the nurse and the patient' (Holmes, 1992, p. 941). A rather different approach, arguing that aesthetics and praxis offer alternative ways of conceiving practice, has been the subject of some interesting exchanges (De Raeve, 1998; Edwards, 1998; Van Hooft et al., 1998).

Another way of conceiving nursing as praxis is in terms of its normative or ethical dimension, which we have emphasised in our preceding outline, and praxis has indeed been linked by some scholars to concepts of nursing as caring (Owen-Mills, 1995; Thorne and Hayes, 1997; Bent, 1999). We wish merely to emphasise here how nursing can simultaneously embody both clinical expertise and ethical beliefs in ways that are liberating and authenticating, and constitute a form of 'ethical praxis.' A nurse who exercises his/her clinical skills without them being linked to a set of ethical principles would be like a sophisticated machine, practising without caring, making judgements without concern for their ethical assumptions or consequences. In reality, nurses always practice from a set of more or less consciously structured ethical principles, usually involving such notions as duty, rights, goodness, and caring. In ethical praxis, clinical expertise embodies these principles and become a vehicle for their expression and fulfillment. Clinical nursing practice sets the nurse ethicist apart from the nurse practitioner, the latter being both a practitioner and an ethicist, engaged in the reflexive dialectic that is ethical praxis. Taking this argument one step further, Warelow (1997) argues that using reflection and developing self-determination allows nurses who have previously functioned as objects in their practice worlds, to transform themselves into pro-active participatory subjects who then challenge the status quo.

Street (1991) depicts this as a journey, suggesting that praxis and/or reflection should include the past and the future in the present, and contain a journey inward and outwards. The 'inner journey' uncovers our values, feelings, language (or 'discourse'), embodiment and ontology, whilst the 'outward' trip involves challenging our findings with an alternative perspective and consequently revising the situation as an emancipatory opportunity.

Conclusion

On its own, this paper sits inert and useless; it will take the imagination and responsiveness of particular readers to incorporate it into a transformatory process. To do this is to take the first steps along that path by which to realise the main objective of the nurse-scholar (to become a theoretico-practical being), and of the nurse practitioner (to become a practico-theoretical being). As we are referring to normative ideals, it is a matter of making progress toward these states, and we all can be located somewhere along the path. Our aim in this paper has been to alert readers to particular windows of opportunity offered under the normative nature and structure of praxis.

REFERENCES

Arendt H. 1958. *The human condition.* University of Chicago Press: Chicago.

Bent KN. 1993. Perspectives on critical and feminist theory in developing nursing praxis. *Journal of Professional Nursing* 9: 296–303.

Bent KN. 1999. The ecologies of community caring. *Advances in Nursing Science 21:* 29–36.

Carr W and S Kemmis. Year?. *Becoming critical: Knowing through action research,* 2nd edn. Geelong, Victoria: Deakin University Press.

Crocker D. 1983. *Praxis and democratic socialism: The critical social theory of markovic and stojanovic.* Atlantic Highlands, New Jersey: Humanities Press.

De Raeve L. 1998. The art of nursing: Aesthetics or praxis? *Nursing Ethics 5:* 401–11.

Edwards SD. 1998. The art of nursing. *Nursing Ethics 5:* 393–400.

Freire P. 1972. *Pedagogy of the oppressed.* Harmondsworth: Penguin.

Freire P. 1973. *Education for critical consciousness.* New York: Continuum.

Goffman E. 1961. *Encounters.* Indianapolis: Bobbs-Merrill.

Grundy S. 1987. *Curriculum: Product or praxis?* London: Falmer Press.

Habermas J. 1972. *Knowledge and human interests.* Boston: Beacon Press.

Holmes CA. 1992. The drama of nursing. *Journal of Advanced Nursing 17:* 941–50.

Holmes CA. 1993. Praxis: a case study in the depoliticization of a concept in nursing research. *Scholarly Inquiry for Nursing Practice 7:* 3–12.

Lutz KF, KD Jones and J Kendall. 1997. Expanding the praxis debate: contributions to clinical inquiry. *Advances in Nursing Research 20:* 23–31.

Markovic M. 1974a. *From affluence to praxis: Philosophy and social criticism.* Ann Arbour: University of Michigan Press.

Markovic M. 1974b. *The contemporary Marx: Essays on humanist communism.* European Socialist Thought series no. 3. Nottingham: Spokesman Books.

Owen-Mills V. 1995. A synthesis of caring praxis and critical social theory in an emancipatory curriculum. *Journal of Advanced Nursing 21:* 1191–5.

Penney W and P Warelow. 1999. Understanding the prattle of praxis. *Nursing Inquiry 6:* 259–68.

Rolfe G. 1993. Closing the theory-practice gap: A model of nursing praxis. *Journal of Clinical Nursing 2:* 173–7.

Stojanovic S. 1981. *In search of democracy in socialism: History and party consciousness.* Buffalo, NY: Prometheus Press.

Street A. 1991. *From image to action: Reflection in nursing practice.* Geelong, Victoria: Deakin University Press.

Thorne SE and VE Hayes, eds. 1997. *Nursing praxis: Knowledge and action.* Thousand Oaks, CA: Sage.

Van Hooft S, L De Raeve and P Nortvedt. 1998. The art of nursing: aesthetics or praxis? A response to Steven Edwards. *Nursing Ethics 5:* 545–52.

Warelow P. 1997. A nursing journey through discursive praxis. *Journal of Advanced Nursing 26:* 1020–7.

The Authors Comment

Nursing as Normative Praxis

In this article, we tried to encapsulate our long-held beliefs about the nature of nursing and the need to conceive it within a broad sociopolitical framework that can successfully depict a constructive relationship between theory, practice, and values. Although its idealism will find little sympathy among postmodernists, we believe that praxis is a realistic ideal that challenges orthodox accounts of nursing's value orientation and offers a useful way to bring that to bear on issues of theory and practice. We especially like the praxis approach because it suggests ways in which personal and communitarian ethics can be reconciled within a general account of action. We hope that others will take up the challenge and explore praxis as a framework within which to theorize aspects of the discipline of nursing.

—COLIN ADRIAN HOLMES
—PHILIP JOHN WARELOW

Future Directions for Nursing Theory

This unit builds upon the writings presented in previous units, to further extend and challenge the reader's developing perspectives on nursing theory. Traditional philosophic views about knowledge development, nursing science, practice, and technology are turned upside down. New philosophies and paradigms are proposed, as are creative conceptions of pattern, client, and nursing. Several authors advance philosophic views that go beyond postmodernism. Overall, the articles contained in this unit span one decade of writing, with the oldest (chronologically speaking) having been written in 1992 by the visionary Martha Rogers. The most recent were published only a few months ago. Although few of the ideas presented in these articles are actively practiced within nursing today, these ideas and the new thinking they will generate among readers promise to soon permeate mainstream nursing.

CHAPTER 55

The Unrecognized Paradigm Shift in Nursing: Implications, Problems, and Possibilities

Ann L. Whall
Frank D. Hicks

An important paradigm (or worldview) shift is occurring in science that affects the nature of nursing education, practice, and research. The shift from positivism to postmodernism and now to neomodernism has received little attention in US nursing and as such may forestall many opportunities related to such change. The nature of this paradigm shift and its effects on selected aspects of nursing education, practice, and research are described, and related implications, problems, and possibilities are explored. Neomodernism is discussed as one future for nursing that encompasses aspects of both positivism and postmodernism but yet goes beyond these to include important meta-narratives as traditional values and beliefs of nursing. The work of Laudan and Lakatos are explored as supportive of this neomodernist approach.

In the last decade of the 20th century, discussions of philosophic issues foundational to the discipline of nursing were infrequently published in nursing journals, although there were several noteworthy exceptions.[1-4] This seeming inattention was, for the most part, characteristic of the US nursing journals and became more apparent in the last decade because of the level of attention focused on other issues, such as nursing praxis, best practices, and evidenced-based practice. It appeared that topics garnering the most disciplinary attention in the United States were not seen as philosophically based and/or related to a worldview (or para-

About the Authors

ANN L. WHALL is a native Michiganian and three-time graduate of Wayne State University in Detroit. She is an Advanced Nurse Practitioner in Michigan and has completed postdoctoral studies in geropsychiatry and neuroscience and, most recently, as a Fulbright Distinguished Scholar in the United Kingdom, examining expert nurses' use of implicit memory in dementia care. Throughout her career, Dr. Whall has been "driven by the desire to explicate the depth and exquisite nature of nursing knowledge, which has historically been unrecognized exterior to nursing." As a diploma graduate, she was denied admittance to graduate programs that were exterior to nursing on the belief that nursing was "manual art, not a science." Her works have since been published widely, and she has held several visiting professorships and completed multiple research studies and related publications, often with an identifiable emphasis upon the metatheoretical nature of nursing knowledge. Dr. Whall enjoys classical music, golfing, interacting with her 3 children, and developing international connections within nursing.

FRANK HICKS is an Associate Professor of Adult Health Nursing in the College of Nursing at Rush University. In addition to his interest in philosophy of science and theory development, Dr. Hicks conducts research into aspects of patient decision making.

digm) shift affecting most disciplines, that is, a shift from positivism to postmodernism and increasingly to a neomodernist perspective. It is important that nursing not overlook the nature of the present paradigm shift, for nursing did not focus on (or perhaps understand) the nature and importance of a paradigm shift that occurred just a few decades ago.[5]

An interesting aspect of this situation was the leadership shown by nursing outside the United States in the discussion of this paradigm shift. A search of nursing publications for the term "postmodernism" in the last decade reveals many articles of Canadian and some of European origin,[1,6-8] with relatively fewer of US origin. This may suggest more recognition in nursing communities exterior to the United States of the importance of philosophic and paradigmatic issues for the profession. The reasons for this difference are not clear but may represent a view in the United States that the paradigm shift either does not exist or is unimportant.

The thesis of this article is that an important paradigm shift is taking place that affects the nature of nursing education, practice, and research but that little notice appears to be taken of this change within US nursing. Lack of attention to the implications, problems, and possibilities related to such change may forestall many opportunities. This article addresses selected ways in which this paradigm shift affects aspects of nursing practice, education, and research and addresses opportunities related to such changes.

Positivism: Gone—Or Is It?

Positivism, one variation of which was logical positivism, dominated scientific thought from the mid-19th century. Related to Kant's attempt to delineate the seemingly impenetrable boundaries between science, morality, and art,[9] positivism was committed to objectively observing phenomena. With this commitment, proponents often projected an intense disdain for metaphysical topics and issues.[10] One of logical positivism's major tenets that had great relevance for nursing was the verification principle, which posited that phenomena were scientifically meaningful only if they were empirically verifiable via sense experience and/or via logical proofs and mathematics.[10]

As nursing has historically dealt with patient values and meanings (eg, spiritual desires, cultural beliefs), the verificationist perspective was seen by many as greatly restrictive and was not generally embraced in nursing education.[11] Although shunned by many sciences today, selected aspects of positivism continue to influence scientific development in many fields, such as education, psychology, sociology, and notably nursing.[1,12-15] This continued influence in nursing is not surprising since one "way of knowing" includes empirics.[16] Although empirics in nursing can take many forms (and generally is not reflective of a strict verificationist perspective), positivism's influence affects segments of nursing practice, education, and research.

Whereas positivism's lingering influence on nursing practice is variable, positivistic views in medical science appear strong and enduring and in interdisciplinary practice these views may greatly affect nursing. Nurse practitioners, for example, who follow a medical model (many times with little choice) may be forced to limit their patient contact to a 10-minute visit. Almost by necessity, these nurses practice in a rather positivistic manner. The focus is on the presenting problem and little else. Laboratory tests often define health, and patient reports of the context of the problem are often discouraged as "not focusing on the problem." A nurse who spends more than 10 minutes per patient may be sanctioned as inefficient and unproductive, and exceeding this 10-minute limit may negatively influence the nurse practitioner's performance evaluation. Such restrictions support a "context stripping" approach in which various aspects of the situation that the patient finds important are not discussed or jointly evaluated. It is little wonder in such situations that missed signs of depression and a related high suicide rate in the elderly are continuing problems for primary care providers.[17-19]

Recently, in a discussion of how physicians viewed optimal interdisciplinary practice, a physician presented this example: "The physician is the master mechanic with his/her head under the hood of the car. The grease-monkeys assist the physician and stand-by to deliver the tools and diagnostics needed by the physician." The approach in this scenario is not only mechanistic but focused solely on procedure and not the patient. Moreover, the physician's estimation of the problem is made on the basis of his or her views alone, without the input of the robot-like "grease monkeys" or the patient. Almost all the characteristics of this situation portray a positivistic paradigm view. The irony is that the nurses who were working to develop the interdisciplinary team held a decidedly postmodern view, that is, one in which all opinions are considered equally important.

In nursing education, the influence of the medical model may persist in curricular design, and when it does, a positivistic approach is often an outcome. Nurse educators who use lists of objectives, diagnoses, interventions, and outcomes in a manner devoid of contextual aspects and patient input are ignoring the traditional contextual focus of nursing practice.[20] Despite cries for curricular revisions in nursing education,[21] the approach often remains greatly influenced by ways of thinking that are clearly positivistic. The primacy of such an approach and an overreliance on evidence-based practice may portend an atheoretical future devoid of the influence of traditional nursing values.[22] These and other examples are plentiful in nursing education and support the view that positivism is alive and well today in many situations.

Postmodernism: Present But Often Unappreciated

Postmodern thinking was, in the main, a reaction to the restrictive views found in positivism. It was also a result of multiple other cultural and philosophical influences, many European in origin. Postmodernism made its appearance in scientific discussions sometime around the beginning of the 20th century, although it was not recognized or seen as influential in nursing until approximately the last decade of the 20th century. Today, many Western sciences, nursing in particular, are significantly influenced by the philosophic shift toward postmodernism, although, as with positivism, its influence is variable, often unrecognized, and/or seen as unimportant. Postmodernists as a group criticized the universal totality claims of the positivists, as well as their claims regarding rationality and scientific truth.[8,23] Postmodernists often characterized positivists' research methods as "context stripping." This term denoted an inattention to the reciprocal relationships between individuals and their many environments and/or objectifying the observed and ignoring reciprocal relationships between the observer and the observed. The context could not, however, be ignored for clinical nursing research, because the clinical situation is often chaotic and characterized by multiple, diverse, and simultaneous interactions that, for the most part, are virtually uncontrollable. Because clinical nursing research was an early and continuing focus in nursing, the lack of control evident in clinical situations was problematic for those with positivistic views; postmodernism, however, allowed for more latitude for consideration of such contexts.

Several characteristics of the newer postmodernist paradigm were very congruent with traditional nursing values and experiences. Not only was the context important in research efforts for the postmodernist, but other freedoms were inherent within the new paradigm that were more consistent with the historical but often overlooked experiences of nursing. Nursing was a suspect entry into the hallowed halls of positivist researchers, often because nurse researchers deviated in both educational background and research training from that of other scientists. However, with a postmodernist view, expanded research training as well as newly accepted topics for research and expanded methods afforded nurse researchers possibilities not available in a positivistic world. In addition, nursing, under the influence of postmodernism, was free to explore the importance of cultural diversity for education, research, and patient care.

Postmodernism is not, however, without criticism. Certain characteristics of postmodernism, such as relativism; irrationalism, nihilism, and a deconstructionist methodology,[2,24] have been problematic for nursing. The tendency for postmodernists to overanalyze and deconstruct and yet provide little alternatives for reconstruction led some to nihilistic conclusions. One outcome of such a nihilistic attitude was the acceptance of all viewpoints as having equal merit/nonmerit. Someone once characterized the ultimate postmodern attitude as taking pleasure in the bottomless nature of a swamp of ever-inadequate knowledge.[6]

In nursing education, postmodernism was reflected by an era in which repeated analysis and evaluation of grand theories was addressed with use of truth criteria that may or may not have been appropriate. This repeated deconstruction of grand theories may have led to the nihilistic feelings inherent in the cry: "Let's get rid of all nursing theory."[25] Likewise, a tendency to eliminate "Philosophic Foundations of Nursing Theory" courses in master's and doctoral programs may be related to such nihilistic feelings and/or an era in which philosophic underpinnings of nursing education, practice, and research are unrecognized. Such outcries and movements in nursing rival the nihilism of the best postmodernists in any discipline.

Another example of the deconstructionist influence in nursing education is preference for a curricular structure that supports a "high wall" between specialties. At the master's level, in particular, faculty often cannot teach across divisional boundaries when a deconstructed view of knowledge prevails. An example of this, cited by the Bureau of Health Professions, is nurses with expertise in elder care (who are in short supply) who are not allowed to use this expertise across master's level specialties.[26]

Thus the influence of positivism and postmodernism remains variable both from discipline to discipline and within disciplinary segments, varying from almost total domination of either paradigm to a sometimes unrecognized allegiance to either of these approaches. In academia, unrecognized allegiance to either approach may have far-reaching and profound effects for nursing, with the selection of nursing faculty, as well as promotion and tenure decisions, riding on unspoken and often unrecognized paradigm assumptions.

Neomodernism as an Alternative Future

Exterior to nursing, the relative influence of and variable shift in the scientific paradigm (from positivism to postmodernism and to neomodernism) have been major topics of discussion for several years. These discussions range from the early views of Kuhn[27] to the more relevant views of Laudan[28] and Lakatos.[29] In an early but still influential view, Kuhn observed that the development of science was neither linear nor neat and that the process was not a smooth one from discovery to discovery, nor was scientific knowledge necessarily cumulative. Likewise, newer (or in his view, revolutionary) theses were not logically and systematically considered and were either not accepted or were discarded on the basis of the adequacy of scientific evidence. Rather, "phage groups" sought to interrupt the influence of new ideas, which might diminish their influence.

Revolutions in science, according to Kuhn, occurred because a particular worldview (or paradigm) delineating the theories and methods by which the discipline did its work was found to be no longer useful in addressing perplexing problems. When the accepted paradigm failed to sufficiently address phenomena relevant to the discipline, a revolution (ie, a gestalt switch) occurred that achieved a better way of viewing scientific problems. Ultimately, Kuhn[27] believed that the new paradigm supplanted the former in a radically different way. The switch was so drastic that the new view (as well its theories and methods) were incommensurable with the old view.

The incommensurability thesis was one of the most problematic aspects of Kuhn's theory,[10] because it suggested that a smooth transition and/or communication among scientists in different paradigms was impossible. Thus, in Kuhn's view, a neomodernist approach including both positivistic and postmodern views would be impossible, because these scientists could not communicate and essentially lived and worked in very different worlds.

Laudan[28] and Lakatos[29] challenged Kuhn's[27] views regarding this transition, including noncoherence of scientific bodies of knowledge and research traditions. Laudan[28] saw science as progressing along research traditions, with a collection of assumptions, tools, methods, and axioms guiding that science. Within these traditions, many theories resided that could change remarkably over time but commonalities remained that were sometimes grounded in the former research traditions. It is clear that Laudan's views are more descrip-

tive of the state of the discipline of nursing, including that science is seen as a rational process used to solve problems. The hallmark of scientific progress in such a world would be the transformation of anomalous and unsolved problems into solved ones.

In nursing today, we see that the complete paradigm shift that Kuhn described has not occurred. There are nursing scientists (e.g., physiologists) still working within a positivist paradigm and other scientists (e.g., nurse anthropologists) who have never adopted a positivistic approach and essentially have always posited postmodernist views. These scientists manage to work side by side in a sometimes uneasy alliance, perhaps willing and able to let their views coexist because of some postmodern influence, such as tolerance for diversity.

Benner et al,[20] Reed,[2] and others have suggested several alternatives by which nursing may capitalize on the more useful aspects of both positivism and postmodernism but which go beyond both philosophic stances. Reed[2] has termed these "above and beyond efforts" *neomodernism* or an approach to nursing science in which a deliberative effort is made to use important traditional metanarratives to address current problems of nursing science. In Reed's view, this neomodernist approach includes the freedom to explore and propose alternative ways and methods for nursing science while taking into account important historic values and traditions. Neomodernism, therefore, offers an even more inclusive and seemingly a more liberated path than that of postmodernism.

Examples in nursing of cross-university research, wherein scientists from various philosophic backgrounds work to solve a specific scientific problem, are representative of a neomodernist perspective. In dementia research, bench scientists (who primarily use a positivist view) work with neomodernist nurse researchers to understand the nature of need-driven but dementia-compromised behavior in a cross-university effort.[30] There are many other examples of such interactive and integrative projects in nursing today. Nursing's scientific progress in the last two decades, therefore, appears more congruent with Laudan's perspective, which ultimately may lead to recognition of the importance of a neomodernist approach for nursing education, practice, and research.

Lakatos'[29] views are likewise congruent with both nursing history and perspective, in that he advocated a shift to holism by making a series of theories, or what he terms "research programs," the object of evaluation. Arguing that research traditions do not produce scientists committed to addressing "timeless" questions, Lakatos believed that scientists strove to solve those problems that they found perplexing. In so doing, their research programs reflected a diversity of theory and method oriented toward problem solution. The rationality of these theories and methods pertained to the consistent goals of research programs and not necessarily to the paradigm within which such research was developed. Given the complexity of phenomena that nurse scientists study, it would seem advisable that an approach embracing diversity of theory and method would more likely result in solutions to problems. Such a view would be applicable across situations and more consistent with the goals of nurse scientists seeking answers to difficult questions (an approach reflective of neomodernist influences).

In nursing there has been debate about the incommensurable nature of the profession's grand theories, in that some may be interpreted as having their basis on either a simultaneity or a totality view. For both Laudan and Lakatos, such distinctions tend to be overly exclusive and thus less useful. Toulmin[31] also stressed that despite notable differences, opposing worldviews are likely to overlap to some degree and such overlap should not necessarily lead to "inescapable incomprehension." This, then, would support inclusion of various views within a given discipline in a neomodernist era.

Summary

Clearly, positivism and postmodernism have contributed to the development of nursing science. Neither, however, is a panacea for scientific truth or consensus given the multifaceted, complex, and dynamic phenomena with which nurses deal in practice, education, and research. Although questions of what constitutes scientific merit and scientifically acceptable explanations continue to arise, it seems apparent that nurse scholars should strive to examine these from a variety of paradigmatic perspectives, especially from a more inclusive neomodernist approach. Ignoring the complexity of nursing phenomena and/or ascribing to only one view will likely lead to an incomplete nursing science. Perhaps nursing can avoid a seemingly inescapable incomprehension by socializing the next generation of nurse scholars into a more flexible and inclusive view of science and scientific knowledge. A more productive neomodernist approach might center on explicating the commonalities of warrantable evidence, scientific progress, and progression toward goal achievement. This seems a viable alternative for nursing, but first the present paradigm shift would need to be recognized and the problems and possibilities addressed.

We thank Dr Pamela Reed of the University of Arizona and Dr Patricia Benner of the University of California at San Francisco for their review of and suggestions for this manuscript.

REFERENCES

1. Forbes D, King K, Kushner K, Letourneau N, Myrick A, Profetto-McGrath J. Warrantable evidence in nursing science. *J Adv Nurs* 1999;29:373–9.
2. Reed PG. A treatise on nursing knowledge development for the 21st century: beyond postmodernism. *Adv Nurs Sci* 1995;17:70–84.
3. Silva MC. Scholarly dialogue. The state of nursing science: reconceptualizing for the 21st century. *Nurs Sci Q* 1999;12:221–6.
4. Jacox A, Webster G. Competing theories of science. In Nicoll L, editor. Perspectives on nursing theory. 3rd ed. New York: Lippincott; 1997, p. 423–31.
5. Letourneau N, Allen, M. Post-positivist critical multiplism: a beginning dialogue. J Adv Nurs 1999;30:623–31.
6. Rolfe G. The pleasure of the bottomless: postmodernism, chaos, and paradigm shifts. *Nurs Educ Today* 1999;19: 668–72.
7. Van der Zalm J, Bergum V. Hermeneutic-phenomenology: providing living knowledge for nursing practice. *J Adv Nurs* 2000;31:211–8.
8. Schrag CO. The self after postmodernity. New Haven: Yale University Press; 1997.
9. Scriven M. The legacy of logical positivism. Baltimore: Johns Hopkins Press; 1969.
10. Phillips D. Philosophy, science, and social inquiry: contemporary methodological controversies in social science and

related applied fields of research. New York: Pergamon; 1987.

11. Whall A. The influence of logical positivism on nursing practice. *Image J Nurs Sch* 1989;21:243–5.

12. Giroux H. Ideology, culture, and the process of schooling. Philadelphia: Temple University Press; 1981.

13. Halfpenny P. Positivism and sociology. London: Allen & Unwin; 1982.

14. Lincoln YS, Guba E. Naturalistic inquiry. Newbury Park (CA): Sage; 1985.

15. Gortner SR. Nursing's syntax revisited: toward a science philosophy. *Int J Nurs Stud* 1993;30:447–88.

16. Carper B. Fundamental patterns of knowing in nursing. *Adv Nurs Sci* 1978;1:13–23.

17. Garrard J, Rolnick S, Nitz N, Luepke L, Jackson J, Fischer L, et al. Clinical detection of depression among community-based elderly people with self-reported symptoms of depression. *J Gerontol* 1998; 53A:M92–101.

18. Morris L. For elderly, relief for emotional ills can be elusive. New York Times. 2001 Mar 21:76.

19. Whall A, Colling KB. Suicide in the elderly: could missed identification be associated with postmodernism? *Refl Nurs Lead* 2001;27:8–9, 45–6.

20. Benner P, Hooper-Kytiakidis P, Stannard D. Clinical wisdom and interventions in critical care: a thinking-in-action approach. Philadelphia: WB Saunders; 1999.

21. Diekelmann N. The nursing curriculum: lived experiences of students. Curriculum revolution: reconceptualizing nursing education. 1989. p. 25–41. National League of Nurses Publication No.: 15–2280.

22. Fawcett J, Watson J, Neuman B, Hinton Walker P, Fitzpatrick J. On nursing theories and evidence. *Image J Nurs Sch* 2001;33:115–9.

23. Abbey R. Charles Taylor: philosophy now. In: John Shand, series editor. Philosophy now. Princeton (NJ): Princeton and Oxford Press; 2000.

24. Best S, Kellner D. Postmodern theory: critical interrogations. New York: Guilford; 1991.

25. Whall A. Let's get rid of all nursing theory! *Nurs Sci Q* 1993;6:164–5.

26. Klein S. A national agenda for geriatric education: white papers. New York: Springer; 1997.

27. Kuhn TS. The structure of scientific revolutions, 2nd ed. Chicago: University of Chicago Press; 1970.

28. Laudan L. Progress and its problems. Los Angeles: University of California Press; 1977.

29. Lakatos I. The methodology of scientific research programmes. In Currie JWG, editor. Philosophical papers. Vol. 1. Cambridge (UK): Cambridge University Press; 1977.

30. Algae D, Beck C, Kolanowski A, Whall A, Berent S, Richards K, et al. Framing an understanding of disruptive behavior in dementia. *Am J Alzheimer Dis* 1996;11:10–9.

31. Toulmin S. Human Understanding, Vol. 1. Princeton (NJ): Princeton University Press; 1972.

The Authors Comment

The Unrecognized Paradigm Shift in Nursing: Implications, Problems and Possibilities

While teaching the philosophic and theoretic foundations course in the doctoral program at the University of Michigan School of Nursing, we reviewed Reed's 1995 article concerning nursing knowledge moving beyond postmodernism. Students always comment that this movement, although extremely important, is the basis for multiple misunderstandings within nursing and is essentially "unrecognized" within the discipline. Frank Hicks, as a Postdoctoral Fellow at the University of Michigan School of Nursing and member of the course, proposed that we write a response to this student concern. This article is a result of that joint effort.

—Ann L. Whall
—Frank Hicks

A Treatise on Nursing Knowledge Development for the 21st Century: Beyond Postmodernism

Pamela G. Reed

This article explicates a framework for nursing knowledge development that incorporates both modernist and postmodernist philosophies The framework derives from an "open philosophy" of science, which links science, philosophy, and practice in development of nursing knowledge. A neomodernist perspective is proposed that upholds modernist values for unified conceptualizations of nursing reality while recognizing the dynamic and value-laden nature of all levels of theory and metatheory. It is proposed that scientific inquiry extend beyond the postmodern critique to identify nursing metanarratives of nursing philosophy and nursing practice that serve as external correctives in the critique process. Philosophic positions related to the science, philosophy, and practice domains are put forth for continued dialogue about future directions for knowledge development in nursing.

Key words: knowledge development, metatheory, philosophy of science, postmodernism.

Among the transitions currently facing nursing is the ending of what someday will be referred to as 20th-century nursing theorizing. For the past several years, nurses have been feeling the ground shift with the re-forming of philosophic ideas that launched nursing as a science. Not since the advent of modernism and the birth of modern nursing at the end of the 19th century has nursing science been faced with such a wealth of possibilities for knowledge development. These possibilities have their roots in modernism to be sure, but they also are nurtured by the current dialogue postmodern thought has precipitated.

Postmodernism has engaged nursing in a dialogue to reconcile a basic awareness about the uniqueness

Advances in Nursing Science, 17(3), 70–84. Copyright © 1995 Aspen Publishers, Inc. Reproduced with permission of Lippincott Williams & Wilkins.

About the Author

PAMELA G. REED was born in Detroit, MI, in June 1952 and grew up in an environment enriched by the sociopolitical and musical events of Motown. She is a three-time graduate of Wayne State University in Detroit, receiving a BSN in 1974, an MSN in 1976 (with a double major in child-adolescent psychiatric mental health nursing and teaching), and her PhD, with a major in nursing (focus on lifespan development and aging, nursing theory) in 1982. She worked as a psychiatric-mental health clinical nurse specialist and was an Instructor in Nursing at Oakland University, Rochester, MI, from 1976 to 1979. From 1983 to the present, she has been on the faculty at the University of Arizona College of Nursing in Tucson, including 7 years serving as Associate Dean for Academic Affairs. With her doctoral work, she pioneered nursing research into spirituality and its role in well-being. Dr. Reed has developed a theory of self-transcendence and two widely used research instruments, the *Spiritual Perspective Scale* and the *Self-Transcendence Scale*. Her publications reflect her three main passions and contributions to nursing: the conceptual and empirical bases of the significance of spirituality in health experiences, a lifespan developmental perspective of well-being in aging and end of life, and the philosophic dimensions of the development of the discipline. Dr. Reed also enjoys classical music, hiking in the Grand Canyon, swimming, and raising her two daughters, Regina and Rebecca, with her husband, Gary.

and differences in human beings and health, with basic beliefs in universals and values about human phenomena. It is a struggle, as a philosopher characterized that of feminism, to "modify the Enlightenment in the context of late modernity but not to capitulate to the postmodern condition."[1(p195)]

This article presents a framework that will help nursing science bridge modernist and postmodernist philosophies as nursing clarifies contemporary approaches to knowledge development. The framework builds on accomplishments of modernist nursing while exploiting opportunities of the postmodern context and, in this sense, is "neomodernist." The framework reaches beyond postmodern prescriptions for nursing science and proposes a neomodernist perspective on knowledge development that incorporates meta-narratives of nursing philosophy and nursing practice into scientific inquiry.

Historical Background: Modernism and Postmodernism

From premodern to postmodern times, paths to knowledge have crossed through the Age of Faith, the Age of Reason, to the Culture of Critique. The once dominant religious and metaphysical approach to reasoning about reality was transformed into avenues to truth that separated philosophic "beliefs" from empiric "knowing." Empiricism supplanted the Aristotelian emphasis on rationality that had inspired early modernists. Although modern science enlightened the world and enhanced everyday life, its approach failed to deliver the anticipated empirical base for ultimate meaning and truth about human beings and their world. Also, as philosopher Popper[2] helped scientists realize during the decline of positivism, knowledge development could not be purged of biases, contradictions, and values. Theories, like the fisherman's net, inevitably influenced what data were caught by the scientist. Postmodern thought helped move scientists toward the realization about the embeddedness of research data and the transitory nature of theory.

Postmodernism is a social movement and philosophy that originated among French literary theorists in the 1960s, although postmodern ideas were expressed prior to this time.[3] Postmodernism is a perspective or intellectual style of creating art, of theorizing, of doing science. And it is influencing nursing's approach to knowledge development.

Postmodernism challenges the modernist idea of a single, transcendent meaning of reality and the importance of the search for empirical patterns that correspond to and represent ultimate meaning. Metanarratives, grand or high theories, or other overarching discourses that identify essential truths and propose to re-present reality are not recognized as valid. The "postmodern condition"[4] is a "crisis of confidence in the narratives of truth, science and progress that epitomized modernity"[5(p98)]—a time of paradigms lost. Instead, there is focus on understanding multiple meanings, with the belief that every representation conceals and reveals meanings and that an inextricable link exists between meaning and power.[6] Whereas modernists fragmented the whole to study parts in the attempt to ultimately unify knowledge about the world, postmodernists fragment and dissolve unities, universals, and metanarratives believed to be entangled with values and beliefs that oppress people and fabricate reality. In postmodern thought, problems are not "solved," they are "deconstructed."

Postmodernists generally deny the existence of an essence of human beings, and they have incited ardent debate on the relevance of philosophy for science, given that a central purpose of philosophy is to examine questions about the intrinsic nature of human beings and the world, truth, and knowledge.[7] In postmodern thought, then, there is no autonomous subject to study; the subject is myth. What is studied is what the culture has inscribed on the object of study; in this sense, the focus of study is text. Meaning derives from the relationship between the text and the reader, and the content is not related to an external narrative. There is no transcendent referent for the knowledge builder and no source of meaning about human beings to be discovered and re-presented to others. So, in a phrase, the gods have fled. Any truths that appear to exist have come about not through historical teleologic progress, but as a product of time and chance, contingent on someone re-describing nature in a way that is temporarily useful to the current culture and context.[8,9] Thus, there is an epistemologic shift from concern over the truth of one's findings to concern over the practical significance of the findings.

Framework for Knowledge Development

Postmodernism's iconoclastic and pluralistic attitudes are dislodging nursing from cherished norms about knowledge development that tended to dichotomize essential units of inquiry: research and practice, inductive and deductive reasoning, qualitative and quantitative data. Twenty-first century approaches to developing knowledge will transcend these dichotomies.

Nursing's knowledge development activities have not been daunted by the shifts in philosophic thought, but instead are evolving out of both modernist and postmodernist influences. Nursing is embracing a broadened definition of scholarship that employs various key sources for development of nursing knowledge. These sources derive from the empirical, conceptual, and practice activities of nurses.[10-12] However, consistent with modern science, these domains have been regarded as independent throughout most of 20th-century nursing.

Science, philosophy, and practice have typically represented "orthogonal subspaces" of a discipline; each domain exists in its own dimension and has no image or projection in the plane of the other.[13] The schisms between these subspaces are a problem inherent in knowledge development. Yet despite the orthogonality and despite even the dominance of the scientific over the spiritual or philosophic modes of thought, none has been eliminated. It is as though each subspace represents some irreducible or essential basis of knowledge development. However, the independence between the domains, as enforced by modernists, proved to be an unsatisfactory approach to inquiry.

What instead may be needed for 21st-century nursing theory development is what Polis[13] labeled an "open philosophy," which deliberately links phenomenon with noumenon and links empirical concepts that can be known through the senses with theoretical concepts of meaning and value that can be known through thought. The postmodern critique of modernism compels nursing to revisit the potential "openness" or linkages between scientific inquiry and the metanarratives of nursing philosophy and nursing practice as a means of both reforming and reaffirming nursing's approaches to knowledge development.

Nursing Science: Modern and Postmodern Influences

A nursing scientist uses valid and reliable systems of inquiry to gain understanding of phenomena of human health and healing processes. The scientist links empirical findings to a conceptual level to create a theoretical story that satisfies certain epistemic criteria, such as predictive accuracy and internal coherence.[14] Nursing science's approach to linking the empirical and theoretical has changed over the history of its science.

Traditional empiricists, of which Nightingale was one, restricted their theorizing to observable processes. Nineteenth-century nursing theorizing did not include much movement up the ladder of abstraction to link empirical and theoretical. Rather than generalizing by abstraction (vertical movement), Nightingale tended to generalize by analogy (horizontal movement). For example, Nightingale's canon about the unhealthful effects of noise on sick people derived from drawing analogies across her observations of disturbing noises, such as rustling dresses, whispered conversations, musical wind instruments, and styles of speaking and reading to patients.[15] Nightingale's theorizing generated empirical generalizations. However, knowledge development by analogy left a gap between the empirical event and theoretical explanation; although this form of knowledge had some predictive power and was used to guide the practitioners of Nightingale's era, it had limited explanatory power.

Prior to and during the half-century hiatus in nursing scientific work between Nightingale and Peplau, a shift in axiology occurred in the scientific community that altered approaches to knowledge development. The shift was precipitated by scientists' growing need to theorize about entities too slow, too small, or otherwise unobservable but inferable from the empirical world, such as gravity or electromagnetism. Hypothetico-deductive logic emerged, whereby vertical links were made between the theoretical and empirical. In this modernist period of science, theory and research were linked through idealized systems of inquiry designed to keep research untainted of values and everyday life and independent of the religious and philosophic roots that once dominated knowledge development.

Peplau's[16] seminal work helped transform nursing from a "science of doing" to a "science of knowing" by reestablishing creative links between theory and research. Her mid-20th century theorizing employed deductive and inductive reasoning, moving up and down the ladder of abstraction to construct nursing knowledge, and produced a nursing practice theory on interpersonal relations.

Today, knowledge is regarded as process and product, as an open system rather than as a fixed set of propositions with truth flowing in top-down fashion, according to Aristotle's ideal of axiomatization.[7] Nursing scientists today are beginning to embrace all three forms of Peirce's[17] system of reasoning—abduction, deduction, and induction—without fragmenting the process. In *abduction* (a term coined by Peirce and similar to retroductive reasoning), the scientist makes a conceptual leap from experience, beliefs, and a preknowledge of patterns to arrive at an educated guess or theory about a phenomenon; the nursing scholar draws from clinical, conceptual, and empirical knowledge to do this. Through *deduction,* the scientist derives empirical events that may occur, given the theory. This deduction is put forth in the form of a hypothesis, research question, grand tour question, or other statement for inquiry. *Induction,* then, refers to the process of subjecting the theoretical ideas to empirical testing. All three forms of reasoning play important roles in knowledge development. Yet postmodernism has introduced some twists to this reasoning process that are relevant to clarifying contemporary approaches to development of nursing knowledge.

First, postmodern thought has sensitized scientists to the primacy of abductive reasoning. Abduction initiates the reasoning processes[18] and, by definition, introduces values and preunderstandings into science. No data can be free of values and biases.

Second, "empirical testing" is acquiring a broadened definition, whereby the postmodern "empirical" extends beyond the meaning of modernist empiricism.

Empirical testing may interface with the practice realm to an extent greater than modernists could tolerate. The "test" of a theory, for example, is not demonstrated primarily (or at all, according to postmodern purists) by correspondence of the empirical with the theoretical but more by the correspondence between the practical and theoretical. The merit of a theory is found in its practical implications and usefulness in solving problems of the discipline.[19,20] Empirical includes the practical.

Third, what qualifies as empirical data has gone beyond empiricism. According to emerging nursing epistemology, acceptable data vary in observability. They include biologic indicators and self-reports, investigator perceptions and informant projections, motor behavior, and personal stories. The modernist distinction between qualitative and quantitative data is blurred for, as is implicit in abduction, no data, whether verbal or numeric symbols, are independent of theory.

Last, scientific work is broader than empirical work. Empirical and nonempirical (or conceptual) knowledge is not hierarchically ordered. Postmodern awareness of the intersubjectivity of knowledge invalidates such ordering and opens the door for valuing contributions to knowledge that are not empirically verifiable in the modernist sense. Nonempirical activities enhance scientific understanding by exposing new and unexpected ideas about a theory or clinical situation in the form of "conceptual innovations."[21] For example, the conceptual innovation from Freudian theory of the "unconscious" revolutionized science and practice of mental health disciplines. Newman's[22] "pattern recognition" and Orem's[23] "self-care" are other conceptual innovations that have attained significance through their meaning in practice as well as their inspiration for theory development.

In the absence of metanarratives about a transcendent truth, postmodernism has further blurred the distinction between the nonempirical and empirical, theory and fact. Theory is regarded as a "forestructure of what form of truth the data will take; theory has priority over what are taken to be facts."[19(p413)] Theory, then, does not represent truth, it creates truth. What Britt[24] stated in reference to the artist and his or her art also applies to the postmodern scientist: Modernists contemplated the meaning of the world and their place in it; postmodernists remake the world as their science demands it.

The Critical Stance: A Call to Armchairs

Given postmodernist influences on the process of knowledge development, the significance of the social critical perspective for science becomes apparent. Data alone do not yield up the theory any more than brushes and paint will produce a painting. Whether qualitative or quantitative, data reside in the researcher's theoretical context. This fact is not a caveat of knowledge development. It is the nature of science, for "when theory does not play a selective role in research, data-gathering activities belong to the realm of journalism."[21(p794)]

Given the subjective and personalized context of theorizing, a critical stance in inquiry helps the scientist develop knowledge that potentially will be more meaningful and useful. More bluntly, some believe that the postmodern critique is a way of salvaging the empiricist tradition.[19,25] The critique serves to keep check on inherent biases and constraints—introduced by the researcher and research focus, the method, theoretical interpretation, and so on—that are not in the best interest of the subject and may oppress or constrain human potential in some way. Neither intuition and empathy nor scientific expertise and statistical significance are enough to reveal the full meaning of the data. A "call to armchairs"[26] is needed, whereby time is sanctioned for reflection and critique to examine one's assumptions and interpretations through discussion, debate, argument, and compromise with colleagues and participants—all who are affected by the knowledge developed.

Whether science is done using modernist methods, empiric-analytic or historist-hermeneutic, science is incomplete without a critical approach to one's work. Thus, the framework proposed in this article endorses a view put forth by Habermas[27] and other contemporary philosophers[1] that does not advocate the overthrow of modernism, but rather the modification of modernism by integrating the critique and communicative model of reasoning into empirical inquiry. But critique alone is not enough.

Beyond the Critique: A Neomodernist View

The neomodernist framework proposed here extends beyond the critique. The postmodern critique, with its methods of reflexivity and analysis to examine the process and products of the scientist, is not sufficient for knowledge development. Because the one who critiques is part of the culture being critiqued, complicity exists, as critics of postmodernism have explained.[1,28] And the critique cannot serve as its own external corrective; it describes a process but does not provide substance. Thus, it is suggested here that the nursing scientist's critique process be linked to a substantive overarching "ideal" or metanarrative. The metanarrative provides a base for examining knowledge as related to the context of a given discipline.[1] It functions as a "narrative foil"[28] against which scientists critique their work to form and reform knowledge.

Nursing knowledge development need not abandon completely modernist views about high theory or universal ideas. Rather than capitulate entirely to postmodernism, nurses can knowingly involve in their science the realm of perspectives and values, initially put forth by modernist nurses, that distinguish nursing knowledge and the caring application of that knowledge. In adopting a neomodernist view, nursing scientists would draw from the metanarratives of nursing for their critique. Metanarratives of nursing are found in nursing philosophy and nursing practice, as these two domains interface with nursing science in the development of knowledge.

Nursing Philosophy: Metanarratives for Knowledge Development

Philosophy, by definition, goes beyond analysis and critique by assigning values to human experiences.[29] In so doing, philosophy is a source for explicating the metanarratives of a discipline. Nursing philosophy is a statement of foundational and universal assumptions, be-

liefs, and principles about the nature of knowledge and truth (epistemology) and about the nature of the entities represented in the metaparadigm (ie, nursing practice and human healing processes [ontology]). A variety of philosophic schemes have been identified for understanding the nature of nursing phenomena.

One major scheme derives from philosopher Stephen Pepper's[30] widely recognized 1942 work in which he explicated what he conceived were the major bases of truth about the world. Three of his six worldviews, particularly as modified slightly by Lerner[31] and other developmental psychologists, predominantly have been used by scientists, including nursing scientists,[32] to frame philosophic assumptions of their discipline. Pepper's work predates philosophic schemes identified in nursing, and it likely provided a basis for conceptualizing the nursing worldviews and paradigms.[32-35] These extant nursing schemes, along with Pepper's original worldviews, are useful in organizing basic assumptions about nursing phenomena and in deriving a nursing metanarrative from philosophy for knowledge development. The three predominant worldviews are the mechanistic, organismic, and developmental–contextual, the latter previously labeled the "contextual–dialectic" worldview.[36]

Within the *mechanistic* worldview, the metaphor for human beings is the machine, composed of parts that can be measured, controlled, predicted, and added together to understand the whole. The whole is equal to the sum of the parts. Human beings are viewed as inherently at rest. Stability is assumed. Any change that occurs results from external forces and is deterministic and reversible, not developmental. The goal of change is to return to a state of equilibrium and balance. The individual's relationship with the environment is reactive. The unit of study is the part, devoid of context.

Within the *organismic* worldview, the metaphor for human beings is the biologic organism, composed of a complexity of interrelated parts. The parts are understood from the perspective of the whole, and the whole is represented in terms of the biologic organism itself. The environment assumes a more passive role, with the organism viewed as active on the environment.

There is interactionism, primarily in the sense that the parts within the person interact and contribute to qualitative, developmental changes. Change is probabilistic and directed toward an end goal.

Within the *developmental–contextual* worldview, the metaphor for human beings is the historic event; that is, the individual is embedded in a context that is dynamic. Change, in both the human being and the environment, is ongoing and irreversible, innovative and developmental. Change occurs not as a result of the person's reaction to or action on the environment, but through a dialectic and interactive relationship with the environment. Change occurs in accord with Werner's[37] "orthogenetic principle" by which living systems develop through patterns of increasing complexity accompanied by increasing organization. Chaos and conflict can provide energy for progressive change. There is no one ideal goal for development that lasts a lifetime; each developmental phase (however defined) is qualitatively different and possesses its own ideals. The whole or basic unit of study is any living structure that manifests developmental patterns of change. Study of the person necessarily involves study of contextual factors.

Various philosophic systems have been put forth by nursing scholars, such as Hall's[33] change and persistence worldviews; Parse's[35] totality and simultaneity paradigms; Newman's[34] particulate–deterministic, inter-active–integrative, and unitary–transformative worldviews; and Fawcett's[32] reaction, reciprocal interaction, and simultaneous action worldviews. These schemes reflect Pepper's[30] different depictions of reality and also extend his ideas by constructing worldviews that speak more directly to nursing and its phenomena of concern.

Some nursing scientists have appropriated worldviews from other disciplines, such as medicine and psychology. Medicine has advanced through three paradigms, namely the biomedical, biopsychosocial, and most recently the psychoneuroimmunologic paradigm.[38] Psychology's models of research and practice have evolved across behavioristic, psychodynamic, humanistic, and transpersonal schools of thought.[28,39]

The status quo in nursing seems to be that knowledge developers embrace the diversity of worldviews in critiquing knowledge and clarifying basic beliefs and assumptions about what are relevant and plausible issues of research and practice.[40] While this "plethora of paradigms"[41] available to nurses may be viewed in a positive way, it also may contribute to the potential for fragmentation within the discipline. This concern has been debated.[40,42] In the spirit of postmodernism, nurses must question the status quo and continue to debate the logic of diversity in worldviews underlying nursing knowledge development. From a neomodernist perspective, this kind of diversity may not be entirely desirable.

Diversity or Fragmentation?

Diversity at the level of the worldview may inhibit clarification of a nursing philosophy[43] and nursing metanarrative for research and critique. The worldviews within each philosophic scheme define and interrelate the nursing metaparadigm concepts in radically different ways. Sanctioning all available worldviews for nursing in one sense reflects the postmodernist retreat from conceptualizing the whole and identifying unifying ideals. In attempting to achieve unity by preserving disparate worldviews, as some advocate,[40] nursing may be sacrificing coherence for diversity.

Does the diversity offer important distinctions in worldviews, each of which has a rightful role in guiding inquiry and critique within a discipline? Or might the diversity in philosophic schemes represent progress in knowledge about the nature of the world, such that some provide for fuller understanding than others? The former position seems less likely. Diversity does not mean that all points of view are equally valid and acceptable for a given context or discipline.[43] Moreover, preserving differences through compromise or coexistence rather than striving to resolve differences in ontology, values, and goals—a purpose of philosophy[44]—blocks dialogue and opportunities to further develop knowledge. Opposing beliefs about the nature of human health and nursing goals can perpetuate even more differences in nursing's epistemic and ethical claims and research funding priorities, "bringing about more confusion in our discipline rather than creating a sense of coherence necessary for its development."[45(p26)]

In addition to the question of the merits of diversity in worldviews for the discipline's progress, there is the more urgent question as to whether entertaining disparate worldviews best serves patients' well-being. Diplomacy and discourse aside, when choices available are between a mechanistic and developmental worldview, or between a paradigm in which the nurse and not the patient possesses the knowledge and authority and a paradigm in which patients are knowledgeable and knowing participants in their own healing process, is not one paradigm more emancipating (for patient and nurse) and more re-presentative of the nature of nursing than the other? The commitment for unity in diversity[42] may not be status quo but may be most appropriate in a postmodern world that tends to fragment focuses of inquiry, human beings, and their world.

To that end, then, the metanarrative of human developmental potential, transformational and self-transcendent capacity for health and healing, and recognition of the developmental histories of persons and their contexts is offered here as an external corrective of choice. It is a metanarrative originating in Lerner's[31] developmental–contextual worldview and congruent with the philosophic ideas expressed in Newman's[34] unitary–transformative paradigm and Parse's[35] simultaneity paradigm.

Given the alternatives, this metanarrative may be the best commitment to be made by the scientist and practitioner, at least at this point in the development of nursing knowledge. In proposing this metanarrative, however, one must acknowledge that inherent in this neomodernist framework is the realization that even metanarratives are temporary and "for the moment."[46] Although metanarratives by definition are more stable than lower levels of theory, their depictions of truth and reality are not fixed and must be open to developmental change themselves, subject in part to influences from the dynamic science and practice dimensions of nursing.

Nursing Practice: A Metanarrative for Knowledge Development

As if anticipating postmodernist values for the reality found in the culture and context of everyday life experiences, nurses have renewed focus on practice as connected to science. Nursing practice is regarded not only as a place of applying knowledge, but also as a place to generate and test ideas for developing knowledge. Early on, Peplau[47] identified practice as the context in which scientific knowledge was transformed into nursing knowledge. Linkages between science and practice help nursing move beyond grand theorizing and operationalize the metanarrative of "responsible participation and consideration of culture and context"[48(pviii)] and the emancipatory potential of nursing knowledge.

From a revisionist perspective of the early nursing theorists such as Peplau[47] and Paterson and Zderad,[49] it can be seen that nursing began moving beyond the reductionist and mechanistic approaches of modernism even before nursing recognition of postpositivism. As a result, nursing practice gave to nursing research a metanarrative that was patient oriented, context sensitive, pattern focused, and participatory. In her practice theory of interpersonal relations, for example, Peplau[47] incorporated practice and theory into her ideas of research. Resembling the hermeneutic circle, Peplau's research process began in practice, spiraled up, drawing in theories—or as she stated, "peeling out theories"—to explain the phenomenon, then returned to practice to examine the new knowledge in light of the experiences and reality of practice.

Paterson and Zderad[49] described a method of "nursology" as the study of nursing practice. They outlined five phases of phenomenologic nursology in which the practitioner role informed the research process: (1) preparing oneself to be an open window, (2) intuiting the rhythm of the other, (3) knowing the other scientifically, (4) synthesizing differences and similarities, and (5) arriving at a conception of the situation that has some universal meaning across many nursing practice situations.

More recently, Newman[50] described research as praxis, meaning an approach to research that takes the form of nursing practice in the researcher's relationship to the participant and in the enactment of values for human transformation through pattern recognition. Similarly, Parse[51] put forth a research methodology based on her "theory of human becoming." One essential step in the research process is "dialogical engagement," which involves establishing a therapeutic presence between researcher and participant.

These and other theorists' models of nursing depict ways in which doing science itself can be linked to the ideals and meta-narratives of practice. Guidelines for evaluating the emancipatory potential of the research process and product have been detailed.[52] Nursing practice frameworks are evolving scientific methods that are tailored not only to elicit desired data while protecting research participants' rights, but also to be therapeutic.

The Esthetic Order and Nursing Practice

Postmodernism has stimulated greater awareness among nurses of the culture of practice as a source of ultimate meaning about the object of that practice, human beings' health and healing. Concomitantly, there has been increased interest in research on nursing care processes ranging from nursing care systems to nursing caring behaviors, intuition, nursing presence, and the nurse-patient relationship. Rather than characterize this focus as a return to the mid-20th century focus of research on nurses, it may be more accurately viewed as a focus of inquiry influenced in part by the postmodern emphasis on context. In postmodernism, the ultimate locus of meaning is the culture or context of the object of inquiry.[2] Professional practice is a nursing context. And nursing practice increasingly is being viewed as a legitimate source of knowledge, in part because it is regarded as an esthetic order of nursing, imbued with meaning and beauty.[53]

Amidst the postmodern emphasis on culture and context as something external to the person, nursing must not lose sight of the other context of healing—the patient. The postmodern notion of context must be broadened in nursing to include, if not to emphasize, the patient as a context of health and healing. Human beings' inner healing nature cannot be dismissed, as postmodernists might have it.[38] Patient as environment was first conceptualized by several nurse theorists (eg, Levine,[54] Orem,[23] Paterson and Zderad,[49] and Neuman[55]) who wrote about the "internal environment" of the person as an inner reality and innate resource for health and development. The significance of an inner healing environment is supported by current worldviews about inner human potential and transformative capacity.[28,30,34,35] A basic assumption of Nightingale was that the natural source of healing resided in the patient.[15] And Rogers[56] wrote emphatically about the coexistence of person and environment, regarding the two as one "person–environment mutual process."

Thus, it is proposed that the esthetic in nursing practice refers not only to the meaningful and beautiful experienced through nursing practice by the nurse, but also, and perhaps more appropriately, to that experienced through nursing practice by the patient. As Kim stated in describing one perspective of esthetics, "Certain aspects of nursing practice may be considered 'art' insofar as they communicate aesthetic ideas to perceivers, especially *clients.*"[57(p281)]

This perspective on the esthetics of nursing practice is contrary to the more commonly held view of the esthetic experience residing primarily in the nurse.[56] However, esthetic experience is not found primarily in the type of brushes the painter uses, or the way a musician holds an instrument, or the style of the conductor or poet. Rather, the esthetic is the beauty that is experienced in seeing the painting, hearing the music, and in reading or reciting the poem. Analogously, in nursing, the esthetic is not primarily that experienced by the practitioner; the esthetic is found in the beauty and meaning associated with the patient's experiences of health and healing—the phenomena of concern to nursing. The esthetic is what is desired, meaningful, beautiful—whether it is experienced through the art of a painter, a musician, or a nurse. Given the esthetic order underlying the nurse's art, then, nursing practice is recognized as possessing powerful metanarratives about health and the processes of healing.

Nursing Conceptual Models: Archetypes of Nursing Practice

The nursing conceptual models are a mechanism of translating the metanarrative of nursing practice for knowledge development. Nursing conceptual models broadly refer to extant conceptual and theoretical systems that describe the nature of nursing practice, patients as human beings, and health. Nursing conceptual models, their biases and preunderstandings notwithstanding,[58] "articulate disciplinary perspectives and underlying philosophical assumptions."[46(p56)] In the modernist era, these models were regarded as ideas to be revered, preserved, unaltered, and used in their entirety. More recently, Whall[59] noted, some are disparaging the conceptual models, reasoning that nursing has matured beyond needing the conceptual models for knowledge development and practice. This reasoning is specious. All levels of theory are needed in generating knowledge for theory-based practice.

The disregard for extant conceptual and theoretical models of nursing may be influenced in part by postmodernists' disinterest in grappling with the wholes that grand-level theories address. In their retreat from dealing with the complexity of a phenomenon, postmodernists fragment objects of inquiry by breaking them into smaller pieces and denying the need to conceptualize the whole.[1] However, from the neomodernist stance proposed in this article, unified conceptualizations of nursing and nursing practice are valued. Nursing conceptual models are more than a modernist artifact; they are archetypes of nursing practice.

Further, these archetypes are dynamic, unlike the archetypes of modernist science. Like the reality they depict, the practice and research contexts in which they are used, the theories they inspire, and the metaparadigm they represent, nursing conceptual models must be allowed to be open and alterable. As systems of knowledge, they must evolve, lest they move from being extant to becoming extinct. Other conceptual models will likely emerge out of the vestiges of earlier models and the new insights of creative nursing scientists, philosophers, and practitioners who grapple with the whole.

Nursing: A Postcritical Discipline

The neomodernist perspectives on knowledge development presented here build on modernist and postmodern ideas. Characteristic assumptions of postmodernism that all methods and sources of knowledge development are value laden and that the process of constructing and perceiving reality is a dynamic, relational endeavor undergird the framework. It is also recognized that knowledge development is more than science, science more than the empirical, and the empirical more than empiricism. Philosophic and practice dimensions in nursing generate open metanarratives for scientific inquiry that serve as external correctives to the critique of knowledge development. Postmodernism alone can never be a critical theory. As first proposed by Plato, critique of the particulars requires grounding in the universals. Metanarratives provide this grounding and are essential in intellectual pursuits.[2]

Postmodernists have challenged the metanarratives, referring to them as "totalizing discourses" that are fabrications and not representations of reality.[38] Other scholars have explained that science cannot exist in the absence of metanarratives, and they repudiate the notion that there are no legitimated metanarratives.[1,3,5] Language is not so slippery nor meanings so unstable that underlying patterns of individuals and groups cannot be identified. In failing to identify meaningful patterns in the ongoing change of person and environment, science becomes merely history. Thus, nursing, proposed here as a neomodernist science, has identified discourses of nursing philosophy and practice that converge on themes of healing environments, inner human potential, and the developmental–contextual nature of health.

The neomodernist framework proposed here also departs from postmodernism in that the object of inquiry—human processes of health and healing—is regarded as more than a "text" to be deconstructed or disentangled of the discourses that authority figures have inscribed on it.[38] Human beings are more than bodies inscribed by their context. There is text, or meaning, beyond the text that informs and stimulates scientific inquiry. The neomodernist retains a belief in an underlying esthetic order in nursing. This order is revealed through nursing practice processes that enhance healing and development.

Nursing can never return to a pre-postmodern era to regain lost and lofty assumptions about knowledge development and nursing. But nursing still possesses the innovativeness and imagination to continue progressing in the metanarrative Nightingale originally established—empowerment of human beings' natural potential for health and healing.

Nursing, by nature, is a postcritical discipline: Self-reflection, personal autonomy, innate developmental potential, connections between truth and life, emancipatory practice and research, and chaos as opportunity are all valued. These are values and conceptual orientations that distinguish the discipline from others.

Yet within this shared focus, there is a diversity in approaches to knowledge development. As a feminist philosopher recently implied, totality does not have to mean totalitarianism; unity does not mean uniformity.[1] A postcritical discipline values challenges to the status quo and critiques and exposes oppressive discourses. And a post-critical discipline is not timid in committing to an overarching discourse that enables and liberates patients and other persons.

Nursing is a metanarrative that shapes the broader scientific community's understanding of human beings. It is a metanarrative needed in health care reform. And, like all discourse, it warrants ongoing critique. A neomodernist perspective of knowledge development provides for this critique while also fostering the grounding and vision to continue scientific inquiry. An open philosophy that exercises connections between science, philosophy, and practice will help ensure that nursing's metanarratives do not become closed ideologic systems, and it will help ensure that the dialogue on knowledge development continues into the 21st century.

REFERENCES

1. Waugh P. *Postmodernism.* New York, NY: Routledge, Chapman and Hall; 1992.
2. Popper KR. *Conjectures and Refutations: The Growth of Scientific Knowledge.* New York, NY: Harper & Row; 1963.
3. Doherty J, Graham E, Malek M, eds. *Postmodernism and the Social Sciences.* New York, NY: Macmillan; 1992.
4. Lyotard J. *The Postmodern Condition: A Report on Knowledge.* Minneapolis, Minn: University of Minnesota Press; 1979.
5. Burman E. Developmental psychology and the postmodern child. In: Doherty J, Graham E, Malek M, eds. *Postmodernism and the Social Sciences.* New York, NY: Macmillan; 1992.
6. Foucault M. *The Order of Things.* London, England: Tavistock; 1974.
7. Philipse H. Towards a postmodern conception of metaphysics: on the genealogy and successor disciplines of modern philosophy. *Metaphilosophy.* 1994;25:1–44.
8. Rorty R. *Philosophy and the Mirror of Nature.* Oxford, England: Blackwell; 1980.
9. Rorty R. *Contingency, Irony and Solidarity.* Cambridge, NY: Cambridge University Press; 1989.
10. Carper BA. Fundamental patterns of knowing in nursing. *ANS.* 1978;1(1):13–24.
11. Chinn PL, Kramer MK, *Theory and Nursing: A Systematic Approach.* 3rd ed. St. Louis, Mo: Mosby; 1991.
12. Schultz PR, Meleis AI. Nursing epistemology: traditions, insights, questions. *Image J Nurs Schol.* 1989;20:217–221.
13. Polis DF. Paradigms for an open philosophy. *Metaphilosophy.* 1993;24:33–46.
14. Howard GS. Culture tales: a narrative approach to thinking. *Cross-Cultural Psychol Psychother.* 1991;46:187–197.
15. Nightingale F. *Notes on Nursing: What It Is, and What It Is Not.* New York, NY: Dover; 1969.
16. Peplau HE. The art and science of nursing: similarities, differences, and relations. *Nurs Sci Q,* 1988;1:8–15.
17. Peirce CS: Hartshorne C, Weiss P, eds. *Charles Sanders Peirce: Collected Papers.* Cambridge, Mass: Harvard University Press; 1934:5.
18. Staat W. On abduction, deduction, induction and the categories. *Transactions Charles S Peirce Soc.* 1993;29:225–237.
19. Gergen KJ. Exploring the postmodern: perils or potentials? *Am Psychol,* 1994;49:412–417.
20. Laudan L. *Progress and Its Problems: Toward a Theory of Scientific Growth.* Berkeley, Calif: University of California Press; 1977.
21. Kukla A. Nonempirical issues in psychology. *Am Psychol.* 1989;44:785–794.
22. Newman M. *Health as Expanding Consciousness.* 2nd ed. New York, NY: National League for Nursing; 1993.
23. Orem DE. *Nursing: Concepts of Practice,* 4th ed. St. Louis, Mo: Mosby; 1991.
24. Britt D, ed. *Modern Art: Impressionism to Post-Modernism.* Boston, Mass: Little, Brown: 1989.
25. Allen DG. Using philosophical and historical methodologies to understand the concept of health. In: Chinn PL, ed. *Nursing Research Methodology.* Rockville, Md: Aspen Publishers; 1986.
26. Omer H. London P. Metamorphosis in psychotherapy; end of the systems era. *Psychotherapy.* 1988;25:171–180.
27. Habermas J. Lawrence FG, trans. *The Philosophical Discourses of Modernity.* Oxford, England: Polity; 1987.
28. Wilber K. *A Sociable God.* New York, NY: McGraw-Hill; 1983.

29. Sahakian WS. *History of Philosophy.* New York, NY: Barnes & Noble; 1968.
30. Pepper SP. *World Hypotheses: A Study in Evidence.* Berkeley, Calif: University of California Press; 1942.
31. Lerner RM. *Concepts and Theories of Human Development.* 2nd ed. New York, NY: Random House; 1986.
32. Fawcett J. *Analysis and Evaluation of Nursing Theories.* Philadelphia, Pa: F. A. Davis; 1993.
33. Hall BA. The change paradigm in nursing: growth versus persistence. *ANS.* 1981;3(4):1–6.
34. Newman MA. Prevailing paradigms in nursing. *Nurs Outlook.* 1992;40:10–13.
35. Parse RR. *Nursing Science: Major Paradigms. Theories, and Critiques.* Philadelphia, Pa: W. B. Saunders; 1987.
36. Reed PG. Toward a nursing theory of self-transcendence: deductive reformulation using developmental theories. *ANS.* 1991;13:64–77.
37. Werner H. The concept of development from a comparative and organismic point of view. In: Harris DB, ed. *The Concept of Development.* Minneapolis, Minn: University of Minnesota Press; 1957.
38. Fox NJ. *Postmodernism, Sociology, and Health.* Toronto, Canada: University of Toronto Press; 1994.
39. Lundin RW. *Theories and Systems of Psychology,* 2nd ed. Lexington, Mass: Heath; 1979.
40. Barrett EAM. Response: disciplinary perspective: unified or diverse? Diversity reigns. *Nurs Sci Q.* 1992;5:155–157.
41. Fawcett J. From a plethora of paradigms to parsimony in world views. *Nurs Sci Q.* 1993;6:56–58.
42. Northrup DT. Commentary: disciplinary perspective: unified or diverse? A unified perspective within nursing. *Nurs Sci Q.* 1992;5:154–156.
43. Kikuchi JF, Simmons H, eds. *Developing a Philosophy of Nursing.* Thousand Oaks, Calif: Sage; 1994.
44. Moccia P. A critique of compromise: beyond the methods debate. *ANS.* 1988;10(4):1–9.
45. Laurin J. A philosophy of nursing: commentary. In: Kikuchi JF, Simmons H, eds. *Developing a Philosophy of Nursing.* Thousands Oaks, Calif: Sage; 1994.
46. Smith MC. Arriving at a philosophy of nursing: discovering? constructing? evolving? In: Kikuchi JF, Simmons H, eds. *Developing a Philosophy of Nursing.* Thousand Oaks, Calif: Sage; 1994.
47. Peplau HE. Interpersonal relations: a theoretical framework for application in nursing practice. *Nurs Sci Q.* 1992;5(1):13–18.
48. Chinn PL. A window of opportunity. *ANS.* 1994;16(4):viii.
49. Paterson JG, Zderad LT. *Humanistic Nursing.* New York, NY: Wiley; 1976.
50. Newman MA. Newman's theory of health as praxis. *Nurs Sci Q.* 1990;3:37–41.
51. Parse RR. Parse's research methodology with an illustration of the lived experience of hope. *Nurs Sci Q.* 1990;3:9–17.
52. DeMarco R, Campbell J, Wuest J. Feminist critique: searching for meaning in research. *ANS.* 1993;16(2):26–38.
53. Katims I. Nursing as aesthetic experience and the notion of practice. *Schol Inq Nurs Pract.* 1993;7:269–278.
54. Levine M. *Introduction to Clinical Nursing,* 2nd ed. Los Angeles, Calif: F. A. Davis; 1973.
55. Neuman B. *The Neuman Systems Model.* 3rd ed. Norwalk, Conn: Appleton-Lange; 1994.
56. Rogers ME. Nursing: a science of unitary man. In: Riehl JP, Roy C, eds. *Conceptual Models for Nursing Practice.* 2nd ed. New York, NY: Appleton-Century-Crofts; 1980.
57. Kim HS. Response to "Nursing as Aesthetic Experience and the Notion of Practice." *Schol Inq Nurs Pract.* 1993;7:279–282.
58. Thompson JL. Practical discourse in nursing: going beyond empiricism and historicism. *ANS.* 1985;7(4):59–71.
59. Whall AL. Let's get rid of all that theory. *Nurs Sci Q.* 1993;6:164–165.

The Author Comments

A Treatise on Nursing Knowledge Development for the 21st Century: Beyond Postmodernism

I wrote this article to articulate a philosophic position for reforming nursing's approach to knowledge development. I integrated the best of modernist and postmodernist thinking, without succumbing to the narrow view of reality that each alone conveys. The approach acknowledges the wealth of knowledge found in our canon of conceptual models and, at the same time, requires a critical perspective of any nursing metanarratives. I tried to extend the traditional views about science, nursing practice, and conceptual models in proposing a "neomodernist" stance for knowledge development. The "open philosophy" proposed in the article will hopefully encourage students to be innovative in thinking about how knowledge is developed in their discipline.

——PAMELA G. REED

CHAPTER 57

Nursing Science and the Space Age

Martha E. Rogers

This article presents the basic elements of Rogers' science of unitary human beings. It defines science, explicates nursing as a science and an art, addresses the meaning of the principles of homeodynamics, and discusses the building blocks of these principles. Several theories arising from the science of unitary human beings are elaborated, and noninvasive therapeutic modalities are discussed as part of nursing practice.

Key words: Nursing Science, Rogers' Framework

Humankind is on the threshold of a new cosmology transcending an earthbound past. In less than a decade the 21st century will arrive, accompanied by many manifestations of accelerating change. Futurists prophecy multiple scenarios, often in conflict with one another. Genetic engineering engenders a mechanistic explanation of life and spawns ethical issues that far exceed Huxley's (1932) *Brave New World*. Economics, education, health, world affairs, lifestyles, as well as robots, computers, environment, and space travel are just a few of the areas undergoing scrutiny. Interplanetary and intergalactic communication with intelligent life beyond the present purview portends new meanings for citizenship in a space-encompassing world society. These new worldviews also take into account the extraterrestrial.

Nursing Science Quarterly, 5(1), 27–34.

About the Author

MARTHA E. ROGERS was born on May 12, 1914, in Dallas, TX. She received her nursing diploma in 1936; a BS in Public Health from George Peabody College in Nashville, TN; an MA in Public Health Nursing Supervision (1945) from Teacher's College, Columbia University, NY; and an MPH (1952) and an ScD (1954) from Johns Hopkins University in Baltimore, MD. Rogers' early nursing practice was in public health nursing in Michigan, and later she established the Visiting Nursing Service in Phoenix, AZ. Dr. Rogers was Professor and Head of the Division of Nursing at New York University for more than 20 years. She was adamant that nursing be recognized as a science with a unique body of knowledge. Dr. Rogers' revolutionary ideas, as expressed in her *Science of Unitary Human Beings* and other writings, have inspired nurses throughout the world. In 1979, Dr. Rogers became Professor Emerita of Nursing at New York University. She was an active member of the nursing community until her death on March 13, 1994. Her vision for nursing continues to play a major role in the evolution of the discipline.

The science of unitary human beings encompasses this human advent into outer space. Today's astronauts are envoys to the human space-directed future. Astronauts, the precursors of spacekind, portend an outward emigration by Homo sapiens and, what is more, their transcendence by Homo spatialis. This transcendence will be an evolutionary, not an adaptive process.

Planet earth is integral with the larger world of human reality. Thus, the space future will not consist of how to use planetary knowledge and skills in space, but an elaboration of a new worldview in which new knowledge and modalities raise new questions, provide new answers, and signify different evolutionary norms. According to Robinson and White (1986), Homo spatialis will transcend Homo sapiens in approximately two generations of space living (about 50 years). Particulate phenomena such as physiological norms are already inadequate for judging the parameters of humankind in space. Even more, the so-called pathology on earth today may signify health for the space-bound.

Homo spatialis looms on the horizon as moon villages, space towns, and Martian communities foretell a new world. Moon-mining and gravity-free manufacturing in space are anticipated within this century. Galactic grocery stores, educational centers, health services, and recreational opportunities are each inevitable inclusions in a space-bound world society.

Increasing space travel capabilities are already manifest in many countries; a new oneness attends planet earth's integration into the space world, a new synthesis in which spinoffs from space exploration mark planet earth's future.

Should all of this seem impossible, one need only recall that in February 1957, Lee DeForest, father of modern electronics, stated: "To place a man in a multistage rocket and propel him into the controlling gravitational field of the moon . . . will never occur regardless of all future scientific endeavors." He compared these proposals to the wildest dreams of Jules Verne (Friedman, 1989). DeForest made this statement just 12 years before the Apollo moon landing.

A New Worldview for Nursing

Nursing's transition from prescience to science has also accelerated, but it must become explicit if nurses are to provide knowledgeable innovative services in a spacebound world society. The explication of an organized body of abstract knowledge specific to nursing is indispensable. The need for such a body of knowledge can be identified in an escalation of science and technology coordinate with public demands for health services of a nature, and in an amount, scarcely envisioned by either the consumers or providers.

A new worldview compatible with the most progressive knowledge available (Lauden, 1977) has become a necessary prelude to studying human health and to determining modalities for its promotion both on this planet and in outer space. The science of nursing is rooted in this new worldview, a pandimensional view of people and their world.

Traditionally nursing's goals have encompassed both the sick and the well, and the consideration of environmental factors has also been integral to nursing's efforts. Education and practice in nursing have been directed toward promotion of health without interruption. The recognition of people as distinct from their parts has characterized nursing from the time of Florence Nightingale to the present.

The introduction of systems theories several decades ago set in motion new ways of perceiving people and their world. Since then, science and technology have escalated. The exploration of space has revised old views, and thus new knowledge has merged with new ways of thinking. Nothing less than a second industrial revolution has been initiated, far more dramatic in its implications and potentials than the first. The pressing need to study people in ways that would enhance their humanness has coordinated with the accelerating technological advances and forced a search for new models. A major hindrance to the evolution of viable models, however, was noted by Capra (1982) when he wrote about the difficulty encountered while trying to apply the concepts of an outdated worldview to a reality that could no longer be understood in terms of these concepts.

The science of nursing was arrived at by the creative synthesis of facts and ideas and is an emergent, a new product. These principles and theories were derived from the abstract system and were tested in the ordinary world. The findings of this research have accumulated and changed commensurate with the new knowledge. A science is open-ended. The elaboration of a science emerges out of scholarly research. Thus, the findings of research are fed back into the system, whereby the system undergoes continuous alteration, revision, and change. A science then, exists only in its entirety, it bespeaks wholeness and unity, and it provides a way of perceiving people and their environment.

The science of unitary human beings has not derived from one or more of the basic sciences. Neither has it come out of a vacuum. It flows instead in novel ways from a multiplicity of knowledge, from many sources, to create a kaleidoscope of potentialities. In turn, fundamental concepts are identified and significant terms are defined congruent with the evolving system. A humane and optimistic view of life's potentials grows as a new reality appears. Then, people's capacity to participate knowingly in the process of change is postulated.

Since nursing is a learned profession, it is both a science and an art. The uniqueness of nursing, like that of other sciences, lies in the phenomenon central to its focus. For nurses, that focus consists of a long established concern with people and the world they live in. It is the natural forerunner of an organized, abstract system encompassing people and their environments. The irreducible, indivisible nature of individuals is different from the sum of their parts. Furthermore, the integrality of people and their environments coordinates with a pandimensional universe of open systems, points to a new paradigm, and initiates the identity of nursing as a science. The purpose of nurses is to promote health and well-being for all persons wherever they are. The art of nursing, then, is the creative use of the science of nursing for human betterment.

A theoretically sound foundation that gives identity to nursing as a science and an art requires an organized abstract system from which to derive unifying principles and hypothetical generalizations. Through basic and applied research, theories are tested, new understandings emerge, and new questions arise. As a result, description and explanation take on new meanings, and a substantive body of knowledge specific to nursing takes form.

A science may be defined as an organized body of abstract knowledge arrived at by scientific research and logical analysis. This knowledge provides a means of describing and explaining the phenomena of concern. A science can also have more than one paradigm or abstract system, but the phenomena of concern remain constant. A worldview is a paradigm from which one can derive principles and theories that may guide practice. More specifically, however, nursing is postulated to be a basic science. Surely, this science does not come out of a vacuum. Neither does it derive from other basic or applied sciences, nor is it a summation of knowledge drawn from other fields. Nursing, instead, consists of its own unique irreducible mix.

Since science is open-ended and change is continuous, new knowledge brings new insights. Thus, the development of a science of unitary human beings is a never-ending process. This abstract system first presented some years ago has continued to gain substance. Concomitantly, early errors have undergone correction, definitions have been revised for greater clarity and accuracy, and updating of content is ongoing. Basic theoretical research, then, continues to be essential for the ongoing development of this field of study.

Both basic and applied research are necessary to nursing's future; basic research provides new knowledge while applied research tests the new knowledge already available. Multiple methodologies that may be used in the pursuit of the new knowledge include quantitative and qualitative methods and encompass philosophic, descriptive, and other approaches. The application of the science of unitary human beings to nursing, from a holistic worldview, also demands new tools and new methods. Moreover, it is only through research that the theoretically sound foundation can continue to evolve.

Historically the term "nursing" has been used as a verb signifying "to do," rather than as a noun meaning "to know." When nursing is identified as a science the term "nursing" becomes a noun signifying a "body of abstract knowledge." Consequently, theories deriving from a science of unitary human beings are specific to nursing, just as theories deriving from biology are specific to biological phenomena, theories deriving from sociology are specific to sociological phenomena, and theories of physics are specific to the physical world.

The study of nursing is not the study of the biological world any more than the study of biology is the study of the physical world. Further, the study of nursing is not the study of nurses and what they do any more than biology is the study of biologists and what they do. Nursing instead, is the study of unitary, irreducible, indivisible human and environmental fields: people and their world. The complexity of investigatory methodology is not a substitute for substantive content in any field. Downs notes " . . . our research efforts are replete with sophisticated methods applied to unsophisticated content" (Downs, 1988, p. 20). The education of nurses gains its identity by the transmission of nursing's body of theoretical knowledge. The practice of nurses, therefore, is the creative use of this knowledge in human service. Research methods are empty without substance to study. Thus, research in nursing specifies a body of knowledge specific to nursing, and research in other fields is not a substitute.

The uniqueness of nursing, like that of any other science, lies in the phenomenon central to its purpose; people and their worlds in a pandimensional universe are nursing's phenomena of concern. The irreducible nature of individuals as energy fields, different from the sum of their parts and integral with their respective environmental fields, differentiates nursing from other sciences and identifies nursing's focus.

Unitary human beings are specified to be irreducible wholes. A whole cannot be understood when it is reduced to its particulars. The use of the term unitary human beings is not to be confused with the current popular usage of the term holistic, generally signifying a summation of parts, whether few or many. The unitary nature of environment is equally irreducible. The concept of field provides a means of perceiving people and their respective environments as irreducible wholes.

The Science of Unitary Human Beings

The significant postulates fundamental to the science of unitary human beings include energy fields, openness, pattern, and pandimensionality. The development of a science portends the emergence of abstract concepts and a corresponding language of specificity. Scientific language evolves out of the general language. Additionally, terms specific to the system are defined for clarity, precision, and communication so that rigorous research can be pursued and replicated. Terminology, except that defined specifically to the system, is interpreted in its general language meaning (see Table 57-1).

Theory concerning a universe of open systems has been gaining support for three quarters of a century. Since the introduction of the theory of relativity, of quantum theory, and of probability, the prevailing absolutism, already shaken by evolutionary theory, has received a critical blow. By the 1920s Selye had proposed adaptation, and by the 1930s von Bertalanffy introduced the idea of negative entropy (Rogers, 1970). Soon after Cannon advanced the idea of homeostasis. Space exploration began in the 1950s, and by the 1960s some physiologists suggested replacing the term homeostasis with the term homeokinesis. As this new knowledge escalated, the traditional meanings of homeostasis, steady-state, adaptation, and equilibrium were no longer tenable. The closed-system, entropic model of the universe began to be questioned and evidence has continued to accumulate in support of a universe of open systems (see Table 57-2).

In a universe of open systems, causality is not an option. Energy fields are open, not a little bit or sometimes, but continuously. A universe of open systems explains the infinite nature of energy fields, how the human and environmental fields are integral with one another, and that causality is invalid. Change, then, is continuously innovative and creative. Moreover, association does not mean causality.

New worldviews abound. Synthesis and holism are predominant among these views. Lovelock (1988) proposed a scientific synthesis in harmony with the Greek conception of the earth as a living whole, as Gaia. Fuller (1981) has argued that earth is a spaceship, and Kenton (1990) emphasizes the fallacy of depending on well-meaning actions and good intentions while people continue to operate with a paradigm that views reality as fragmented. Holistic new worldviews are being proposed by such persons as Bohm (1980), Capra (1982), Sheldrake (Weber, Bohm, & Sheldrake, 1986), and Weber (1986). In addition, Rogers' work focuses on developing a pandimensional worldview by proposing a science of unitary, irreducible human beings that is coordinate with a worldview that includes outer space.

Within this pandimensional view, energy fields are postulated to constitute the fundamental unit of both the living and the nonliving. Field, then, is a unifying concept and energy signifies the dynamic nature of the field. Energy fields are infinite and pandimensional; they are in continuous motion. Two energy fields are identified: the human field and the environmental field. Specifically, human beings and the environment *are* energy

Table 57-1
Key Definitions Specific to the Science of Nursing

Energy Field:	The fundamental unit of the living and the non-living. Field is a unifying concept. Energy signifies the dynamic nature of the field. A field is in continuous motion and is infinite
Pattern:	The distinguishing characteristic of an energy field perceived as a single wave.
Pandimensional:*	A non-linear domain without spatial or temporal attributes.
Unitary Human Being: (Human field)	An irreducible, indivisible, pandimensional energy field identified by pattern and manifesting characteristics that are specific to the whole and which cannot be predicted from knowledge of the parts.
Environment: (Environmental field)	An irreducible, pandimensional energy field identified by pattern and integral with the human field.

*Formerly titled four-dimensional and multidimensional.
Reprinted with permission from the National League for Nursing, *Visions of Rogers' science-based nursing,* 1990, p. 9. Update 1991.

Table 57-2
Some Differences Between Older and Newer Worldviews

Older Views	Newer Views
cell theory	field theory
entropic universe	negentropic universe
three-dimensional	pandimensional
homeostasis	homeodynamics
person/environment: dichotomous	person/environment: integral
causation: single and multiple	mutual process
adaptation	mutual process
closed systems	open systems
dynamic equilibrium	innovative growing diversity
waking: basic state	waking: an evolutionary emergent
being	becoming

Initial development 1968; update 1991.

fields; they do not *have* energy fields. Moreover, human and environmental fields are not biological fields, physical fields, social fields, or psychological fields. Nor are human and environmental fields a summation of biological, physical, social, and psychological fields. This is not a denial of the importance of knowledge from other fields. Rather, it is to make clear that human and environmental fields have their own identity and are not to be confused with parts. Human and environmental fields are irreducible and indivisible. What may be quite valid in describing biological phenomena does not describe unitary human beings, any more than describing a molecule tells you about laughter.

A science of unitary human beings is equally as applicable to groups as it is to individuals. The group energy field to be considered is identified. It may be a family, a social group, or a community, a crowd or some other combination. Regardless of the group identified, the group field is irreducible and indivisible. The group field is integral with its own environmental field. The environmental field is unique to any given group field. The principles of homeodynamics postulate the nature of group field change just as they postulate the nature of individual field change. They are equally relevant for Homo sapiens, Homo spatialis, and beyond. Furthermore, these principles have validity only within the context of the science of unitary human beings,

their meaning has specificity within their definitions, and together they postulate the nature and direction of change.

Pattern is a key postulate in this system (see Table 57-3). It is defined as the distinguishing characteristic of an energy field perceived as a single wave. Pattern is an abstraction, its nature changes continuously, and it gives identity to the field. Moreover, each human field pattern is unique and is integral with its own unique environmental field pattern. In fact, the term "pattern" is used only to refer to an energy field. The characteristics of unitary human beings are specific to unitary human beings. Pattern is not directly observable. However, manifestations of field patterning are observable events in the real world. They are postulated to emerge out of the human-environment field mutual process (see Box 57-1).

Change is continuous, relative, and innovative. The increasing diversity of field patterning characterizes this process of change. Individual differences serve only to point up the significance of this relative diversity. For example, changing rhythmicities possess individual uniqueness. The transition from longer sleeping, to longer waking, to beyond waking is highly variable between individuals. Moreover, further diversity is manifested in so-called "day people" and "night people" as well as in other examples of rhythmical diversity.

Table 57-3
Principles of Homeodynamics

Principle of Resonancy:	Continuous change from lower to higher frequency wave patterns in human and environmental fields.
Principle of Helicy:	Continuous, innovative, unpredictable, increasing diversity of human and environmental field patterns.
Principle of Integrality:	Continuous mutual human field and environmental field process.

Reprinted with permission from the National League for Nursing, *Visions of Rogers' science-based nursing*, 1990, p. 8.

Field pattern has been a central idea in this system from its inception over 25 years ago. It is interesting to note that Ferguson (1980) wrote in her book *The Aquarian Conspiracy* that "synthesis and pattern seeing are survival skills of the 21st Century." Ferguson's comment is certainly apropos to the science of unitary human beings. Pattern reveals itself through its manifestations. These manifestations are continuously innovative while the evolution of life and non-life is a dynamic, irreducible, non-linear process characterized by increasing complexification of energy field patterning. The nature of change is unpredictable and increasingly diverse. The rhythms and motion that "seem continuous" refer to a wave frequency so rapid that the observer perceives it as a single, unbroken event. Not only is field pattern diversity relative for any given individual, but there is also a marked increase in diversity between individuals. The implications of this for increased individualization of nursing services are explicit.

Pandimensionality

A universe of open systems underwrites the growing diversity of people and their environments. Pandimensionality characterizes these human and environmental fields and all reality is postulated to be pandimensional. Within this postulate the relative nature of change becomes explicit. The use of the term "pandimensional" to replace the terms "four dimensional" and "multidi-

BOX   57–1

Manifestations of Field Patterning in Unitary Human Beings

The evolution of unitary human beings is a dynamic, irreducible, nonlinear process characterized by increasing diversity of energy field patterning. Manifestations of patterning emerge out of the human/environment field mutual process and are continuously innovative. Pattern is an abstraction that reveals itself through its manifestations.

The nature of unitary field patterning is unpredictable and creative. Change is relative and increasingly diverse. Some manifestations of relative diversity in field patterning are noted below.

lesser diversity	greater diversity	
longer rhythms	shorter rhythms	seems continuous
slower motion	faster motion	seems continuous
time experienced as slower	time experienced as faster	timelessness
pragmatic	imaginative	visionary
longer sleeping	longer waking	beyond waking

■ Reprinted with permission from The National League for Nursing, *Visions of Rogers' science-based nursing*, 1990, p. 9.

mensional" does not represent any change in definition. One does not move into or become pandimensional. Rather, this is a way of perceiving reality. Efforts to select words best suited to portray one's thoughts are at best difficult because words are often inadequate to fully communicate the meaning of a particular postulate. One useful analogy of pandimensionality, however, can be found in Abbott's (1952) *Flatland*. Here, the term pandimensional provides for an infinite domain without limit. It best expresses the idea of a unitary whole, and it is defined as a nonlinear domain without spatial or temporal attributes.

The abstract system exists as an irreducible whole; principles and theories derive from this irreducible whole. The nature of change finds expression in the principles of homeodynamics. New knowledge is contributing continuously to revisions of thinking. A significant change in one word in the principle of helicy occurred. Interestingly enough this change from probability to unpredictability is consistent with the abstract system, and new knowledge supports it. Some clarification is in order. The reader is familiar with the currently accepted transition from absolutism to probability. The literature now points up that unpredictability transcends probability. Mallove (1989) in the May/June 1989 issue of *The Planetary Report* writes, "To find in the late 20th Century that unpredictability plays a significant role in the orderly celestial arena is not only a surprising development but a revolutionary one in the history of science" (p. 12). Moreover, Peterson (1989) in the July 15, 1989, issue of *Science News* discussed further the unpredictability of self-organizing critical systems.

The deletion of probability from the abstract system underlying the science of unitary human beings and the addition of unpredictability strengthen consistency and support the nature of change proposed in the principles of homeodynamics. This continuous change emerges out of nonequilibrium and exhibits punctualism not gradualism. In addition, change is accelerating. Chaos theory, too, is transforming the way we think of the world (Crum, 1989; Peterson, 1989; Percival, 1989; Stewart, 1989).

Theories in the Science of Unitary Human Beings

A theory of accelerating evolution deriving from the science of unitary human beings puts in different perspective today's rapidly changing norms in blood pressure levels, children's behavior, longer waking periods, and other events. The higher frequency wave patterns manifesting growing diversity portend new norms to coordinate with this accelerating change. Labels of pathology that are based on old norms may generate hypochondriasis and iatrogenesis in patients. Normal means average. Normal (average) blood pressure readings in all age groups are notably higher today than they were a few decades ago. Not only has the average waking period lengthened, but sleep/wake continuities are increasingly diverse. Interestingly, gifted children and the so-called hyperactive not uncommonly manifest similar behaviors. It would seem more reasonable, then, to hypothesize that hyperactivity was accelerating evolution, rather than to denigrate rhythmicities that diverge from outdated norms and erroneous expectations.

Manifestations of the speeding up of human field rhythms are coordinate with higher frequency environmental field patterns. Humans and their environments evolve and change together. Therefore, radiating increments of widely diverse frequencies are common household accompaniments of everyday life. Environmental motion has quickened, while atmospheric and cosmological complexity continue to grow.

Accelerating change characterized by higher wave frequency field patterns might be expected to manifest itself in new norms with a wider range of distribution of differences among individuals. The doomsayers who claim that people are destroying themselves are in error. On the contrary, there is population explosion, increased longevity, escalating levels of science and technology, the development of space communities, and multiple other evidences of human potential in the process of actualization.

With increased longevity, there are growing numbers of older persons. And contrary to a static view engendered by a closed system model of the universe that postulates aging to be a decline, the science of unitary human beings postulates aging to be a continuously creative process. Aging evolves from conception through the dying process. The aging of a unitary human field is not a running down. Rather, field patterns become increasingly diverse as older people need less sleep, and sleep-wake frequencies become more varied. Higher frequency patterns give meaning to multiple reports of time perceived as racing.

The pandimensional nature of reality is of further relevance. A nonlinear domain points up the invalidity of chronological age as a basis for differentiating human change. In fact, as evolutionary diversity continues to accelerate, the range and variety of differences between individuals also increase; the more diverse field patterns evolve more rapidly than the less diverse ones. Populations defy so-called normal curves as individual differences multiply.

In spite of this, the emergence of paranormal phenomena as valid subjects for serious scientific research has been handicapped by a paucity of viable theories to explain these events. The nature of the science of unitary human beings provides a framework to examine such theories. Pandimensional reality as conceptualized is a factor in deriving testable hypotheses.

The ability to explain precognition, deja vu, and clairvoyance becomes a rational process in pandimensional human and environmental fields. Within this science such occurrences become "normal" rather than "paranormal." The implications for creative health services under these conditions are notable. As a result, alternative forms of healing have become increasingly popular and some forms are surprisingly effective. Meditative modalities, for example, bespeak "beyond waking" manifestations, and the use of therapeutic touch has been documented as efficacious.

Theories continue to be derived from this science. As these theories are tested some will be supported; others will not. Replication and testing of theories by research methods will contribute to one's level of confidence in a given theory. Thus, everyday events, examined through this new worldview, will provide a fresh perspective, raise new questions, and allow new explanations.

Research results from studies concerned with unitary human beings and their environments support the nature of change postulated in the principles of homeodynamics (Barrett, 1990; Malinski, 1986; Sarter, 1988). New tools of measurement have become essential adjuncts to studying questions that arise out of a worldview quite different from the prevalent view. The research potentials of this new system are infinite. It is logically and scientifically tenable, flexible and open-ended. It is a new reality and encompasses new ways of thinking, new questions, and new interpretations. It also requires consistency with the system if one is to study it. The practical implications for human betterment are demonstrable.

The Science and Art of Nursing Practice

Seeing the world from this viewpoint requires a new synthesis, a creative leap, and the inculcation of new attitudes and values. The guiding principles of this science are broad generalizations that require imaginative and innovative modalities for their implementation. The science of unitary human beings identifies nursing's uniqueness and signifies the potential of nurses to fulfill their social responsibility in human service.

Nursing, therefore, is inseparable from the new worldview and the process of change. A new vision of a world encompassing far more than planet earth is in the making. The science of nursing emerges out of this space-age world-view. The evidence of diversifying wholeness is substantial. For instance, the pace of evolution from clans to tribes, to city-states, to nation-states, to one planet is accelerating.

The future, as well, is one of growing diversity, of accelerating evolution, and of nonrepeating rhythmicities. As such, it demands new visions, flexibility, curiosity, imagination, courage, risk taking, compassion, and above all, an excellent sense of humor.

The science of unitary human beings sparks new modalities that evolve as life evolves from earth to space and beyond. Spin-offs from space study and travel can lead to more effective services for Homo sapiens on planet earth. A positive attitude toward change will be generated while vision and imagination grow.

The purpose of nursing is to promote human betterment wherever people are, on planet earth or in outer space. As diversity increases, so too will individualization of services. How can nurses best demonstrate imagination and ingenuity in helping people design ways to fulfill their different rhythmic patterns? One method is to provide community-based health services. Community-based health services must take precedence over shrinking hospital-based sick services. Moreover, the term community-based takes on enhanced meaning as it is defined to include multiple extraterrestrial centers. Supportive services such as hospitals provide an orientation toward pathology, not toward health. Although both community agencies and hospitals provide meaningful services, it is the broad community-based health promotion services that provide the umbrella. As a defined orientation toward health takes place, fewer and fewer people will need the same type of sick services that currently exist. Nevertheless, nothing in this science suggests that humans will be freed from all "disease" and live happily ever after. Disease and pathology are value terms applied when the human field manifests characteristics that may be deemed undesirable. One of today's major health problems is nosophobia, a morbid dread of disease.

Autonomous nursing practice directed by nurses holding valid baccalaureate and higher degrees with an upper division major in nursing science is central to the future. Noninvasive therapeutic modalities are emphasized in this new reality (Barrett, 1990). The practice of therapeutic touch, developed by Krieger (1981), is already in use in many places around this planet. The use of humor, sound, color, and motion also continue to undergo investigation. Additionally, the concept of unconditional love is receiving attention. Attitudes of hope, humor, and upbeat moods have often been documented as better therapy than drugs. Imagery and meditative modalities have much to offer as well. Continued emphasis on human rights, client decision-making, and noncompliance with the traditional rules of thumb are also necessary dimensions of the new science and art of nursing. In addition to this, the noninvasive therapeutic modalities, increasingly emphasized by a range of health care workers, mark the future of nursing practice on this planet and in outer space.

The outcomes of the research in the science of nursing have been reported in the literature and are now finding their way into the practice arena wherever people are (Barrett, 1990; Malinski, 1986; Sarter, 1988). Such research enables one to understand better the nature of human evolution and its multiple, unpredictable potentialities. Description, explanation, and vision strengthen a nurse's ability to practice according to the level and scope of preparation and knowledge in the science of nursing. What is more, holistic trends open up new ways of thinking and spell new worldviews. Other new modalities will emerge out of this evolution toward spacekind that will spark more effective modalities for earthkind.

Caring is one practice modality getting much attention from nurses today. However, as such, caring does not identify nurses any more than it identifies workers from another field. Everyone needs to care; the nature of caring in a given field depends entirely on the body of scientific knowledge specific to the field. Caring is simply a way of using knowledge. Nurses care on the basis of ways they use the science of unitary, irreducible human beings.

Since today's world is rapidly becoming an entrepreneurial society, and nurses continue to move into its mainstream, a substantive knowledge base in a science of nursing has become indispensable. In addition, there is as well a critical need for mutual respect and valuing of differences between all health personnel: between nurses, between health fields, and between the fields of science.

Human beings are on the threshold of a fantastic and unimagined future. In light of this, the potential for human service is greater than it has ever been before. Many nurses have been moving apace to assure that there will be a substantive body of theoretical knowledge specific to nursing to underwrite the practice of nursing. The science of unitary human beings portends a new world in space, the next frontier.

REFERENCES

Abbott, E. A. (1952). *Flatland.* New York: Dover.

Barrett, E. A. M. (Ed.) (1990). *Visions of Rogers' science-based nursing.* New York: National League for Nursing.

Bohm, D. (1980). *Wholeness and the implicate order.* Boston: Routledge & Kegan Paul.

Capra, F. (1982). *The turning point.* New York: Simon and Schuster.

Crum, R. (1989). Why Johnny kills. *New York University Magazine, 4*(2), 34.

Downs, F. (1988). Nursing research: State-of-the-art. *Journal of the New York State Nurses Association, 19* (3), 20.

Ferguson, M. (1980). *The aquarian conspiracy.* Los Angeles: Tarcher.

Friedman, S. T. (1989). Who believes in UFO's? *International UFO Reporter, 14* (1), 6–10.

Fuller, R. B. (1981). *Critical path.* New York: St. Martin's Press.

Huxley, A. (1932). *Brave new world.* New York: Modern Library.

Kenton, L. (1990). Member forum. *Noetic Sciences Bulletin, 5* (1), 6.

Krieger, D. (1981). *Foundations for holistic health nursing practices: The renaissance nurse.* Philadelphia: Lippincott.

Lauden, L. (1977). *Progress and its problems: Toward a theory of scientific growth.* Berkeley: University of California Press.

Lovelock, J. (1988). *The age of Goia.* New York: Norton.

Malinski, V. M. (Ed.) (1986). *Exploration on Martha Rogers' science of unitary human beings.* Norwalk, CT: Appleton-Century-Crofts.

Mallove, E. T. (1989, May-June). The solar system in chaos. *The Planetary Report,* pp. 12–13.

Percival, I. (1989). Chaos: A science for the real world. *New Scientist, 123,* 42–47.

Peterson, I. (1989, July). Digging into sand. *Science News, 136,* 40.

Robinson, G. S. & White, H. M. (1986). *Envoys of mankind.* Washington, D.C.: Smithsonian Institute Press.

Rogers, M. E. (1970). *An introduction to the theoretical basis of nursing.* Philadelphia: Davis.

Sarter, B. (1988). *The stream of becoming: A study of Martha Rogers' theory.* New York: National League for Nursing.

Stewart, I. (1989). *Does God play dice?: The mathematics of chaos.* Cambridge, MA: Brasil Blackwell, Inc.

Weber, R. (Ed.). (1986). *Dialogue with scientists and sages: The search for unity.* New York: Routledge & Kegan Paul.

Weber, R., Bohm, D., & Sheldrake, R. (1986). Matter as a meaning field. In R. Weber (Ed.), *Dialogue with scientists and sages: The search for unity* (pp. 105–123). New York: Routledge & Kegan Paul.

Comments for Author

Nursing Science and the Space Age

Martha intended this article to be an up-to-date summary of her work, and that is what it represents. It is comprehensive and includes her most recent thinking. In writing this article, Martha updated her work from the time of her early 1970s book. She was clear that her revisions through the years did not reflect changes in her basic ideas; rather, she said that she just learned better ways of expressing and elaborating on this basic science. Martha often said that there were many pages in the 1970 purple book that she would like to tear out; she hoped that her most recent thoughts would be the ones people used instead of referring back to the 1970 book and some of its outdated terminology. Although Martha did not write another book, she did want this 1992 article to be used to pull together the most important and current ideas in the *Science of Unitary Human Beings.* Although it is not the last thing Martha published, it is her last major treatise on Rogerian Science.

—ELIZABETH ANN MANHART BARRETT

CHAPTER 58

The Pattern That Connects

Margaret A. Newman

Debate over whether nursing is an art or a science culminates in the need for integration of the two as a guide to practice. The historical development of nursing knowledge reveals a spectrum of evolution from physical care to interpersonal relationships to an integrative approach and, most recently, to a unitary perspective. The author proposes pattern as the integrating factor that eliminates the dichotomies of traditional art and science and transforms nursing knowledge to a higher dimension that includes and transcends the knowledge that has gone before. Nursing praxis is presented as integrated theory-research-practice that is consistent with a unitary perspective.

Key words: evolution of nursing theory, integration of theory, nursing art, nursing praxis, nursing science, pattern

It is urgent that we clarify the *nature* of nursing knowledge. Some view it as an art, others as a science, and some, unfortunately, cannot distinguish nursing knowledge from medical knowledge. The time is past due to recognize the substance of the discipline and the relatedness of art and science, especially in a practice discipline such as nursing.[1-3] Johnson[1] described five separate views of what she considered to be the *art* of nursing, characterized as the nurse's ability to: (1) grasp meaning in patient encounters, (2) establish meaningful connection with the patient, (3) skillfully perform nursing activities, (4) determine an appropriate course of action, and (5) act morally. Nursing scholars, in Johnson's view, have not recognized that different conceptions of nursing art exist. Further, I submit, there is little recognition that these same realms—pattern

Advances in Nursing Science, 24(3), 1–7, Copyright © 2002 Aspen Publishers, Inc. Reprinted with permission of Lippincott Williams & Wilkins

About the Author

MARGARET A. NEWMAN was born in Memphis, TN, on October 10, 1933. She received her first degree (BSHE, 1954) in home economics at Baylor University. She entered nursing at the University of Tennessee, Memphis, in 1959 and received a BSN in 1962. Her graduate study included an emphasis on medical-surgical nursing at the University of California, San Francisco (MS, 1964) and a further emphasis on rehabilitation nursing and nursing science at New York University (PhD, 1971). Except for a short tenure as director of nursing for the clinical research center at the University of Tennessee, the emphasis of her work has been in education (at New York University, Penn State University, and the University of Minnesota). The focus of her scholarship has been on theory development in nursing. The books *Health as Expanding Consciousness* (1986, 1994) and *A Developing Discipline* (1995) represent her major contribution to nursing theory. She is an avid fan of live theater and music, with subscriptions to two local theater groups' offerings and the St. Paul Chamber Orchestra.

recognition, connectedness, technical skill, rational action, and moral imperative—represent knowledge that has been pursued within the context of nursing *science*. Practitioners are faced with a vast array of paradigms, theories, and approaches to practice, but little that pulls it all together. The need for a comprehensive theoretical guide for nursing practice is paramount.

I would like to present the thesis that attention to *pattern* constitutes the unitary grasp of knowledge the discipline seeks. Premises on which this thesis is based include the following:

- Development of nursing knowledge has evolved from an emphasis on parts to a focus on the unitary pattern of the whole, a direction that parallels the development of theory in general.
- Praxis research with the intent of pattern recognition reveals the nature of nursing practice.
- Focus on pattern represents a shift to a higher dimension, which includes and transcends previous nursing knowledge.

The Development of Nursing Knowledge

A brief retrospective review of the development of nursing knowledge provides the background for examining its position in relation to the development of knowledge in general. The early development of nursing knowledge focused primarily on physical environmental factors affecting the health of the patient. From there the emphasis was on actions of the nurse to stabilize and assist patients in circumstances of physical disability. Next, attention was turned to the interpersonal process of the nurse-patient relationship. As nursing began to focus on the person rather than the disease or disability, research was directed to physical and behavioral correlates of health, meaning health as absence of disease.[4] The separation of mind and body in most of these approaches reflected reliance on a traditional science of observables. A holistic perspective was acknowledged as important to nursing, but was considered unscientific, and research proceeded in a correlational, integrative attempt to construct the whole. Martha Rogers[5] introduced a major shift from a particulate approach to a unitary, dynamic perspective of the human being in an undivided universe. Even so, research lagged in its attempts to capture the whole.[6] Eventually the transformative potential of a holographic, dynamic model of nursing practice emerged as it became clear that the whole of the nursing phenomenon would have to be grasped simultaneously as unitary and transformative.[4,7,8]

Midway in the development of nursing knowledge, a movement to establish the concept of nursing diagnosis gained momentum. Nursing theorists were convened to examine the data of nursing practice to try to identify an organizing framework.[9] The product of this effort in the late 1970s emerged as a philosophical set of assumptions identified by the theorist task force reflecting a unitary view of the pattern of person-environment interaction. At the same time, broad dimensions of person-environment relating based on practitioners' observations were identified. The empirical data of nursing practice covered a full spectrum of physical, interpersonal, and inner experiences of relatedness. Though emanating from different paradigmatic views, the philosophical framework and the dimensions of relating contributed to the conceptualization of *pattern* as the basis for nursing diagnosis.[10,11] The direction posed by the North American Nursing Diagnosis Association (NANDA) nurse theorist group pointed toward integration of the various realms of nursing knowledge as the pattern of the whole. The structure of the framework was adopted, but the unitary nature of the phenomenon was obscured as the work of NANDA proceeded by looking at the parts in an effort to construct the whole.

Another step in the explication of nursing knowledge was taken by nursing theorists to delineate the differences in perspective within the nursing community.[7,8,12] The intent was to clarify the assumptions underlying the different paradigms[13]; the effect was to imply the views as separate and, in some instances, to create a competitive arena within the discipline.[14,15] In retrospect, the paradigms were described individually but were not intended to represent separate knowledge. There was intuitive recognition that nursing theory was evolving from particulate to reciprocal to unitary ways of knowing. The misconception of separateness may have arisen out of a need to respect each type of theory. In actuality we were seeing the unitary paradigm as inclusive of and moving beyond the other perspectives.

A current task is to reconcile the seemingly contradictory points of view. Just as relativity theory includes mechanistic theory as special cases, the unitary perspective includes the more particulate view. For example, a three-dimensional perspective includes two-dimensional phenomena, but the Flatlander, the person living in a two-dimensional world, cannot imagine a world of three dimensions.[16] The growth in understanding is unidirectional. When Sime, Corcoran-Perry, and I[7] began to describe different perspectives (with each of us representing a different point of view), we first thought of them as separate, but more and more we found ourselves on common ground, that of the more inclusive unitary, transformative view that not only transcends the former views but also includes the knowledge of those perspectives. Nursing knowledge development is a *process* of the patterning of the whole. It is important that the practitioner of nursing incorporate knowledge of prior realms of knowledge as special cases of the pattern of the whole. At the same time, it is important to recognize that the pattern of the whole *already contains* knowledge of the parts. It is not a matter of adding to or summing up.

Wilber[3] called for the integration of the arts, ethics, and science and illustrated that evolution of theory in general has moved from *matter* to *body* to *mind* to *spirit* with each subsequent realm of knowledge *transcending and including* the realm that preceded it. He referred to this progression as a holarchy (rather than hierarchy), with each level being whole within itself but also a part of a larger whole. A holarchical progression of nursing knowledge has moved from emphasis on *physical* care to *interpersonal* process to an *integrative* approach to a *unitary* perspective. Each succeeding level *transcends and includes* the previous ones. So having reached the unitary perspective, we do not discard the physical, interpersonal and integrative knowledge. All are vital to the greater whole.

Praxis Research on Pattern Recognition

One of the essential aspects of scientific inquiry is the injunction that takes the form of "If you want to know this, do this."[3] So, if you want to know nursing, you engage in nursing practice. In efforts to explicate theory of nursing practice it became apparent that findings from objective, controlled studies, although related to nursing, were not sufficient to provide a comprehensive guide for practice.[17-19] Nursing situations are often ambiguous and characterized by uncertainty—characteristics not usually associated with science. If the phenomenon of our inquiry is unitary and dynamic—common nursing assumptions—then the method of our research must capture those characteristics. It must capture the essence of the nurse-client encounter in relation to the health experience of the client without breaking it apart.

With pattern as a basic assumption of a unitary, transformative perspective, a method was sought to identify a person's unitary, evolving pattern within the context of the mutual process of the nurse-client relationship.[20] The dialogue between nurse-researcher and client-participant became focused on the meaningfulness of events in the client's life. Meaning in a person's life is not only critical but also a way of identifying pattern. A pattern possesses meaning. As meaning is discovered, the pattern becomes apparent (and vice versa).

This research takes on the form and purpose of practice (ie, a shift from observation of "the other" to "we" knowledge) with the intent of assisting clients to get in touch with the meaning of their health experience and thereby get insight into the pattern of the process and its potential for action. The nurse comes to the situation with a theoretical perspective that then becomes a part of the process. Transformation occurs in the interpenetration of the client's and the nurse's patterns, which includes the client's concept of health and the nurse's theoretical understanding. The theory illuminates the meaning of the experience and is in turn illuminated by the data of the experience.

The process of pattern recognition evolving from an authentic, mutual relationship makes a meaningful difference in the experience of the participants. The dialogue of the encounter follows the lead of the client. The significant events described by the client are viewed as configurations (patterns) of relatedness over time. In the process of this dialogue, insight regarding the client's evolving pattern occurs. The clients grasp greater understanding of themselves and their relationships. The process is directly, immediately applicable as nursing practice, and one that is illuminating to both the researched and the researcher.[21,22]

Lather[23] described this process as *research as praxis,* a mutual process that makes a difference in the lives of the participants; one in which the theory is active a priori, and one that enriches the theory but does not necessarily fulfill the expectations of the theory. Others working in collaborative inquiry have further elaborated this type of research as *transformative,*[24] *process wisdom,*[25] and *practice wisdom.*[26] This hermeneutic, dialectic process focuses on the nurse-client relationship and incorporates latent knowledge of other domains. It has the capacity to guide nursing practice. Nursing praxis integrates theory, research, and practice. It is art, science, and practice.

For example, within the context of the theory of health as expanding consciousness, Litchfield[26] participated in the process of pattern recognition and transformation in her relationship with a family who were participants in her research. Epilepsy occupied a major focus in the family since both the mother and the child experienced epileptic seizures that disrupted their lives. Their concept of health initially was a medical perspective of the causation and treatment of epilepsy, in which the father perceived that he had no part. As the nurse-client dialogue about their health circumstances unfolded, the father began to grasp the rhythmic dissonance of the patterns of a stay-at-home mother, a hyperactive son, and the fast-paced father, who was accustomed to the activity of his work world. He saw the role he could play in offering opportunities that would allow the mother the time and space to exercise her own rhythmic (transforming) pattern while providing new father-son opportunities to exercise their own patterns. A new pattern of family relating evolved, one that incorporated the medical meaning of epilepsy within a family-oriented concept of health. This insight was accomplished by the caring dialectic and pattern recognition that took place in the nurse-client dialogue about the family's health circumstances. The dialogue, fundamental to nursing praxis, contained statements of the nurse-researcher merged with statements from the family reflecting their emerging enlightenment. Research as praxis "enables people to change by encouraging self-reflection and a deeper understanding of their particular situations."[23(p263)] A person comes into a higher stage by being known. The nurse becomes the means whereby clients emerge as a transformation of themselves.

Pattern as a Shift to a Higher Dimension

Many theorists echo the call for integration of knowledge: the physical and the non-physical, the parts and the whole, the local and the non-local.[17-19,27,28] Bernstein's emphasis is particularly relevant to nursing: "I argued for a new sensibility and universe of discourse . . . one which sought to integrate dialectically the empirical, interpretive, and critical dimensions of a theoretical orientation that is directed toward practical activity."[29(px)]

Similarly Fawcett and associates[30] called for the integration of the ways of knowing identified by Carper[31] (empirical, ethical, personal, and aesthetic) as a knowledge base for nursing. Further, Smith acknowledged that knowing is holistic and integrative and may have multiple dimensions "but the process and experience is a unity that transcends them."[32(p2)]

Integration is a step in the overall cyclic scheme of things, *but not enough.* Just as one cannot understand the whole of a person by integration of the parts, we cannot understand the unity of nursing knowledge by an integration of the parts. In a hologram, each part contains the whole; each part is reflective of the whole. Mind and matter are not separate, interactive parts; they are different dimensions of the whole and unbroken movement of reality. The common ground of these various manifestations of reality is found in a *higher dimension.*

What is needed is transformation to another realm: a shift to a more inclusive level of wholeness. I submit that the transformation comes about by attending to *pattern.* The concept of pattern is integral to nursing. It is based on relationships, it includes the focus (ie, the client) and the environment, and its meaning permits a jump from what is seen and heard to the larger context and from the explicit to the implicit. The data of pattern are the stories of people and their connectedness with their environment, reflecting the complexity of continuing change. The "*pattern which connects*" was Bateson's[33] central thesis; he emphasized pattern as meaning within context over time. Pattern transcends the boundaries of different types of knowledge and is inclusive of the realms that have gone before. (For example, a pattern of movement includes knowledge of aesthetics, neurophysiology, kinesiology, interpersonal relations, and so on and at the same time transcends them all.)

In eliminating the false dichotomies of the sciences, we capture the dynamic nature of the living process, what Bernstein referred to as "the dialogical character of our human existence."[29(pxv)] It is not enough to describe the unitary pattern of a person at various points over time. We need to learn how to enter into the evolving patterning process with the client.[34] Litchfield[26] addressed this need by focusing her research on the process of nurse-client relating in recognizing pattern and envisioning new avenues of action. Endo[35] followed with an elaboration of the phases of the process, illustrating how the nurse facilitates the breakthrough of satori (insight, freedom) on the part of clients and their subsequent enlightened actions and new relationships. Cowling[36,37] elaborated a process of pattern appreciation that incorporates multiple ways of knowing and ties together theory, research, and practice. Pharris (see the article in this issue entitled "Coming To Know Ourselves as Community through a Nursing Partnership with Adolescents Convicted of Murder") is beginning to show the relatedness of individual pattern to environmental pattern with important implications for community health. These and many other studies stemming from a unitary perspective illustrate the relevance of patterning as the dimension that pulls it all together.

Conclusion

We need to move to a realm of nursing knowledge that *includes and transcends* all of the realms that have gone before. Nursing praxis based on pattern recognition illumines the process engaged in by the nurse and client and transforms the various realms of knowledge into a dynamic pattern of the whole. It transcends separate realms of knowledge. Concentrating on the evolving pattern of this process provides an integrating shift to a more inclusive domain of knowledge.

REFERENCES

1. Johnson JL. A dialectical examination of nursing art. *Adv Nurs Sci,* 1994;17(1):1–14.
2. Alligood MR. Toward a unitary view of nursing practice. In: Madrid M. Barrett EAM. eds. *Rogers' Scientific Art of Nursing Practice.* New York: National League for Nursing: 1994.
3. Wilber K. *The Marriage of Sense and Soul.* New York: Random House: 1998.
4. Newman MA. The continuing revolution: a history of nursing science. In: Chaska N. ed. *The Nursing Profession: A Time To Speak.* New York: McGraw-Hill; 1983.
5. Rogers ME. *An Introduction to the Theoretical Basis of Nursing.* Philadelphia: F. A. Davis: 1970.
6. Newman MA. Review of Barrett EAM, ed. *Visions of Rogers' Science-Based Nursing. Nurs Sci Q.* 1991;4(1):41–42.
7. Newman MA, Sime AM. Corcoran-Perry SA. The focus of the discipline of nursing. *Adv Nurs Sci.* 1991;14(1):1–6.
8. Parse RR. *Nursing Science: Major Paradigms, Theories and Critiques.* Philadelphia: W. B. Saunders: 1987.
9. Roy C, Rogers M, Fitzpatrick J, Newman M, Orem D. Nursing diagnosis and nursing theory. In: Kim M, Moritz D, eds. *Classification of Nursing Diagnosis.* New York: McGraw-Hill; 1982:215–231.
10. Newman M. Nursing diagnosis: looking at the whole. *Am J Nurs.* 1984;84(12):1496–1499.
11. Newman MA. Nursing's emerging paradigm: the diagnosis of pattern. In: McLane AM, ed. *Classification of Nursing Diagnosis.* St. Louis: Mosby; 1986:53–60.
12. Fawcett J. From a plethora of paradigms to parsimony in worldviews. *Nurs Sci Q.* 1993;6(2):56–58.
13. Cody WK. About all those paradigms: many in the universe, two in nursing. *Nurs Sci Q.* 1995;8(4):144–147.
14. Leddy SK. Toward a complementary perspective on worldviews. *Nurs Sci Q.* 2000;13(3):225–229.
15. Thorne SE. Are egalitarian relationships a desirable ideal in nursing? *West J Nurs Res.* 1999;21(1):16–34.
16. Abbott EA. *Flatland.* New York: Dover: 1952.
17. Boyd C. Toward a nursing practice research method. *Adv Nurs Sci.* 1993;16(2):9–25.
18. Kim S. Challenge of new perspectives: moving toward a new epistemology for nursing. Presented at Knowledge Conference: Developing Knowledge for Nursing Practice; October 4–6, 1996; Boston, MA.
19. Chinn PL, Kramer MK. *Theory and Nursing: Integrated Knowledge Development.* St. Louis, MO: Mosby; 1999.
20. Newman MA. Newman's theory of health as praxis. *Nurs Sci Q.* 1990;3(1):37–41.
21. Newman MA. *Health as Expanding Consciousness.* St. Louis. MO: Mosby: 1986.
22. Newman MA. *Health as Expanding Consciousness,* 2nd ed. Sudbury. MA: Jones & Barlett (NLN Press): 1994.
23. Lather P. Research as praxis. *Harvard Educ Rev.* 1986;56(3):257–277.
24. Heron J. Philosophical basis for a new paradigm. In: Reason P, Rowan J, eds. *Human Inquiry: A Sourcebook of New Paradigm Research.* New York: Wiley; 1981.
25. Vaill P. Process wisdom for a new age. *Re-Vision,* 1984–1985;7(2):39–49.
26. Litchfield M. Practice wisdom. *Adv Nurs Sci.* 1999;22(2):62–73.
27. Im E-O, Meleis AI. Situation-specific theories: philosophical roots, properties, and approach. *Adv Nurs Sci.* 1999;22(2):11–24.
28. Walker L. Is integrative science necessary to improve nursing practice? *West J Nurs Res.* 1999;21(1):94–102.
29. Bernstein R. *Beyond Objectivism and Relativism: Science, Hermeneutics, and Praxis.* Philadelphia: University of Pennsylvania; 1983.
30. Fawcett J, Watson J, Neuman B, Walker PH, Fitzpatrick J. On nursing theories and evidence. *J Nurs Sch.* 2001;33(2):115–119.
31. Carper BA. Fundamental patterns of knowing in nursing. *Adv Nurs Sci.* 1978;1(1):13–23.
32. Smith MC. Is all knowing personal knowing? *Nurs Sci Q.* 1992;5(1):2–3.
33. Bateson G. *Mind and Nature: A Necessary Unity.* New York: Bantam; 1979.
34. Newman MA. Experiencing the whole. *Adv Nurs Sci.* 1997;20(1):34–39.
35. Endo E. Pattern recognition as a nursing intervention with Japanese women with ovarian cancer. *Adv Nurs Sci.* 1998;20(4):49–61.
36. Cowling WR. Unitary pattern appreciation: the unitary science/practice of reaching for essence. In: Madrid M, ed. *Patterns of Rogerian Knowing.* New York: National League for Nursing; 1997.
37. Cowling WR. Unitary appreciative inquiry. *Adv Nurs Sci.* 2001;23(4)32–48.

The Author Comments

The Pattern That Connects

Three decades later (from the 1972 "Nursing's theoretical evolution" article), I am still trying to explicate the connections that define the discipline of nursing. Pattern is recognized as integral to nursing knowledge. In this article, I propose the concept of pattern as an integrating dimension that includes and transcends all forms of nursing knowledge.

—MARGARET A. NEWMAN

Middle Range Theory: Spinning Research and Practice to Create Knowledge for the New Millennium

Patricia Liehr

Mary Jane Smith

The foundation of middle range theory reported during the past decade was described and analyzed. A CINAHL search revealed 22 middle range theories that met selected criteria. This foundation is a firm base for new millennium theorizing. Recommendations for future theorizing include: clear articulation of theory names and approaches for generating theories; clarification of concept linkages with inclusion of diagrammed models; deliberate attention to research-practice connections of theories; creation of theories in concert with the disciplinary perspective; and, movement of middle range theories to the front lines of nursing research and practice for further analysis, critique, and development.

Key words: *middle range theory, theory, 21st century perspective*

A spinner prepares wool by combing, to discard debris and align the strands of a matted mass in much the same way as content is sifted to tease central ideas out of extraneous ones. Just as the spinner twirls strands to compose a single thread; the nurse theorist spins central ideas into a synthesized thread for research and practice. Twisting single threads with each other enhances the strength of the product; as does the crafting of research-practice links in the creation of strong middle range theory. The beauty of any woven article is dependent on its warp and weft; likewise, the esthetics of the discipline is dependent on its theories. Spinning, like theorizing, is rigorous work aimed at creating esthetic, useful products. This article describes and analyzes a

Advances in Nursing Science, 21(4), 81–91. Copyright © 1999, Aspen Publishers.
Reprinted with permission of Lippincott Williams & Wilkins.

About the Authors

PATRICIA LIEHR was born in Pittsburgh, PA, and received her first nursing education at Ohio Valley General Hospital, School of Nursing in Pittsburgh; her baccalaureate education at Villa Maria College in Erie, PA; and her master's in education at Duquesne University in Pittsburgh. Her doctorate in nursing was completed at the University of Maryland, and she did postdoctoral study as a Robert Wood Johnson Scholar at the University of Pennsylvania. She has been a nursing faculty member at the University of Texas, Health Science Center at Houston, since 1989. Over time, in her scholarly work, she has woven the threads of theory, practice, and research together to enhance her understanding of each. Interestingly, she is a weaver with little time for warp and weft these days...but still a weaver in her heart. Her scholarly endeavors focus on human language, including and extending beyond words and on the scientific structures, which guide nurse-person dialogue.

MARY JANE SMITH was born in Johnstown, PA, and earned a BSN and an MNEd from the University of Pittsburgh and a PhD from New York University. She has taught nursing theory to master's-level students for 25 years and, more recently, to doctoral students. She has been on the faculty at West Virginia University since 1981, during the past 4 years as Associate Dean for Graduate Academic Affairs. The focus of her scholarly work is gathering and analyzing the stories of becoming pregnant for teenaged high school students, time-pressured busyness for graduate students, and intervening in drinking/driving situations for rural youth. She likes to cook, garden, and dance.

decade of middle range theory products that establish a foundation for the new millennium. This foundation highlights the current structure of middle range theory and offers direction for 21st century spinning.

The Historical Context of Middle Range Theory

Modernism, postmodernism, and neomodernism are historical descriptors that represent change in the course of a developing discipline by influencing thinking and scholarship. Modernism espouses beliefs about human beings that affirm a unidimensional and stable existence, while post modernism adheres to views that affirm multidimensional, ever-changing, and complex human unfolding existence.[1] Watson[2] identified the postmodern for nursing as reconnecting with "the truths of unfoldment, an expansion and fusing of horizons of meaning, an attending to the authenticity, ethos, and ethic of caring relations, context, continuity, connections, aesthetics, interpretation and construction."[2(p63)] She concludes that these postmodern di-

mensions tie directly to developing the art and science of nursing as a caring-healing transformative praxis paradigm. Reed[3] moves beyond postmodernism to neomodernism and calls for a synthesis of modernism and postmodernism. She describes the synthesis as a metanarrative reflecting the human developmental potential, transformation, and self-transcendent capacity for health and healing, including a recognition of the developmental histories of persons and their contexts.[3] It is expected that theories that offer direction for the new millennium will emerge from the historical context that defines the time. The current context urges a focus on the human developmental potential of health and healing and supports a nursing knowledge base that synthesizes art and science; practice and research. Theories at the middle range level of discourse are in keeping with the historical context launching the new millennium.

Merton describes theories of the middle range as those

that lie between the minor but necessary working hypotheses that evolve in abundance during day-today research and the all-inclusive systematic efforts to develop unified theory that will explain all the observed uniformities of social behavior, social organization and social change.[4(p39)]

He goes on to describe the principal ideas of middle range theory as relatively simple. Simple, in this sense, means rudimentary straightforward ideas that stem from the perspective of the discipline. An example of such an idea is that when individuals tell their story to one who truly listens, a change takes place. This idea is central to the middle range theory of attentively embracing story.[5] The ideas of middle range theory are simple yet general and are more than mere empirical generalizations.

In keeping with the views of Merton,[4] the following descriptions of middle range theory are found in the nursing literature: testable and intermediate in scope,[6] adequate in empirical foundations,[7] neither too broad nor too narrow,[8] circumscribed and substantively specific,[9] and more circumscribed than grand theory but not as concrete as practice theory.[10] In 1974, Jacox[11] described middle range theories as those including a limited number of variables and focused on a limited aspect of reality. Each of these descriptions highlights a scope somewhere in the middle, allowing for broad definitions. Lenz[12] addresses the issue of definitional clarity and believes that although the definitions of middle range theory are consistent, theories of varying scope have been labeled middle-range and the discipline may be well served by recognizing levels of theory within the middle range. She states the challenge for the discipline will be to not generate a plethora of middle range theories, but to develop a few that are empirically sound, coherent, meaningful, useful, and illuminating.[12] To meet the challenge set by Lenz in the next century, it is essential that middle range theories emerge from the twisting of research and practice threads by nurse scholars who are building on the work of others and creating the future direction of the discipline. The spinning of middle range theory in the next century will be guided by the existing middle range theory foundation.

The Existing Middle Range Theory Foundation

To assess the current foundation of middle range theory, a CINAHL search of the past 10 years of nursing literature was done entering middle range theory, mid-range theory, and nursing as search terms. The search was conducted independently in two institutions. All papers written in English that surfaced from the combined search were evaluated for inclusion in the foundation list of middle range theories (Table 59-1). Criteria for inclusion were

1. The theory was identified as middle range by its author;
2. The theory name was accessible in the paper;
3. Concepts of the theory were explicitly identified or implicitly identified in propositions; and
4. The development of the theory was the major focus of the paper.

These criteria represent an intent to be inclusive, providing the broadest view of available middle range nursing theory. However, some papers excluded were primarily methodological in focus.[13,14] These were identified in the literature search but did not meet the criteria. Table 59-1 describes the middle range theory foundation that has emerged during the past decade. Along with including identifying and locating information about the theory, it notes the inclusion of a diagrammed model and the approaches for theory generation identified by the author.

Analysis of the Middle Range Theory Foundation

The Middle Range Theories

There are 22 middle range theories proposed as the current foundation. Two theories, Unpleasant Symptoms[7,15] and Balance between Analgesia and Side Effects,[16,17] are accompanied by two citations. Unpleasant Symptoms is the only theory to have documented, ongoing development in the past decade. The second citation for Balance between Analgesia and Side Effects provides

Table 59-1
Middle Range Theories Over the Decade: 1988–1998

Year Published	Author(s), Journal	Name of Theory	Inclusion of Model		Theory Generating Approach
			Yes	No	
1988	Mishel *Image*	Uncertainty in Illness	X		Empirical research, literature synthesis from nursing and other disciplines
1989	Thompson, et al. *Journal of Nurse Midwifery*	Nurse Midwifery Care		X	Philosophy of nurse-midwifery profession, survey data, patient-nurse practice video-tapes, empirical research
1990	Kinney *Issues in Mental Health Nursing*	Facilitating Growth and Development		X	Middle range model from Erickson's Modeling and Role Modeling theory, practice
1991	Reed *ANS*	Self-Transcendence		X	Literature reviews, clinical experience, empirical research, deductive reformulation of life span theories from developmental psychology with Rogers Conceptual System
1991	Burke, Kauffmann, Costello, Dillon *Image*	Hazardous Secrets and Reluctantly Taking Charge	X		Grounded theory
1991	Thomas *Issues in Mental Health Nursing*	Women's Anger	X		Existential and cognitive-behavioral theories, literature review, clinical knowledge, intuition, logic
1991	Swanson *Nursing Research*	Caring		X	Phenomenological studies
1994	Powell-Cope *Nursing Research*	Negotiating Partnership		X	Extending Swanson's Caring theory using grounded theory
1995, 1997	Lenz, et al. *ANS*	Unpleasant Symptoms	X		Empirical research, clinical observation, concept analysis, collaboration
1995	Jezewski *ANS*	Cultural Brokering	X		Concept analysis, ethnography, grounded theory, practice experience, literature synthesis
1995	Tollett, Thomas *ANS*	Homelessness-Hopelessness	X		Testing Miller's Patient Power Resources Model using a quasi-experimental study
1996, 1998	Good, Moore, Good *Nursing Outlook*	Balance between Analgesia and Side Effects	X		Clinical practice guidelines; empirical research
1997	Auvil-Novak *Nursing Research*	Chronotherapeutic Intervention for Postsurgical Pain	X		Chronobiologic theory, literature synthesis, empirical research
1997	Olson, Hanchett *Image*	Nurse-Expressed Empathy and Patient Distress	X		Orlando's nursing model, empirical research
1997	Brooks, Thomas *ANS*	Interpersonal Perceptual Awareness	X		Concept analysis to extend King's Interacting System framework

(Continues)

Table 59-1
Middle Range Theories Over the Decade: 1988–1998 *(Continued)*

Year Published	Author(s), Journal	Name of Theory	Inclusion of Model		Theory Generating Approach
			Yes	No	
1997	Polk *ANS*	Resilience	X		Concept synthesis using literature from other disciplines, Roger's *Science of Unitary Beings*
1997	Gerdner *Journal of American Psychiatric Nurses' Association*	Individualized Music Intervention for Agitation	X		Clinical practice, literature review, pilot study
1997	Acton *Journal of Holistic Nursing*	Affiliated Individuation as a Mediator of Stress	X		Middle range model from Erickson's Modeling and Role Modeling theory, Empirical research
1998	Eakes, Burke, Hainsworth *Image*	Chronic Sorrow	X		Concept analysis, literature review, qualitative research
1998	Huth, Moore *Journal of the Society of Pediatric Nurses*	Acute Pain Management	X		Clinical practice guidelines
1998	Levesque, et al. *Nursing Science Quarterly*	Psychological Adaptation	X		Middle range theories from other disciplines, empirical research, collaboration, Roy's Adaptation Model
1998	Ruland, Moore *Nursing Outlook*	Peaceful End of Life	X		Standards of care

examples of use of the theory for research but does not alter its original structure. Powell-Cope,[18] using Swanson's[19] theory of Caring—with the intent of extending it—derived yet another theory, Negotiating Partnerships. This was the only instance of one middle range nursing theory generating another. However, Levesque et al.[20] report that a foundation of middle range theories from other disciplines was the basis of their work.

Several theories that have been labeled middle range by persons who are not the primary author of the theory do not appear in the middle range foundation list. For instance, Fawcett[9] labels Orlando's Deliberative Nursing, Peplau's Interpersonal Relations, and Watson's Human Caring theory as middle range; however, none of these came up in the literature search for middle range theory. Nolan and Grant[21] labeled Chenitz's theory of

Entry into a Nursing Home as Status Passage as middle range and reported a test of the theory with a respite care sample. Review of Chenitz's theory[22] indicated that it was labeled practice theory by the author even though it may be at the middle range level of discourse. There are other theories that seem to be at the middle range level of discourse but have not been so identified by the primary author. One example is the work of Beck, who has developed a theory of postpartum depression that includes initial quantitative inquiry[23] followed by qualitative study.[24-26] Although this body of work is at the middle range level of discourse, Beck has not labeled it as middle range theory.

Based on the identified foundation of middle range theory, as the decade unfolded, there appeared to be increased willingness to label theory as middle range.

Seven of the theories in Table 59-1 were proposed in the 4-year span between 1988 and 1992 and 15 were proposed in the most recent 4 years of the decade, since 1994, with six middle range theory papers published in 1997 alone. Some of the 1997 proliferation can be attributed to an issue of *Advances in Nursing Science* devoted to middle range theory. Three of the middle range theories listed in 1997 were published in this issue. In her editorial for the issue, Chinn[27] highlighted a shift in nurses' scholarly endeavors to create possibilities for healing science-art as evidenced by the issue's middle range theories, which, she noted, defy a single, limited perspective definition. The question about what constitutes theory at the middle range is not a black and white issue for which a precise and clear definition can be offered. Middle range theory holds to a given level of abstraction. It is not too broad nor too narrow, but somewhere in the middle. It is expected that finding the middle will come as theory in the middle range is spun in the next millennium.

Naming the Theory

Theory, especially at the middle range, is known to practitioners and researchers by the way it is named. It is essential that theories at the middle range be named in the context of the disciplinary perspective and at the appropriate level of discourse. Figuring out the name is a process of creative conceptualization that moves back and forth between putting together and pulling apart until the right name is found. Implicit in naming is a search for a conceptual structure as the theorist remembers and relives practice and research experiences, reflecting on proposed meaning in relation to the literature. This is a creative, energy-demanding process intended to uncover the heart of the theory. The central theory core is molded by the conceptual structure that exposes it and is articulated at the middle range level of abstraction as the name of the theory.

A theory name was accessible in each of the papers in Table 59-1, although some names were more accessible than others. A few theorists announced the presentation of a middle range theory and provided a name in the title of the paper,[7,15,28-31] while others embedded the name in the body of the paper. Facilitating Growth and Development[32] and Affiliated Individuation[33] both emerge from Modeling and Role-Modeling theory.[34] While each is described as a model at the middle range level of abstraction, distinguishing the unique name from the parent theory was difficult. The challenge of naming a middle range theory resides in determining the middle as sufficiently abstract to allow a breadth of application yet narrow enough to permit guidance in research and practice. Table 59-2 organizes the existing middle range theories into the high-middle, middle, and low-middle level of abstraction, using the theory name. The theories were grouped, relative to each other, based on the generality or scope of the theory indicated by the name. Using the theory name to distinguish the level of abstraction has inherent limitations because the name may not reflect theory content. However, the theory name is its guiding label and this analysis highlights the importance of the theory name. It also highlights the existence of multiple levels of abstraction within the middle range, a fact introduced by Lenz,[12] for further recognition and development. To name a middle range theory is to locate it at an appropriate level of abstraction and to commit to a conceptual structure. Capturing a conceptual structure and expressing theory at the middle range level of abstraction will enable 21st century scholars to recognize, use, and critique the theory for practice and research applications.

Inclusion of a Model

Chinn and Kramer[35] define theory as "a creative and rigorous structuring of ideas that projects a tentative, purposeful, and systematic view of phenomena."[35(p106)] They include purpose, concepts, definitions, relationships, structure, and assumptions as components of theory suggested by their definition, noting that purpose and assumptions may be implicit rather than explicit. So, concepts with their definitions—and relationships expressed as structure—are the core components expected to be made explicit regardless of the theory's level of abstraction. One of the criteria for theories in the foundation list was the presentation of concepts. The relationship and structure components were evalu-

Table 59-2
Middle Range Nursing Theories by Level of Abstraction

High Middle	Middle	Low Middle
Caring		Uncertainty in IllnessHazardous Secrets and Reluctantly Taking Charge
Facilitating Growth and Development	Unpleasant Symptoms	Affiliated Individuation as a Mediator of Stress
Interpersonal Perceptual Awareness	Chronic Sorrow	Women's Anger
Self-Transcendence	Peaceful End of Life	Nurse Midwifery Care
Resilience	Negotiating Partnerships	Acute Pain Management
Psychological Adaptation	Cultural Brokering	Balance between Analgesia and Side Effects
	Nurse-Expressed Empathy and Patient Distress	Homelessness-Helplessness
		Individualized Music Intervention for Agitation
		Chronotherapeutic Intervention for Post-Surgical Pain

ated by determining whether the theorist included a diagrammed model in the paper. Of the 22 theories in the foundation list, only 5 did not diagram a model.[18,19,32,36,37] Three[18,19,36] did not explicitly address relationships between concepts. One[37] specified relationships through propositions; one[32] described middle range relationships between concepts of a parent theory. All middle range theories since 1995 have included a diagrammed model.

Approaches for Generating Middle Range Theory

Lenz[12] has identified six approaches for generating middle range theory; these were used to categorize the methods used by the creators of the 22 theories identified in the foundation. The categories are not mutually exclusive because theorists often used more than one approach. Lenz's approaches are

1. inductive theory building through research,
2. deductive theory building from grand nursing theories,
3. combining existing nursing and non-nursing theories,
4. deriving theories from other disciplines,
5. synthesizing theories from published research findings, and

6. developing theories from clinical practice guidelines.

A review of the foundation theories indicates that fourteen* appeared to use inductive theory building through research. Three derived the theory from grand nursing theory,[20,29,43] two combined nursing and non-nursing theories,[30,37] four derived theories from those of other disciplines,[20,28,37,44] and two[16,45] developed theory from practice guidelines. The approach of synthesizing theories from published research identified by Lenz was difficult to determine when categorizing the theories. No middle range theory was cited that was generated only by published research. Even when not stated explicitly, there were implicit indications that every theory had referred to published research when generating the theory. Two theories[32,46] fit into none of the approaches described by Lenz. Ruland and Moore[46] recently have proposed using standards of care to generate middle range theory and Kinney[32] describes a practice example to demonstrate a middle range model. Including Kinney, seven theories[7,15,32,36,37,40,42,44] explicitly cited personal practice experiences as contributing to middle range theory development. Only four[7,15,36,40,42] of the seven also described research threads, thus enabling the spinning of research with practice in the building of middle range theory.

The analysis of approaches for generating middle range theory suggests that Lenz's listing generally is comprehensive. The elimination of the approach noting synthesis from published research findings may be appropriate, and an expansion of "clinical practice guidelines" to "practice guidelines and standards" will cover the recent work by Ruland and Moore.[46] Inclusion of the practice thread is critical for 21st century spinning. Therefore, the following five approaches are proposed for middle range theory generation in the new millennium:

1. induction through research and practice;
2. deduction from research and practice applications of grand theories;
3. combination of existing nursing and non-nursing middle range theories;
4. derivation from theories of other disciplines that relate to nursing's disciplinary perspective; and
5. derivation from practice guidelines and standards rooted in research.

It is unlikely that any of these theory generation approaches will stand alone as nursing moves into the next century. Each will need to be combined to most effectively guide the discipline. Guidance for the new millennium is most likely to emerge from theories that spin research and practice to focus on the human developmental potential of health and healing.

Juxtaposition with Grand Nursing Theory

As middle range theory is generated for the new millennium, it is essential that it move beyond the polarities often created between it and grand theories. The all-embracing grand theories were espoused by individuals who attempted to create a view of the whole of nursing. Groups have developed into small circles of schools of thought in which an all-or-nothing adherence to the perspective is advocated strongly. This approach has advanced the discipline through generation of scholarly pursuits and offers a grounding for middle range theory. It is not separate nor antithetical to middle range theory

development. Merton[4] identifies the following criticisms of middle range theory leveled by those who advocate grand approaches: (1) conceptualizing middle range theory is low in intellectual ambitions; (2) it completely excludes grand theory; (3) it will fragment the discipline into unrelated special theories; and (4) a positivist conception of theory will be the result. There is no evidence that these criticisms have been realized. Nursing's current middle range theory foundation: reflects scholarly work conceptualized at a lower level of abstraction that rises to intellectual challenge; builds on grand theory that continues to offer a foundation for development; and projects a historical context to begin the millennium with theories at the middle range in the perspective of the discipline.

Disciplinary Perspective of the Middle Range Theory Foundation

An association between the existing middle range theory foundation and the disciplinary perspective synthesized as a caring, healing process in which the human developmental potential for health and transformation emerge[2,3] is depicted in Table 59-3. Through the reflective process of dwelling with the essence of the disciplinary perspective and the middle range theories as named, two themes surfaced. These themes were caring—healing processes and transforming struggle-growth. These themes offer a view of the existing middle range theory foundation in the context of a disciplinary perspective as well as an integrated paradigm for spinning middle range theory in the new millennium.

The Future: Where Does Nursing Theory Go From Here?

In conclusion, a lot of thoughtful spinning of middle range theory has been done in the past decade; and although knots and tangles have been created along the way, one must remember that spinning theory is a creative human endeavor that can best be described as a

Table 59-3
Middle Range Theories by Disciplinary Themes

Caring—Healing Process	Transforming Struggle—Growth
Caring	Self-Transcendence
Facilitating Growth and Development	Resilience
Interpersonal Perceptual Awareness	Psychological Adaptation
Cultural Brokering	Uncertainty in Illness
Nurse-Expressed Empathy and Patient Distress	Unpleasant Symptoms
Nurse Midwifery Care	Chronic Sorrow
Acute Pain Management	Peaceful End of Life
Balance between Analgesia and Side Effects	Negotiating Partnerships
Individualized Music Intervention for Agitation	Hazardous Secrets and Reluctantly Taking Charge
Chronotherapeutic Intervention for Post-Surgical Pain	Affiliated Individuation as a Mediator of Stress
	Women's Anger
	Homelessness-Helplessness

work in progress. It is expected that the knots and tangles will be sorted out with the spinner's persistence and careful attention to creating and combining fibers. Based on the description and analysis of the current middle range theory foundation, several recommendations are presented for developing middle range theory in the future. The recommendations are that the creators of middle range theory:

1. take care to clearly articulate the theory name and approaches used for generating the theory;
2. strive to clarify the conceptual linkages of the theory in a diagrammed model;
3. give deliberate attention to articulating the research-practice links of the theory;
4. create an association between the proposed theory and a disciplinary perspective in nursing; and
5. move middle range theory to the front lines of nursing practice and research for further analysis, critique, and development.

Twenty-first century theorists are offered the challenge of these recommendations. The challenge is to move nursing theory forward by spinning research and practice in the creation of middle range theories congruent with the current historical context. It is this forward movement that will give substance and direction to the discipline. Middle range theory will create the disciplinary fabric of the new millennium as nurse theorists spin and twist fibers from the past-present into the future.

REFERENCES

1. Anderson TA. Post modern person. *Noetic Sciences Review.* 1998;45:28–33.
2. Watson J. Postmodernism and knowledge development in nursing. *Nurs Sci Quarterly.* 1994;8:60–64.
3. Reed PG. A treatise on nursing knowledge development for the 21st century: beyond postmodernism. *ANS.* 1995;17:70–84.
4. Merton RK. On sociological theories of the middle range. In: *Social Theory and Social Structure.* New York: Free Press: 1968.
5. Smith MJ, Liehr P. Attentively embracing story: a middle range theory with practice and research implications. *Sch Ing Nurs Prac.* In press.
6. Suppe F. Middle range theory—Role in nursing theory and knowledge development. In: *Proceedings of the Sixth Rosemary Ellis Scholar's Retreat, Nursing Science Implications for the 21st century.* Cleveland. OH: Frances Payne Bolton School of Nursing, Case Western Reserve University: 1996.
7. Lenz ER, Suppe F, Gift AG, Pugh LC, Milligan RA. Collaborative development of middle-range nursing theories: toward a theory of unpleasant symptoms. *ANS.* 1995;17:1–13.
8. Reed P. toward a nursing theory of self-transcendence: deductive reformulation using developmental theories. *ANS.* 1991;12:64–74.
9. Fawcett J. *Analysis and Evaluation of Nursing Theories.* Philadelphia, PA: F. A. Davis: 1993.
10. Morris D. Middle range theory role in education. In: *Pro-*

ceedings of the Sixth Rosemary Ellis Scholar's Retreat, Nursing Science Implications for the 21st century. Cleveland, OH: Frances Payne Bolton School of Nursing, Case Western Reserve University; 1996.

11. Jacox A. Theory construction in nursing: an overview. *Nurs Res.* 1974;23:4–12.

12. Lenz E. Middle range theory—Role in research and practice. In: *Proceedings of the Sixth Rosemary Ellis Scholar's Retreat, Nursing Science Implications for the 21st century.* Cleveland, OH: Frances Payne Bolton School of Nursing, Case Western Reserve University; 1996.

13. Dluhy NM. Mapping knowledge in chronic illness. *J Adv Nurs.* 1995;21:1051–1058.

14. Jenny JJ, Logan J. Caring and comfort metaphors used by patients in critical care. *Image.* 1996;28:349–352.

15. Lenz ER, Pugh LC, Milligan RA. Gift AG, Suppe F. The middle range theory of unpleasant symptoms: an update. *ANS.* 1997;19:14–27.

16. Good M, Moore SM. Clinical practice guidelines as a new source of middle range theory: focus on acute pain. *Nurs Outlook.* 1996;44:74–79.

17. Good M. A middle range theory of acute pain management use in research. *Nurs Outlook.* 1998;46:120–124.

18. Powell-Cope GM. Family caregivers of people with AIDS: negotiating partnerships with professional health care providers. *Nurs Res.* 1994;43:324–330.

19. Swanson KM. Empirical development of a middle range theory of caring. *Nurs Res.* 1991;40:161–166.

20. Levesque L, Ricard N, Ducharme F, Duquette A, Bonin J. Empirical verification of a theoretical model derived from the Roy Adaptation Model: findings from five studies. *Nurs Sci Q.* 1998;11:31–39.

21. Nolan M. Grant G. Mid-range theory building and the nursing theory-practice gap: a respite care case study. *J Adv Nurs.* 1992;17:217–223.

22. Chenitz WC. Entry into a nursing home as status passage: a theory to guide nursing practice. *Geriatric Nurs.* 1983; Mar/Apr: 92–97.

23. Beck CT, Reynolds MA, Rutowski P. Maternity blues and postpartum depression. *JOGNN.* 1992;21:287–293.

24. Beck CT. The lived experience of postpartum depression: a phenomenological study. *Nurs Res.* 1992;41:166–170.

25. Beck CT. Teetering on the edge: a substantive theory of postpartum depression. *Nurs Res.* 1993;42:42–48.

26. Beck CT. Postpartum depressed mothers' experiences interacting with their children. *Nurs Res.* 1996;45:98–104.

27. Chinn P. Why middle range theory? *ANS.* 1997;19:viii.

28. Auvil-Novak SE. A mid-range theory of chronotherapeutic intervention for postsurgical pain. *Nurs Res.* 1997;46:66–71.

29. Olson J, Hanchett E. Nurse-expressed empathy, patient outcomes, and development of a middle-range theory. *Image.* 1997;29:71–76.

30. Polk LV. Toward a middle range theory of resilience. *ANS.* 1997;19:1–13.

31. Eakes GG, Burke ML, Hainsworth MA. Middle-range theory of chronic sorrow. *Image.* 1998;30:179–184.

32. Kinney CK. Facilitating growth and development: a paradigm case for modeling and role-modeling. *Issues Ment Health Nurs.* 1990;11:375–395.

33. Acton GJ. Affiliated-individuation as a mediator of stress and burden in caregivers of adults with dementia. *J Holistic Nurs.* 1997;15:336–357.

34. Erickson HC, Tomlin EM, Swain MAP. *Modeling and Role-Modeling: A Theory and Paradigm for Nursing.* Englewood Cliffs, NJ: Prentice-Hall; 1983.

35. Chinn PL, Kramer MK. *Theory and Nursing: A Systematic Approach.* St. Louis, MO: Mosby; 1995.

36. Thompson JE, Oakley D, Burke M, Jay S, Conklin M. Theory building in nurse-midwifery: the care process. *J Nurs-Midwifery.* 1989;34:120–130.

37. Reed PG. Toward a nursing theory of self-transcendence: deductive reformulation using developmental theories. *ANS.* 1991;13:64–77.

38. Mishel MH. Uncertainty in illness. *Image.* 1988;20:225–232.

39. Burke SO, Kauffmann E, Costello EA, Dillon MC. Hazardous secrets and reluctantly taking charge: parenting a child with repeated hospitalizations. *Image,* 1991;23:39–45.

40. Jezewski MA. Evolution of a grounded theory: conflict resolution through culture brokering. *ANS.* 1995;17:14–30.

41. Tollett JH, Thomas SP. A theory-based nursing intervention to instill hope in homeless veterans. *ANS.* 1995;18:76–90.

42. Gerdner L. An individualized music intervention for agitation. *J Am Psych Nurs Assoc.* 1997;3:177–184.

43. Brooks EM, Thomas S. The perception and judgment of senior baccalaureate student nurses in clinical decision making. *ANS.* 1997;19:50–69.

44. Thomas SP. Toward a new conceptualization of women's anger. *Issues Ment Health Nurs,* 1991;12:31–49.

45. Huth MM, Moore SM. Prescriptive theory of acute pain management in infants and children. *JSPN.* 1998;3:23–32.

46. Ruland CM, Moore SM. Theory construction based on standards of care: a proposed theory of the peaceful end of life. *Nurs Outlook,* 1998;46:169–175.

The Authors Comment

Middle Range Theory: Spinning Research and Practice to Create Knowledge for the New Millennium

We wrote the Spinning article because we were entrenched in making sense of middle-range theory. Our graduate students repeatedly told us that it was challenging to attempt to figure out what theory was middle range. When sent to the literature in search of meaningful middle-range theory, the students returned with questions and quagmire. We thought it was important to make some sense of the existing literature on middle-range theory if the discipline ever expected to use it as a base for practice and research. We believe that middle-range theory offers a promising direction for the next generation of nursing scholars. We have recently coedited a book, *Middle Range Theory for Nursing,* which extends the knowledge developed in the Spinning article and describes eight middle-range theories useful for nursing practice and research.

—Patricia Liehr
—Mary Jane Smith

An Integrative Framework for Conceptualizing Clients: A Proposal for a Nursing Perspective in the New Century

Hesook Suzie Kim

Key words: client domain, human living construct, paradigms, pluralism

It is exciting to view the year 2000 as the beginning for a new century and a new millennium that can be based on a new resolve and a refreshing insight. In thinking and reflecting about what aspects of nursing and nursing knowledge development that should be the focus for formulating such a new resolve or a refreshing insight, pluralism comes to mind as one of the critical issues that is both important and troublesome. Nursing has pursued multiple paths to develop knowledge with different commitments to philosophies and epistemological orientations during the past three decades. The resulting pluralism is evident not only in philosophical orientations regarding human nature and nursing, but also in theories, scientific explanations, and methods of inquiry adopted in nursing science.

During the past three decades we have put a great deal of our scientific effort into developing nursing knowledge in terms of (a) conceptualizing the key and essential phenomena of concern, (b) identifying the nature of nursing problems and different ways of solving such problems, (c) understanding fundamental human processes associated with health and illness through development of multiple theories, (d) identifying the impact of environment on human functioning and health,

Nursing Science Quarterly, *Vol. 13 No. 1, January 2000, 37–44 Copyright © 2000 Sage Publications, Inc.*
Reprinted with permission.

About the Author

HESOOK SUZIE KIM was born in Korea and came to the United States as an undergraduate student at Indiana University. She received a BS in nursing and an MS in nursing education from Indiana University and an MA and a PhD in sociology from Brown University. She has been in Rhode Island since 1964 and has been a faculty member at the University of Rhode Island College of Nursing since 1973, having taught mostly in the graduate programs. Her scholarly work has focused on metatheoretical questions in nursing, and she considers her two books, *The Nature of Theoretical Thinking in Nursing* (2nd edition published in 2000) and *Nursing Theories: Conceptual and Philosophical Foundations* (edited with Ingrid Kollak, published in 1999), to be her major contributions to the discipline. Her empirical research has been on nursing practice issues from the cross-national perspective, including research on collaboration, pain assessment, clinical decision making, and the nature of nursing practice carried out in Finland, Japan, Korea, Norway, the United States, and Sweden. She reads (Günter Grass is her favorite author), listens to jazz, plays golf, and skis for sheer enjoyment and relaxation.

and (e) advancing technical supports that enhance human health. These efforts have resulted in truly pluralistic knowledge development in nursing in terms of theories, empirical findings, and practical approaches, along with differences in philosophical and value orientations. A rich array of scientific results has provided the foundation to move nursing practice to be grounded in scientific knowledge. On the other hand, multiple theories, conflicting findings, and competing approaches to patient care have created confusion as well as a heightened sense of separation and schism between science and practice in nursing.

One of the most critical aspects of such pluralism is in regard to theories and conceptualizations about phenomena in the client domain. Client domain, identified as one of the four domains of nursing's subject matter (Kim, 1987), refers to the key area of nursing's concern for knowledge development. There has been a long-standing presumption that through the understanding and explanation about client phenomena, nursing could develop its approaches, that is, therapeutics and strategies of care regarding clients' problems. The conceptual works of early nurse scholars helped to shift nursing's orientation from medicine and pathologies to human needs. In the ensuing decades, the relevance of these frameworks as a basis for the practice of

nursing became apparent, and a series of grand theories concerned with the knowledge domain of the client were proposed and studied.

Rogers's (1970, 1992) science of unitary human beings, Roy's (Roy & Andrews, 1997) adaptation model, Orem's (1995) self-care model, Neuman's (1995) systems model, and Parse's (1998) theory of human becoming are the major grand frameworks in nursing that try to formulaté and explain client domain phenomena from generalized conceptualizations of humanity and health. These and related nursing models can be categorized into six major types according to their views on humanity and health: (a) holistic processes as the modes through which humans coexist within their environment, (b) balance as the essential human characteristic that expresses human condition, (c) configuration of structural and functional aspects as an integrative basis for human functioning, (d) aggregation of parts as revealing states of the human condition, (e) experiencing as the basic form of human existence, and (f) meaning-making as the essential feature of human life.

This categorization suggests that in nursing there is diversity in the way clients and client phenomena are conceptualized and that there is no generally endorsed unified perspective regarding humans. It would be quite premature to state that nursing has firmly established specific paradigms or schools of thought based on these differing conceptualizations of humans and grand theories. However, these grand theories persist as the bases for empirical work and research, middle-range theory development, nursing curricula, and nursing practice models. In addition, knowledge development in nursing regarding client phenomena, particularly during the past decade, has also been rich and active not only in association with nursing's grand theories but in relation to general theoretical orientations such as biobehavioral, cognitive, psychosocial, and phenomenological frameworks. Multiple paradigmatic orientations are certainly in place in nursing and are viewed to be viable and necessary aspects of nursing knowledge development and practice (Gortner, 1993; Nagle & Mitchell, 1991).

Nevertheless, there are differing philosophical positions regarding this apparent pluralism in nursing. Many scholars seem to adhere to the notion that it is both acceptable and to some degree necessary to have multiple conceptualizations of persons and different grand theories in nursing. Others argue that for multiple paradigms and grand theories to be viable as the basis for scientific knowledge development, it is necessary to have a unifying perspective that provides the focus of the nursing discipline. It is from this second position that I propose a revisioning for the knowledge domain of client as necessary to establish firmly the unique focus of nursing in the larger context of healthcare. The conceptualization of the client domain as human living is presented as both a unifying perspective and a unique focus for nursing in the new century.

Human Living as a Metaparadigm Concept

From the 1960s and throughout the ensuing decades, nursing's focus has been to meet patients' needs related to maintaining health or to assist individuals in their responses to health and illness. As stated in the American Nurses' Association's (1980) first social policy statements, nursing is defined as "the diagnosis and treatment of human responses to actual or potential health problems" (p. 9). This view places an emphasis on clients' problems that are specified as *reactions* and *concerns* attendant with health problems. These widely accepted orientations have firmly grounded nursing to focus on states of clients, rather than on clients as humans. These client states are not only specified in the languages of the grand theories but also in the works of nursing diagnoses classifications and other concept developments such as deficiencies, deficits, adaptation/maladaptation, balance/imbalance, homeostasis, or disturbances. Such seemingly unwitting focus on states of clients also has led nursing to view time as a discrete entity tied to states of responses and occurrences, rather than as a continuum in terms of history and trajectories, and in so doing has imposed an artificial interruption in connected human experience.

Furthermore, I believe this orientation and its subsequent developments have resulted in overemphasis on technical treatment of patients' problems, thereby shadowing the essential nursing philosophy of client care. Consequently, either by design or under pressure, professional nursing began handing over the care of certain states of clients traditionally associated with nursing to other healthcare workers and assistive healthcare personnel, while taking on tasks and responsibilities of other client states that were formerly within the professional domain of physicians. Often this reshaping of nursing's realm of responsibilities, which is usually considered unsatisfactory to us, has been attributed to political and economic pressures within the dynamics of the healthcare system. However, as Kitson (1997) states, it may also have resulted from nursing's "ineptitude and lack of appreciating what matters to us" (p. 114).

Hence, the heart of the matter is in articulating clearly what the essential and central focus of nursing is, so that it becomes the guiding post not only for knowledge development but also for nursing practice. It is not satisfactory just to say that nursing contributes to patient outcomes differently from medicine and other healthcare professionals, or to say that nursing is oriented to the promotion of health and to the care of people in illness. It is this ambiguity that needs to be addressed to avoid continued diffusion of nursing's unique contribution to healthcare. Therefore, I propose human living as the revisioning orientation of the knowledge domain of client for nursing in the new century. By orienting its mission to clients' living rather than limiting its focus to clients' states, nursing can clarify its distinctive role within the community of healthcare providers, formulate client-centered outcomes that are uniquely related to its knowledge-based practice, and ensure public recognition of its distinctive professional contribution in healthcare.

Dimensions of the Human Living Concept

Although I believe that as a profession nursing has been always concerned with clients' living, I do not believe that it has been articulated clearly as the central focus of the discipline. The following discussion is aimed at achieving this necessary articulation. Human beings are biological and symbolic entities entrusted with bodies, selves, and histories, intertwined to carry on living by continuing, responding to happenings, appropriating and accommodating, and controlling. The concept of human living is based on ontological assumptions that accept humanness in terms of its biology, personhood, and sociality. And living as it is embedded in situations cannot be clearly viewed or fully understood out of context. Given these assumptions of biology, personhood, sociality, and context, human living constitutes three dimensions—living of oneself, living with others, and living in situations—which are coalesced through integration and intersection. These three dimensions are not partitioned sectors of living or even different aspects of living, but are integrative orientations that make human living what it is.

The essential features of humanness that frame human living are body and personhood as aspects of human selves. A human body entrusted with its appearance, makeup, concreteness, and boundedness is, to begin with, biological. But this human entity is also existential, because it exists only through what is experienced in time and space. Furthermore, a human body can be considered as a vehicle through which humans are social beings, capable of symbolizing and interacting. Thus, a human body or entity is both biological/materialistic and symbolic/cultural. On the other hand, personhood is a specification of symbolic self constructed through reflexivity, consciousness, and meaning-making, which are uniquely human qualities. Hence, human living of oneself refers to body and personhood intricately connected and mediated to project the nature of living that is uniquely human. For example, eating as one particular form of human living is not simply an act of getting food but is an act having specific personal meanings and modes of operation established through personal, social, and cultural habits and desires. Living of oneself, then, is oriented to aspects of one's life related to rhythms, intactness and appearance, capacities and limitations, body feelings and sensations, history and genealogy, desires and wants, dreams and hopes, ideas and opinions, choices, habits, and knowing. For a nursing perspective, living of oneself has a specific meaning in terms of how clients' living needs to be supported and/or guided when it is constrained by various sorts of health-related threats to the integrity of body and personhood or to the modes of living itself.

The second dimension, human living with others, is based on the sociality of humans and refers to communality of human existence. Living with others (i.e., with family, friends, colleagues, neighbors, countrymen, and citizens of the world—both intimates and strangers) involves coexisting, communicating, coordinating, exchanging, and interacting as human selves, sometimes by choice and design and other times through accidents or force, both natural and instrumental. Living with others pertains to relating one's instrumental, symbolic, and affective needs with those of others, and to making connections with others for sharing humanness. Living with others is intrinsically tied to living of oneself, in that for one to live of oneself, it is necessary instrumentally to live with others in specific ways. From the nursing perspective, living with others may be viewed to have potential for being constrained or needing to be arranged differently because of clients' health status or healthcare experiences.

Living in situations refers to the idea that living takes place in contexts and that modes of living are adjusted and modified to address contextual requirements of human existence. Situations of living may vary from ordinary life situations such as family, work, and community settings to more specialized situations such as hospitals or prisons. Situations also can be considered to be stable and continuous over time, or to be transient and changing. Living in situations involves responding to, accommodating and adapting to, managing of, engaging in, and choosing and creating contexts of one's existence. From the nursing perspective, living in situations raises questions regarding clients' relationships with their environment and accommodations or variations necessary in clients' living that are necessary, inescapable, or desirable because of situational contingencies accompanying health problems or healthcare.

Relevance for Theory and Practice

Focusing on human living as nursing's orientation gives a possibility to articulate nursing's unique contribution in healthcare. I believe nursing's orientation to human responses and conditions arising from actual or potential health problems, and resulting formulations in many of nursing's grand theories that emphasize clients' states, have limited the scope of that contribution. Revisioning nursing's focus emerges from shifting an attention on states to an attention on living, especially in response to the outcomes-based culture of healthcare practice. Nursing's concern with client outcomes, then, can focus on, for example, how well the client is living in this situation of healthcare, how the client is progressing with his or her living throughout this episode of care, how well the client is managing his or her living in the context of given health-related threats or problems, or with what sorts of continuity or alignment the client is carrying on his or her living. Nursing is primarily concerned with helping people to live as well as they can, whether they are experiencing acute episodes of illness or trauma, chronic disease trajectories, transient or persisting disabilities, or terminal illness. Nursing is also concerned with helping people to live as well as they can as they engage in anticipated developmental

human living experiences such as giving birth, aging, and dying. Diagnosing and treating conditions, difficulties, and disturbances must not be an end in themselves but must be oriented to supporting and helping clients to find ways of living through these experiences—ways of living more creatively, more wisely, more meaningfully, and with more personal control.

The human living concept, elaborated in this way as a unifying focus for the discipline, is metaparadigmatic and hence is not tied to any specific theoretical formulation. Extant nursing theories and conceptualizations regarding clients and client phenomena, therefore, need to be reframed in relation to human living as an essential metaparadigm concept and knowledge domain in nursing. For many decades, nurse scholars have considered health, person, environment, and nursing as the essential metaparadigm concepts for nursing (Fawcett, 1984; Yura & Torres, 1975). However, as concepts these are so nonspecific that they have not been used to identify a distinctive nursing focus as a discipline and an area of study. Human living as an explication of the metaparadigm concept concerned with client and client phenomena can stipulate nursing to be concerned primarily not with health problems such as diseases, illness, or disability but with living in the context of health problems and healthcare. As shown in Figure 60-1, human living as a metaparadigm concept can embrace many theoretical concepts and phenomena of clients, which can be elaborated in terms of specific theoretical orientations.

Explanations and understanding about human responses, behaviors, processes, functioning, and subjectivity can thus be formulated, developed, and empirically examined from various theoretical orientations, such as from different grand theories of nursing as well as other theoretical frameworks. When such theoretical frameworks are interpreted within nursing practice, it would be necessary to frame nursing therapeutics in terms of the three dimensions of human living, considering it as an essential metaparadigm concept of nursing. For example, the phenomenon of being diagnosed with a chronic disease such as diabetes can be examined from various theoretical

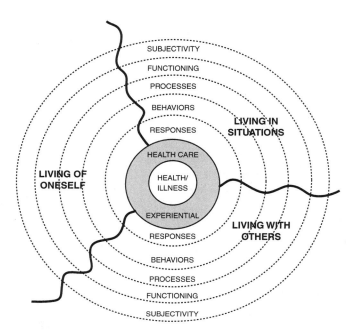

Figure 60-1   *Three Dimensions of Human Living as a Metaparadigm Concept in Nursing.*

perspectives (adaptation, cognitive, or phenomenological). Ultimately, any theoretical explanation about this phenomenon must address possible ways of helping individuals who are diagnosed with chronic disease. At this point, the question of what nursing can do and needs to do for such clients must be framed in regard to human living in terms of living of oneself, living with others, and living in situations. This orientation means that nursing will focus on client outcomes of its practice in terms of promoting quality in human living that is understood as it is experienced—continuous, transitional, and trajectorial.

Conclusions

In this exposition, I have suggested that it is necessary to reposition nursing's focus within healthcare and uphold human living as its primary orientation. I have argued from the perspective of a pluralistic approach that allows for multiple paradigms and theories in nursing that is grounded in a unifying focus in the metaparadigm domain of client. Human living has been explained as a three-dimensional integrative dynamic of biology, personhood, and sociality. This unifying focus on human living provides a new, fresh image of nursing that can redefine and direct our role within healthcare in the emerging century. The vision it gives us is a vitalized sense of mission for nursing, through which nursing can uniquely contribute to the lives of its clients. During the past decades, nursing has established a firm alliance with the culture of science and technology, which is primarily oriented to controlling health problems. Without diminishing our involvement in the scientific problem-solving traditions, we can renew our commitment to a human-practice perspective through a unifying disciplinary focus that orients our practice to helping clients in their living within the context of health and healthcare in the new century.

REFERENCES

American Nurses' Association. (1980). *Nursing: A social policy statement.* Kansas City, MO: Author.

Fawcett, J. (1984). The metaparadigm of nursing: Present status and future refinements. *Image: Journal of Nursing Scholarship, 16,* 84–87.

Gortner, S. R. (1993). Nursing's syntax revisited: A critique of philosophies said to influence nursing theories. *International Journal of Nursing Studies, 30,* 477–488.

Kim, H. S. (1987). Structuring the nursing knowledge system: A typology of four domains. *Scholarly Inquiry for Nursing Practice: An International Journal, 1,* 111–114.

Kitson, A. L. (1997). Johns Hopkins Address: Does nursing have a future? *Image: Journal of Nursing Scholarship, 29,* 111–115.

Nagle, L. M., & Mitchell, G. J. (1991). Theoretic diversity: Evolving paradigmatic issues in research and practice. *Advances in Nursing Science, 14,* 17–25.

Neuman, B. (1995). *The Neuman systems model* (3rd ed.). Norwalk, CT: Appleton & Lange.

Orem, D. (1995). *Nursing: Concepts of practice* (5th ed.). St. Louis, MO: Mosby.

Parse, R. R. (1998). *The human becoming school of thought: A perspective for nurses and other health professionals.* Thousand Oaks, CA: Sage.

Rogers, M. E. (1970). *An introduction to the theoretical basis of nursing.* Philadelphia: F. A. Davis.

Rogers, M. E. (1992). Nursing and the space age. *Nursing Science Quarterly, 5,* 27–33.

Roy, C., & Andrews, H. A. (1997). *The Roy adaptation model: The definitive statement.* Norwalk, CT: Appleton & Lange.

Yura, H., & Torres, G. (1975). *Today's conceptual frameworks with the baccalaureate nursing programs* (NLN Pub. No. 15-1558, pp. 17–75). New York: National League for Nursing.

The Author Comments

An Integrative Framework for Conceptualizing Clients: A Proposal for a Nursing Perspective in the New Century

Throughout the years, I have become increasingly concerned with the apparent difficulty nursing continues to have in articulating its independence of and separation from medicine in terms of the aspects of clients with which nursing is concerned. I believe this results from nursing's continuous emphasis on clients' conditions, states, responses, and behaviors, which are the ways client phenomena are conceptualized within many of the major nursing theories. I believe nursing must shift its major mission to focus on people's living and helping people to live well in the context of health and illness rather than dealing with and solving problems associated with clients' conditions, responses, and behaviors. Such a shift will certainly require rethinking regarding clients' problems that nursing should be concerned with, as well as the nature of nursing diagnoses. Hopefully, this shift in thinking will lead to new ways of conceptualizing and theorizing about clients and client phenomena in this new century and firmly establish the nursing perspective.

—Hesook Suzie Kim

CHAPTER 61

Philosophy of Technology and Nursing

Alan Barnard

This paper outlines the background and significance of philosophy of technology as a focus of inquiry emerging within nursing scholarship and research. The thesis of the paper is that philosophy of technology and nursing is fundamental to discipline development and our role in enhancing health care. It is argued that we must further our responsibility and interest in critiquing current and future health care systems through philosophical inquiry into the experience, meaning and implications of technology. This paper locates nurses as important contributors to the use and integration of health care technology and identifies nursing as a discipline that can provide specific insights into the health experience(s) of individuals, cultures and societies. Nurses are encouraged to undertake further examination of epistemological, ontological and ethical challenges to arise from technology as a focus of philosophical inquiry. The advancement of philosophy of technology and nursing will make a profound contribution to inquiry into the experience of technology, the needs of humanity and the development of appropriate health care.

Key words: technology, nursing, philosophy of technology, philosophy, medical technology, health care.

Meaning in Technology

Technology embodies our desire to influence the world around us. At its most obvious, technology manifests itself as current, antiquated and failed objects and re- sources (e.g., stethoscopes, pharmaceuticals, machinery and devices) that are designed to enhance healthcare treatment through nursing and medical practice. In ad- dition, technology manifests as knowledge and skills as- sociated with the use and application of resources and

Blackwell Science Limited, copyright © 2002. Nursing Philosophy, 3, *15–26.*

About the Author

ALAN GORDON BARNARD was born in Australia and has qualifications in nursing, psychology, and education and holds a PhD. He has been involved in clinical practice and nurse education for more than 20 years and has extensive research and scholarly experience. Dr. Barnard has held positions in three Australian universities and has a professional commitment to qualitative method/methodology and furthering the theoretic basis of nursing. His research and scholarly interests relate to human experience of health care technology and the education of nurses, with particular emphasis on critical examination of beliefs and assumptions that inform the relations between technology and health care delivery. Dr. Barnard currently is currently the Course Coordinator for the Bachelor of Nursing Program, Queensland University of Technology, Australia.

objects that nurses maintain and assess on a daily and ongoing basis. Finally, modern technology manifests increasingly within a technological system (technique) in which politics, organizations and humans are brought together with a primary aim of maximizing efficient and rational order. The relation of objects and resources to health-care practice is linked to the history of nursing practice and introduces patterns of activity that by their very nature influence patient care, values, knowledge, skills, political agendas, roles and responsibilities (Sandelowski, 1997; Barnard & Gerber, 1999b; Fairman & D'Antonio, 1999; Barnard, 2001c).

Technology is a word that engenders both confusion and meaning, and is used often to engender an aura of professionalism. The word is a commonplace descriptor for specialist and pseudo-specialist knowledge and skills (e.g., food technology, medical technology) that are influential in the ongoing development of specializations within healthcare and nursing. Its meaning is subject to historical and socio-cultural bias and is associated increasingly with sophisticated machinery, industrial objects, computerized or electronic automata, scientific knowledge and technical skills.

In recent years the dominant hierarchical model that treated technology as applied science has been replaced by a model that identifies science and technology as two separate bodies of knowledge and skills. It has been recognized that technology often creates, develops and modifies existing technology using specific knowledge and skills and has a varied historical relation with science. In addition, numerous technological advances have originated from little or no understanding of science, and technological advances have preceded scientific knowledge and rationale. The development of the first aircraft and the steam engine are two commonly cited instances of technology developing separate from scientific explanation (Mumford, 1934; Ellul, 1964; Ihde, 1993).

Although science has provided technology with knowledge and insights for ongoing development, science should not be conceived of as essential for technological advancement from either an historical or a pre-conditional perspective (Barnard, 1996). Notwithstanding, throughout the last century science and technology combined increasingly to a point where both are interlinked in the process of discovery and development. Ihde (1993, p. 78) notes that technology and science now combine regularly to assist with modern research and development. Recent advancements are described best as techno-science because more than ever before, they rely on a fusion of scientific and technological knowledge and skills.

Technology has direct association with historical, scientific, philosophical and social precepts that are embodied in our lives, culture, politics, work, professions, language, values, education, knowledge and skills. Nurses are more than at any time before, required to undertake roles and responsibilities associated with the application and interpretation of health-care technology. Therefore, our involvement brings with it new epistemological, ontological and ethical challenges and raises numerous questions such as: What are the effects of technological development on patient care? What effect(s) does efficiency have on clinical practice? What is reality in clinical environments dominated by screens and monitors? Is there technology-related knowledge specific to nursing? It is appropriate, therefore, given the influence and complexity of technology, that we examine philosophy of technology and nursing as a domain of inquiry that focuses on the experience, meaning and implications of the relations between technology and nursing.

Philosophy of Technology

Philosophy of technology is an attempt to interpret contemporary phenomena within the light of our praxes and technologies (Ihde, 1993; Ferre, 1995). It is an approach to contemporary challenges that emphasizes philosophical reflection and critique of technology. It respects the complexity of technology as more than a means-end tool and a neutral phenomenon. Technology becomes a focal point of cultural, ethical, professional, political, human and social significance that receives concerted and consistent reflection and debate.

Philosophy of technology is a relatively recent focus of inquiry and has developed over the past 200 years. Prior to this period, technology was considered a part of science and attracted minimal philosophical interest. Understanding of technology was influenced significantly by classical Platonic philosophy that emphasized separation of body and material presence from mind and soul. The creation of a separation between thought and action continued up to, and included, its manifestation in positivist philosophy within philosophy of science. There was a particular emphasis on the advancement of pure theory (*theoria*) or thinking. Discussion of technology was almost non-existent and there was a tendency to assume modern technology is derived from modern science. Ihde (1995) argues that even though Plato may seem a long way from philosophy of technology, the way of thinking has downgraded the material and elevated contemplative theory to a higher status.

However, since the industrial revolution and the writings of Karl Marx (1818–1883) and Ernst Kapp (1877) (who first used the term philosophy of technology, *Technikphilosopie*) there has been increasing philosophical interest in technology as a phenomenon worthy of serious and disciplined critical reflection. According to both Ihde (1993) and Ferre (1995) the development of philosophy of technology as a subcategory of philosophy (as is, for example, *philosophy of* science or medicine) was realized following the social changes that arose from the 20th century world wars and the emergence of technology as a phenomenon too important to ignore. European and American philosophers began to make technology and technological civilization(s) a primary theme of reflection (e.g., Martin Heidegger, John Dewey) and interdisciplinary groups such as the Society for Philosophy of Technology [HTTP://HTTP://www.spt.org/] were established during the 1970s as forums for critical debate and advancement of inquiry.

Although developments in the field have been slow, the principal aim has been to describe and illuminate the central features of technology as a phenomenon, and to improve our understanding of the way(s) that technology is manifest in our ideas, values, politics, history, environment, actions and culture(s) (Borgmann, 1984; Winner, 1986; Ihde, 1990; Ferre, 1995; Feenberg, 1999). The outcome of continued reflection has seen the development of two perspectives that are manifested as a binary approach to interpreting the development of philosophy of technology (i.e., engineering versus humanities-based philosophies of technology) (Mitcham, 1994; Ihde, 1995).

Philosophy of Technology: The Engineering Perspective

Engineering philosophy of technology explains the nature of technology in terms of technical use, concepts, methods, design and objective presence. The principal aim has been to identify the nature of technology as it is manifested through human affairs. The perspective tends toward a pro-technology approach to philosophy of technology. Non-human and human worlds have a tendency to be explained in technical terms and variation in human experience is acknowledged yet minimized as a manifestation of technology. Technology is examined from a mechanistic or functional viewpoint and the world is judged in terms of an instrumental consciousness. Mitcham (1994, p. 62) notes that early engineering philosophers of technology argued: 'culture is a form of technology' (Ernst Knapp); 'the state and economy should be organized according to technological principles' (Peter Engelmeier and Thorstein Veblem); and 'religious experience is united with technological creativity' (Friedrich Dessauer and Juan David Garcia Bacca).

The engineering perspective distinguishes between levels of technological operation in terms of engineers, managers, experts, technicians and technologists as indicated by characteristic roles such as the operation of machinery, design, testing or assembling devices. Although the engineering perspective raises materiality to a higher role than has been achieved in traditional philosophy (Ihde, 1995), there is a tendency toward positive affirmation of technological development and the furthering of an essentialist perspective. Essentialism holds that there is one true *essence* of technology. Essentialist perspectives emphasize a dualistic approach to the examination of technology (analytically splitting conceptual issues into two halves). For example, a renal dialysis machine would be interpreted as a device that is separate, at least conceptually, to the values and experiences of the person to whom it is attached. The device belongs to the sphere of technology and the person (other) belongs within the sphere of lifeworld meaning. There is a philosophical distinction between the operation and design of technology(ies) and human experience within the environments that they inhabit. An ontological separation emerges between technology and the society(ies) in which they exist/operate, in order to create a disconnection between boundaries such as technical–experiential, technical–meaning and technical–lifeworld practice(s) (Feenberg, 1999).

Serious consideration of experiential, ethical and political dimensions of technology within the engineering philosophy of technology perspective have been sporadic. There has been a tendency to be reactive rather than proactive in assessing the philosophical implications of technology for human experience, values, gender and culture (Ihde, 1993; Mitcham, 1994; Feenberg, 1999).

Philosophy of Technology: The Humanities Perspective

Humanities philosophy of technology interprets technology as not only what we do, but in relation to how the world is experienced by individuals, groups and cultures. The perspective accepts the engineering perspective, but expands on it to include not only the object or agent of use, but understanding of technological events. Mitcham (1994, p. 63) notes that early examples of humanities philosophy of technology examined technology as: 'a special myth' (Lewis Mumford); 'self-determination' (Jose Ortega); 'posing ontological questions' (Martin Heidegger); and 'a risk-fraught attempt at total control' (Jacque Ellul).

Humanities philosophy of technology aims at further insight into the meaning of technology and its relationship to the world. It draws on alternative frameworks or philosophical perspectives such as substantivism and more recently, varying aspects of social constructivism to inform critical inquiry. Although interested in the function and use of machinery, automata and equipment, technology is examined in relation to non-technical aspects of the lifeworld.

Substantivism argues that fundamental to the development of technology is a bias towards domination and control. It is argued that the further we advance, the further we progress towards a situation that is mediated increasingly by technology. The perspective attributes a substantive role to technical mediation. That is, technology embodies inherent gender, cultural and political values that influence practice(s), experience and perspectives. Technology is interpreted as a non-neutral phenomenon because of its inherently transformative influence in seeking increasing efforts towards efficiency and rational control. Technology becomes more than a mere instrumental phenomenon. It is understood as *the* characteristic of modern society over and above political and economic ideology. In its extreme form it too fulfils the definition of being an essentialist perspective, because it is argued that technology is responsible for all the major challenges that afflict contemporary western societies (Feenberg, 1999).

Social constructivism focuses on social alliances that are important to technical choices. It is argued that different social groups (e.g., nurses, doctors, manufacturers, specialists) come together in one way or another in order to make choices and influence the use and development of technology. They influence the manifestation and/or experience(s) of technology through processes such as the supplying of resources, participation in its use, political support, financial support, etc., in the interests of differing groups, individuals and networks, who participate (or do not participate) in the process of accepting, rejecting and fostering technology. Technology is understood to be neither neutral nor autonomous. Technology reflects the outcome of a process of development that fixes the way it manifests and the social interests that may (not) accept a stake in its eventual form and influence (Feenberg, 1999).

Regardless of whether one assumes a substantivist, essentialist or social constructivist perspective (or a position somewhere in between), humanities philosophy of technology emphasizes critical examination of technology, and is positioned in opposition to the more hard-edged economic and technocratic view of the world that dominates much of current research and literature. It survives, somewhat tenuously, despite attempts to label it as anti-technology or unenlightened. The approach highlights nontechnical criteria in the interpretation of technology in order to develop a level of awareness that emphasizes human experience, values and understanding (i.e., the subject being dealt with, in addition to the object or agent of use). Contemporary humanities-orientated philosophers of technology such as Albert Borgmann, Andrew Feenberg, Don Ihde and Langdon Winner, confirm it is equally important to investigate the use and design of material artifacts as it is to understand machinery and equipment in terms of human experience, gender, politics and culture. The perspective confirms that technology needs to be interpreted as more than material presence and/or instrumental action because technology embodies change, and is significant to interpreting gender, culture, traditions, action, values and praxis (Mitcham, 1994; Ihde, 1995; Feenberg, 1999).

Philosophy of Technology and Nursing

Bringing Forth Technology and Nursing Knowledge

The need to think about and find meaning in technology is evident increasingly in the practice development and future direction(s) of nursing. The task of understanding technology within nursing is both important and challenging due to its ubiquitous nature. Technology is everywhere we practice, yet we are not always aware of it. It seems at once to be both with us and yet not at the forefront of our experience. We use hundreds, if not thousands, of machines, pieces of equipment, tools, automata, policies and procedures in any one day, yet many of these things and activities go unnoticed as ordinary or commonplace. The technology of nursing is concealed often from our reflection, even though we have witnessed significant developments in technology and science. In fact, it is not until technology is revealed for its lack of utility and/or failure to respond in a desired manner that we notice it. In such cases, we may even award it a role in determining our life: 'the intravenous infusion pump will not work,' 'my watch has stopped' or 'the fridge is acting up.' Technology has seemingly a life of its own that we occasionally notice and engage with in a reflective way.

However, despite its quality of remaining hidden, it is important to recognize that nurses have always used tools and techniques in valued ways in order to achieve valued ends. Before the 20th century, nursing was a craft practised by individuals, of whom the vast majority were women who had gained experience in caregiving through religious orders and/or through families. Knowledge and skill developed by trial and error and were passed down through generations. Nursing practice relied on experience, intuition and faith, and was isolated to groups of individuals and geographical areas. Nurses relied less on scientific knowledge than on a personal and intuitive understanding and techniques developed and refined through practice (Abel-Smith, 1960; Reverby, 1987; Baly, 1995; Barnard, 2001b).

By the 1940s, nurses in developed countries were experiencing rapid expansion of knowledge and skills as a direct result of the development of medical science and technology. The rapid expansion led to the development of specialist wards/units/community services within environments that are noteworthy for their increasing patient acuity, changing values, computerization, unresolved ethical dilemmas, and changing economic, political, human and gender relations. In addition, nurses have accepted roles and responsibilities that have originated from the reassignment of medical and administrative duties (i.e., deputized to enact certain roles and responsibilities on their behalf). The deputation process (Barnard, 2001b) is ongoing and is characterized by an expansion of technical and administrative roles and responsibilities with varying degrees of nursing governorship (i.e., medicine often retains a supervisory and ownership role) (Reiser, 1978; Reverby, 1987; Brown, 1992; Walters, 1994; Fairman & Lynaugh, 1998; Barnard, 2001b).

The rapid growth of techno-science and the deputation of nurses has fostered the introduction of sophisticated technologies under the practice ambit of nurses. The process described has been central to our current position as a major contributor in the use of medical technology for health care delivery. Nurses accept a primary role for the use and integration of significant amounts of medical technology in health care in addition to the daily care of people in hospitals and the community. Therefore, nurses are positioned at an axis point between technology, individuals, clinical environments and communities and have a responsibility to take a primary role in interpreting and influencing the relationship(s) between technology, health care praxis and human experience.

Since the development of theories of nursing from the 1960s onwards, technology has become a focus of serious reflection. Nurse authors have focused on machinery and equipment use, alteration to skills and knowledge, nurse education, patient care outcomes and technology assessment as primary foci of concern (Carnevali, 1985; Jacox et al., 1990; McConnell, 1991; Calne, 1994; Locsin, 1995; McConnell, 1995; Pelletier, 1995; Hawthorne & Yurkovich, 1995; Bernardo, 1998). Nurse scholars have attempted to situate the outcomes of technological development and change within the contexts of nursing practice and care. They have stressed the need to develop technological intervention within various health care environments and in relation to changing health care practices.

In addition, there have been early advances in humanities-type perspectives that emphasize conceptual debate, historical analysis and critical inquiry. Literature has stressed the need for understanding of the relations between technology and the experience(s) of individuals and groups, nursing precepts, the future direction(s) for nursing practice, and conceptual/philosophical development (Ray, 1987; Allan & Hall, 1988; Fairman, 1992; Walters, 1995; Barnard, 1997; Sandelowski, 1997; Rudge, 1999; Purkis, 1999; Marck, 2000; Sandelowski, 2000; Barnard, 2001a, 2001c).

These developments represent a small yet growing collection of nursing research and scholarship that highlights technology as a principle focus of attention. Other developments important to furthering inquiry into technology and nursing have been, for example, the 1998 special edition of the journal *Holistic Nursing Practice 12*(4), the 1999 special edition of the Australian journal *Nursing Inquiry 6*(3), and the recently published books by Margarete Sandelowski (2000) entitled *Devices and Desires: Gender, Technology and American Nursing,* and Rozanno Locsin (2001) entitled *Advancing Technology, Caring, and Nursing.*

Technology: A Phenomenon Worthy of Philosophical Wonder

Technology is an important phenomenon and is worthy of significant philosophical reflection. Such worthiness demands a sustained focus on associated epistemological questions of knowledge, both in its modern reciprocal relations to science but also as a consequence of its relations with nursing. In addition, technology brings with it also evolving axiological challenges in nursing related to values and (non)legitimate use of ends and means. In fact, Ferre (1995, p. 11) confirms that technology is the offspring in praxis of the relations between knowledge and values and highlights that:

> Aristotle pointed out, one can only deliberate about what is within one's power to do. Since it is the nature of technology to increase the range of human powers, the associated range of questions for which human beings must assume responsibility varies with the available technology, and ethics for the philosophy of technology becomes an exciting dynamic field for thought and application.

Finally, technology raises metaphysical issues specific to nursing. Technology influences our perception and understanding of reality. We engage on a daily basis in technology-human-means-ends relations in which questions arise as to whether humans and/or technology are responsible for determining or manipulating human thoughts and decisions. Technology brings challenges for reflection that are associated with, for example, personal identity, life and death, changing beliefs, ideas and practices, and altering conceptions of society, healthcare and nursing. There are any number of epistemological, metaphysical, axiological and ethical challenges confronting nursing. Examples of foci requiring philosophical inquiry, research and reflection include: What is the role of the nurse? How are technological activities and actions related to thought? How is nursing action and knowledge related to values? How can a focus on humanity be expressed within environments that stress increasing efficiency and objective measures? What are nursing responses to aesthetic and ethical questions related to right and wrong, good and evil, means and ends? Can caring be enacted in technologically complex environments or are nurses merely machines? What is quality nursing care?

To these ends, there has been a tendency to juxtapose technology against nursing and thus approach questions and issues from a dualistic perspective. For example, technology has been conceived to be in opposition to therapeutic touch (Mackey, 1995; Bernardo, 1998) and in opposition to caring (Ray, 1987; Cooper, 1994; Locsin, 1998). A body of nursing literature has evolved that presents strategies such as the use of complementary therapies in clinical practice (Mackey, 1995; Engebretson, 1999), improved educational strategies to enhance technology use (Hawthorne, 1995) and spiritual renewal that emphasizes the importance of human life (Donley, 1991), as ways to curb *negative* outcomes that arise from medical technology. Whilst not wishing to de-emphasize the strategies suggested, Barnard & Sandelowski (2001c, p. 368) argue that:

> . . . recent scholarship suggests a more complicated relationship, as what any technology is at any moment in time is increasingly understood to depend on the eye of the beholder, the hand of the user, and the technological systems that influence integration and use.

Philosophical inquiry will assist to inform understanding and changes in our practice and assist to focus nursing care, skills and knowledge. For example, Pacey (1983, p. 72) argued that the reduction in infant mortality in England during the 20th century was due primarily to public health reform with specific emphasis on the application of technology . . . improvement of water supply and sanitation and the hygienic bottling of milk. It was observed that technology is less likely to produce desired outcomes without appropriate understanding of the relations between technology and healthcare, adequate education and enhancement of knowledge and skills. Pacey (1983) demonstrated that the outcomes of technology are not understood nor assessed adequately when they are interpreted as merely outcomes of the use of isolated objects, tools and machines.

Philosophical inquiry will assist also with moral and ethical dilemmas confronting nurses and other healthcare practitioners. It can inform issues related to individual rights, ends-means decisions and values clarification, and begin the process of finding meaning through debate, theory development and practice advancement. For example, a frequent complaint of workers involved with industrial technology is the problem of personal autonomy. There are often competing interests and pressures on workers to meet various goals that are embodied in technology because of efforts to maximize efficiency and rational order. Experiences associated with varying levels of personal autonomy have been associated with surgical nurses working in busy surgical wards/units (Barnard, 1999b, 2000a). Research demonstrated that nurses in busy environments can not use technology without also, to some extent, being influenced by its use. The inclusion of machinery and equipment (e.g., oxygen saturation machines, intravenous pumps, enteral feeding pumps, telephones, intravenous medications, digital monitors) in clinical practice engages each nurse automatically in a reciprocal relationship that places demands on both the nurse and technology. Despite the best efforts of many surgical nurses, the demands placed on them by technology in the form of alarms, flashing lights, reading screens, recording outputs, modifying functions and fixing faults, sometimes orientates their attention and practice away from many other important roles and responsibilities:

> Whether it be, for example, the act of fixing an intravenous infusion pump instead of spending time with a patient, or leaving a patient to answer a buzzer or telephone, there can be an associated feeling of making a bitter sweet choice between two actions, that has no strict objective or imperative principle except that they are the reality of nursing. (Barnard, 2000a, p. 1141)

Introducing new or updated technological objects into clinical practice places renewed demands on clinical skills, knowledge and time. They can introduce new patterns of clinical activity and a likelihood of modified practices, values and expectations. Although change is often to the advantage of treatment and care, sometimes the total demands of technology can alter a nurse's ability (personal autonomy, volition, will) to express her or his desire to care for people on an individualized basis, despite prior experience, educational preparation, or will to do so (Brunt, 1985; Walters, 1995; Barnard,

1999b, 2000a). Therefore, appropriate examination of the influence of technology on nursing and patient care is made best through considered reflection on all the means used in an environment, rather than specific machinery or equipment.

Technology can be sensitive to the needs of society and cultural groups, and the values and precepts of nursing if its design engenders all these needs and precepts. Contemporary nursing will benefit from philosophical inquiry that places technology as a primary focus of attention. The continuing focus will enable us to broaden our predominantly instrumental understanding of technology in order to foster clinical orientations and practices that enhance a deeper vision of technology and health care (Harding, 1980; Fairman, 1996; Barnard, 1996, 1997, 2001c; Fairman, 1999; Sandelowski, 1999a; Fry, 1999; Purkis, 1999; Marck, 2000).

Future Directions

So far in this paper I have tried to identify what philosophy of technology is and suggested the reasons for its continued development within the domain of nursing. I have noted that it is an important perspective on contemporary problems, and one that has seeds of development already within nursing research and scholarship. Although there are many issues related to technology that need to be addressed by nurses, four key areas for future development are identified in relation to philosophy of technology and nursing. First, we need to develop nursing and healthcare practitioner-specific perspectives that interpret technology based on a range of philosophical frameworks. At the present time there is a predominance of essentialist interpretation that seeks singular characteristics and an essence of technology. In order to broaden interpretation there is a need to foster substantivist, social constructivist and interpretive frameworks that assist in the development of alternative philosophy(ies) of technology and nursing.

Secondly, there is a need to find balance between hyped utopian and dystopian perspectives that characterize much nursing literature. More particular, specific and refined analyses are required that rely less on generalizations about dehumanization, alienation or uncritical celebration of technology, than on considered critical reflection on specific relations between technology(ies), nursing care and healthcare practice(s). Broadening of interpretation is required that not only seeks macro examination of the relations between nursing and technology, but specific examination of discrete interventions and technology(ies). For example, there are domains of nursing practice that involve technologies that are subject commonly to cultural, gender and evolutionary alteration (e.g., care of the body, birthing practices). What was appropriate in the 1970s can bear little resemblance to our present time. In addition, technology manifests in certain social relations and is a reflection of cultural orientation, symbolism, technological systems and division of power. The use of technology can lead to 'positive' or 'negative' outcomes, but will most certainly not lead to outcomes that are neutral or do not require critical examination and reflection (Harding, 1980; Sandelowski, 2000; Marck, 2000; May et al., 2001; Barnard, 2001c; Barnard, 2001a).

Thirdly, philosophy of technology encourages us to reflect on technology from perspectives that are wider than the relation between technology and western culture. There are many countries that do not experience the same levels of techno-scientific development in healthcare services and nursing practices, although they are increasingly influenced by technical rationality. Therefore, for example, what are the implications of increasing technology in developing countries for current and future nursing practice and education? What lessons can be learned from contemporary nursing practice that may be instructive for healthcare provision and development?

Fourthly, it has been argued outside of nursing that issues related to cultural and global environments are of central and crucial concern, and the environmental movement is a potential source for the development of new healthcare perspectives (Ihde, 1993; Ferre, 1995). Foci specific to the environmental movement have potential for assisting with the development of nursing,

particularly in relation to the use and disposal of health-related products and our role in the promotion of healthcare practices and lifestyles that are environmentally sensitive, appropriate and responsive to socio-cultural contexts. Ferre (1995) argues that the ecology movement has potential to provide assistance in 'postmodern' (alternative) interpretation(s) of technology. The movement has scope for greater synthesis of ideas and thinking that draws on the benefits of modern scientific analysis but is free to establish coherence in thinking that is not bound to the physics-based technological models of the pre- and current modern world. There is opportunity for scientific work that draws on the purposes and values of cultures, people, individuals and groups and emphasis on stability, durability, sustainability and satisfaction as dominant considerations rather than maximization of use, efficiency and rationalism. There is scope also to see nature and the human world as fundamentally intertwined with the objective world of technology and science. There are opportunities to make a significant contribution to thinking that seeks to correct what are according to Ferre (1995) the two great failures of modern technology: incoherence, or the failure to achieve synthesis for understanding, and inadequacy, or the failure to include subtle data in the powerful but ideally simplified concepts and models it uses.

Technology and Philosophical Reflection: Great Advance or Great Refusal

What is, and/or could be, the future for philosophy(ies) of technology and nursing? Can it assist nurses to interpret and engage with contemporary changes as they evolve rather than responding to them *post hoc?* Ihde (1993) notes that the use of philosophy/philosophers in applied ethics contexts such as medicine and healthcare comes too late. Philosophies are required to fix up or inquire into changes and developments that have occurred already in practice and contexts. Ihde (1993) emphasizes that even better assistance could be provided by philosophy through its inclusion in development processes. For example, it would be beneficial for nurses to be involved further in examining tele-medicine/nursing as approaches to the provision of health-care services. May et al. (2001) note that although access to healthcare services is a primary reason for the development of tele-medicine, in the United Kingdom the reasons for its development are increasingly associated with economic/risk management. The technologies involved are seen increasingly as a political/technological fix to solving inequalities and the criteria used to assess the effectiveness of services are based commonly on objective measures such as efficiency, lowering costs, confidentiality and access to information. Whilst these measures are important, there are other measures of quality care that nurses would seek to include such as human-focused care, holistic treatment, the limitations of a lack of a physical presence in care, and the limitations of relying on digital information when undertaking healthcare assessment. These issues, and many more, require development and critique that arise from various philosophical perspectives.

The viewpoints expressed in this paper are predicated on the belief/assumption that the nursing discipline wants to progress understanding of technology that is based not only on dominant instrumentalist perspectives, but on critical analysis, reflection and evidence. To date, there has been a tendency within nursing and society(ies) to interpret technology based on inadequate and commonplace assumptions, and to foster a dominant agenda that has accepted technological development as a platform for professional advancement and prestige (Barnard, 1996, 1999b, 2000b, 2001c; Sandelowski, 1997; Purkis, 1999; Marck, 2000).

Professional advancement in association with technology is appropriate, but advancement must include active participation in seeking to optimize both health care intervention and understanding. The challenge is commonplace to society (and nursing) and was identified by Ellul (1997, p. 41) who noted that:

> People will ask, then, is a pure intellectual work what is needed? In a certain measure, yes. And it seems to me quite vain to want to dispense with intelligence in order to direct the action and to want to act right away and at any price, without knowing

what one is going to do, without previously having sat down to count the cost. Now this is very characteristic of the utopia and of technical solutions: one applies no serious intellectual method, and one seeks immediately to govern the action.

We need nursing practices that are culturally sensitive, individually aligned to specific needs, able to promote resistance and acceptance of technology(ies), and are reflective of adequate clinical reflection and judgement. If it is the case that we are not seeking to advance understanding of technology past instrumental action and application, then perhaps Marcuse (1964, p. 257) was correct when he argued that even if our thinking is judged by others to be incorrect or subversive, at minimum it is 'loyal to those who, without hope, have given there life to the great refusal.'

Conclusion: Technology and an Invitation to Inquiry

Philosophical and conceptual development that seeks to explain technology within the domain of nursing will assist to improve clinical practice, patient care and health care. Walters (1995, p. 339) highlighted its importance when he stated that:

> As nursing is practised in the midst of technology, acknowledging the material world of health care involves developing an understanding of technology used by nurses in their daily practice.

There is a need to (re)examine the relations between nursing and technology from not only an instrumental action but also from humanities-based perspectives that emphasize society, cultures and human experience. We require a type of technological thinking that seeks to examine our ambivalence towards technology with specific reference to its manifestation as 'both objective, material force and as a socially constructed and chameleon-like entity' (Barnard, 2001c, p. 372).

To these ends, there is need to critique rudimentary and popularized assumptions (popularized meaning: to make popular, especially by writing about (a subject) in a way that is understandable to most people) (Barnhart & Barnhart, 1994, p. 1622) associated with technological determinism, faith in technological progress, and conceiving technology to be a neutral influence on the outcomes of care (i.e., nurses can always master (control) all the actions and outcomes to arise from technology) (Barnard, 1997, 1999a; Sandelowski, 1997, 1999b; Fairman, 1999; Purkis, 1999). An alternative interpretation of technology is required that emphasizes new visions and ways of understanding technology and nursing. Critical debate and philosophical inquiry is required for the future development of nursing practice within healthcare contexts that are increasingly complex and technological (Sandelowski, 1997; Fairman, 1999; Purkis, 1999; Barnard, 2001c).

Philosophy of technology and nursing requires us to make technology a foreground of critical reflection. Responsibility for the future of nursing and healthcare involves more than learning to use machinery and equipment and a momentum in which acceptance of change is a logical aspiration. Although Ihde (1993) highlights that philosophy of technology can lead to changes in practice(s) by informing practitioners of ways to understand and respond to challenges and dilemmas, Mitcham (1994) notes that it is not clear how philosophy of technology contributes to immediate decision making that is undertaken under pressure. However, he emphasizes that informed decisions need to be undertaken. He notes that the need for decisiveness should not be confused with decisiveness about needs. We need to examine nursing practice and healthcare policy and direction regularly in order to identify, prompt and respond to philosophical questions, existing ideas, emerging concepts and alternative ways to consider and develop an understanding of technology and nursing. Philosophy of technology and nursing is emerging at a timely period and offers opportunities for enriched insight into questions and challenges related to the nature and scope of technology and nursing practice. It will provide an avenue to combine technological knowledge, skills and activity with the development of a technological consciousness specific to nursing. It is an opportunity to turn towards the meaning of technology, to examine the technological systems that enrol us, and to act in defence and facilitation of meaningful and worthwhile healthcare practice(s). Philosophy of technology and nursing has the potential to make a profound contribution to nursing, healthcare and philosophical inquiry.

REFERENCES

Abel-Smith, B. (1960). *A History of the Nursing Profession.* Heinemann, London.

Allan, J. D. & Hall, B. A. (1988). Challenging the focus on technology: a critique of the medical model in a changing health care system. *Advances in Nursing Science, 10,* 22–34.

Baly, M. E. (1995). *Nursing and Social Change.* Routledge, London.

Barnard, A. (1996). Technology and nursing: an anatomy of definition. *International Journal of Nursing Studies, 33,* 433–441.

Barnard, A. (1997). A critical review of the belief that technology is a neutral object and nurses are its master. *Journal of Advanced Nursing, 26,* 126–131.

Barnard, A. (1999a). Nursing and the primacy of technological progress. *International Journal of Nursing Studies 36,* 435–442.

Barnard, A. (2000a). Alteration to will as an experience of technology and nursing. *Journal of Advanced Nursing, 31,* 1136–1144.

Barnard, A. (2000b). Technology and the Australian nursing experience. In: *Contexts of Nursing: an Introduction* (eds J. Daly, S. Speedy & D. Jackson), pp. 163–176. Maclennan & Petty, Sydney.

Barnard, A. (2001a). On the relationship between technique and dehumanization. In: *Advancing Technology, Caring and Nursing* (ed. R. Locsin), pp. 96–105. Auburn House Westport.

Barnard, A. & Cushing, A. (2001b). Technology and historical inquiry in nursing. In: *Advancing Technology, Caring and Nursing* (ed. R. Locsin), pp. 12–21. Auburn House, Westport.

Barnard, A. & Sandelowski, M. (2001c). Technology and humane nursing care: (ir) reconcilable or invented difference? *Journal of Advanced Nursing, 34,* 367–375.

Barnard, A. & Gerber, R. (1999b). Understanding technology in contemporary surgical nursing: a phenomenographic examination. *Nursing Inquiry, 6,* 157–170.

Barnhart, C. & Barnhart, R. (1994). *The World Book Dictionary.* Scott Fettzer, Chicago.

Bernardo, A. (1998). Technology and true presence in nursing. *Holistic Nursing Practice, 12,* 40–49.

Borgmann, A. (1984). *Technology and the Character of Contemporary Life.* Chicago University press, Chicago.

Brown, J. (1992). Nurses or technicians? The impact of technology on oncology nursing. *Canadian Oncology Nursing Journal, 2,* 12–17.

Brunt, H. J. (1985). An exploration of the relationship between nurses empathy and technology. *Nurse Administration Quarterly, 9,* 69–78.

Calne, S. (1994). Dehumanisation in intensive care. *Nursing Times, 90,* 31–33.

Carnevali, D. L. (1985). Nursing perspectives in health care technology. *Nursing Administration Quarterly, 9,* 10–18.

Cooper, M. C. (1994). Care: antidote for nurses' love-hate relationship with technology. *American Journal of Critical Care, 3,* 402–403.

Donley, R. (1991). Spiritual dimensions of health care: nursing mission. *Nursing and Health Care, 12,* 178–183.

Ellul, J. (1964). *The Technological Society.* Alfred A. Knopf, New York.

Ellul, J. (1997). Needed: a new Karl Marx! In: *Sources and Trajectories* (ed. M. J. Dawn), pp. 29–48. Eerdmanns, Grand Rapids, Michigan.

Engebretson, J. (1999). Alternative and complimentary healing: implications for nursing. *Journal of Professional Nursing, 15,* 214–223.

Fairman, J. (1992). Watchful vigilance: nursing care, technology, and the development of intensive care units. *Nursing Research, 41,* 56–60.

Fairman, J. (1996). Response to tools of the trade: analysing technology as object in nursing. *Scholarly Inquiry for Nursing Practice: an International Journal, 10,* 17–21.

Fairman, J. & D'Antonio, P. (1999). Virtual power: gendering the nurse-technology relationship. *Nursing Inquiry, 6,* 178–186.

Fairman, J. & Lynaugh, J. E. (1998). *Critical Care Nursing: a History.* The University of Pennsylvania Press, Philadelphia.

Feenberg, A. (1999). *Questioning Technology.* Routledge, New York.

Ferre, F. (1995). *Philosophy of Technology.* The University of Georgia Press, London.

Fry, S. T. (1999). The philosophy of nursing. *Scholarly Inquiry for Nursing Practice, 13,* 5–15.

Harding, S. (1980). Value laden technologies and the politics of nursing. In: *Nursing: Images and Ideals* (eds S. E. Spicker & S. Gadow), pp. 49–75. Springer, New York.

Hawthorne, D. L. & Yurkovich, N. J. (1995). Science, technology, caring and the professions: are they compatible? *Journal of Advanced Nursing, 21,* 1087–1091.

Ihde, D. (1990). *Technology and the Life World: from Garden to Earth.* Indiana University Press, Bloomington.

Ihde, D. (1993). *Philosophy of Technology: an Introduction.* Indiana University Press, Indiana.

Ihde, D. (1995). Philosophy of technology, 1975–95. *Techne, 1,* 1–6.

Jacox, A., Pillar, B. & Redman, B. (1990). A classification of nursing technology. *Nursing Outlook, 38,* 81–85.

Locsin, R. (1995). Machine technologies and caring in nursing. *Image: Journal of Nursing Scholarship, 27,* 201–203.

Locsin, R. (1998). Technologic competence as caring in critical care. *Holistic Nursing Practice, 12,* 50–56.

Locsin, R. (2001). *Advancing Technology, Nursing and Caring.* Auburn House, Westport, Connecticut.

Mackey, R. B. (1995). Discover the healing power of therapeutic touch. *American Journal of Nursing, 95,* 27–32.

Marck, P. B. (2000). Recovering ethics after 'technics': developing critical text on technology. *Nursing Ethics, 7,* 5–14.

Marcuse, H. (1964). *One-Dimensional Man.* Beacon Press, Boston.

May, C., Gask, L., Atkinson, T., Ellis, N., Mair, F. & Esmail, A. (2001). Resisting and promoting new technologies in clinical practice: the case of telepsychiatry. *Social Science & Medicine, 52,* 1889–1901.

McConnell, E. (1995). How and what staff nurses learn about the medical devices they use in direct patient care. *Research in Nursing and Health, 18,* 165–172.

McConnell, E. A. (1991). Key issues of devise use in nursing practice. *Nursing Management, 22,* 32–33.

Mitcham, C. (1994). *Thinking Through Technology: the Path Between Engineering and Philosophy.* University of Chicago, Chicago.

Mumford, L. (1934). *Technics and Civilisation.* Harcourt Brace, New York.

Pacey, A. (1983). *The Culture of Technology.* MIT Press, Massachusetts.

Pelletier, D. (1995). Diploma-prepared nurses' use of technological equipment in clinical practice. *Journal of Advanced Nursing, 21,* 6–14.

Purkis, M. E. (1999). Embracing technology: an exploration of the effects of writing nursing. *Nursing Inquiry, 6,* 147–156.

Ray, M. A. (1987). Technological caring: a new model in critical care. *Dimensions of Critical Care Nursing, 6,* 166–173.

Reiser, S. J. (1978). *Medicine and the Reign of Technology.* Cambridge University Press, Cambridge.

Reverby, S. (1987). *Ordered to Care: the Dilemma of American Nursing, 1850–1945.* Cambridge University Press, Cambridge.

Rudge, T. (1999). Situating wound management: techno-science, dressings and 'other' skins. *Nursing Inquiry, 6,* 167–177.

Sandelowski, M. (1997). (Ir) Reconcilable differences? The debate concerning nursing and technology. *Image: Journal of Nursing Scholarship, 29,* 169–174.

Sandelowski, M. (1999a). Culture, conceptive technology, and nursing. *International Journal of Nursing Studies, 36,* 13–20.

Sandelowski, M. (1999b). Nursing, technology and the millennium. *Nursing Inquiry, 6,* 145.

Sandelowski, M. (2000). *Devices and Desires: Gender, Technology and American Nursing.* University of North Carolina, Chapel Hill.

Walters, A. J. (1994). An interpretative study of the clinical practice of critical care nurses. *Contemporary Nurse, 3,* 21–25.

Walters, A. J. (1995). Technology and the lifeworld of critical care nursing. *Journal of Advanced Nursing, 22,* 338–346.

Winner, L. (1986). *The Whale and the Reactor.* University of Chicago, Chicago.

The Author Comments

Philosophy of Technology and Nursing

Technology is significant to the history, contemporary practice, and future of nursing. Although nurses do an outstanding job at the delivery end of technology implementation, we have been less noteworthy in our critical examination of the relations between technology, nursing practice, and human experience. The article before the reader argues that theoretic/philosophic interpretation of technology is central to the future development of nursing as a profession. As we move forward into our new century, it is important that all nurses engage more with understanding the relations between technology and health care not only to provide care but also to determine appropriate care that is informed by debate and understanding. Philosophy of technology has the potential to assist us to raise our expectations and critically examine the many assumptions that inform clinical practice, research, and the education of nurses.

—ALAN GORDON BARNARD

CHAPTER 62

What Is Nursing Science?

Elizabeth A. M. Barrett

The enigma of defining nursing science is preceded by defining nursing, science, research, and nursing theory-guided practice. The context for exploring the meaning of nursing science is provided through examination of the totality and simultaneity paradigms. Differing views of nursing as a discipline are discussed. The position is taken that nursing is a basic science with various nursing schools of thought that constitute the substantive knowledge of the discipline. Finally, a definition of nursing science is presented that is broad enough to encompass all disciplinary knowledge. Despite current challenges, an optimistic vision is emerging. The nurse theorists and other nurse scholars who are furthering the development of this work are considered to be the cultural creatives of nursing and contributors to a larger movement toward wholeness in science and in society.

Key words: *discipline of nursing, nursing research, nursing science, nursing theory, nursing theory-guided practice*

Definition of Nursing

What is nursing science? Although the term is quite familiar to many nurses, its definition remains an enigma. Trying to capture the meaning accurately is perhaps almost as difficult as trying to define love, because it is interpreted in many ways. At various times as I was pulling my thoughts together to answer what at first seemed like such a simple question, I began to think this was an impossible mission.

Nursing Science Quarterly, 15*(1)*, *51–60. Copyright © 2002, Sage Publications. Reproduced with permission.*

About the Author

ELIZABETH ANN MANHART BARRETT was born in Hume, IL. She holds a PhD in nursing science from New York University, a master of science in nursing, a master of arts, and a bachelor of science in nursing, summa cum laude, from the University of Evansville, Evansville, IN. She has 5 children and 15 grandchildren. Dr. Barrett is Professor Emerita of Nursing, Hunter College, City University of New York. Currently, she maintains a private nursing practice of health patterning in New York City and is also a research consultant. The primary focus of Dr. Barrett's research and other scholarly activities is *Rogers' Science of Unitary Human Beings*. Reflecting Rogers' worldview, she developed a theory of power, an instrument to measure the power construct, and the practice methodology of Health Patterning.

Trying to define nursing is an age-old dilemma. Traditionally, *nursing* has been defined as a verb, meaning *to do*. Fawcett (2000a) defines the metaparadigm concept of nursing as "the actions taken by nurses on behalf of or in conjunction with the person, and the goals or outcomes of nursing actions" (p. 5). King (1981/1990) says nursing is "a process of action, reaction, and interaction" (p. 2). Orem (1997) views nursing as "a triad of interrelated action systems" (p. 28) that compose nursing agency (Fawcett, 2000a).

Rogers (1992), on the other hand, defines *nursing* as a noun meaning *to know*. She proposes that nursing is a basic science whose phenomenon of concern is unitary human beings in mutual process with their environments. She says, "The practice of nursing is not nursing. Rather, it is the use of nursing knowledge for human betterment" (Rogers, 1994, p. 34). Parse (1997) says "nursing is a discipline, the practice of which is a performing art" (p. 73). Most commonly, *nursing* is defined as both a noun and a verb. Orem also notes that in addition, *nursing* can be defined as a participle, as in *I am nursing* (Fawcett, 2000a).

I view nursing as a scientific art, which may seem like an oxymoron. However, I believe that the art cannot exist without the science. I define nursing as a basic science and the practice of nursing as the scientific art of using knowledge of unitary human beings who are in mutual process with their environments for the well-being of people. Personal definitions of nursing are quite varied, as they reflect our unique professional identities, as well as our philosophies of nursing and our paradigmatic propensities. This seems evident in the way nursing has been defined by the various nurse theorists as well as by other nurses. At this point, I need to make explicit what has been implicit, and that is that I speak through the bias of my own perspective.

Definition of Science

If these are some ways to look at defining nursing, what then is science? King (1997a) says *science* is *to know*. Parse (1997) defines *science* as "the theoretical explanation of the subject of inquiry and the methodological process of attaining knowledge in a discipline; thus, science is both product and process" (p. 74) and is arrived at through "creative conceptualization and formal inquiry" (p. 75). Others view science as product only, and propose that "science is a coherent body of knowledge composed of research findings and tested theories for a specific discipline" (Burns & Grove, 2000, p. 10). Science, as scientific knowledge, represents best efforts toward discovering truth. It is open-ended, evolving, and subject to revision and occasionally unfolds in dramatic shifts in thought.

Research is how we create science. *Research*, according to Parse (1997), is "the formal process of seeking knowledge and understanding through use of rigorous methodologies" (p. 74). Taking a narrower view, the National Institutes of Health propose that "research means a systematic investigation designed to develop or contribute to generalizable knowledge" (Daniel Vasgird, personal communication, November, 21, 2000).

What is Nursing Science? Prelude

After this brief look at *What is nursing?* and *What is science?* we return to the question, *What is nursing science?* Although the term *nursing science* is used liberally throughout the literature, there are few definitions. Likewise, there are also few definitions of *nursing research*. It was amazing to discover this in computer searches and in a variety of books on nursing research and nursing theory. In other words, the majority of these authors do not differentiate nursing science from science produced by nurses, or nursing research from research conducted by nurses. This is the crux of the matter.

For most sources that do offer definitions, they may not be universally acceptable, nor can they be if they represent a particular philosophy, rather than the various philosophies that guide multiple schools of thought within the discipline. Failure to define key terms and failure to specify philosophical underpinnings are grave errors in building a unique body of disciplinary knowledge, which by definition reflects more than one paradigm (Parse, 1997). In addition, definitions need to be congruent with the philosophical underpinnings. To illustrate this point, in Fitzpatrick's (2000) *Encyclopedia of Nursing Research,* nursing science is not listed in the index, nor is nursing research. What is listed is *nursing care research,* and it is defined as "research directed to understanding the nursing care of individuals and groups and the biological, physiological, social, behavioral, and environmental mechanisms influencing health and disease that are relevant to nursing care" (p. 507). This reflects a particular worldview and does not reflect the discipline as a whole.

Context of Nursing Science

Munhall (1997) makes the important point that definitions require examination within their context and re-flect assumptions as well as philosophical, political, and practical dimensions. Indeed, it is context that explains why different authors define and use the same nursing terms differently, and why many terms cannot be defined universally.

In attempting to rise above the bias of personal perceptions, it is indeed a formidable task to answer the question, What is nursing science? Nevertheless, this collegial journey is justified because, as Watson (1999) says so clearly, without a language, we are invisible. Nursing will remain invisible as a distinct discipline and be viewed as a subset of medical science or social science until we have clearly defined and embraced our unique identity. Yet, in many nursing circles, this conversation is dismissed as valueless.

Before nursing science can be defined, the point about context must be addressed. Fortunately, there are several ways to contextualize nursing science, including paradigmatic schemas developed by Fawcett in 1993, and Newman, Sime, and Corcoran-Perry in 1991. In 1984, Parse (as cited in Parse, 2000) designed the original, and most widely used, paradigmatic organization of nursing knowledge based on a conceptual differentiation of the totality and simultaneity paradigms (see Table 62-1). Each of these two paradigms is a worldview that expresses a philosophical perspective about the nursing discipline's unique phenomenon of concern; all nursing knowledge is connected with this phenomenon in some way (Parse, 1997). Nursing's phenomenon of concern focuses on the human as a whole being, the environment, and health. Some authors add other concepts, such as nursing and caring.

In general, there is agreement on nursing's phenomenon of concern, expressed by Parse (1997, 2000) as the human-universe-health process. However, the definitions of these terms differ according to paradigms, thereby serving to clarify rather than confuse, since the philosophical context is now explicated. The contrast between worldviews is often explained by the two paradigmatic views of the human as a whole person, although this is only one example of difference. The totality paradigm views the whole human as a biopsycho-socioculturalspiritual being who can be un-

Table 62-1
Comparison of Nursing Paradigms

| | Simultaneity | | |
	Science of Unitary Human Becoming	Human Beings	All Totality Theories
Human being	Open being cocreating meaning in multidimensional mutual process with the universe recognized by patterns of relating	Energy field in mutual process with environmental field	Biopsychosociospiritual organism interacting with environment
	Freely chooses in situation	Participates knowingly in change	Interacts by coping with or managing the environment
Health	Cocreated process of becoming as experienced and described by the person, family, and community	A value	Physical, psychological, social, and spiritual well-being as defined by norms
Central phenomenon of nursing	Unitary human's becoming	Unitary human beings	Self-care, adaptation, goal attainment, or caring
Goal of the discipline of nursing	Quality of life	Well-being and optimal health	Promotion of health and prevention of disease
Mode of inquiry	Qualitative: Parse's research method; human becoming hermeneutic method	Quantitative and qualitative methods	Extant quantitative and qualitative methods
Mode of practice	True presence in all-at-once illuminating meaning through explicating, synchronizing rhythms through dwelling with, mobilizing transcendence through moving beyond	Patterns manifestation appraisal; pattern profile—perceptions, expressions, experiences; deliberative mutual patterning	Nursing process with nursing diagnoses

NOTE: From *The Human Becoming School of Thought* (p. 11), by R. R. Parse, 1998, Thousand Oaks, CA: Sage. © 1998 by Sage. Reprinted with permission.

derstood by studying the parts, yet is more than the sum of parts. The person is separate from the changing environment, but interacts continuously with it. Health exists on a wellness-illness continuum. Most authors include King (1981/1990), Orem (1995), Roy (1997), Betty Neuman (1996), Peplau (1952), Leininger (1995), and others as totality paradigm theorists.

In the simultaneity paradigm *whole* means unitary, and the unitary human has characteristics that are dif-ferent from the parts and cannot be understood by a knowledge of the parts. Moreover, the human cannot be separated from the entirety of the universe, as both change continuously in innovative, unpredictable ways, and together create health, a value defined by people for themselves (Parse, 1997, 1998, 2000; Rogers, 1992). The simultaneity theorists include Rogers (1994), Parse (1998), Margaret Newman (1990), and some, including myself, would say Watson (1999).

Although the two paradigms of nursing are different, neither is superior, and it is important to remember that a discipline requires more than one worldview of the phenomenon of concern (Parse, 1997). These differences give rise to different methods of inquiry and practice and provide sufficient scope to encompass all disciplinary activities.

Schools of Thought

Parse (1997) has advanced the conceptualization of schools of thought and proposes that each paradigm is composed of philosophically congruent schools of thought based on similar beliefs about the essential phenomenon of concern of nursing. She states, "Each school of thought is a knowledge tradition that includes a specific ontology (belief system) and congruent methodologies (approaches to research and practice)" (p. 74). In other words, schools of thought comprise the substantive knowledge of the discipline (Parse, 1997). Figure 62-1, developed by Parse, illustrates Orem's (1995) school of thought as one example from the total-

ity paradigm and Parse's (1998) school of thought as one example from the simultaneity paradigm.

The ontology consists of the assumptions, postulates, and principles of the framework or theory. The epistemology flows from the ontology and gives rise to both research methods and practice methods that are congruent with the framework or theory.

Nursing frameworks and theories have birthed numerous research instruments to measure constructs operationally defined to provide consistency with the particular framework or theory. Such instrumentation is essential to advance nursing knowledge in some frameworks and theories, notably in the totality paradigm. Rogerian science may be the only framework or theory in the simultaneity paradigm that endorses quantitative as well as qualitative methods. At least 32 instruments have been developed specifically to measure constructs reflecting eight (King, 1981/1990; Neuman, 1996; Orem, 1995; Pender, 1996; Peplau, 1952; Rogers, 1994; Roy, 1997; Watson, 1999) nursing science frameworks and theories (Young, Taylor, & Renpenning, 2001).

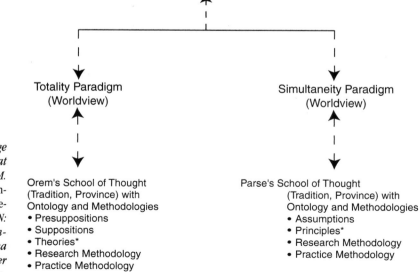

Figure 62-1 *From "The Language of Nursing Knowledge: Saying What We Mean," by R. R. Parse, in I. M. King and J. Fawcett (Eds.), The Language of Nursing Theory and Metatheory (p. 76), 1997, Indianapolis, IN: Sigma Theta Tau International Center Nursing Press. © 1997 by Sigma Theta Tau International Center Nursing Press. Reprinted with permission.*

Unique Research and Practice Methodologies

Of even greater significance is the development of unique research methodologies. Table 62-2 shows Fawcett's (2000b) listing of those methods. They are all qualitative in nature. Fawcett insists that

> we must extricate ourselves from the research methods of other disciplines, such as the phenomenological methods that have their roots in psychology, the grounded theory method that comes from sociology, and the randomized, controlled trials methodology that originated in agriculture and now is frequently used by pharmacologists and physicians. (p. 5)

Fawcett does, however, endorse reformulation of a method within the parameters of a nursing framework or theory. For example, Leininger (1995) reformulated ethnography, a method from anthropology, within the view of her nursing theory, and thereby created the ethnonursing method (Fawcett, 2000b).

In 1998, I (Barrett) proposed that unique research methods are one direct route to moving nursing toward further disciplinary definition. These methods "facilitate creation of knowledge for colleagues who practice nursing in the new way" (Barrett, 1998, p. 95). Those who use them are on the cutting edge, experiencing the passion of blazing a new trail as they sing the diversity chant of pioneers on the nursing road less traveled (Barrett, 1998).

Nursing practice methodologies are another aspect of a school of thought and are essential for making the leap from the theoretical to the practical, and clearly demonstrating the practical nature of nursing theories. Fawcett (2000b) noted that Johnson (1992), King (1981/1990), Levine (1996), Margaret Newman (1990), Orem (1995), Rogers (1994), and Parse (1998), or scholars working with those frameworks and theories, have developed practice methodologies consistent with their work that can also form the basis for research methodologies. In other words, Fawcett (2000b), and earlier Newman (1990), proposed that information obtained during the practice of nursing can be regarded as research data.

Nursing Theory–Guided Practice

The American Academy of Nursing's Expert Panel on Nursing Theory-Guided Practice developed the following definition:

Table 62-2
Nursing Discipline–specific Research Methodologies

Conceptual Model or Theory	Research Methodology
Rogers' Science of Unitary Human Beings	Bultemeier's Photo-Disclosure Method Butcher's Unitary Field Portrait Research Method Cowling's Unitary Pattern Appreciation Case Method Carboni's Rogerian Process of Inquiry
Leininger's Theory of Culture Care Diversity and Universality	Ethnonursing Research Method
Newman's Theory of Health as Expanding Consciousness	Research as Praxis Method
Parse's Theory of Human Becoming	Parse's Method of Basic Research Cody's Human Becoming Hermeneutic Method of Basic Research Parse's Preproject-Process-Postproject Descriptive Qualitative Method of Applied Research

NOTE: From "The State of Nursing Science: Where Is the Nursing in the Science," by J. Fawcett, 2000b, *Theoria: Journal of Nursing Theory, 9*(3), p. 4. © 2000 by the Swedish Society for Nursing Theories in Practice, Research, and Education. Reprinted with permission.

Nursing theory-guided practice is a human health service to society based on the discipline-specific knowledge articulated in the nursing frameworks and theories. The discipline-specific knowledge reflects the philosophical perspectives embedded in the ontological, epistemological, and methodological processes that frame nursing's ethical approach to the human-universe-health process. (Parse et al., 2000, p. 177)

Nursing frameworks and theories provide two avenues to nursing practice by way of nursing theory–guided practice. The totality paradigm allows for adoption of evidence-based practice, defined differently in nursing than in medicine, particularly when it is nursing theory–guided. In medicine, the gold standard for evidence-based practice is outcomes of randomized controlled trials. Evidence-based nursing, linked with the current buzzword in medicine, refers to research usage, but Ingersoll (2000) proposes a definition of evidence-based nursing that, unlike medicine's definition, does include theory. Her definition states, "Evidence-based nursing practice is the conscientious, explicit and judicious use of theory-derived, research-based information in making decisions about care delivery to individuals or groups of patients and in consideration of individual needs and preferences" (p. 152).

Nursing theory–guided evidence-based nursing differs from evidence-based nursing in that the practice is guided by the discipline-specific knowledge reflected in the schools of thought within the totality paradigm. King (2000) has provided an example using her conceptual system. Her "theory of goal attainment within which a transaction process model was derived results in the following: Goals set lead to transactions which lead to goal attainment (outcomes) which is evidence-based practice" (p. 8).

Within the simultaneity paradigm, practice is simply nursing theory–guided or nursing science–guided. Evidence-based nursing is not compatible because it is philosophically incongruent. Its problem-oriented focus on diagnosis, interventions, and outcomes reflects the natural science approach, rather than the human science approach of the simultaneity paradigm.

Nursing as a Discipline

If nursing is a discipline, what then is a discipline? Parse (1997) describes a discipline as "a branch of knowledge ordered through the theories and methods evolving from more than one worldview of the phenomenon of concern" (p. 74). Her schema of worldviews in nursing, presented in Table 62-1, clarifies why the same words have different definitions and rather than serving to confuse, the different definitions serve to clarify when viewed within their appropriate place in the disciplinary domain.

To make matters more confusing, nursing is often called a practice discipline, or as Donaldson and Crowley described it in 1978, a professional discipline. Twenty-five years ago, many of us were still debating whether or not nursing was a profession, and we began to see these attributes on a continuum. Rather than asking if nursing was a profession, we started asking, "How professionalized is nursing?" But nursing has moved on and now the debate centers on the extent to which we are a discipline. Those who specify nursing as a professional discipline emphasize that nursing has a "social mandate to develop, disseminate, and use knowledge. In contrast, academic disciplines, such as physics, physiology, sociology, psychology, and philosophy, are mandated only to develop and disseminate knowledge" (Fawcett, 2000a, p. 692). The knowledge of academic disciplines can be practiced in a corresponding profession.

According to Newman et al. (1991), a discipline is

distinguished by a domain of inquiry that represents a shared belief among its members regarding its reason for being. . . . A professional discipline is defined by social relevance and value orientations. The focus is derived from a belief and value system about the profession's social commitment, the nature of its service, and an area of responsibility for knowledge development. (p. 1)

Fawcett's (2000a) description of the discipline, as she presented it in Figure 62-2, presents nursing science and the nursing profession as the two major dimensions. Nursing research is the means for developing the knowledge of nursing science, and the product of the research is all the knowledge that has been developed and disseminated. The nursing profession, in a reciprocal relationship to nursing science, is actualized in nursing practice, with the major activities being use and evaluation of the knowledge previously developed and disseminated (Fawcett, 2000a).

Fawcett (2000a) summarizes the thinking of several nurse scholars when she says that "the responsibility and goal of the professional discipline of nursing is to conduct discipline-specific research using discipline-specific methodologies and to engage in discipline-specific practice" (p. 693). She echoes Parse (1999), who notes that nothing less will establish nursing as an autonomous profession and define the unique gift that we contribute to the healthcare system. Leininger (1995) also argues that professional decisions and actions by nurses require substantive disciplinary knowledge.

What Nursing Science Is Not

Before proposing a working definition of nursing science, it seems important to ask, "What is it, then, that nursing science is not?" Rogers (1992), Parse (2000), and Fawcett (2000a) are all clear that research by nurses that generates or tests theories from other disciplines is not nursing research. Furthermore, findings of such research build the knowledge base of the other disciplines. Since most nursing research falls into this category, the premise is that we are using precious resources to build a knowledge base with strong roots in other disciplines. This is not to say this research should not be done. Scholars are free to pursue whatever route to knowledge that they choose. Yet, can we call it nursing knowledge if its origins are in other disciplines? One cannot help but wonder what progress could be made in developing the nursing discipline if all nursing research, by definition, was guided by the extant nursing frameworks and theories.

This is not to say that the knowledge of other disciplines is not valuable and is not used by nurses. Of course it is. It is simply knowledge required of a learned person. Likewise, nursing knowledge can be used by others. Knowledge, per se, does not belong to anyone. It is not a commodity to be bought and sold, even though in the not too distant past, access to medical knowledge, for example, was much more difficult to obtain. We simply need to be clear on what is nursing knowledge and what is not. However, there is a difference between access to information and the use of the discipline-specific knowledge to provide a professional service that constitutes the practice of a particular discipline. Furthermore, knowledge that is not nursing knowledge simply does not reflect the uniqueness of what nurses and nursing are about. In contrast, it is nursing knowledge from both paradigms that allows us to build our discipline so that nursing services reflect nursing's distinctive schools of thought.

Public's View of Nursing

Perhaps one reason the public is often unclear in defining what is unique about nursing is related to the fact that they may not have experienced the *real thing*. In other words, they may not have experienced being honored and cared for knowledgeably as humans who are whole and who are living life in an ever-changing and all-encompassing environment. Equally as important, they may not have experienced that their nurse caregivers are themselves humans who are aware of their

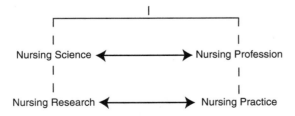

Figure 62-2 *From* Analysis and Evaluation of Contemporary Nursing Knowledge: Nursing Models and Theories *(p. 692), by J. Fawcett, 2000, Philadelphia: F. A. Davis.* © *F. A. Davis. Adapted with permission.*

wholeness and of living their life in an ever-changing and all-encompassing environment. The mutuality of the experience is what distinguishes this from the usual experience of clients who receive less than this standard of care. Instead, for the most part, the public views *nursing* as a verb that means doing, and nurses as those who carry out tasks of a certain nature. What nurses do is based on what nurses know. It is time to ask, "What is the foundational knowledge that drives the modus operandi of nursing practice?" Nursing theory-guided practice allows the discipline to escape from its low profile and create waves that demonstrate to the public why nursing services are essential to health and well-being.

What Is Nursing Science? Revisited

Finally, we return to the question, *What is nursing science?* The definition, I propose, must be broad enough to encompass all disciplinary knowledge and cannot focus on only one paradigm. Nor can the primary focus be on the activities of our science, such as theory development and research; rather, the essential focus is on knowledge. The most definitive perspective that was located appeared in the Scholarly Dialogue column of *Nursing Science Quarterly* in 1997 when nurse scholars (Daly et al., 1997) from Australia, Canada, Finland, Great Britain, Italy, Japan, Sweden, and the United States answered the question, *What is nursing science?* Only a few of their answers can be presented here. Daly (as cited in Daly et al., 1997), from Australia, said, "Nursing science is an identifiable, discrete body of knowledge comprising paradigms, frameworks, and theories" (p. 10). Mitchell (as cited in Daly et al., 1997), representing Canada, said, "Nursing science represents clusters of precisely selected beliefs and values that are crafted into distinct theoretical structures" (p. 10). Cody (as cited in Daly et al., 1997), from the United States, had this to say about the discipline and nursing science:

> The discipline encompasses all that nursing is and all that nurses do, overlaps with other disciplines, and is more than the theory and research base. The discipline of nursing requires knowledge and methods other than nursing science, but nursing science is the essence of nursing as a scholarly discipline; without it there would be no nursing, only care. (p. 12)

The nursing theory movement is a global endeavor. It is important to recognize that nurse theorists in other parts of the world are developing their formulations of nursing science. The Roper-Logan-Tierney (Roper, Logan, & Tierney, 2000) model, originating in Scotland, dates back to the 1970s and Gustafsson and Porn's (as cited in Gustafsson, 2000) sympathy-acceptance-understanding-competence model, originating in Sweden, emerged in the 1990s.

The structure of the definition of nursing theory-guided practice as defined by the American Academy of Nursing's Expert Panel (Parse et al., 2000) was used as a guide to formulate the following definition as a work in progress:

> Nursing science, a basic science, is the substantive discipline-specific knowledge that focuses on the human-universe-health process articulated in the nursing frameworks and theories. The discipline-specific knowledge resides within schools of thought that reflect differing philosophical perspectives that give rise to ontological, epistemological, and methodological processes for the development and use of knowledge concerning nursing's unique phenomenon of concern.

The critical dimensions of this definition guide nursing's ongoing search for substantive disciplinary knowledge.

The Significance of Nursing Science

It is not enough to ask, *What is nursing science?* An equally important question is, *What is the significance of nursing science?* Cody (as cited in Daly et al., 1997) warned that nursing's difficulty in articulating our uniqueness in the healthcare arena has put the survival of nursing as a distinct discipline at risk. In a similar vein, Nagle (1999) says our future is "a matter of extinction or distinction" (p. 71). She notes that in view of fiscal constraints, the increasingly technological work environment, healthcare restructuring, the introduction of generic workers, and a dependent mode of practice, the viability of nursing seems less likely. She points out that practice defined by tasks that do not necessitate discipline-specific knowledge will not differentiate nurses' work. She wonders if we can answer the question, "What distinguishes the practice of nurses from that of a provider by any other name?" (Nagle, 1999, p. 76). The answer to that question can be found in nursing's schools of thought. Yet, it is absolutely imperative that we articulate our uniqueness to the public and other healthcare personnel, as well as articulating differences in nursing practice expected from the different paradigms.

Perhaps the strongest voice warning nurses of the consequences of what she sees as the impending demise is Fawcett (2000b), who recently asked, when considering the state of nursing science, *Where is the nursing in the science?* She analyzed 116 articles published in 1999 by *Nursing Research, Research in Nursing and Health,* and the *Western Journal of Nursing Research.* Only 4% were grounded in an existing conceptual model of nursing. Only 24% were testing an existing nursing theory. No studies were designed to generate a new nursing theory based on a nursing conceptual model. Interestingly, 39% were grounded in theories and conceptual models from other disciplines. The remaining 33% were not based on any theory or conceptual model. Over two thirds had nothing to do with nursing science as defined by nursing's schools of thought.

Truly, one begins to wonder if the adjective *nursing* in nursing science and nursing research, as it is used in mainstream nursing, is a euphemism disguising what our scholarship is really all about. Perhaps the terminology of nursing science has simply become jargon. For some, the coupling of the words *nursing* and *science* would seem a contradiction in terms. Others pay lip service to nursing science, and that is as far as it goes. Others use the words, but define them in ways that do not relate to nursing frameworks and theories, or simply do not define them distinctively from science in its general sense.

The Courage of Nurse Scholars

Orem (1995) urged nurse scholars to "have the courage to take a position about why people need nursing and about what nursing can and should be" (p. 414). This is surely necessary if we are to realize the vision of King (1997b), who has "a dream that nurses will be at the center of healthcare delivery in the 21st century" (p. 16). Nursing frameworks and theories provide the power that gives the vision substantive form. Fawcett (2000a), summarizing the words of Orlando (1987) and Allison and Renpenning (1999), says,

> The development, dissemination, utilization, and clinical evaluation of explicit nursing discipline-specific conceptual-theoretical-empirical systems will end the journey on the dependent path . . . and will facilitate . . . the journey along the independent path of professional nursing (Orlando, 1987, p. 412). . . . [This is] the only way that nursing can move from a "silent service" recognized primarily by its absence (Allison & Renpenning, 1999, p. 26) to a very public service, the need for which is widely recognized. (Fawcett, 2000a, p. 697)

Cody (as cited in Daly et al., 1997) believes that "in these frameworks lies the hope of clarifying nursing's unique contribution to healthcare in an important way and thus further enhancing nursing as a scholarly discipline" (p. 13). Moreover, this exemplifies the freedom and autonomy of distinctive nursing territory that Watson (1999) describes in her portrayal of nursing-qua-nursing as opposed to nursing-qua-medicine and provides a language that makes nursing visible to the public and other professionals (Orem, 1997; Watson, 1999). So, as I see it, nursing frameworks and theories as the basis of the definition of nursing science are essential ingredients in the survival of the discipline. They are perhaps the sine qua non of nursing.

Present Challenges

Indeed, the challenges to all registered nurses are daunting. Yet, nurse educators, in particular, have great power to turn the tide away from an atheoretical focus on skills (Fawcett, 2000b) or technical competencies based on knowledge derived from other disciplines (Nagle, 1999). A large volume of literature explaining how various nursing conceptual models and theories can be applied in nursing situations is available (Fawcett, 2000a). Unless the tide turns, students cannot learn enough to identify and study phenomena central to nursing's concern or to build practices that allow for delivery of discipline-specific care (Fawcett, 2000b). Cody (as cited in Daly et al., 1997) laments the continued identification of nursing with medicine and warns that "vast numbers of nurses continue to emerge from entry-level programs with only an applied-science knowledge base for nursing" (p. 13). The increased emphasis on theory and research in the mainstream of nursing education, unfortunately, often does not concern nursing discipline-specific theory or discipline-specific research. Until this situation changes, the future of our discipline is at risk.

It is of absolute importance that we foster scholars and identify students and nurses with the potential to become scholars. What appears to be nursing's lack of substantive scholarship has created a brain drain. The bright ones are going elsewhere, because nursing is often perceived as an occupation with minimum educational requirements for licensure. Of employed registered nurses, 58% have less than a bachelor of science in nursing, and only 0.6% hold earned doctorates (American Association of Colleges of Nursing, as cited in Phillips, 2000). Anderson (2000) asks, "Why would a young person choose nursing?" She answers:

> Nursing does not reward education either with salary or role differentials, nursing does not have a clearly articulated career path aligned with education, nursing is dominated by people without a college education, and nursing departments are administered by persons who have less education than their fellow administrators. Finally, and importantly, nurses are not valued within the institutions in which they practice except when they are, as they are now, in short supply. So, who is it we *can* recruit? (p. 257)

It is predicted that by 2020 there will be a dire shortage of nurses (O'Neill, 2000). According to O'Neill, unless nursing is viewed as a substantive scientific discipline, today's bright Generation Xers, who could solve the longstanding issues that Anderson (2000) discussed, will not be attracted.

Anderson (2000) suggests, as others have before her, that the only long-range solution is to require a postbaccalaureate degree for entry into practice. Although this is a worthy proposal, the futility of the 1985 proposal requiring a baccalaureate for entry into practice has not faded from memory. In the meantime, it is crucial that nurse scholars from the various frameworks and theories collaborate to develop a description of nursing portraying the substantive nature of the nursing discipline. Videos, films, novels, compact disks, and other media, such as lay publications, can be used to present a realistic portrayal of nursing scholarship, a counterpoint to anti-educationism and anti-intellectualism so often associated with the profession.

Future Optimism

Although many have lamented the demise of nursing, and Wieck (2000) even considered a future where there may be no nurses at all, I remain optimistic. This optimism flows from the incredible changes in nursing science that have transpired in the last 50 years along with the movement of nursing education into institutions of higher learning. In 1964, Rogers proclaimed that "nursing is a learned profession" (p. 31) and that "scholarship is the hallmark of higher education" (p. 63). In 1952, Peplau published *Interpersonal Relations in Nursing,* the first book describing a nursing theory, and nursing science has been evolving ever since. Rogers (1970) laid out the blueprint for a science of nursing in *An Introduction to the Theoretical Basis of Nursing.* In the past 25 years, major milestones have been achieved through the creative work of the nurse theorists and other nurse scholars who are participating in the ongoing scholarship of nursing science. We enter the 21st century with a strong global effort to actualize nursing's potential for delivering discipline-specific care to all people. This progress has been so noticeable that perhaps it has created a countermovement. For those who discard nursing science as insignificant, I reply that nursing science is a force to be reckoned with, and it is here to stay. Devaluing nursing science is devaluing nursing. Yet, we must honor those in nursing with different views, lest we fall into the trap so often experienced by nurses, the trap of destroying ourselves from within. We can respect and appreciate differences, rather than being threatened by them. Beginning with Nightingale's lamp, it has always been better to light one candle than to curse the darkness. Perhaps pre-science nursing has entered the dark phase of obsolescence; perhaps nursing science is a light shining into that darkness, transforming nursing's identity.

I am encouraged, rather than discouraged, that more than one fourth of the articles published in 1999 in three major nursing research journals were nursing theory–guided. I am encouraged that since 1988, *Nursing Science Quarterly* has provided an avenue in which all articles link to nursing frameworks and theories. I am encouraged by other nursing theory journals such as the Swedish publication, *Theoria: Journal of Nursing Theory,* and *Visions: The Journal of Rogerian Nursing Science.* I am encouraged by the project of Roy and colleagues that identified, critically analyzed, and synthesized the contributions of 163 published studies, dissertations, and theses that were completed between 1970 and 1995 and based on Roy's adaptation model (Roy, 1997). Roy's (1999) book that presented this work, *The Roy Adaptation Model-Based Research: 25 Years of Contributions to Nursing Science,* won a very prestigious science award, the Alpha Sigma Nu National Jesuit Book Award. This is the first time the award has been given to the discipline of nursing (Callista Roy, personal communication, November 6, 2000). I am encouraged by the many other nursing theory–guided books too numerous to name.

I am encouraged by the movement in other disciplines toward a science of wholeness. Nursing's paradigms view wholeness as a basic axiom of the human-universe-health process, our disciplinary phenomenon of concern. At the turn of the century, there was a paradigm shift from classical physics to modern physics. In nursing, Rogers (1970) took a quantum leap from the medical model and created a similar paradigm shift from a particulate view to a unitary worldview of people and their environments.

Cultural Creatives of Nursing

Ray and Anderson (2000), a sociologist-psychologist team who conducted 13 years of research on more than 100,000 Americans, described the emergence over the last generation of the *cultural creatives.* Beginning to grow more rapidly in the 1960s to now 50 million adults in this country, this group of people have shifted their values and their worldviews, and they may be shifting the culture itself. The cultural creatives have a more holistic orientation toward health and care deeply about ecology; about social justice, peace, and relationships; and about spirituality, self-actualization, and self-expression. They are both socially concerned and inner-directed. They are activists, volunteers, and participants in worthy causes. They often use the perspective of whole systems, see *the big picture,* and believe the world is too complex for linear, analytic thinking. Ray and Anderson propose that the cultural creatives have been relatively invisible, but that they will have an enormous impact on society, once they realize their numbers. They say that this creative minority can carry us away from a fall and toward a renaissance. This is exactly how I see the persons in the nursing theory movement.

In nursing, the nurse theorists were the original cultural creatives. Starting with Nightingale, they have changed the nursing world, leaving their distinctive marks on the discipline. This minority of nurse theorists, many who could not be mentioned in this article, and those who learn, use, and expand their work, are creating a shift that will radically change the face of nursing in the 21st century. Particularly if they unite as a group with each other in support of the various world-views, frameworks, and theories that constitute the *big picture* of nursing science, their power will be exponential. Like Robert Frost (1967) describing the traveler who comes to a fork in the road, it will make all the difference which way the men and women of nursing turn. Those who embrace nursing frameworks and theories are bringing more nurses along with them on the road less traveled. This path is antithetical to traditional definitions of nursing, nursing care, and the nursing knowledge base. The implications of the nursing theory movement are heresies of the first order. For example, will the diffusion of these nursing knowledge innovations become nursing's legacy to revolutionary health-care reform?

Yes, those in the nursing theory movement are a minority on the road less traveled. Although the possibility cannot be ruled out that history will reveal that they are lone voices crying in the wilderness, I believe that will not be the case because this group is part of a larger movement in science, in society, in the universe. Nurse scholars who work within the new way of thinking about nursing are the cultural creatives of the discipline. You will be hearing more from them in the future. As the saying goes, *You haven't seen anything yet.* Those who walk down that road less traveled would do well to remember Margaret Mead's (as cited in Barrett, 1990) prophetic insight: "Never doubt that a small group of thoughtful, committed citizens can change the world; indeed it's the only thing that ever has" (p. xxi).

REFERENCES

Allison, S. E., & Renpenning, K. (1999). *Nursing administration in the 21st century.* Thousand Oaks, CA: Sage.

Anderson, C. A. (2000). The time is now. *Nursing Outlook, 48,* 257–258.

Barrett, E. A. M. (1990). Preface. In E. A. M. Barrett (Ed.), *Visions of Rogers' science-based nursing* (pp. xxi-xxiii). New York: National League for Nursing.

Barrett, E. A. M. (1998). Unique nursing research methods: The diversity chant of pioneers. *Nursing Science Quarterly, 11,* 94–96.

Burns, N., & Grove, S. K. (2000). *The practice of nursing research: Conduct, critique, & utilization* (4th ed.). Philadelphia: Saunders.

Daly, J., Mitchell, G. J., Toikkanen, T., Millar, B., Zanotti, R.,

Takahashi, T., et al. (1997). What is nursing science? An international dialogue. *Nursing Science Quarterly, 10,* 10–13.

Donaldson, S. K., & Crowley, D. M. (1978). The discipline of nursing. *Nursing Outlook, 26,* 113–120.

Fawcett, J. (1993). From a plethora of paradigms to parsimony in world views. *Nursing Science Quarterly, 6,* 56–58.

Fawcett, J. (2000a). *Analysis and evaluation of contemporary nursing knowledge: Nursing models and theories.* Philadelphia: F. A. Davis.

Fawcett, J. (2000b). The state of nursing science: Where is the nursing in the science? *Theoria: Journal of Nursing Theory, 9*(3), 3–10.

Fitzpatrick, J. J. (Ed.). (2000). *Encyclopedia of nursing research.* New York: Springer.

Frost, R. (1967). The road not taken. In R. Frost (Ed.), *Complete poems of Robert Frost* (p. 131). New York: Holt, Rinehart & Winston.

Gustafsson, B. (2000). The SAUC model for confirming nursing. *Theoria: Journal of Nursing Theory, 9*(1), 6–21.

Ingersoll, G. L. (2000). Evidence-based nursing: What it is and what it isn't. *Nursing Outlook, 48,* 151–152.

Johnson, D. E. (1992). The origins of the behavioral system model. In F. N. Nightingale (Ed.), *Notes on nursing: What it is, and what it is not* (Commemorative ed., pp. 23–27). Philadelphia: J. B. Lippincott.

King, I. M. (1990). *A theory for nursing: Systems, concepts, process.* Albany, NY: Delmar. (Original work published 1981)

King, I. M. (1997a). Knowledge development for nursing: A process. In I. M. King & J. Fawcett (Eds.), *The language of nursing theory and metatheory* (pp. 19–25). Indianapolis, IN: Center Nursing Press.

King, I. M. (1997b). Reflections on the past and a vision of the future. *Nursing Science Quarterly, 10,* 15–17.

King, I. M. (2000). Evidence-based nursing practice. *Theoria: Journal of Nursing Theory, 9*(2), 4–9.

Leininger, M. (1995). Culture care theory, research and practice. *Nursing Science Quarterly, 9,* 71–78.

Levine, M. E. (1996). The conservation principles: A retrospective. *Nursing Science Quarterly, 9,* 38–41.

Munhall, P. L. (1997). Deja vu, parroting, buy-ins, and an opening. In I. M. King & J. Fawcett (Eds.), *The language of nursing theory and metatheory* (pp. 79–87). Indianapolis, IN: Center Nursing Press.

Nagle, L. M. (1999). A matter of extinction or distinction. *Western Journal of Nursing Research, 21,* 71–82.

Neuman, B. M. (1996). *The Neuman systems model* (3rd ed.). Norwalk, CT: Appleton & Lange.

Newman, M. A. (1990). Newman's theory of health as praxis. *Nursing Science Quarterly, 3,* 37–41.

Newman, M. A., Sime, A. M., & Corcoran-Perry, S. A. (1991). The focus of the discipline of nursing. *Advances in Nursing Science, 14*(1), 1–6.

O'Neill, E. (2000, November). *Workplace Issues in Nursing.* Paper presented at the annual conference of the American Academy of Nursing, San Diego, CA.

Orem, D. E. (1995). *Nursing: Concepts of practice* (5th ed.). St. Louis, MO: Mosby.

Orem, D. E. (1997). Views of human beings specific to nursing. *Nursing Science Quarterly, 10,* 26–31.

Orlando, I. J. (1987). Nursing in the 21st century: Alternate paths. *Journal of Advanced Nursing, 12,* 405–412.

Parse, R. R. (1997). The language of nursing knowledge: Saying what we mean. In I. M. King & J. Fawcett (Eds.), *The language of nursing theory and metatheory* (pp. 73–77). Indianapolis, IN: Center Nursing Press.

Parse, R. R. (1998). *The human becoming school of thought: A perspective for nurses and other health professionals.* Thousand Oaks, CA: Sage.

Parse, R. R. (1999). The discipline and the profession. *Nursing Science Quarterly, 12,* 275.

Parse, R. R. (2000). Paradigms: A reprise. *Nursing Science Quarterly, 13,* 275–276.

Parse, R. R., Barrett, E., Bourgeois, M., Dee, V., Egan, E., Germain, C., et al. (2000). Nursing theory-guided practice: A definition. *Nursing Science Quarterly, 13,* 177.

Pender, N. J. (1996). *Health promotion in nursing practice* (3rd ed.). Stamford, CT: Appleton & Lange.

Peplau, H. (1952). *Interpersonal relations in nursing.* New York: Putnam.

Phillips, J. R. (2000). Rogerian nursing science and research: A healing process for nursing. *Nursing Science Quarterly, 13,* 196–203.

Ray, P. H., & Anderson, S. R. (2000). *The cultural creatives: How 50 million people are changing the world.* New York: Harmony Books.

Rogers, M. E. (1964). *Reveille in nursing.* Philadelphia: F. A. Davis.

Rogers, M. E. (1970). *An introduction to the theoretical basis of nursing.* Philadelphia: F. A. Davis.

Rogers, M. E. (1992). Nursing science and the space age. *Nursing Science Quarterly, 5,* 27–34.

Rogers, M. E. (1994). The science of unitary human beings. *Nursing Science Quarterly, 7,* 33–35.

Roper, N., Logan, W., & Tierney, A. J. (2000). *The Roper-Logan-Tierney model of nursing.* New York: Churchill Livingstone.

Roy, C. (1997). Future of the Roy model: Challenge to redefine adaptation. *Nursing Science Quarterly, 10,* 42–48.

Roy, C. (1999). *The Roy adaptation model-based research: 25 years of contributions to nursing science.* Indianapolis, IN: Center Nursing Press.

Watson, J. (1999). *Postmodern nursing and beyond.* New York: Churchill Livingston.

Wieck, K. L. (2000). A vision for nursing: The future revisited. *Nursing Outlook, 48,* 7–8.

Young, A., Taylor, S. G., & Renpenning, K. (2001). *Connections: Nursing theory, research, and practice.* St. Louis, MO: Mosby.

The Author Comments

What Is Nursing Science?

An Open Letter to Nurses of the 21st Century

In the second half of the 20th century, nurse theorists created a radical shift and developed discipline-specific knowledge that has boundless potential to radically change the face of nursing in the 21st century. I saw a need for a definition of nursing science that would encompass the work of theorists from the differing paradigms and guide the ongoing search for knowledge of nursing's unique phenomenon of concern, the human-universe-health process. Now, at a time when the world is moving so quickly that tomorrow is almost history, it is up to the students of today, who will soon be the nursing leaders of the future, to embrace, further develop, and use this knowledge for human betterment. Will you, the nurses of the 21st century, knowingly participate in continuing this revolution? You have power. Use it!

—ELIZABETH ANN MANHART BARRETT

Author Index

Subject Index